Common Foundation Studies in Nursing

2

04

Illustrations: Robert Britton
Gecko Studios

For Churchill Livingstone:

Commissioning Editor: Ellen Green
Project Manager: Valerie Burgess
Project Development Editor: Mairi McCubbin
Design Direction: Judith Wright
Project Controllers: Pat Miller
Copy-editor: Carrie Walker
Indexer: Nina Boyd
Sales Promotion Executive: Hilary Brown

Common Foundation Studies in Nursing

Edited by

Neil Kenworthy MBA BEd RGN RMN
Management and Training Consultant, PNK Associates,
Lincoln, UK
Formerly Vice Principal, Mid Trent College of Nursing and Midwifery

Gillian Snowley MEd BSc(Hons) DipNurs(Lond) RGN
Dean, School of Health, University of Hull, Hull, UK
Formerly Deputy Director, Humberside College of Health,
Hull, UK

Cynthia Gilling MA BEd(Hons) RGN RM RNT
Head of School of Health and Community Studies, King Alfred's College of Higher
Education, Winchester, UK

SECOND EDITION

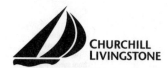

CHURCHILL
LIVINGSTONE

NEW YORK EDINBURGH LONDON MADRID MELBOURNE SAN FRANCISCO TOKYO 1996

CHURCHILL LIVINGSTONE
Medical Division of Pearson Professional Limited

Distributed in the United States of America by Churchill
Livingstone Inc., 650 Avenue of the Americas, New York,
N.Y. 10011, and by associated companies, branches and
representatives throughout the world.

First edition 1992
Second edition 1996

ISBN 0 443 05280 8

British Library of Cataloguing in Publication Data
A catalogue record for this book is available from the British
Library.

Library of Congress Cataloging in Publication Data
A catalogue record for this book is available from the
Library of Congress

Note
Medical knowledge is constantly changing. As new
information becomes available, changes in treatment,
procedures, equipment and the use of drugs become
necessary. The editors/authors/contributors and the
publishers have, as far as it is possible, taken care to ensure
that the information given in this text is accurate and up to
date. However, readers are strongly advised to confirm that
the information, especially with regard to drug usage,
complies with latest legislation and standards of practice.

The
publisher's
policy is to use
**paper manufactured
from sustainable forests**

Produced by Longman Singapore Publishers (Pte) Ltd
Printed in Singapore

Contents

Contributors

Alison Barnes BA RGN RM RHY
Regional Nurse Manager, Marie Curie Cancer
Care, London
19 Care of the dying and bereaved

Andrew M. Betts MEd RMN AdvDipCouns CPNCert CertEd
Specialist Subject Leader, School of Nursing and
Midwifery, University of Nottingham,
Nottingham
17 The nurse as communicator

Helen Caulfield LLB MA
Solicitor, Royal College of Nursing, London
13 Legal aspects of nursing

Margaret Clarke RGN RNT BSc(Hons) MPhil
Emeritus Professor of Nursing Studies,
University of Hull, Hull
4 Stress and the individual

Terttu (Tepi) Corbett MEd BA RGN DipN(Lond) CertEd
RNT
Lecturer in Nursing Studies, University of Hull,
Hull
3 The sociological self

Peter Draper PhD BSc RGN CertEd RNT ENB 249
Lecturer in Nursing Studies, Institute of Nursing
Studies, University of Hull
14 Concepts of individual care

Roger B. Ellis BSc MEd DipStudCouns
Independent Counsellor, Supervisor, Consultant
and Trainer, Frogs Leap, 615 Newark Road,
Lincoln
2 The psychological self

Jon Evans MA MIHSM
Consultant in Health Services Management,
Shrewsbury Cottage, Nettleham Road, Scothern,
Lincoln
9 Health care provision

Diana Forster BA(Hons) MSc RGN RM RHVT RNT
Independent Writer and Consultant in Health
Psychology and Health Promotion, London
6 Normal health
7 Health promotion

Eva Garland RGN NDN
Director of Nursing, Marie Curie Cancer Care,
London
19 Care of the dying and bereaved

Bob Gates MSc BEd(Hons) DipNurs(Lond) CertEd RNT RNMH
RMN
Lecturer in Nursing and Deputy Head of
Department, Institute of Nursing Studies,
University of Hull;
Head of Profession for Learning Disability
Nursing, The Hull and Holderness NHS Trust,
Hull
22 Learning disability

Cynthia Gilling MA BEd(Hons) RGN RM RNT
Head of School of Health and Community

Studies, King Alfred's College of Higher
Education, Winchester
16 The professional role of the nurse

Christopher J. Goodall RGN DipN RNT
Visiting Lecturer, North Yorkshire College of
Health Studies, York
5 Pain

J. Jane Hodges BSc(Hons) DipNurs(Lond) CertEd RGN RCNT
Nurse Lecturer, Nursing Studies,
European Institute of Health and Medical
Sciences, University of Surrey, Guildford
20 Adults

Sally Huband SRN RSCN SCM RNT BA(Hons)
Formerly Senior Lecturer Paediatrics,
Sussex and Kent Institute, Brighton
21 Children

Neil Kenworthy MBA BEd RGN RMN
Management and Training Consultant,
PNK Associates, Lincoln
Formerly Vice Principal, Mid Trent College of
Nursing and Midwifery, Lincoln
9 Health care provision

Stephanie Kirby MA(Lond) RGN RNT
Senior Lecturer, Redwood College of Health
Studies, South Bank University, London
11 The development of the nursing profession

Rob Newell BSc RGN RMN RNT ENB650
Lecturer in Nursing, Institute of Nursing
Studies, University of Hull, Hull
23 Mental health

Peter J. Nicklin MEd MBA DipEd(Lond) RGN RMN RNT
MHSM
Director, Managing and Continuing Education

Studies, Department of Health Studies,
University of York, York
10 Providing a quality service

Gill Pharaoh SRN
Regional Care Advisor, Motor Neurone Disease
Association, London
19 Care of the dying and bereaved

Pam Smith PhD BNurs RGN RNT
Visiting Research Fellow, School of Health,
University of Greenwich
Formerly Lecturer, Institute of Advanced
Nursing Education, Royal College of Nursing,
London
15 Research and its application

Gillian Snowley MEd BSc(Hons) DipNurs(Lond) RGN
Dean, School of Health, University of Hull, Hull
Formerly Deputy Director, Humberside College
of Health, Hull
1 The physiological self

Mary Walker MA RGN RM MFPHM(Hons)
Research Administrator, Department of Public
Health and Primary Care, Royal Free Hospital
School of Medicine, London
8 Patterns of ill health

Mary Watkins DipN DipNEd RGN RMN MN PhD
Head of Institute of Health Studies,
University of Plymouth, Plymouth
18 The nurse as educator

Isabelle Whaite MA DPSN Cert Ed RGN RM RCNT
Operational Manager Nursing, Health and
Social Policy, Lancashire College of Nursing and
Health, Ormskirk
12 Ethics

Preface

It is now some 10 years since the UKCC published its report *Project 2000 – A New Preparation for Practice*. During the intervening period a major transformation has taken place in the way that student nurses are prepared for entry to the professional register.

All pre-registration courses are now at diploma level and are provided within universities or other higher education institutions.

The concept of the nurse as a 'knowledgeable doer' is still relevant, and the nature of the relationship between the practice setting of the NHS and the academic ethos of the university is critical in the provision and development of today's registered nurses. Emphasis is very much on students taking more responsibility for their own studies, and teachers/lecturers have to create opportunities for enhancing and facilitating student-centred learning.

As with the first edition of this text the contributors are, in the main, people closely involved in the preparation and delivery of nursing courses. Those that are not are specialists in their own field and their contribution gives the text an added dimension so necessary in extending the knowledge base of nurses.

Before this second edition entered the planning stage the views and opinions of a large number of students and teachers were sought about the content, style and level of the first edition and many of their comments have guided the editors in compiling this new text.

The two major concepts of the first edition are retained: that nursing must recognise the *individuality* of both patient and nurse and that nursing must be *health* focused rather than illness driven.

Whilst the overall structure of the book remains unchanged there is now a chapter on legal issues in nursing. The topics of pain and stress have been extended and other chapters have been rigorously updated in the light of the NHS reforms and the developments in nursing education.

Section 1 The individual: self and society explores the individual from three aspects: physiological, psychological and sociological. It then considers how the individual responds to stress and pain, together with the implications of this for nursing care.

Section 2 Concepts of health commences at the 'normal health' end of the health-illness continuum and discusses the promotion of health before considering patterns of ill health.

Because resources for the provision of health care are finite, the student must understand how health-care services are organised and what factors are involved in determining the amount, range and quality of such services. This section of the book ends by enabling the student to see how health services are provided, with particular emphasis on improving the quality of service.

Within these two major themes of individuality and health, the book goes on to present some fundamental principles within nursing, as well as descriptions of important nursing roles.

Section 3 Nursing: fundamental principles and skills explores the development of nursing and the role of the nurse as communicator, educator and researcher, alongside some of the more emotive issues facing nurses in relation to ethical, moral and professional values.

Section 4 An introduction to the main client groups During the Common Foundation Programme students will observe and sample nursing care being provided in each of the four 'branch' areas, that is, adult care, child care, care of those with leaving disabilities and care of the mentally ill. The final section of the book takes this into account. It provides the student with an overview of each of the four 'branch' groups and examines some of their nursing needs while identifying issues of current concern and exploring likely future developments.

Other features

No book will succeed, no matter how well planned, unless the needs of the reader are taken into account. We have therefore paid considerable attention to the book's presentation: it is well illustrated and the page layout is attractive and inviting to the reader. There are numerous headings, making it easy for the student to read, refer to and remember.

In addition, there are a number of case studies and examples which should help 'bring to life' some of the more abstract concepts which underpin nursing. The text is also enhanced by the inclusion of open-learning style activities, which will encourage students to apply their knowledge in their own way and in their own situation.

Finally, each chapter ends with lists of references and further reading, which remind students of the essential requirement to develop their knowledge beyond the bounds of this single text.

This last point is particularly important, since the editors and contributors share the view that this book is a beginning, not an end. It should give new students an indispensable and comprehensive introduction to the core subjects of the Common Foundation Programme while at the same time providing a springboard for the acquisition of further knowledge.

1996   N. K.
                                              G. S.
                                              C. G.

ACKNOWLEDGEMENT

The editors would like to extend particular thanks to Sheenan Kindlen BSc SRD LRS, Coordinator, Biological Sciences (Health and Nursing) and Lecturer in Physiology/Clinical Physiology, Queen Margaret College, Edinburgh, for her valuable advice on the following chapters: *1 The physiological self, 4 Stress and the individual* and *5 Pain*.

1

The individual: self and society

The first section acknowledges the importance of *individuality* in nursing, from the standpoint of both the nurse and the patient. It addresses the concept of individuality from physiological and psychological perspectives before exploring how the person fits into and interacts with the environment.

The environment is a major source of physical and emotional stress and pain for the individual although internal factors may also be significant contributors.

1

The physiological self

Gillian Snowley

CHAPTER CONTENTS

In one chapter, it is impossible to convey more than some basic principles and objectives for understanding the physiological self. This chapter attempts to lead the reader towards the underlying purpose of body function – the constant endeavour by the body to remain physically and chemically 'balanced' or homeostatic. In doing this, the text aims to:

- introduce the basic physiology of the cell
- outline, with specific examples, the principles of cell division and inheritance
- describe the production of energy in the cell

- **explore homeostasis, focusing on specific body systems and using examples relevant to nursing practice to explain how problems may arise and the role of health professionals in re-establishing the balance.**

Much of physiology is an account, largely in terms of physics and chemistry, of *what* happens *where* in the body. In the past, detailed information about the minute structure of the cell was considered to be of academic interest only, but it is now evident that cytology (the study of the cell) is of major significance to physiology and pathology (the study of disease) and hence to health care. The other main area of physiology deals with the coordination of the individual parts of an organism to form an efficiently functioning whole: how the whole is greater than the sum of its parts, and how the parts behave as if they knew of the existence of each other and of the whole.

RECURRING PRINCIPLES OF PHYSIOLOGY

To attempt to cover, completely, the depth and the mysteries of the 'physiological self' in one chapter is not only an impossibility but also a belittling of the subject and of those who have studied it and made such knowledge available. However, certain principles or themes recur throughout the study of physiology, which may be summarised as follows.

Function is based on structure. Human movement, for example, depends on the structure of muscles, bones and nerves, and on their anatomical interrelationship. The dependence becomes even more evident when microscopic and more intricate structures are studied. One of the most intensively studied tissues is skeletal muscle, whose ultrastructure is revealed by electron microscopy and provides an explanation of muscular contraction.

The principle that function depends on structure applies also to biochemical events. For example, changing the shape of an enzyme molecule by heating it to above 40°C may render it biologically non-functional.

Genetics determines biological function. It is generally agreed that the information content of a DNA (deoxyribonucleic acid) molecule is responsible for the structure, function, behaviour and survival of a species. DNA carries the genetic code, and every part of body structure and function is determined by this code. Every detail of structure and function, every second of chemical activity, is ultimately subservient to the transmission of the genetic code to the germline (reproductive cells) for the survival of the species. Physiology is the discipline whose study reveals how this is achieved.

Homeostasis ensures survival. All organisms survive, in their lifetime, because of their ability to maintain a constant environment for their cells and tissues. In human beings, this environment is the fluid that surrounds the body cells (tissue fluid). The content of this fluid must be regulated to provide adequate nutrients to the cells (and to remove toxic waste) at the correct rate and temperature and within a narrow range of acidity/alkalinity. Much of the study of physiology is the study of how systems work to produce homeostasis.

These principles are explored further in this chapter. It has not been possible to provide an explanation of basic biochemical principles, nor is basic anatomy of tissues, organs and systems dealt with in any detail, but the microstructure of cells and molecules is outlined where this is essential to an understanding of physiology. (See the further reading list for helpful texts.)

The cell, its boundaries and its DNA are described in the first section. This enables the reader to move on to a brief exploration of heredity. The second section introduces some aspects of basic biochemistry, as well as factors that affect the sustenance of life at cellular and whole-body levels. The third section is devoted to the concept of homeostasis and how all the major body systems function towards its achievement. Throughout the chapter, examples are given of the relevance of physiology to nursing, health, and disorders of health. The following quotation explains why all nurses should have some knowledge of physiology:

When a physiological response is observed, one generally proceeds to ask the questions 'How' and 'Why'? The first is a physiological one; it means: 'what are the mechanisms responsible for the change; what is the sequence of events between the stimulus and the response?' The second question is not really physiological at all; it is an appeal to the idea of purpose . . . but can be very useful. Most people asking 'Why?' mean 'In what way does the response help to preserve the integrity and the efficiency of the organism, or to protect it from changes in the environment, either external or internal?' We reasonably take it for granted that unless an organism were equipped to make such responses it would never have survived. (Wright 1965)

THE CELL

The structure of a typical cell is shown in Figure 1.1.

Human beings are made up of cells, but there is a high degree of differentiation whereby these cells perform a variety of specialised functions, as befits a sophisticated animal such as a human being. With the exception of red blood cells, all human cells contain at least one nucleus surrounded by a mass of cytoplasm, which may contain a variety of cellular sub-units or organelles. Probably of greatest importance in appreciating the place of the cell in the overall physiology of the body is an understanding of the nature and purpose of the cell membranes, the nucleus and its genetic importance, and the biochemical cycle of events that produces energy.

THE CELL AND NUCLEAR MEMBRANES

The limiting boundary of the cell is the plasma membrane (cytoplasmic membrane or cell membrane). The plasma membrane acts as a permeability barrier that regulates the entry and exit of materials. It is composed of a double layer of phospholipids – fats – with protein molecules floating in a 'fatty' sea. Thus, the membrane structure is far from rigid, and the protein molecules are believed to be mobile within it, some extending all the way through it (protein bridges or channels). No holes or pores have been identified in the plasma membrane, and it is believed that the protein bridges allow fat-insoluble substances, for example, glucose, to cross the membrane. Fat-soluble substances, for example, alcohol, can, obviously, pass through the lipid layer.

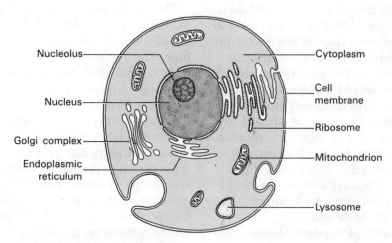

Nucleolus

Nucleus

Golgi complex

Endoplasmic reticulum

Cytoplasm

Cell membrane

Ribosome

Mitochondrion

Lysosome

Figure 1.1   A typical animal cell.

Transport across membranes

There are several mechanisms by which substances gain entry to or leave a cell:

- diffusion
- osmosis
- facilitated diffusion
- active transport
- phagocytosis and pinocytosis.

Diffusion is the passive movement of a substance from an area of high concentration to an area of low concentration of that substance. The substance may be water or a solute, such as glucose or sodium (Na^+). Diffusion requires no energy expenditure by the cell. Only small molecules make the transfer in this way.

Osmosis is the flow of a solvent (water, in the body) across a semi-permeable membrane (the cell membrane) from a weaker to a more concentrated solution, i.e. from a high water concentration to a low water concentration. This process will continue until the solutions on either side of the membrane are of equal concentration.

Facilitated diffusion is the method by which molecules become attached to carrier molecules within the membrane itself. The carrier molecule is specific for the transported substance, and there must still be a concentration gradient for facilitated diffusion to occur. Glucose is a substance transported across a muscle cell membrane in this way. No cell energy is expended to achieve such transport. The limiting factor for transport is the number of free carrier molecules.

Active transport is the process by which substances transfer across the plasma membrane when there is no concentration gradient, or against the gradient, i.e. from an area of low concentration to an area of high concentration. Cell energy is expended for this to occur. Active transport is an essential mechanism for the maintenance of constant cell composition within a changing extracellular environment (see 'Homeostasis and the body systems).

Phagocytosis and pinocytosis. Some substances or larger particles may enter cells by becoming engulfed (phagocytosis for particles, pinocytosis for water). The plasma membrane enfolds them, and they become enclosed in a fluid-filled vesicle. This method is regularly used by the mobile white blood cells that engulf bacteria. Once inside the cell, the engulfed substance undergoes chemical breakdown by intracellular enzymes. The soluble end-products then diffuse into the cytoplasm whilst indigestible remains are released into the surrounding environment by the reversal of phagocytosis.

THE NUCLEUS AND GENETIC MATERIAL

The most prominent feature of a cell, when viewed under the microscope, is the nucleus. It is separated from the cytoplasm by a double membrane. Transport mechanisms through the nuclear membrane are not as well understood as are those of the cytoplasmic membrane, and during the process of cell division the membrane disappears altogether, to re-form later.

Electron micrography reveals irregular masses of material, called chromatin, in the nucleus. Chromatin is a mixture of protein, deoxyribonucleic acid (DNA) and ribonucleic acid (RNA). When the cell reproduces itself, the chromatin becomes clearly visible in threads known as chromosomes. Also within the nucleus are one or two denser areas known as nucleoli. These are known to be rich in RNA.

The chromosomes contain the genetic information for the whole body, but, in any one cell, not all of this information will be active all of the time. The key molecule that carries the 'genetic code' is the DNA molecule (Fig. 1.2). Genetic information (genes) determines all parts of our make-up, from the colour of our eyes to the way we walk. The particular sequencing of bases within the DNA molecule determines the synthesis of a particular protein within a cell and thus controls cellular function. RNA, found within the nucleus and the cytoplasm, is a molecule that is able to transmit the genetic information from gene to ribosomes, which is where proteins are made (Box 1.1).

With the exception of the germ cells in the ovaries and testes, i.e. ova and spermatozoa, all

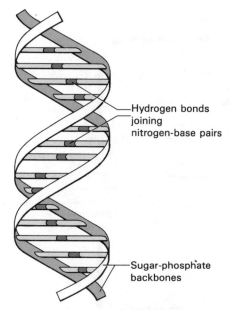

Hydrogen bonds joining nitrogen-base pairs

Sugar-phosphate backbones

Figure 1.2   The Watson and Crick model for DNA.

the nucleated cells of the human body contain 46 chromosomes, in 23 homologous pairs. Of each pair, one chromosome is derived from the person's mother and the other from the father. (The actual number of genes carried on these 46 chromosomes is at present unknown.) The chromosomes of a homologous pair are alike in size and shape, and can line up together as exactly as the two halves of a zip. There is one exception to this ruling, which is the pair of sex chromosomes. Of this pair, one is the X chromosome and the other may be the different Y chromosome, whose presence means that the person will be genetically male. An appreciation of the processes of cell division is the first step to understanding how characteristics are inherited.

CELL DIVISION

Mitosis

Man consists of approximately 10^{16} cells, but each individual is developed from a single cell. Not only must the 10^{16} cells be formed as the body grows and matures, but they must also be replaced in regeneration and repair. The type of

Box 1.1 **DNA and the genetic code**

DNA is a massive molecule (molecular weight in the millions) whose now well-known structure was identified by Watson and Crick in the 1950s.

It is composed of two molecular chains, which are intertwined in a helical configuration. The 'backbone' of each chain is made of sugars and phosphates. Protruding at regular intervals along the chain is one of four nitrogen base materials. Each chain of the double helix links with the other by a 'loose' chemical combination of the opposing nitrogen base (see Fig. 1.2).

It is the particular order of the bases in the two chains that determines the genetic information encoded in the DNA. It is important to remember that the base on one chain can only ever combine with one other base on the opposite chain. The four bases are:

- **adenosine**, which always links with **thymine**
- **guanine**, which always links with **cytosine**.

It is the sequencing of the nitrogen bases on one strand of the DNA double helix which conveys the genetic code. A DNA molecule is capable of reproducing itself exactly, according to the sequencing of bases on each strand. This is what happens during mitosis: as the chromosomes replicate, so does the DNA. In meiosis, as the chromosomes' strands become intertwined and partially exchanged, so do the strands of DNA, leading to genetic variation in the gametes and, therefore, the offspring.

The actual genetic code is now known to be a triplet code. A sequence of three bases on a DNA strand recognises one amino acid, so successive triplets specify amino acid sequence and hence protein structure. The codes for all 20 known amino acids are now well understood. Since proteins are made of amino acids, sometimes many thousands of triplet codings are necessary for the 'blueprint' of a single protein.

cell division that provides for this growth and repair is mitosis. The special significance of mitosis is that it ensures a continuous succession of cells with 46 chromosomes and the same genetic endowment.

During mitosis, the nucleus of the parent cell divides into two identical nuclei, after which the cytoplasm of the cell divides. In the early stage of mitosis each chromosome is duplicated so that the nucleus contains two identical complete sets of genes on identical pairs of chromosomes. Each chromosome is connected to its duplicate at one point called the centromere. Each identical portion of chromosome is known as a chromatid. The stages of mitosis are shown in Figure 1.3.

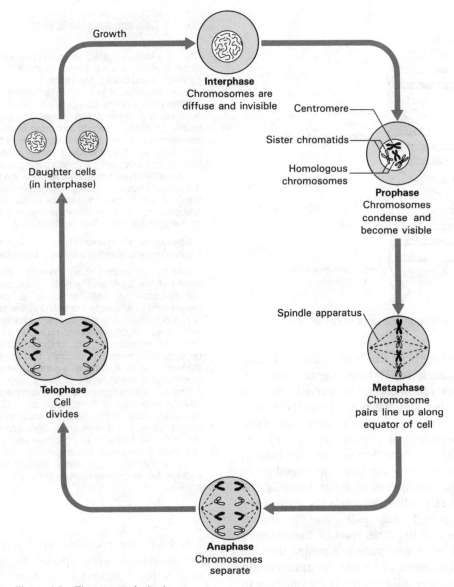

Figure 1.3   The stages of mitosis.

Although the process of mitosis produces millions of cells carrying identical sets of genes, it is important to remember that the resultant cells undergo specialisation by using only part of their inherent genetic code; for example, some cells in the pancreas produce insulin while nerve cells conduct electrical impulses. However, this feature of specialised cells doing specialised things is, itself, coded for in the DNA.

Meiosis

Some cells become specialised to form the reproductive cells or gametes. The female gamete is the ovum, and the male gamete is the sperm. Meiosis is the cell division that produces gametes. If gametes were produced by mitosis, the human egg and sperm would each contain 46 chromosomes. The fertilised egg, formed by their union, would then contain 92 chromosomes, as would the gametes produced by the resultant adult. Thus, with each new generation, the chromosome number would double. Meiosis prevents this from happening. The two most significant outcomes of meiosis are that:

- 23 single chromosomes occur in the gamete
- genes may have switched between paired chromosomes prior to their separation at actual cell division.

The process of meiosis is illustrated in Figure 1.4. (It should be noted that genetic switching occurs in the first division stage.) The resulting cells contain a mixture of maternal and paternal chromosomes because their segregation at anaphase is entirely random. Further randomness of gene inheritance in the gametes is produced by the 'crossing-over' of genetic material between chromatids. Since the resultant cells contribute through fertilisation to the next generation, sexual reproduction ensures the production of individuals who are different from their parents and from each other. (The exception here is identical twins, who are formed by a mitosis of the fertilised egg.)

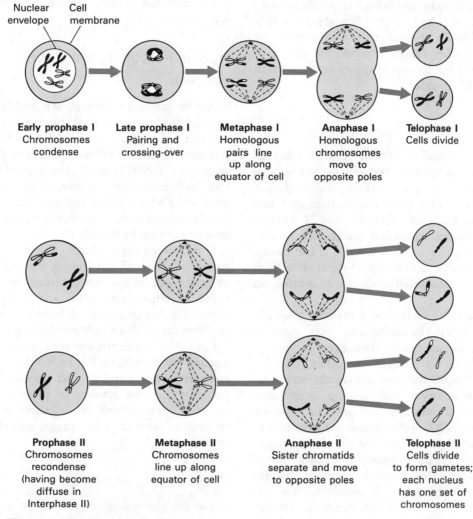

Figure 1.4 The stages of meiosis.

INHERITANCE

Meiosis provides a general picture of how the basic physiological process of inheritance works. It is the process whereby genetic material passes from one generation to the next. The foundations for the study and development of genetics and inheritance were laid by an Austrian monk, Gregor Mendel, in 1866. Mendel's work was brilliant and classical, and is still highly regarded as the first fundamental study of inheritance. However, he knew nothing of chromosomes and DNA, let alone cell structure, mitosis and meiosis. This makes his work all the more remarkable. The modern study of genetics, however, has shown that human inheritance is infinitely more complex than is laid out in Mendel's laws. It is not possible in this chapter to include any details of human inheritance and the theory of genetics, but the following topics are important for nurses to consider.

Factors affecting sex determination

In human beings, the female has 22 pairs of ordinary chromosomes (known as autosomes) and one pair of similar sex chromosomes (two X chromosomes, one from the mother and one from the father). The male also has 22 pairs of ordinary chromosomes but has a pair of dissimilar sex chromosomes (one X chromosome from the mother, and one Y chromosome from the father). Sex inheritance is illustrated in Figure 1.5.

The possibility of having a male or a female child is equal according to this normal, chromosomal inheritance. However, the sex of an individual is subject to other possible variables, despite the person's sex chromosome. All human embryos will develop as females, irrespective of whether the sex chromosome construction is XX or XY, unless male hormones are produced and function at early stages of embryonic development (usually about 6 weeks after fertilisation). It has been thought that a gene controlling male development exists and is located on the Y chromosome, but this has yet to be confirmed. The role of the

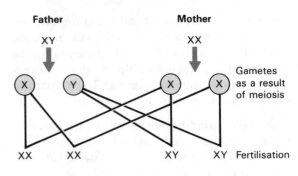

Figure 1.5 Sex inheritance.

Y chromosome in determining maleness is not well understood.

Human hereditary disorders

Mutations

By understanding what a gene is and how genes specify the formation of proteins, it is not difficult to appreciate how alteration to gene coding, for whatever reason, alters the functioning of a cell. Indeed, it is remarkable that this happens so infrequently. Changes in genes are known as mutations and may be responsible for altered function, disease or disability, which may or may not be inherited.

If mutations occur during the production of gametes (germinal mutations), the mutant gene or genes will be inherited. Mutations may also occur in other body cells, and these mutant genes will not be inherited (somatic mutations: e.g. skin cancer due to ultraviolet radiation).

Causes of mutations are always the subject of research investigations, but known causes include environmental, physical and chemical factors; possibly the best known of these is ionising radiation, the subject of extensive studies in relation to nuclear power plants and childhood leukaemia.

Chromosomal abnormalities

These are the results of too many or too few chromosomes being present in egg or sperm prior to fertilisation. The embryo produced will then have an abnormal number of chromosomes, which may or may not be compatible with life. The most common cause of chromosomal abnormality is failure of chromosome segregation in meiosis.

X-linked inheritance

This is a special kind of inheritance of a mutant gene, because it is carried on the X chromosome, and thus its pattern of inheritance is said to be sex-linked. This is because the opposing Y chromosome does not carry any genes to complement those carried on the X, so a male needs to inherit only one, possibly recessive, gene to exhibit the characteristic. If the gene happens to be a disease-causing one, the male then has the disease. X-linked inheritance, therefore, usually affects only males (Box 1.2).

There is now considerable debate around the suggestion that some serious mental illnesses (such as schizophrenia) are genetically attributable (and inheritable) because of mutations. (See Table 1.1 for examples of human hereditary disorders.)

THE SUSTENANCE OF LIFE

If human physiology is a study of *what* happens *where* in the body, there needs to be an understanding of the processes by which everything keeps going. This means that some appreciation of energy in the body is necessary. The cells of the body require energy for:

Box 1.2 Haemophilia as an example of sex-linked inheritance

Genes that are located on the X chromosome are said to be sex-linked, because usually only the male is affected by them. A female can also have a sex-linked characteristic, providing that both her X chromosomes carry the recessive gene. Probably the most well-known and serious sex-linked inherited disorder is the blood clotting disorder haemophilia. It has been famous as an inherited disorder in Queen Victoria's family, and, with intermarriage with European royals, the disorder has been inherited in these families. The disease has not been transmitted to living descendants of the English royal family.

Because of the different structures of X and Y chromosomes, a male (XY) will have haemophilia even if he carries only one recessive gene on his X chromosome. There is no opposing or complementary gene on the Y chromosome. A female must carry two recessive genes (one on each X chromosome) to have haemophilia. A female who is heterozygous for the condition is said to be a **carrier** although she will not have haemophilia.

When a carrier female (X*X) and a normal male (XY) have children, the following hereditary pattern is possible:

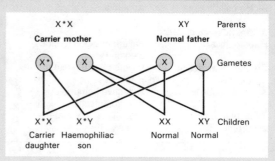

Below is a family pedigree for haemophilia. Can you determine why the blood-clotting status of one of the women in the second generation is unknown?

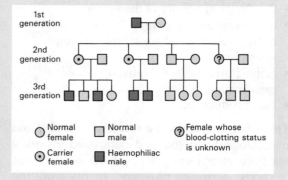

Table 1.1 Some well-known human hereditary disorders and diseases and their consequences

Disease	Major consequences
Chromosome abnormalities	
Down's syndrome	Mental retardation
Klinefelter's syndrome	Sterility, occasional mental retardation
Turner's syndrome	Sterility, lack of sexual development
Autosomal dominant mutations	
Achondroplasia	Dwarfism
Retinoblastoma	Blindness
Porphyria	Abnominal pain, psychosis
Huntington's chorea	Nervous-system degeneration
Neurofibromatosis	Growths in nervous system and skin
Polydactyly	Extra fingers and toes
Autosomal recessive mutations	
Cystic fibrosis	Respiratory disorders
Xeroderma pigmentosum	Skin cancers
Albinism	Lack of pigment in skin and eyes
Phenylketonuria	Mental retardation
Homocystinuria	Mental retardation
Sickle-cell disease	Anaemia
X chromosome mutations	
Haemophilia	Failure of blood to clot, bleeding
Duchenne muscular dystrophy	Progressive muscular weakness
Agammaglobulinaemia	Defective immune system, infections
Testicular feminising syndrome	Sterility, lack of male organs

- the synthesis of large molecules, such as proteins, from smaller ones (which happens in growth)
- the electrical activity of the nerves
- the activation of the contractile machinery of muscle cells to produce contraction and movement
- active transport (see 'Transport across membranes,' above)
- heat production.

These five functions, the result of complex and meticulously ordered and controlled chemical reactions at cell level, support the whole range of body activities. All are energy-requiring reactions, the energy being supplied by energy-releasing reactions, of which cellular respiration is the most significant. Cellular respiration makes a sixth function, which is the result of complex and controlled intracellular chemistry, and completes the list of life-sustaining processes. However, without it, none of the other five would ever happen at all; thus cellular respiration merits consideration at this early stage.

ENERGY FROM CELLULAR RESPIRATION

Cellular respiration is the production of energy as a result of the oxidation of food material such as glucose. Since the production of energy does not necessarily correspond with the body's needs at any given moment, the body requires a mechanism for storing energy. Stored energy is the outcome of cellular respiration. The unit of stored energy is known as adenosine triphosphate (ATP). This molecule is able to release energy, when required, and it then changes into adenosine diphosphate (ADP), having lost a phosphate group.

Cellular respiration is the process by which energy-laden molecules of ATP are made. The basic ingredients for cellular respiration are food material (such as glucose) and oxygen. A large number of reactions is involved in the full breakdown of glucose to produce energy. Every stage requires the presence of its own specific enzyme, and oxygen is required for the final stage of this chain reaction. This makes cellular respiration an aerobic reaction (requiring the presence of oxygen), although, if the oxygen supply is limited, a less efficient form of cellular respiration occurs. This process, known as anaerobic respiration, produces less energy. (A byproduct of anaerobic respiration is lactic acid, which produces the well-known symptom of 'cramp' in the muscles of weary athletes.)

The way in which cellular energy production is expressed is in units of ATP, the unit of stored energy. Cells can 'manage' with a limited supply of oxygen, but their ability to carry out the full range of energy-requiring chemical activities is much diminished by a reduction in oxygen, and cells cannot function for more than a few minutes if the oxygen supply is completely blocked for any reason. Nervous tissue is particularly sensitive to oxygen deficit and will not maintain its function after a maximum of about 3 minutes of anoxia (lack of oxygen).

Although glucose is the major food molecule used in cellular respiration, almost all cells, with the exception of nervous tissue, are able to use fats for energy production. Fats, when oxidised in cellular respiration, produce large numbers of ATP molecules, but unfortunate byproducts are also produced. These are acidic substances, which, if produced unchecked because of a shortage of glucose, can cause highly acidic body fluids, a situation that eventually leads to death. Fats are metabolised only if there is a shortage of glucose or if glucose use is impaired, as in diabetes. Similarly, proteins can be used to produce energy, but the output is small. Proteins are used for energy production only in cases of extreme lack of glucose (such as during starvation), and, if this happens, the main protein stores (muscles) are much reduced and severe weight loss ensues.

Most of the reactions of cellular respiration occur in the mitochondria of the cells. Enzymes coat the inner, folded lining of the mitochondria. The number and inner complexity of the mitochondria increase markedly in a cell that is highly active in producing energy. Cells in the most metabolically active organ in the body, the liver, have large numbers of complex mitochondria.

It may not be necessary for the reader to know any greater detail than this about the chemistry of energy production. Much more specific detail is known, and there is a great deal of information available for the interested student. In the early stages of nursing studies, however, it will not normally be necessary to take this topic any further.

THE IMPORTANCE OF ENZYMES IN CELL CHEMISTRY

To be alive means to be producing energy by the oxidation of carbon compounds, such as glucose. Without this basic cell chemistry, nothing else will happen. Although glucose (or some other food molecule) and oxygen are primary require-ments for energy production, of equal significance are the enzyme molecules that must be present for even the simplest of the oxidation reactions to take place. All enzymes are proteins and they, themselves, have to be made and replaced. This, too, requires energy. Enzymes, like all proteins, are highly sensitive to changes in their environment, so that minute changes in temperature, acidity/alkalinity and concentrations of components of the cellular fluid around them may reduce or stop altogether the chemical reactions they initiate and control. Their physical, molecular structure is a highly significant factor in their ability to function at all, because of the required physical linkage between the enzyme and the molecule undergoing the chemical reaction (the substrate). This means that even if the basic ingredients for energy production are present, unless the intracellular environment is perfect, cell chemistry will not proceed normally, and life will cease, if imperfections persist.

Factors affecting enzyme action

Each cell contains many different enzymes, each catalysing a specific chemical reaction. Without exception, each species of enzyme molecule is a protein of very specific amino acid composition and sequence. The work of geneticists has demonstrated that proteins, including enzymes, are the primary gene products. Enzymes regulate all the synthesising and metabolising activities of the cell, but enzymes will function only when the following conditions are fulfilled:

1. Enzymes normally function within a very narrow range of pH, although the optimum pH will be different for different enzymes.
2. Enzymes function within a very narrow temperature range. As temperatures rise, enzymes may break down chemically and be permanently denatured. At low temperatures they become inactive but are restored to activity when normal temperature is restored.
3. Frequently, the action of enzymes depends upon the presence of co-factors. Minerals (such as iron, sodium, potassium) and vitamins are co-factors in enzyme function (Table 1.2).

Table 1.2   The vitamins: their actions, sources and results of deficiency (Reproduced from Wilson 1990)

Vitamin	Chemical name	Source	Stability	Functions	Deficiency diseases	Dietary reference values (Department of Health 1991)
Fat-soluble vitamins*						
A	Retinol (carotene provitamin in plants)	Milk, butter, cheese, egg yolk, fish liver oils, green and yellow vegetables	Some loss at high temperatures and long exposure to light and air	Maintains healthy epithelial tissues and cornea. Formation of visual purple	Keratinisation Xerophthalmia Stunted growth Night blindness	1–2 mg
D	Calciferol	Fish liver oils, milk, cheese, egg yolk, irradiated 7-dehydro-cholesterol in human skin	Very stable	Facilitates the absorption and utilisation of calcium and phosphorus = healthy bones and teeth	Rickets Osteomalacia	2–10 µg
E	Tocopherols	Egg yolk, milk, butter, green vegetables, nuts	Destroyed by rancid fat and iron salts	Prevents catabolism of polyunsaturated fats	Anaemia Ataxia Cystic fibrosis Scotomas	15 mg
K	Phylloquinone	Leafy vegetables, fish liver, fruit	Destroyed by light, strong acids and alkalis	Formation of prothrombin and Factors VII, IX and X in the liver	Slow blood clotting Haemorrhages in the newborn	2–10 µg
Water-soluble vitamins						
B_1	Thiamin	Yeast, liver, germ of cereals, nuts, pulses, rice polishings, egg yolk, liver, legumes	Destroyed by heat	Metabolism of carbohydrates and nutrition of nerve cells	General fatigue and loss of muscle tone Ultimately leads to beriberi Stunted growth	1–1.5 mg
B_2	Riboflavin	Liver, yeast, milk, eggs, green vegetables, kidney, fish roe	Destroyed by light and alkalis	Carbohydrate and protein metabolism Healthy skin and eyes	Angular stomatitis Cheilosis Dermatitis Eye lesions	1.5–2 mg
B_6	Pyridoxine	Meat, liver, vegetables, bran of cereals, egg yolk, beans, soya beans	Stable	Protein metabolism Production of antibodies	Very rare	1.5–2.5 mg
B_{12}	Cobalamine	Liver, milk, moulds, fermenting liquors, egg	Destroyed by heat	Maturation of RBCs	Pernicious anaemia Degeneration of nerve fibres of the spinal cord	1–2 µg
B	Folic acid	Dark green vegetables, liver, kidney, eggs. Synthesised in colon	Destroyed by heat and moisture	Formation of RBCs	Anaemia	100–200 µg

Table 1.2 (*cont.*)

Vitamin	Chemical name	Source	Stability	Functions	Deficiency diseases	Dietary reference values (Department of Health 1991)
B	Niacin (nicotinic acid)	Yeast, offal, fish, pulses, whole-meal cereals. Synthesised in the body from tryptophan	Fairly stable	Necessary for tissue oxidation Inhibits production of cholesterol	Prolonged deficiency causes pellagra, i.e. dermatitis, diarrhoea and dementia	15–20 mg
B	Pantothenic acid	Liver, yeast, egg yolk, fresh vegetables	Destroyed by excessive heat and freezing	Associated with amino acid metabolism	Unknown	Unknown
B	Biotin	Yeasts, liver, kidney pulses, nuts	Stable	Carbohydrates and fat metabolism Growth of bacteria	Dermatitis Conjunctivitis Hypercholes-terolaemia	100 µg
C	Ascorbic acid	Citrus fruits, currants, berries, green vegetables, potatoes, liver and glandular tissue in animals	Destroyed by heat, ageing, acids, alkalis, chopping salting and drying	Formation of intercellular matrix Maturation of RBCs	Multiple haemorrhages Slow wound healing Anaemia Gross deficiency causes scurvy	30–60 mg

*Bile is necessary for the absorption of these vitamins. Mineral oils interfere with absorption.

4. Enzymes are very specific in action – each enzyme will catalyse reactions for only chemically related substrates – and act by forming a complex, but temporary, bonding with one of the reacting molecules.
5. Enzymes are swiftly inhibited by the presence of foreign substances. (Minute quantities of some poisons can have a devastating effect by stopping enzyme activity.)
6. Some enzymes have to be stored in inactive form, e.g. a protein-digesting enzyme would, otherwise, destroy the organ in which it is stored.

Because of these demanding requirements to sustain enzyme activity, upon which the life of cells depends, the whole of the rest of human structure and function works to maintain the constancy of the environment for the sake of the enzymes, those fussy proteins that DNA produces. Maintenance of a constant internal environment is called homeostasis.

HOMEOSTASIS AND THE BODY SYSTEMS

Homeostasis is the tendency of the body to maintain the stability of the internal environment in the face of environmental changes and changing internal demands. It enables, for example, the individual to adapt slowly to living at high altitude or to rapidly flee from danger. Two points about homeostasis should be borne in mind throughout the following discussion:

1. Homeostasis is a dynamic process, sometimes referred to as dynamic equilibrium. Everything that happens in the body is monitored constantly, with small adjustments being made. Even during sleep, a great deal happens; for example, sugar levels, blood oxygen levels and body temperature are constantly monitored and adjusted. The body never rests completely, even during sleep.

2. When homeostatic balance is not maintained, the health of the person is threatened, and disease or even death may be the result. Nursing and medical intervention is an attempt to prevent imbalance occurring or to restore homeostasis.

Maintenance of intracellular chemistry, by maintaining a balanced intra- and extracellular environment, is essential to life. The regulation of osmolarity, pH, temperature and the balance of the ions in body fluids is critical for maintaining cell function. Every system in the body has maintenance of this constant internal environment as its ultimate purpose. (The possible exception is the reproductive system, whose sole function is the long-term survival of the species, rather than the short-term survival of the individual – although homeostatic mechanisms will, themselves, ensure correct functioning of this system!)

The body systems, in homeostatic terms, are as follows:

1. *Suppliers, waste disposers and transporters.* These are systems that communicate with the external environment. They supply nutrients, water and oxygen to the tissues, and remove waste. They are the respiratory, gastrointestinal, renal and cardiovascular systems.

2. *Detectors.* These are usually nervous (sensory) receptors, which can detect internal changes of pressure, changes in muscular tone or external dangers, such as heat, cold and physical trauma. Some detectors may be chemical in nature, such as the oxygen- and carbon dioxide-sensitive cells in the brain, which detect abnormally high or low blood gas levels. Some glands also act as detectors, as seen, for example, in the pancreatic β-cells, which monitor blood glucose levels.

3. *Effectors.* These are usually muscular structures (such as in the heart, as well as muscles for breathing, shivering and major body movement) and glands. Muscles and glands act to make changes.

4. *Regulators.* These systems make sure that the detector–effector mechanism is continued, so that the timing, strength and duration of response are appropriate. These systems are the nervous system and the endocrine system.

In any further study about the physiological functioning of the person, the reader should strive to discover how these individual systems contribute to the homeostatic balance of the whole body.

REGULATION MECHANISMS IN HOMEOSTASIS

The regulatory processes depend in many instances on the principle of feedback. A man-made physical system, such as a computer, can be made so accurate that it will produce a predictable result under normal and predictable conditions. Living systems, however, must be able to function to produce a balanced system within narrow limits despite large and unexpected external variations; for example, they must maintain a normal glucose supply to cells during a period of fasting. The means by which the body achieves regulation is feedback.

Most control systems in the body act by negative feedback, which may be represented as in Figure 1.6. An example of such a system is maintaining balanced blood sugar levels. A disturbance, such as the absorption of high levels of glucose into the blood following a meal, 'signals' the sensor in the control system (in this case, cells in the pancreas). The pancreas also acts as the effector by releasing the hormone insulin. Insulin then acts on several body tissues, for example muscle and fat cells, and reduces the blood glucose level by facilitating their uptake of glucose from the blood. The response by the body has been in a negative or opposite direction to the disturbance, to compensate for the abnormality. Such mechanisms are self-regulating and automatic. There is no voluntary control over them, which is just as well because it would be impossible to manage, voluntarily, all the thousands of controlling mechanisms that operate simultaneously within the body. Such feedback mechanisms occur in every compartment of human physiology, including endocrine function, blood circulation, breathing and body

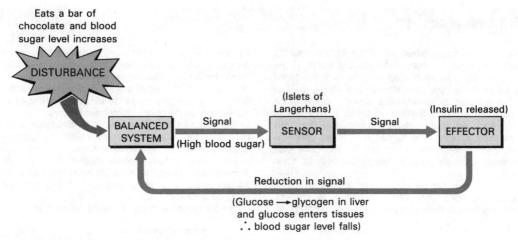

Figure 1.6 Negative feedback mechanism.

temperature. Positive feedback mechanisms are much less frequent. As the name suggests, they act in the direction of the disturbance, thus compounding the situation.

Positive feedback is generally used to produce an explosive or successively catalytic effect. Examples of useful positive feedback mechanisms include uterine contractions at birth (whereby one contraction induces further contractions and so on until the baby is expelled from the uterus) and the less obviously energetic blood-clotting mechanism (Box 1.3). Most positive feedback mechanisms are harmful, even fatal, the most well-known of these probably being progressive shock (Box 1.4).

Although homeostatic regulating mechanisms are automatic, they are not always rapid. This is because they often act via chemical messengers in the blood (hormones) or via slow-acting nerve fibres. There is often a time lapse between stimulus (abnormality) and response (restoration). Therefore, there may be too great a build-up of stimulus, or too great a production of restorative, and perfect balance may take some time to be achieved. This is what leads to fluctuations around the normal value, although these are usually within narrow limits. If the fluctuations increase and remain unrestored, homeostasis is lost, and it is at this stage that medical or nursing intervention may prevent disaster or speed recovery. This is why it is important for nurses to know something about normal levels (and acceptable fluctuations around the normal) of the measurable components of homeostatic mechanisms in human physiology. Of equal importance is the ability to observe and detect any of these dangerous fluctuations. Probably the most obvious measurement a nurse may undertake is the person's body temperature, but the range of disturbances of homeostatic control is as vast as the numbers of chemical reactions and controlling mechanisms that support them.

THE CARDIOVASCULAR SYSTEM AND HOMEOSTASIS

The cardiovascular system – i.e., the heart, blood and the vessels along which the blood moves – has evolved to transport materials to and from all regions of the body. In simple organisms (e.g. yeast cells or amoebae), such a system is unnecessary because the functioning units (the cells) are in direct contact with their nutrient and oxygen supply and their means of waste removal – normally the solution in which they live.

In the human body, the cardiovascular system transports respiratory gases, nutrients, waste products, hormones, antibodies and salts to and from all cells. Blood is a complex tissue and contains many cell types. It acts as a vehicle for many homeostatic agents and is, in fact, one itself.

Box 1.3 **Blood clotting**

Blood clots (or **coagulates**) when the soluble plasma protein **fibrinogen** changes into insoluble **fibrin**. Fibrin forms a webby network of long strands, in which blood cells become trapped. The strands are sticky, so that the clot adheres to surrounding tissues, which plugs any gap and prevents leakage of blood. If exposed to the air, such as at an external wound, the clot dries and hardens. Clotting (the formation of fibrin) concerns the plasma. Plasma without cells will clot: cells play an entirely passive role in being trapped in fibrin strands.

Fibrinogen is a natural constituent of plasma, but it changes into fibrin only when **thrombin** is present. Thrombin is not normally present in plasma, existing only as the precursor substance, **prothrombin**, which is another plasma protein. The conversion of prothrombin to thrombin takes place when activator substances are released from damaged tissues and platelets (**extrinsic factors**) and in the presence of certain other essential substances in the plasma (**intrinsic factors**).

The coagulation mechanism is a 'biological amplifier' (positive feedback), sometimes called a 'cascade' of enzyme-controlled reactions, whereby one substance is activated and, in turn, triggers another action and so on. Thirteen main coagulation factors have now been named. Absence of one or more of them will cause failure (or reduced speed) of clotting.

The full mechanism can be represented thus:

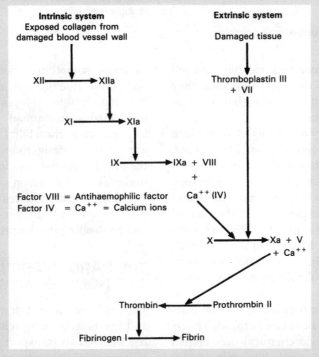

The intrinsic and extrinsic systems join in the final common pathway, which converts prothrombin to thrombin. It will not be necessary to know all of the factors and reactions, but the following simplified version should be learned.

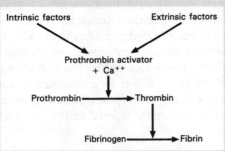

The entire clotting sequence takes about 4–8 minutes (the clotting time). However, once Factor X is activated, the rest takes just a few seconds.

It is important to realise that blood must contain regulators or natural inhibitors of clotting to prevent the clotting mechanism spreading from the point of injury or damage to the entire system. Some of these have been identified, but the whole process is not well understood at the present time.

Box 1.4 **Shock**

'Shock' means a decrease in circulating blood volume, caused by the loss of blood (haemorrhagic or hypovolaemic shock), poor cardiac activity (cardiogenic shock) or severe distress (neurogenic shock). Whatever the cause, the loss of circulating blood volume causes the following sequence of events to occur (at this stage, the reader may not be familiar with all of the terms used, but the important thing is the overall pattern).

Non-progressive shock

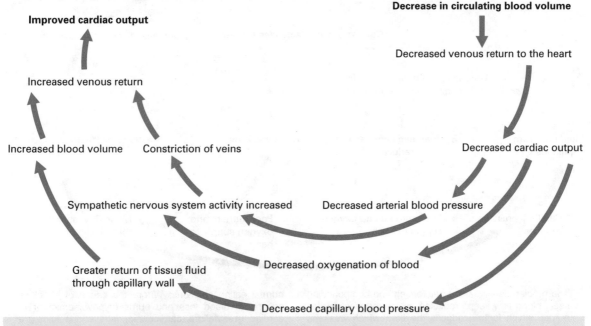

In the illustration above, negative feedback mechanisms, acting through the sympathetic nervous system, produce an increase in the circulating blood volume to improve cardiac output and so restore equilibrium.

Signs and symptoms of shock

Under conditions of shock, the circulation of blood to the vital organs (brain and heart) has priority, with the result that blood supply to the skin, gut, kidneys and skeletal muscle is reduced. Because of this, and taking account of the cycle illustrated above, it is easy to understand the common signs and symptoms observed in a shocked patient:

- Pallor – owing to constriction of peripheral capillaries
- Rapid pulse ⎱ – owing to sympathetic nervous
- Sweating ⎰ stimulation
- Weak pulse – owing to low blood volume and reduced cardiac output
- Oligaemia – owing to reduced kidney function
- Low blood pressure – owing to reduced cardiac output.

(cont'd on p. 20)

Apart from the blood itself, the cardiovascular system consists of:

- the main propulsive organ, the *heart*, which forces blood around the body
- an *arterial system*, which assists in propelling the blood and smoothing the blood flow to the periphery
- *capillaries*, across the walls of which transfer of materials occurs between blood and tissues
- the *venous system*, which acts as a blood reservoir and as a system for returning blood to the heart.

Blood

This is the medium in which all materials are transported around the body. In its passage through the capillaries, its composition changes as components are exchanged across the capillary walls with those of tissue fluid. Thus continuous

Box 1.4 (cont.)

Progressive shock

Here, the cause is so severe (usually severe haemorrhage, extensive fluid loss through burns, or cardiac failure) that the usual negative feedback mechanisms cannot compensate. Thus, the following cycle occurs:

Decreased blood volume

Decreased venous return to the heart

Decreased cardiac output

Mechanisms illustrated above fail to compensate

Blood flow so reduced that...

Poor nutrient and oxygen supply to heart

Heart weakens

Cardiac output decreases further

Venous return diminishes, blood vessels dilate and blood pools in veins

Sympathetic nerve activity reduces

Poor nutrient and oxygen supply to brain

Fluid loss from capillaries

Capillary pressure reduces

The problem is increasing, reinforcing and compounding itself: blood flow keeps reducing, which reduces cardiac output, which further reduces the flow, which weakens the heart further, etc., etc.

Treatment of shock

The priority is to improve the circulating blood volume by giving intravenous fluids, such as plasma, whole blood or normal saline solutions. Where the cause of shock is severe, in blood loss and burns (hypovolaemic) or in cardiac arrest/failure (cardiogenic), intravenous fluids are always given. In neurogenic shock (pain, bad news or other emotional shock), the shock is rarely progressive, and recovery does not normally require fluid replacement, although other care may be required for pain relief, reassurance and rest.

exchange functions to maintain an optimum internal environment for cell and tissue function, and without it homeostasis would not exist.

Plasma

The fluid component of blood, plasma, is the transporting agent for nutrients, hormones, salts (electrolytes) and carbon dioxide. Of special significance in homeostasis at tissue fluid level is the plasma protein content of plasma, which exerts a significant osmotic pressure within blood and assists in the osmotic recovery of water from body tissues. Another particular homeostatic component of plasma is the protein fibrinogen and the other clotting factors, whose cascading interactions cause the formation of blood clots, a protective mechanism of singular significance (see Box 1.3). Many other plasma proteins have the specific function of giving protection against invading foreign proteins, and are known collectively as antibodies.

The cellular components of blood

The cellular components of the blood (Fig. 1.7) are:

- erythrocytes (red blood cells)
- leucocytes (white blood cells)
- thrombocytes (platelets).

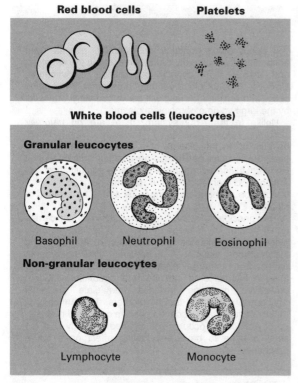

Red blood cells   **Platelets**

White blood cells (leucocytes)

Granular leucocytes

Basophil   Neutrophil   Eosinophil

Non-granular leucocytes

Lymphocyte   Monocyte

Figure 1.7   The cellular components of blood. Adults have close to 30 trillion red blood cells. *Note 1*: There are about 5×10^9 red blood cells and 7.5×10^6 white blood cells in each litre of blood. *Note 2*: Basophils, neutrophils, eosinophils and lymphocytes are sometimes known collectively as polymorphs because of their irregular shape and many-lobed nuclei.

Erythrocytes

These should be considered, in homeostatic terms, for two major reasons:

1. The major constituent of a red blood cell is haemoglobin. This protein molecule, with its constituent iron-containing portion, has a structure that enables it to form a rapid but reversible combination with oxygen. As oxyhaemoglobin, life-sustaining oxygen is collected in the lung tissues and transported to all body cells. The affinity of haemoglobin for oxygen keeps increasing as more oxygen is bound and delivered; this is a positive feedback mechanism that is due to successive minor changes in the configuration of the globin part of the molecule.

Some genetic abnormalities exist that affect the structure of the haemoglobin molecule, thereby affecting its ability to transport oxygen. The best-known disorder is sickle-cell anaemia, which is anaemia (lack of circulating blood oxygen) caused by a mutant kind of haemoglobin.

2. Red blood cells also carry the proteins that are responsible for blood grouping. The blood grouping proteins are known as antigens as they will stimulate antibody production (as would any other foreign protein) if introduced into the blood of a person whose grouping is different. There are a great many antigens carried on the surface of red blood cells, but the most significant to understand are those concerned with the ABO and Rhesus systems: this is because of their potentially devastating effects during blood transfusions. The actual physiological importance of these proteins to the person whose blood cells carry them is unknown: they are significant only when they cause problems, which, fortunately, is rare (Box 1.5).

Leucocytes

The homeostatic significance of leucocytes is discussed in 'The immune system and homeostasis' below.

Thrombocytes

Often known as platelets, these are the smallest cellular components of blood. Their major function is in the arrest of bleeding, by adhesion to the endothelium of a damaged blood vessel. They form a platelet plug, which can stop blood flow (see Box 1.3). In a situation of vessel damage, platelets also produce an activator chemical, which assists in the blood-clotting mechanism. Thrombocytes are significant homeostatic regulators.

The heart

The mammalian heart has evolved to become a sophisticated muscular pump, capable of sustained and untiring activity and able to respond to the changing homeostatic needs of the body. A detailed consideration of the structure of cardiac muscle shows that the tissue has similarities to ordinary skeletal muscle, but that its cells are electrically coupled. Cardiac muscle is capable of spontaneous contraction, even if removed from the body and kept in a warm,

Box 1.5 **Blood groups**

About 12 different blood grouping systems have been identified, the most important of which are the ABO and Rhesus systems. Blood grouping is the result of particular **antigens** carried on the surface of red blood cells. An antigen is any substance that causes the stimulation of an antibody. Blood groups are genetically determined.

The ABO system

Group	Antigens present on red blood cells	Antibodies naturally present in plasma
A	A	Antibody B
B	B	Antibody A
AB	A and B	None
O	Neither	Antibody A and antibody B

If plasma containing Antibody A comes into contact with red blood cells containing Antigen A, the cells clump together and are eventually destroyed. The clumping (**agglutination**) can cause serious blockage in small blood vessels, and red cell destruction causes anaemia and jaundice. Small concentrations of antibody do not cause seriously damaging agglutination. Whilst exactly matched blood is normally provided for transfusion, certain transfusions are possible in emergencies, as in the following:

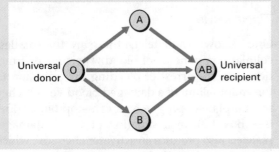

If donor blood contains unfavourable plasma (with antibodies) this is rapidly diluted on entering the recipient, and stands little chance of causing agglutination. However, if donor blood contains unfavourable red blood cells (with antigens), these will be immediately 'attacked' by the large volume of recipient plasma.

Unlike in the ABO system, there are *no naturally occurring Rhesus antibodies*. However, Antibody D will be built up in the plasma of a Rhesus negative (Rh⁻) person who receives Rhesus positive (Rh⁺) blood. A first Rh⁺ transfusion will not normally cause agglutination, but Antibody D remains in the plasma. A second Rh⁺ transfusion is, therefore, dangerous and to be avoided at all costs.

This principle is at work when an Rh⁻ woman carries an Rh⁺ child. Any leakage of fetal cells into the maternal bloodstream stimulates the production of Antibody D in the mother's plasma. A subsequent Rh⁺ fetus is in danger from maternal Antibody D, which may transfer through the placenta into the fetal circulation. Modern preventive medicine includes immediate postnatal Antibody D injections to Rh⁻ mothers. The Antibody D rapidly destroys any escaped positive cells, and no build-up of Antibody D occurs. The injected Antibody D is too small a dose to have any lasting effect on a future pregnancy.

The Rhesus system

Group	Antigen present on red blood cells	Antibodies in plasma
Rhesus positive	Rhesus antigen (D)	None
Rhesus negative	None	None

nutrient- and oxygen-rich solution. Within the body, the muscle is coordinated to contract rhythmically and strongly by the nervous stimulation of the tissue.

The electrical stimulation of the heart is initiated in the pacemaking region, and electrical activity spreads over the heart from one cell to another because of electrical coupling. As the wave of excitation spreads, so the cardiac cells are stimulated to contract. Any interference with this electrical transmission, such as may occur with cardiac tissue death (usually due to a dis-

rupted blood supply to the tissue and called myocardial infarction), can stop the coordinated pumping action of the heart.

The mechanical pumping action of the heart, once initiated by the pacemaker, is a controlled system of fluid flowing through chambers, sustained by the action of valves that prevent backflow and disturbance (see Fig. 1.8). Wear and tear or disease of the valves can affect this smooth flow and lead to mechanical stress on the cardiac muscle, with resultant loss of vigour, accompanied by heart enlargement.

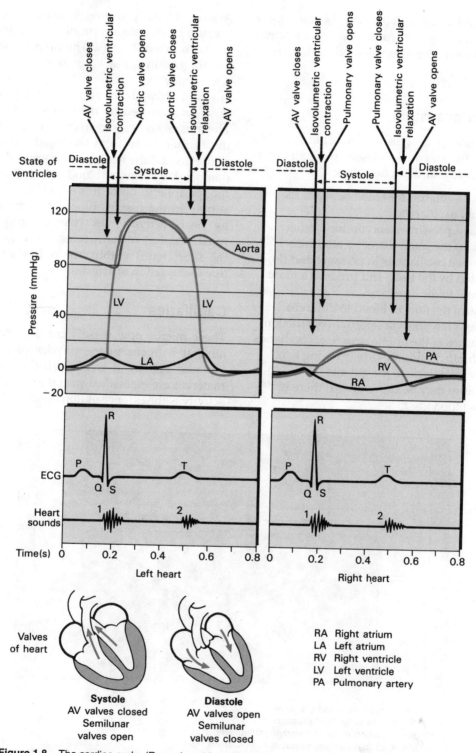

Figure 1.8   The cardiac cycle. (Reproduced from Hinchliff & Montague (1988) with kind permission from Baillière Tindall.)

These mechanical activities may be the subject of careful investigation for sounds of abnormal valve closure or abnormal blood flow sounds in the heart.

The arterial system

This consists of a series of branching vessels whose walls are thick, elastic and muscular. Arteries serve four main functions:

1. To act as a conduit for blood between the heart and capillaries.
2. To act as a pressure reservoir for forcing blood into the small-diameter arterioles.
3. To dampen oscillations in pressure and flow generated by the heart and produce a more even flow to the capillaries.
4. To control the flow of blood to different capillary networks via selective constriction of branches of the arterial tree (e.g. capillaries to the brain, heart and kidneys being kept open, whilst those to the gut and/or extremities may be shut down, if there is serious blood loss).

Arterial blood pressure is controlled, largely because of the proportion of muscle and elastic tissue in arterial walls. The arteries alter their control within quite large ranges of pressure, which may be augmented by increased heart rate and strength or by restriction in capillary flow, or decreased by the opposite phenomena. The muscle and elastic layers alter in proportion the further away from the heart the artery is. Those nearest the heart require great elasticity to dampen the surges of blood, whilst those nearer the periphery need more rigidity to sustain supply to the tissues. Blood pressure is altered by heart activity and changes in peripheral resistance, but remains remarkably constant (in the short term) within one individual, largely due to the action of arteries.

Capillaries

These microscopic vessels are the end-point of all that happens in the physics of the cardio-vascular system. It is through their walls that materials are exchanged with the tissues, and this activity is the essence of homeostasis (Fig. 1.9).

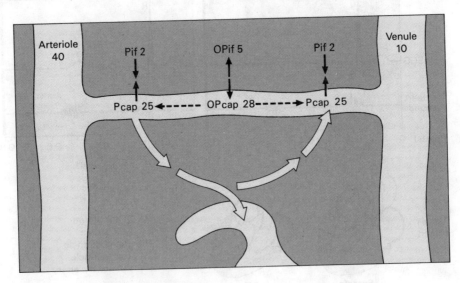

Pcap = capillary blood pressure
Pif = interstitial fluid pressure
OPcap = colloid osmotic pressure in capillary
OPif = colloid osmotic pressure in interstitial fluid

All figures refer to pressure in mmHg

Figure 1.9 The formation and reabsorption of tissue fluid.

Under normal conditions, the volume of the plasma and the volume of tissue fluid that it is supplying change very little, despite massive transfers of substances between the two. This phenomenon is known as the Starling equilibrium of capillary exchange. The physiologist Starling pointed out as long ago as the last century that the direction and rate of transfer of substances between the capillary and the fluid in tissue spaces depended on three things:

1. the hydrostatic pressure on each side of the capillary wall
2. the osmotic pressure of protein in the plasma and in the tissue fluid
3. the properties of the capillary wall (its semi-permeability).

The venous system

This is a large-volume, low-pressure system with vessels of large internal diameter. It acts as a storage reservoir for blood, which is returned steadily to the heart for redistribution.

Blood flow in veins is affected by a number of factors other than contraction of the heart. Activity of limb muscles and pressure exerted within the thoracic and abdominal cavities squeeze veins in those parts of the body. Long, large veins also have pocket valves in their walls; these prevent backflow.

Bleeding depletes the venous blood reservoir, but the smooth muscle tissue in the arteriolar walls is stimulated into action (negative feedback mechanism) to cause some reduction in outflow to the skin and gut and thus help to maintain venous blood pressure.

The lymphatic system

Any consideration of the cardiovascular system would be incomplete without reference to the lymphatic system. This system is a drainage system additional to the veins. Most of the tissue fluid returns to the blood capillaries, but a little remains to be drained by the lymphatic capillaries, which originate as blind-ending, microscopic tubules within the tissues. As well as returning excess fluid to the cardiovascular system (which the lymph vessels join in the large veins of the neck), any leaked plasma proteins readily enter the lymph vessels, whose hydrostatic pressure is very low. Lymphatic capillaries are also important in the absorption of fat from the intestine. The lymphatic system also includes lymph glands, which filter debris and are the main centres of lymphocyte production (see 'The immune system and homeostasis').

THE RESPIRATORY SYSTEM AND HOMEOSTASIS

Oxygen, combined with carbon compounds, is used to produce energy in tissue respiration, as previously described; during this process carbon dioxide is produced as a waste product. The body must, therefore, have a mechanism for transferring oxygen to and removing carbon dioxide from the tissues as quickly and efficiently as possible. Transportation of these materials is carried out by the cardiovascular system, as already described, but the actual exchange of these gases between the external world and the individual is the function of the respiratory system.

In more primitive animals, the gases are exchanged by passive diffusion across the body surface (cf. the moist skin of a frog or earthworm, or the cell membrane of an amoeba). The human gas exchange surface is provided by the microscopic alveoli of the lungs. These provide the following requirements for gaseous exchange:

- The surface area of the exchange membrane is large in comparison with the body volume to be supplied. (Human alveoli would fill a tennis court if spread out.)
- The exchange surface is thin, and permeable. (Alveoli have one-cell-thick walls.)
- The surface is moist to facilitate diffusion. (The lining of the alveoli is always moist.)
- Stagnation of the medium close to the surface of the epithelium is avoided by:
  - movement of air across it by ventilation of the lungs, and
  - removal of diffused materials by circulating blood at the surface of the alveoli: capillary blood supply to the alveoli is rich and intimate (very close and intertwined).

The rate of gas transfer across this respiratory surface depends on the rate of lung ventilation *and* on the blood flow to the surface; these factors, in turn, depend on total ventilation volume and cardiac output. So, lung function and cardiovascular function are here interrelated.

The mechanisms of lung ventilation

The lungs are elastic, multichambered bags that are suspended within an airtight pleural cavity and open to the exterior via a single tube to the trachea (Fig. 1.10). The space between the lungs and the wall of the thoracic cage is lined with a pleural membrane and filled with a thin layer of pleural fluid. This thin cavity provides a flexible, lubricated connection between lung and thoracic wall. When the thoracic cage changes volume, the gas-filled lungs do so also.

During normal breathing, the thoracic cage is expanded and contracted by the action of the muscles in the diaphragm and between the ribs (intercostal muscles). When the diaphragm and intercostal muscles contract, the thoracic cavity enlarges, the lungs expand (because of the pleural membrane attachments) and air is drawn in via the trachea. Expiration is the opposite of this and happens when the respiratory muscles relax. Thus inspiration is *active* and expiration is *passive* (Fig. 1.11).

If the air-tightness of the thoracic cavity is damaged by injury or puncture of the pleural membrane, air enters the pleural cavity and the lung(s) collapse. This is a state known as pneumothorax, and, except in very severe cases, it can be cured by slowly allowing the air to move out of the pleural cavity through a secondary, airtight drainage system.

Contractions of the respiratory muscles are controlled by specialised receptor neurones (central chemoreceptors) in the respiratory centre of the brain stem. These neurones respond to changes in carbon dioxide (CO_2) and oxygen (O_2) levels in the blood, and they control the

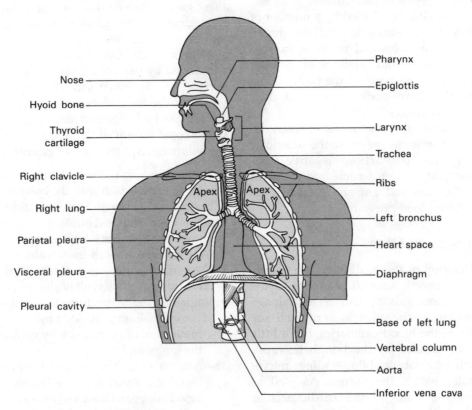

Figure 1.10   The respiratory organs.

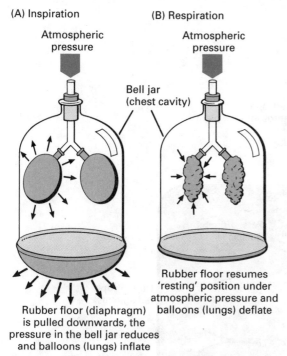

(A) Inspiration

Atmospheric pressure

(B) Respiration

Atmospheric pressure

Bell jar (chest cavity)

Rubber floor resumes 'resting' position under atmospheric pressure and balloons (lungs) deflate

Rubber floor (diaphragm) is pulled downwards, the pressure in the bell jar reduces and balloons (lungs) inflate

Figure 1.11 A model to illustrate the process of inspiration and expiration.

rhythmic nature of breathing. There are also extremely sensitive stretch receptors in the lungs themselves, which prevent over-expansion of the lungs. The neuronal mechanisms causing rhythmic breathing are complex and poorly understood at present.

In addition to these neural mechanisms, which produce normal, rhythmic, quiet breathing, chemoreceptors in the carotid and aortic bodies (on the carotid and aortic arteries) respond to changes in O_2 and CO_2 levels in arterial blood. It is always the CO_2 increase that causes a response before a lowered O_2 level does. Since an increase in CO_2 causes increased acidity of the blood, it is possible that the response is due to the reduced pH rather than the CO_2 itself.

Whatever the combination of mechanisms, the rate and depth of breathing alter unconsciously according to O_2, CO_2, pH, emotions and sleep. Control can be voluntary, too, as in the fine changes needed for the complex human activities of singing, whistling and just talking. The limitations of voluntary control over normal ventilation can be seen, however, in breath-

holding, which is always overcome by the eventual need to breathe!

THE DIGESTIVE SYSTEM AND HOMEOSTASIS

Ingestion

All living organisms depend on external sources for the raw materials and energy needed for their growth, normal functioning and repair. Food, which provides energy as well as material for the production of new tissue, is obtained from a variety of plant, animal and inorganic sources. The chemical energy for fuelling all processes in the animal body comes ultimately from a single source, the sun. Solar energy is not available directly to animals. Only autotrophic (or self-nourishing) organisms, i.e. chlorophyll-containing plants, can harness light energy to produce biochemical molecules for growth and energy conservation.

All animals are heterotrophic: they derive all their energy-yielding and body-building carbon compounds from ingested foodstuffs, which are, ultimately, derived from autotrophic organisms (Fig. 1.12).

Obtaining food

Before food can be used for tissue chemistry, growth and repair, it must first be obtained. Obtaining nutritional essentials is, clearly, a key to the survival of any species. Much of human enterprise is an effort towards finding enough to eat, although in comparison with other animals we have become less in need of the natural mechanisms to 'catch' or gather food, or to prevent ourselves from becoming a meal for predators. However, the complexities of the nervous system, sensory organs and muscular system have, in fact, evolved in part to ensure survival by obtaining sufficient food.

Digestion

Once food is obtained, it must be digested before any of it can be used by body tissues for energy production and body-building. Digestion

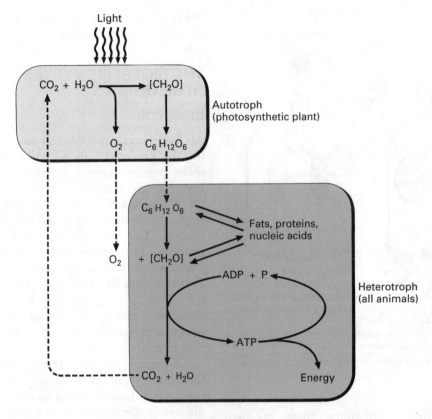

Note: (CH_2O) is an abbreviation formula for carbohydrate

Figure 1.12 Flow of chemical energy in the living world. In plants, high-energy sugars $(C_6H_{12}O_6)$ are made, using light energy, from the raw materials of carbon dioxide and water. In the heterotroph, which eats ready-made high-energy compounds, the sugars and other foodstuffs yield energy when oxidised in the tissues.

is a chemical process in which special digestive enzymes catalyse the breakdown of large food-stuff molecules into simpler compounds that are small enough to diffuse or be transported across cell membranes for incorporation into cell chemistry.

The digestive system itself is a tube, or canal, with a receiving end (the mouth) and a dis-charging end (the anus). Its structure is varied to suit the function of its components (Fig. 1.13). For propelling material along the tube in the stomach and intestine, its walls are muscular. For carrying out enzymatic digestion in the stomach and small intestine, the lining contains enzyme-secreting cells; supplementary digestive glands open into the gut. Where digested

nutrients are transferred into the bloodstream, the lining is deeply folded to increase the absorptive area. Of significant importance in digestion are two functions: the motility of the gut and the secretion of gastrointestinal enzymes.

Motility of the alimentary canal

The muscles in the wall of the gut are arranged in a layer of circular muscle and a layer of longitudinal muscle. All gut muscle is smooth, involuntary muscle. The coordinated contrac-tions of these muscles produce peristaltic waves of constriction, which propel the contents down the length of the tube. Movement of the contents

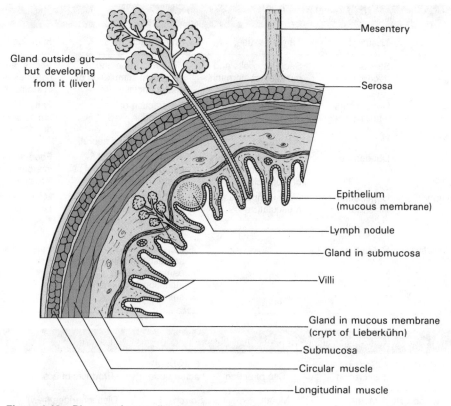

Figure 1.13   Diagram of generalised cross-section of gut.

within the tube is caused by a different sequencing of contractions (circular muscles contract in bands along the gut, causing intermittent segment formation, which squeezes and churns the food). Swallowing involves integrated movements of the tongue and pharynx, as well as peristaltic movements of the oesophagus. These actions move food out of the mouth and down the stomach without the person choking. Once in the stomach, food is mixed and squeezed vigorously by peristaltic activity and is retained in the stomach by closed cardiac and pyloric sphincter muscles at each end of the stomach. Like heart muscle, gastrointestinal muscle is capable of spontaneous contraction, but, in the gut, the automatic contractions are much slower. They are coordinated by a range of influences, including nerve control and hormonal mechanisms, and by the actual presence of food in the stomach and intestine.

Gastrointestinal secretions

The alimentary canal produces both endocrine and exocrine secretions.

Endocrine secretions

Endocrine glands are ductless glands that release their secretions (hormones) directly into the bloodstream for distribution to the target tissues (see 'The endocrine system and homeostasis', below). Some hormones important in the digestive process are also released from special tissues within the gut itself (Table 1.3).

Exocrine secretions

Exocrine glands are very important in the gut. The output of an exocrine gland flows through a duct into a body cavity, such as the mouth, gut,

Table 1.3   The gastrointestinal hormones (Adapted from Eckert 1988)

Hormone	Tissue of origin	Target tissue	Primary action	Stimulus to secretion
Gastrin	Stomach and duodenum	Secretory cells and muscles of stomach	HCl production and secretion; stimulation of gastric motility	Vagus nerve activity; peptides and proteins in stomach
Cholecystokinin-pancreozymin (CCK-PZ)	Upper small intestine	Gallbladder	Contraction of gallbladder	Fatty acids and amino acids in duodenum
		Pancreas	Pancreatic juice secretion	
Secretin	Duodenum	Pancreas; secretory cells and muscles of stomach	Water and $NaHCO_3$ secretion; inhibition of gastric motility	Food and strong acid in stomach and small intestine
Gastric inhibitory peptide (GIP)	Upper small intestine	Gastric mucosa and musculature	Inhibition of gastric secretion and motility; stimulation of Brunner's glands	Monosaccharides and fats in duodenum
Vasoactive intestinal peptide (VIP)	Duodenum		Increase of blood flow; secretion of thin pancreatic fluid; inhibition of gastric secretion	Fats in duodenum

Table 1.4   The digestive enzymes (Adapted from Eckert 1988)

Enzyme	Site of secretion	Site of action	Substrate acted upon	Products of action
Salivary α-amylase	Mouth	Mouth	Starch	Disaccharides (few)
Pepsinogen → pepsin	Stomach	Stomach	Proteins	Large peptides
Pancreatic α-amylase	Pancreas	Small intestine	Starch	Disaccharides
Trypsinogen → trypsin	Pancreas	Small intestine	Proteins	Large peptides
Chymotrypsin	Pancreas	Small intestine	Proteins	Large peptides
Peptidases	Pancreas	Small intestine	Large peptides	Small peptides (oligopeptides)
Lipase	Pancreas	Small intestine	Triglycerides	Monoglycerides, fatty acids, glycerol
Enterokinase	Small intestine	Small intestine	Trypsinogen	Trypsin
Disaccharidases	Small intestine	Small intestine	Disaccharides	Monosaccharides
Peptidases	Small intestine	Small intestine	Oligopeptides	Amino acids

or urinary tract. In the alimentary canal, these secretions are a mixture of water, salts, mucus and digestive enzymes. Their timing and duration of activity is controlled and coordinated by nervous and hormonal collaboration. The main initiating stimulus for the secretion of digestive juices is the presence of food within that portion of the tract. For example, saliva is secreted freely when food is in the mouth; it is impossible to prevent such secretion by volition, and this applies elsewhere in the alimentary tract.

With the exception of bile, all digestive juices contain enzymes that successively break down large food molecules into their smallest and simplest form, ready for absorption into the bloodstream (Table 1.4). Bile contains no enzymes, but it does contain alkaline bile salts that physically break up and disperse fats for their easy digestion by enzymes.

Absorption

Two products of digestion must find their way into all the tissues and cells of the body. The first stage in this process is by transport through the cells that line the gut. Transport is by a mixture of diffusion, facilitated diffusion and active transport. Most nutrients are absorbed across the lining of the small intestine, but a few will be absorbed from the stomach if, for example, like alcohol, they are simple and soluble enough. Once they have left the gut, nutrients move into the blood and lymphatic capillaries with which the gut wall is richly endowed. Digested fats enter the lymphatic capillaries and are then transferred to the venous system (see 'Lymphatic system', above) whilst sugars, amino acids and water more readily enter the blood capillaries.

Defaecation

Most food absorption is complete by the time the gut contents reach the colon. Into the colon move the indigestible remains and water from the food itself and from the digestive juices. Water is gradually absorbed as the contents are moved along the colon, so that what remains for egestion, or defaecation, is a semi-solid mass of largely cellulose material (roughage) and dead bacteria, with some water and bile pigments.

The muscular coordination of defaecation is initiated by an involuntary nervous sensation (often termed 'the call to stool'), which is then usually accompanied by some measure of voluntary effort. Where nervous control is not yet matured (in babies) or has been damaged (e.g. by stroke, or by cerebral or spinal cord trauma), defaecation is not voluntarily controlled; in the latter case, this can cause severe distress to the sufferer and his carers.

THE RENAL SYSTEM AND HOMEOSTASIS

Regulation of a constant internal environment demands that the levels of water and intra- and extracellular solutes are constantly monitored and altered, as necessary, to restore balance. This process is known as osmoregulation. Also, the cellular environment must be freed of potentially toxic wastes that accumulate as a by-product of metabolism. This process is known as excretion. The renal system is the major excretor and osmoregulator in the body. (See Box 1.6 for detail about the production of nitrogenous waste.)

Although there may be hourly and daily variations in fluid (osmotic balance) within the tissues, the healthy body is generally in an osmotically steady state over the long term. Water enters the body with food and drink, and leaves in the urine, faeces, sweat and expired air. The 'fluid balance' (i.e. water in = water out) is relatively straightforward, but osmoregulation also has to maintain a favourable solute (e.g. sodium, potassium, chloride and acid/base) balance within the intra- and extracellular fluids. This balance is required during periods of feeding, fasting, exposure to extreme temperatures, exercising and so on.

All of these activities will also alter the rate at which excretory products (urea, carbon dioxide and water) are manufactured. The renal system is able to regulate body fluids for all these changes. At least one adequately functioning kidney is vital to life. The gross anatomy of the kidney is shown in Figure 1.14. There are normally two kidneys, lying one on each side

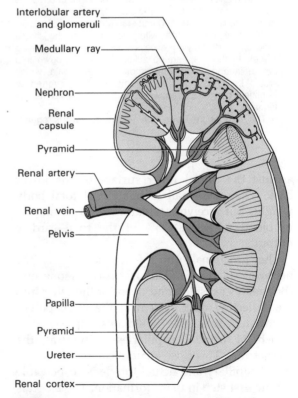

Interlobular artery and glomeruli
Medullary ray
Nephron
Renal capsule
Pyramid
Renal artery
Renal vein
Pelvis
Papilla
Pyramid
Ureter
Renal cortex

Figure 1.14 Anatomy of the kidney. The nephrons lie parallel to one another, with their collecting ducts opening through the papillae into a central cavity (the renal pelvis). The urine passes from the pelvis into the ureter, and from there to the urinary bladder.

Box 1.6 **The liver**

The liver is the largest and probably the most metabolically active organ in the body. It does not belong to any one system as such, yet it is intimately involved in the biochemistry of the whole body. Its cells have abundant mitochondria (always a sign of fiercely active cells), and the liver tissues are heavily supplied with blood. It appears that all liver cells are capable of carrying out all the chemical functions of the liver. These can be summarised as follows:

Functions concerned with blood. The liver plays an important part in the production of erythrocytes in fetal life. It is also the place where old erythrocytes are broken down and their haemoglobin converted to bilirubin, which is excreted within the bile. The liver also manufactures all plasma proteins, except for the immune gammaglobulins. This protein manufacture includes the clotting factors prothrombin and fibrinogen.

Functions concerned with food. The liver stores *carbohydrate* in the form of glycogen. Under the control of hormones, liver glycogen is the main source of blood glucose, whose maintenance is vital to life. Carbohydrate can be manufactured in the liver from non-carbohydrate sources such as fats and proteins. This is an important function in times of fasting and starvation.

Of great importance with foodstuffs is the liver's function in detoxifying excess *protein* products (amino acids). In the liver, amino acids are broken down into ammonia and other compounds. The ammonia, which would be toxic if left to accumulate, is converted to relatively harmless urea, which is then excreted via the kidneys.

The role of the liver with regard to *fats* is equally significant. It produces bile salts, which are stored in the gall bladder and then released onto food in the small intestine. These salts assist in the physical breakdown (emulsification) of fats in food. They act as detergents. Fat-soluble vitamins (A, D, E and K) are stored in the liver. The liver also stores some fats as fatty acids, and these can be metabolised in a variety of ways to produce energy and heat. This metabolism is particularly important in conditions of starvation or when insufficient carbohydrate (glucose) is being absorbed by the tissues. The latter state is the case in diabetes mellitus, in which alternatives to carbohydrate have to be metabolised to maintain life. The breakdown of fats in this case produces waste products called ketones, which can cause acidosis. Fortunately, this condition can now be reversed rapidly, providing that medical and nursing care is sought.

Functions concerned with detoxification. The liver is the most important organ in the metabolism of drugs and alcohol. Most of these substances, if taken in moderation, are modified by the liver, excreted and eventually cleared completely from the body. A few cause lasting damage to the liver cells, which, of course, are then less efficient in their detoxification activity. In particular, high doses of paracetamol, Distalgesic and alcohol are known to cause severe liver damage, which can provoke liver failure.

The biochemistry of drugs and poisons and their metabolism within the liver is the subject matter of pharmacology textbooks. It is not essential to know these complexities, but the principles of assessing potential dangers and therapeutic doses in association with liver functions must always be applied when drugs are prescribed and administered.

---

against the dorsal inner surface of the lower back. They are small (about 1% of total body weight) but receive a remarkably large amount of blood (about 20–25% of the total cardiac output).

The functional unit of the kidney is the nephron (Fig. 1.15). This is closed at one end (Bowman's capsule), and opens at the other into the collecting duct system at the renal pelvis. Associated with the Bowman's capsule is a bunch of arterial capillaries known as the glomerulus. This close anatomical association of blood capillary and actual tubule is responsible for the first step in urine formation. The blood is filtered at the glomerulus, and the filtrate begins its journey along the nephron. Of particular significance to the osmoregulatory function of the kidney is the loop of Henlé and its associated blood capillary supply, which also follows a looping structure.

Formation of urine

There are four processes that contribute to the ultimate composition of urine:

- glomerular filtration
- tubular reabsorption
- tubular synthesis
- tubular secretion.

Glomerular filtration. The blood is, effectively, 'sieved', and the factors determining which substances leave the blood and enter the nephron are molecular size, electrical charge and blood

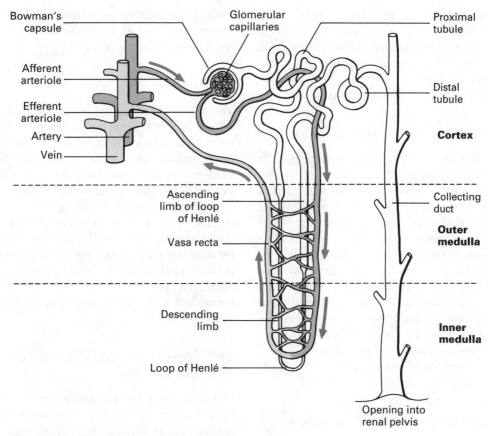

Figure 1.15 The nephron with its blood supply.

pressure. In healthy people, the only substances that do not enter the nephron are blood cells and plasma proteins. Water, Na⁺, potassium (K⁺), chloride (Cl⁻), glucose and urea are all passed into the nephron.

Tubular reabsorption. The original filtrate composition is rapidly modified, so that about 75% of the water is reabsorbed before it gets to the loop of Henlé. Glucose, in healthy people, is reabsorbed completely along the nephron, and water and other solutes are selectively reabsorbed according to their varying concentrations in the blood plasma. Urea is about 50% reabsorbed, and Na⁺, Cl⁻ and H₂O reabsorption levels are critical in maintaining homeostasis. Water and Na⁺ reabsorption are controlled by antidiuretic hormone (ADH) and aldosterone respectively. The structure of the loop of Henlé and related blood vessels is critical in allowing

for the formation of a highly concentrated urine, if necessary, well above the concentration of blood plasma.

Tubular synthesis. Some excretory substances, mainly nitrogenous waste materials that are derived from escaped amino acids in the glomerular filtrate, are produced in the tubule and added to the urine.

Tubular secretion. As urine passes down the renal tubule, exchange of materials between urine and plasma can occur. There is sometimes a need for substances to be secreted from the blood into the urine (the opposite of reabsorption). By secretion, acidic ions (H⁺), uric acid and potassium are removed from the blood for excretion.

All terrestrial animals, including man, are faced with the risk of dehydration. Indeed, for man this becomes a stark reality in desert-like conditions or during periods of water starvation of over 24 hours. The structure of the kidney, with its loop of Henlé, is specific to birds and mammals, which are the only animals able to produce a urine that is more concentrated than blood.

Excretory function of the kidneys

In addition to the vital function of the kidneys in osmoregulation, their excretory function is also life-saving. Nitrogenous waste products, such as ammonia, from the breakdown of proteins are highly toxic if allowed to accumulate. If proteins are eaten to excess (eating too much meat is common in Western society), they cannot be stored, so are converted, by the liver, to urea (see Box 1.6). Urea is excreted via the urine, and although coincidental to the osmoregulatory activity of kidneys, the process is vital nonetheless. Urea excretion by the kidneys is a straightforward passive process of filtration and normal diffusion. Excretion of urea is interrupted if the liver or kidneys are damaged or diseased.

The importance of healthy kidneys

Apart from the acutely life-threatening dangers of cardiovascular or cerebral disorders, the most dangerous diseases are those that affect the kidneys. It is well understood that acute failure of the heart or brain can deprive tissues of oxygen, and that death can result within a few minutes, but renal failure, whilst not usually the cause of immediate death, can produce severe and lasting deviations from normal tissue function because of interruptions to homeostasis. This is equally life-threatening if left untreated, and may require intervention in the form of renal dialysis, in which unwanted substances are removed from the blood, or renal transplant surgery.

The kidneys are also vital for some non-excretory functions. For example, they are believed to produce the hormone erythropoietin in response to a low blood oxygen level (hypoxia) in the renal arteries. Erythropoietin stimulates the production of red blood cells (erythropoiesis)

in the bone marrow and other sites. (For further information, see Hinchliff & Montague 1988 in the 'Further reading' list.)

Micturition

The pelvis of the kidney gives rise to the ureter, which empties into the urinary bladder. The formation of urine is complete as it reaches the renal pelvis, and below the kidney the renal system can be considered as mere plumbing. Fortunately, this plumbing allows for the storage of urine in the bladder, with occasional release. This release is under neural control, which responds to stretching of the bladder wall by relaxing the bladder sphincter muscle: urine is then expelled (micturition). As in defaecation, emptying of the bladder is not voluntarily controlled if the nervous system is immature or damaged.

THE NERVOUS SYSTEM AND HOMEOSTASIS

Nervous systems are undoubtedly the most intricately organised structures to have evolved on earth. The human nervous system contains anything up to 10^9 cells, which, during development in the fetus, become arranged into the neural circuits that make up the system. No part of the body – no system, organ or tissue – is without its own neural circuit. In spite of the complexity of organisation within the nervous system, the large number of nerve cells that comprises it is not accompanied by an equally large number of methods of working.

The function of the nervous system depends almost entirely on the same repertoire of electrical signals produced by the same physical and chemical changes across nerve cell membranes. The sophistication of the nervous system lies in the complexity of its organisation, which results in an immeasurable number of connections.

Neurones. The rapidity of neural communication is due to the structure and function of the individual nerve cells or neurones. Neurones are known as 'excitable' cells because they respond readily to physical or chemical changes in their environment and convert these responses into nerve impulses. Impulses can be transmitted at speeds of up to 120 m/s, and may travel along neurones that are, themselves, up to a metre long (Fig. 1.16).

Transmission of impulses. The physiological behaviour of a neurone depends upon its anatomical form and on the properties of its membranes. For example, the long axon (as in Fig. 1.16) has the ability for rapid conduction of electrical impulses from the cell body to the target structure, which is usually a muscle. The membranes of neurone terminals are specialised for the secretion of transmitter substances into the extracellular fluid between it and the target organ (e.g. muscle) cells, or for electrical transmission to another neurone (Box 1.7).

This highly simplified version of nervous transmission within nervous tissue itself and between neurones and target organs gives an indication of how fully and rapidly the regulating mechanism can operate. To understand how nervous tissue makes and transmits impulses, it is necessary to know about the electrical and biochemical activity of cells. That is beyond the capacity of this chapter but it can be followed up in Cree & Rischmiller (1991) pp 384–394 (see 'Further reading', below).

Components of the nervous system. Anatomically, the nervous system has the following components:

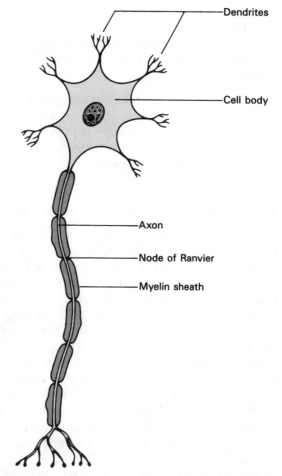

Figure 1.16 Structure of a neurone.

Box 1.7 **Transmission at synapse**

Before the development of electron microscopy in the 1940s, it was uncertain whether the nervous system was a continuous web of tissue, or whether there were distinct 'gaps' between neurones. The latter is now known to be the case and these gaps are called synapses. This discovery means that electrical excitation of a neurone must be transmissible across a gap to another neurone, and/or to the cell of an organ which is being stimulated to act (e.g. a muscle). This transmission may be either electrical or chemical.

Electrical transmission. In this type of transmission, electrical current simply transfers from the pre-synaptic cell membrane to the post-synaptic cell membrane. This permits very rapid transmission and is known to occur within cardiac muscle and smooth muscle cells. It is well suited to rapid transmission in a group of nerve cells or

across a series of cell–cell junctions such as are found in those tissues.

Chemical transmission. The vast majority of synaptic transmissions involve chemical transmitters. The pre-synaptic neurone liberates a transmitter substance that interacts with receptor molecules on the post-synaptic membrane. The post-synaptic cell is usually 'triggered' into action, which may be further transmission of electrical potential towards the next cell, or a different kind of excitation that results in muscular contraction if the next cell is a muscle fibre. Many transmitter chemicals are now identified and research still continues. Both excitatory and inhibitory transmitters are known to exist. The best known neurotransmitters are *acetylcholine* and *noradrenaline*, both of which are released in the autonomic nervous system.

- the central nervous system (CNS), consisting of the brain and spinal cord
- the peripheral nervous system, consisting of cranial nerves, spinal nerves and autonomic nerve fibres.

Although not part of the nervous system as such, special sense organs (eyes, ears, tongue, nose and skin) are richly supplied with specialised receptors and, via these, have direct links with the nervous system.

The processes of nervous regulation

The main sequence of events in nervous regulation is shown in Figure 1.17. A stimulus is anything that excites a neurone. Internally, it may be, for example, raised hydrostatic pressure within tissue fluid, an excess of CO_2 in the blood, or raised body temperature. Externally, it may be sound waves stimulating the nerve endings in the ear, a feather tickling the skin, or acid in a lemon affecting the taste buds. There are many different structural types of sensory receptor responsive to many different kinds of stimulation, but their overall function is to raise awareness in the CNS of a change of circumstances. The excitability of the sensory receptor is translated into electrical impulses transmitted along sensory nerve fibres to the CNS (so-called

afferent nerves). Specialised groups of cells in the brain and spinal cord interpret the received sensory information and, if necessary, initiate a homeostatic response via another kind of nerve cell whose fibres (efferent nerves) terminate in muscles or glands that are required to produce a response (of contraction or secretion). Not all sensory stimulation reaches consciousness. This is because it is interpreted either within the spinal cord with no cerebral (brain) interaction, or because the part of the brain used for interpretation of the signal is not within the consciousness area.

Unconscious nervous homeostasis includes control of breathing, heart rate and force of heart contraction, digestive tract activity, sweating, and vasodilatation in body temperature control. These are all activities controlled by the nervous system and of which we are normally unaware (except for sweating and glowing when hot!). Conscious sensations involve vision, hearing, taste, smell and touch, which special sense organs are responsible for initiating. Whilst, for much of the time, such sensations do not provoke a homeostatic response, there may be occasions when they do, and these are related to basic survival needs to flee from or face danger (the 'flight or fight' response). Their role is considered to be much more significant in more primitive animals.

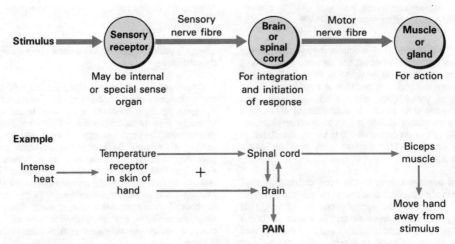

Figure 1.17   The sequencing of nervous regulation.

It will be helpful to know more about the nervous system and its application to nursing (see 'Further reading', below). Its significance in maintaining homeostasis should always be an important consideration, but the nervous system is responsible for many of the less well understood higher-order activities (such as speech and perception) in man.

THE ENDOCRINE SYSTEM AND HOMEOSTASIS

Just as the muscular activity of the body would be impossible without the coordination and control exerted by means of the electrical signals of the nervous system, so also would the metabolic activities of the body (such as growth, maintenance and reproduction) be impossible without the coordination and control exerted by chemical agents. These chemical messengers are known as hormones and are secreted from a number of organs, the major endocrine glands being shown in Figure 1.18. The activity of a number of endocrine glands is regulated through the activity of the hypothalamus in the brain.

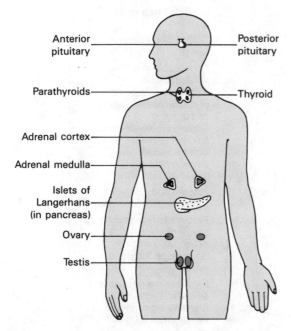

Figure 1.18 The major endocrine glands.

Hormones

A hormone is a chemical released directly into the bloodstream to be carried in the circulation to a distant target tissue. In addition to the hormones secreted by the endocrine glands, other groups of hormones are released into the bloodstream from nervous tissue. The hypothalamic hormones are neurohormones. There is also a group of hormones known as local hormones; these are secreted from various tissues to act on nearby targets, and include histamine and some of the intestinal hormones (Table 1.5).

The term hormone comes from the Greek for 'arouse to activity'. It is known that the hormone molecules react with specific receptor molecules on the surface of their target cells. By an interaction of the hormone molecule with the receptor molecule, a series of cascade-type, enzyme-mediated reactions is initiated within the cell. Although hormone molecules come into contact with all the tissues in the body, only cells that contain the receptors specific for the hormone are affected by that hormone.

The amount of hormone produced by an endocrine gland is very small. Blood concentrations are low and target cells are extraordinarily sensitive to their hormone. The typical blood plasma level of a hormone would be similar to the concentration achieved by dissolving a pinch of sugar in a large swimming pool full of water.

The secretion and circulation of hormones both take place relatively slowly, unlike the rapid reaction times experienced in nervous control activities. Thus the endocrine system is well suited for regulation that is sustained for minutes, hours or days. Such long-term control is required for regulating blood osmolarity (water/salts balance), blood sugar levels, growth and metabolic rate. The reproductive cycle in women also requires cyclical and sustained hormonal control. The quick-acting nervous system and the slower, sustained activity of the endocrine system complement one another in the overall regulation of physiological activity (Table 1.5).

Homeostatic control may be lost if hormones are under- or over-secreted. The normal mechanism for controlling secretion level is by

Table 1.5   The major hormones and their functions

Gland	Hormone	Functions
Anterior pituitary (adenohypophysis)	Thyroid stimulating hormone (THS)	Controls the activity of the thyroid gland
	Adrenocorticotrophic hormone (ACTH)	Controls the activity of the adrenal cortex
	Follicle stimulating hormone (FSH)	Controls the menstrual cycle in females
	Luteinising hormone (LH)	Stimulates sperm production in males
	Growth hormone	Controls physical growth
	Luteotrophic hormone	Controls production and secretion of milk during pregnancy and after childbirth
Middle lobe of pituitary	Melanocyte stimulating hormone	Deposition of melanin pigment in melanocytes in skin
Posterior pituitary (neurohypophysis)	Antidiuretic hormone (ADH)	Regulates reabsorption of water from renal tubules
	Oxytocin	Stimulates uterine contractions during childbirth
		Causes milk ejection from breasts during infant suckling
Thyroid	Tri-iodo thyronine (T_3) Thyroxine (T_4)	Stimulate metabolism in the tissues generally
	Calcitonin	Controls blood calcium levels
Parathyroid	Parathyroid hormone	Controls blood calcium levels
Pancreas (islets of Langerhans)	Insulin Glucagon	Control blood sugar levels
Adrenal cortex	Aldosterone	Controls blood sodium ion (Na^+) levels
	Cortisol	Regulates metabolism of carbohydrates, fats and proteins
		Complex involvement in stress responses
	Sex hormones (androgens and oestrogens)	Control sexual development
Adrenal medulla	Adrenaline Noradrenaline	Prepare body for action: 'fight or flight' response
Ovaries	Oestrogen Progesterone	Produce female secondary sexual characteristics
		Act on uterine lining during each menstrual cycle
Testes	Testosterone	Produces male secondary sexual characteristics
		Stimulates growth of seminiferous tubules
Placenta	Human chorionic gonadotrophin (HCG)	Maintains oestrogen and progesterone production in early pregnancy

negative feedback, as described earlier. Mal-functioning endocrine glands (causes for this not being completely known but including congenital abnormality, heredity and viral infection) upset homeostatic regulation most severely.

THE IMMUNE SYSTEM AND HOMEOSTASIS

The immune system defends the body against a variety of foreign substances, including micro-organisms (which cause infection), transplanted cells, tissues or organs, and irritants such as pollen. The mechanisms involved enable the individual to recognise and respond to the 'foreignness' of a wide range of biological substances that are potentially harmful if present in the body.

There are several important defences that prevent foreign substances from entering the body. The most obvious is the skin, but others include the mucous linings of the respiratory and digestive tracts, which trap foreign particles or stimulate their expulsion by coughing and sneezing. In addition, some body secretions, such as gastric juices, are acidic and therefore destroy disease-producing bacteria.

However, foreign materials can enter the body via damage to the skin, by ingestion or inhalation of pathogens, by deliberate introduction of 'foreign bodies' via transplants or blood transfusions, or by the development of abnormal tissues within the body (e.g. cancerous growths). In every case, the presence of foreign material is likely to provoke an automatic series of responses designed to destroy or contain its damaging effects. Unfortunately, the response mechanisms do not distinguish between harmful 'foreigners' (infections) and potentially life-saving ones (transplants): the nature of the response is geared to neutralise foreign substances that have the potential to interfere with the delicate balance of homeostasis.

How the immune system works

The immune system works in two main ways:

• direct physical attack
• antibody production.

Direct physical attack

When foreign matter penetrates the defences of the skin and mucous membranes to enter the superficial tissues (such as in a spot or boil) or the bloodstream, it encounters special white blood cells known as polymorphs and monocytes. These cells engulf particles, including infectious agents, and destroy them. This is phagocytosis, referred to in 'Transport across membranes' above. These phagocytic cells can carry out their function within the bloodstream, or they can migrate out of the blood vessels into affected tissues in response to a chemical stimulus from the foreign materials. Tissues that have been damaged or which contain foreign substances evoke an inflammatory response (Box 1.8).

Antibody production

A vascular immune response occurs when the phagocytic cells are unable to recognise (chemically) the invading agent, or are unable to engulf foreign particles because they lack the appropriate chemical receptors to do so. In this case, a more subtle and sophisticated type of germ warfare may be engaged, or may occur simultaneously. This is the production of antibodies, i.e. proteins manufactured specifically to attend to and neutralise invading or foreign substances. Substances that stimulate the production of antibodies are known collectively as antigens. The hallmark of the immune system is the specificity of an antibody for a particular antigen.

Antibodies are manufactured by cells called lymphocytes, some of which circulate in the blood and some of which exist in lymphatic tissues within the body. Antibodies act by directly attacking the foreign cells and neutralising them by locking on to their surface, but the special feature of lymphocytes is that they carry genetic information to cope with an almost infinite variety of antigens, i.e. they can produce a protein antibody for any antigen. Once a lymphocyte has been processed to 'recognise' and interact with a particular antigen, it remains in the blood or lymphatic tissue, able to recognise it again should a further invasion occur. The specificity of the antibody/antigen relationship

Box 1.8 Inflammation explained

Inflammation is the protective response of the body to irritation or injury. The word 'inflame' means, literally, 'to set afire', and the suffix '-itis' denotes an inflammatory response as, for example, in appendicitis and arthritis.

Common causes of inflammation

- Mechanical – caused by direct trauma.
- Chemical – corrosion of tissues by direct contact, for example acid burns to the skin or acid reflux from the stomach to the oesophagus.
- Allergenic – for example pollen in hayfever, contact objects causing dermatitis, some foods, insect bites and stings.
- Infective – either external (topical) or systemic.
- Thermal – excessive heat or cold, which causes tissue damage.

Physiology of the inflammatory response

The blood vessels local to the damaged area dilate, increasing blood supply to the area. The dilated vessels become more permeable, and fluid escapes into the surrounding tissues. The escaped fluid, or exudate, contains fibrinogen and immunoglobulins. Polymorphonucleocytes are attracted to the area, where they destroy damaged tissue and invading microbes by phagocytosis. Histamine is released from local tissues.

The local signs of inflammation

These commonly include:

- redness } – due to vasodilatation
- heat
- swelling – due to accumulation of tissue fluid
- pain – due to increased activity, through disturbance, of local pain receptors
- loss of function – due to pain, swelling and protective 'guarding' by adjacent muscles.

The systemic responses to inflammation

These may include:

- a rise in body temperature
- general malaise with poor appetite
- changes in blood electrolyte levels
- changes in plasma protein levels, owing to immune responses
- an increase of white blood cell levels
- increased activity of lymphatic tissue ('swollen glands').

Managing inflammation

Local and simple inflammation requires the relief of pain and management of the swelling. Wherever possible, foreign bodies and pus should be removed. Systemic responses to inflammation, such as with infections, surgery or other internal causes, require more extensive intervention to reduce the stimulus, for example by using antibiotics for infection.

In all cases, the need to achieve restoration of homeostasis is the key component, but the patient may be distressed and will need management of this, alongside attention to physical and social needs.

Anaphylactic shock

In extreme cases, a localised cause of inflammation, such as a bee sting, may cause a rapid and extreme systemic response, leading to a case of allergenic shock, or anaphylactic shock. This is very rare but life-threatening, and requires urgent medical intervention, with intravenous adrenaline and life-sustaining measures such as cardiopulmonary resuscitation.

Anaphylaxis is, fortunately, rare, but it is a clear example of a case where the internal homeostatic mechanisms are unable to meet the unusual demands of an external disruption to a stable internal environment (see Box 1.4).

---

is what makes this recognition possible. A second infection will thus be 'neutralised' rapidly, preventing widespread damage. This is immunity in its simplest explanation. Its discovery led to the development of artificial immunisation against severe infections, whereby a reduced dose is introduced to the individual in order to stimulate production of antibodies against a further attack.

Immunity and immunisation

Immunity has been achieved when an individual is no longer susceptible, or has a reduced susceptibility, to one or more antigens. Gaining immunity to infectious diseases (or other antigens) is an important factor in health care programmes, and nurses need to be familiar with the processes by which immunity may be acquired.

Passive immunity

This occurs when the individual has not produced her own antibodies. The simplest example of such immunity is the natural transfer of antibodies from mother to baby, both prenatally via placental exchange and postnatally through breastfeeding. This 'transfer' of anti-body is mostly extremely beneficial, and confers to the child the ability to fight off early infections until it is able to produce its own antibodies.

Artificial passive immunity is provided when people receive specific antibody injections against infectious diseases. The effect is immediate but shortlived, lasting only until the antibodies are destroyed in the recipient's body. Passive immunisation is reserved for situations where a person is at risk from a dangerous disease but has had no previous opportunity to develop a personal active immunity (i.e. he has had no previous contact with the disease). An important example of passive artificial immunisation is in the prevention of Rhesus incompatibility in pregnancy (see Box 1.5).

Active immunity

This occurs when an individual produces her own antibodies in response to the presence of the specific antigen. Immunity may have been acquired naturally, where the immune system has responded by producing antibodies to fight the antigens of a naturally occurring infection. These antibodies then remain, often for many years, so that a further invasion of the antigen is immediately attacked, and no further disease occurs. A common example of active natural immunity is that which occurs for chickenpox.

Active immunity can also be artificially stimulated. A small, safe dose of the disease-producing organism, or some of its components or products, is given to an individual. Routes of administration vary, according to the disease and vaccine, but many more are now oral prep-arations rather than injections. The recipient's immune system responds by producing anti-bodies that provide protection from the serious disease. This kind of immunity (active artificial) is now widely used in health care programmes. Common illnesses now almost completely preventable by this method include diphtheria, whooping cough, poliomyelitis, tuberculosis, measles and rubella (German measles), because the antibodies are long-lived. Artificial immunity

for influenza is less certain, because the influenza virus repeatedly changes its protein specificity, so needs repeatedly different antibodies for its destruction.

All nurses need to be familiar with the dev-elopment of natural immunity and its exploitation in programmes of immunisation for children, or for any individuals at risk of infection.

Immunological mechanisms are essential for survival, and have formed the basis for significant research in the past few years. With the increas-ing ability of surgeons and medical engineers to undertake transplants, a major problem of tissue rejection (of foreign protein material) has required massive investigation.

A number of illnesses arise because of auto-immunity, when immune reactions are directed against an individual's own cells. Examples include rheumatoid arthritis, some cases of diabetes mellitus and ulcerative colitis. Probably the greatest challenge at the time of writing is the problem of AIDS (acquired immune deficiency syndrome), whose name explains the condition in terms of immunity.

Summary

Underlying all the physiological changes in the body is the principle of homeostasis – the tendency to main-tain the stability of the internal environment in the face of changing internal and external demands. In health, the feedback mechanisms enable this balance to be held, but when it is not maintained, illness threatens. As the aim of health care intervention is to restore the status quo, an understanding of homeostatic mech-anisms is of vital importance in caring for patients.

In this chapter, the functions of each of the body systems are examined, with specific examples illus-trating the application of principles to nursing care, and the interrelationships between all the systems are acknowledged. As each tissue, organ and system has as its basic component the cell, the cell's physiology and genetic importance is also described.

The level of physiology presented is aimed at com-mon foundation programme students, although after this stage, a greater understanding of applied physi-ology will be required in relation to specific client groups. Above all it has been hoped to convey a sense of enthusiasm for how the body works, and to encourage the reader to follow up other sources for a more dedicated study of some important areas.

REFERENCES

Eckert R 1988 Animal physiology, 3rd edn. WH Freeman, Oxford

Wright S 1965 Applied physiology, 11th edn. Oxford University Press, London

FURTHER READING

Cree L, Rischmiller S 1991 Science in nursing, 2nd edn. WB Saunders/Baillière Tindall, Sydney (Helpful for readers who wish to understand more about basic physical sciences and their place in physiology for nurses. Full of nursing examples that illustrate underlying physical principles.)

Edlin G 1990 Human genetics. Jones and Bartlett Publishers, Boston (Very readable and well illustrated; covers the subject in an entertaining way. Useful reading if more information is needed on hereditary diseases, screening and genetic engineering.)

Hinchliff S, Montague S 1988 Physiology for nursing practice. Baillière Tindall, London (Provides extensive description of physiology of all the systems.)

Wilson K J W 1990 Ross & Wilson Anatomy and physiology in health and illness, 7th edn. Churchill Livingstone, Edinburgh (Covers anatomy in good detail. Well illustrated. A good support to any student of physiology.)

2

The psychological self

Roger B Ellis

In the previous chapter the focus was on the body: how cells work, how organs function, how systems interact to make up a whole. As individuals, we use parts of our body (for example our eyes) to observe other parts. Normally we cannot see the interior organs and most of us are quite content to 'leave well alone'. Doctors and nurses clearly have a professional interest in knowing a great deal about the body so that they can give effective care to the patient in distress. Medical researchers continually strive to improve that knowledge.

In this chapter, the focus shifts from the body to the mind, from physiology to psychology.

The chapter will aim to:

- **outline the approaches underlying the science of psychology**
- **consider the role of genetic, environmental and cultural factors in development, and discuss the stages and tasks of development throughout a person's lifespan**
- **look at the way in which we interpret our surroundings and ourselves, and consider psychological reactions to our findings**
- **stress the importance of self-understanding to the nurse, both in terms of her relationship with her patients and her own personal and professional development.**

As with the body, most of us do not want to know how the mind works when we are healthy and functioning normally; there are too many other things to do. However, when we or others became distressed, we are more inclined to be curious and to find out about the psychological self. This knowledge comes from our everyday observations of ourselves and others, and from clinical experience and research.

The material of this chapter is organised around three fundamental questions:

- How did we become what we are?
- How do we make sense of what is happening now?
- Can we predict our own behaviour?

These basic questions have been asked throughout history, and answers have been attempted through myth, literature, religion, art, philosophy and, more recently, science. They are therefore both very old and urgently topical, for to be alive at all is to try to make sense of our experience of ourselves and of other people.

PSYCHOLOGY: WHAT SORT OF SCIENCE IS IT?

We have come to know a great deal about the human body by using the methods of physical science: observation, investigation, experimentation, hypothesis testing, theory and model-making. The scientist uses intellectual tools to understand something that is essentially non-mental. However, in trying to understand the psychological self, we use the mind to understand itself. This poses quite different problems from those of understanding the body.

The oldest method of finding out about the mind is to look inside oneself (introspection) and try to understand one's own experience. 'Why did I get so angry when she suggested I was lazy?' 'What is it that I like about my boss?' Any insights gained in this way can then be assumed to apply to others as well. Or can they?

DIFFERENT APPROACHES TO THE SCIENCE

Psychoanalysis

Sigmund Freud, the father of psychoanalysis, committed himself to this process of self-examination all his professional life and gained considerable insight into his own psyche as a result. In addition, he made careful observations of his individual patients' thoughts, feelings and behaviour in a clinical setting in order to understand the causes of their psychological difficulties, and compared his findings with the results of his own introspection. The word 'idiographic' is applied to this sort of approach because its concern is with the uniqueness of the individual person, an idiograph being a person's private mark or signature.

Behaviourism

Other thinkers, contemporary with Freud in the early part of this century, reacted against such a subjective approach to understanding human psychology. They could see the limitation of views that could not be tested and verified, or shown to be false, in a strictly scientific way. In particular, American psychologists such as J.B. Watson shunned any subjective report of mental processes and studied only what was overt behaviour – hence they were called 'behaviourists'. They studied the relationship between a stimulus being received by an organism and the response that was made, without considering what happened in between. Psychology then became 'the science of mental life', investigated by means of experiments under laboratory conditions, commonly using animals rather than human beings and aiming to formulate general laws of behaviour. This approach is called 'nomothetic', meaning 'law-giving'.

A clear division arose between psychoanalysis and behaviourism, each convinced that its own assumptions and methods would provide definitive knowledge about psychology, thus enabling human behaviour to be understood and predicted. This division goes some way toward explaining why there are so many different ways of thinking about psychological issues. In the medical setting, this gives rise to a variety of treatments of psychological problems, for example behaviour modification, drugs therapy, and psychotherapy. It is useful to clarify this broad distinction between the two approaches (Table 2.1 gives a summary), whilst acknowledging that the methodology of psychology is much more complex than this.

THE NEED TO CONSIDER BOTH APPROACHES

For the newcomer trying to understand the psychological self, it can be confusing and infuriating to receive an indirect or equivocal answer to a question such as 'What caused him to be so depressed?' The answer might be 'What sort of answer do you want?' or 'It all depends on how you look at it.' It is perhaps less surprising that similar answers are given to political or economic questions, in which the reasons for different points of view are more obvious than in psychology. This complexity is unavoidable, but it does turn many people away to more certain areas of knowledge. For others, this open-ended quality is attractive and engages their interest.

This chapter draws on both idiographic *and* nomothetic approaches in an attempt to offer as rich an understanding as possible of our psychological selves, so avoiding the limitations of any one school of thought. This approach involves a tension between opposing views and a willingness to live with that tension.

Consider these three statements:

- I am like all other people
- I am like some other people
- I am like no other person.

These statements are all true, yet superficially they appear to contradict each other. Only by using all sources of information can we do justice to all three and get the fullest picture of an individual. A woman may say in anger, 'I'm not just a mother and wife and daughter. I'm *me*!', while yet being all of these.

Another instance of this integrative way of thinking is the answer to the question 'What is real?' Many people, both inside and outside medicine, still commonly talk of the external world of objects and people as the 'real' world and the internal world as being 'only psychological', implying that it is less 'real'. Yet we live in both worlds simultaneously, and each affects the other in a dynamic way. Thus, both are real, although in different ways.

Table 2.1	Different approaches in psychology
Idiographic	Nomothetic
Focuses on the inner world of personal experience	Focuses on the outer world of observable behaviour
Subjective	Objective
Uses few individuals or case studies	Uses large numbers of subjects
Encourages individual interpretation and intuition	Strictly scientific in method
Few generalisations possible	Aims to generalise to all people
Emphasises the uniqueness of individuals	Emphasises statistical differences between people

HOW DID WE BECOME WHAT WE ARE?

TIME: PAST, PRESENT AND FUTURE

Time is an elusive aspect of our experience, which can pass all too quickly at certain times and painfully slowly at others. We are conceived and born at particular moments, and our lives are lived within the essentially finite and scarce resource we call time. We are locked into a constant present that is immediately past, and the future seems to flow past us as we watch. Because of clocks and calendars and history, we tend to think of time in a linear way, as shown in Figure 2.1.

Our present is sliding along a line, converting future into past, and we are marooned in the present. Externally, physically, this formulation can be a useful one, but, psychologically, we may conceive of time quite differently, as in Figure 2.2.

Our remarkable brains allow us to remember the past and anticipate the future, vastly enriching our present from both directions. The ways in which our past is always present is one of the great psychological discoveries of the last hundred years, and we now understand a little better how we reach out to the future to bring it into the present. Our past rolls up like a carpet behind us (see Fig. 2.2), always at our heels, affecting the way we think, feel and behave right now. We also know that how we *expect* something to happen affects, to some extent, how it *does* happen, especially in the areas of human perception, judgement and feeling; we often call this 'self-fulfilling prophecy'.

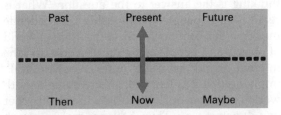

Figure 2.1   Linear time.

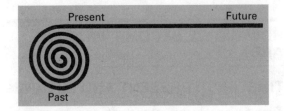

Figure 2.2   Psychological time.

The model of human lifespan development described by Erik Erikson, one of a number of approaches to describing how human beings change over a lifetime, is built on these ideas: what we are in the present is made up in a cumulative way from our experience in the past; in that sense, we are a product of what has happened to us. But we can always make something new of our present and future: we are both product *and* author of our experience (Noonan 1983). These ideas will be considered more fully later in the chapter.

The past

Our bodies are made up of cells in which genetic material is fixed at conception. Just as a large number of our physical attributes are genetically determined, so, it is thought, are many of our psychological aspects. How much our differences in temperament, personality, intelligence and character are determined by genes (nature) and how much by experience in the world (nurture) has been a heated and controversial debate for a long time. It is much more difficult to find clear evidence one way or the other in the psychological sphere than it is in the physical or biological sphere. The current state of the argument is that it is probably best to accept that we are both genetically *and* environmentally determined, that both factors interact and that the weight of the contribution of each is unknowable. Maybe which side any individual tends to support in this debate depends on his personality, which may, in its turn, be a product of both nature and nurture!

The 'nurture' factors that affect individuals are now known to be emotional as well as physical, and are to do with how others relate and treat them over long periods of time rather than in isolated incidents alone. If, for example, people are habitually abused physically, emotionally or sexually, we can expect this to profoundly affect their psychological state over a long period of time. If a person is generally loved, cherished, encouraged and validated, we can expect this to have an equally profound effect.

The present

The factors that affect the way we are in the present are generally more obvious and accessible than those pertaining to the past or future. I may be aware that my reaction to a patient depends on my current mood, how tired I am, whether I am anxious about my skills and how the patient responds to me. However, there are other influences – from the past – of which I might be quite unaware. These are unconscious influences, which are equally powerful but unknowable in normal circumstances. The unconscious mind, the focus of so much attention by psychoanalysts, is still for some a contentious issue. Perhaps it is best seen as a repository of those forces and experiences that affect the way we feel, think and act without us knowing how or why.

My present behaviour, then, depends on me, on the other person with whom I am interacting and on the context in which the interaction takes place (see Fig. 2.3). These three elements affect one another dynamically in a fluent and changing process. The self–other interaction is clearly a central part of any nursing process and is examined in more detail in Chapter 17. The wider issues of how physical and social contexts have an impact on human behaviour is examined in Chapter 3.

The future

Although the future is unknown, we all speculate about it, using our past experience to guide us. Kelly (1955) argues that anticipation is central to our experience and suggests that the way in which people anticipate events channels their behaviour, i.e. how a person expects things to happen will affect how he feels and behaves

towards them. Our task in the world, according to Kelly, is to interpret, theorise and make predictions like a scientist does, and to check whether our predictions match what actually happens. If we are good scientists, adaptable human beings, we will change our view of things under the pressure of any mismatch between the prediction and actual evidence. If not, we will maintain our view in spite of contrary, invalidating experience. Some of the reasons why an individual might resist change, even when it is in his best interests, are examined in 'Self-concept and change', below.

ERIKSON'S LIFESPAN DEVELOPMENT

Erikson (1985) offers a model of human development that gives an overview of what happens to an individual during the course of a whole lifetime – from birth to old age and death. He addresses immediately the tension between a person's uniqueness and his ordinariness. It is as if Erikson gives us a map of the countryside through which the individual can expect to journey, but on which the actual path taken is unmarked, as it depends on many, uniquely personal, factors. Each makes his own way with some detours and set-backs but can get his bearings relative to the large features that the map shows.

The map is built on the principle of **epigenesis**, first observed and formulated in embryology. This principle suggests that the blueprint for the development of an organism throughout its lifespan is given from the beginning. Maturation and development are a matter of the unfolding of potential and are encouraged by the interaction of the organism and the external environment, together with the growth of the organism itself. A human being's capacity to walk or to think in an abstract way or to grow quickly in puberty, for example, exists as potential from the earliest days but happens at the appropriate time, given normal maturation and a supportive environment.

For human beings, the life issues of the future emerge out of the present and the past. These issues are not random but orderly and give rise

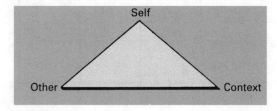

Figure 2.3   The interaction of self, other and context.

to reasonable expectations of how things will be. Of course, the unexpected, such as accidents and sudden illness, can always occur, but these stand out against a background of continuity and gradual change.

Erikson's map consists of eight stages of human development covering the whole normal lifespan, from birth to death in old age, in a rising diagonal as shown in Figure 2.4. Each stage is characterised by tasks of development that are particularly relevant to that stage but which are also anticipated by the previous stage and taken forward to the next. Erikson called these stages 'psychosocial crises', a rather dramatic name but one that suggests that something important has to be done at each stage in our lives to sustain our continued growth and development, both psychologically (in relation to ourselves) and socially (in relation to others). The first stage, for example, is characterised as 'trust v. mistrust', suggesting that the first task in life is centred around the question of whether

a baby's early experience will lead him to adopt a trusting orientation towards life or the opposite. In all eight stages, the first word of the opposites suggests a positive resolution of the psychosocial task and the second a negative outcome. Most of us, in our development, are not clearly located at one end or the other of these polarities but experience the tension that results from some mixture of the two.

Progress through the stages

Erikson's model suggests that the personality develops progressively, according to the epigenetic principle, with the early stages acting as a foundation for all that comes later. If the balance between the opposites is tilted towards the positive, it makes the positive resolution of the next stage more likely. Conversely, if the balance is negative, it makes it more difficult in later stages to achieve a positive outcome. If an individual cannot, for whatever reason, manage

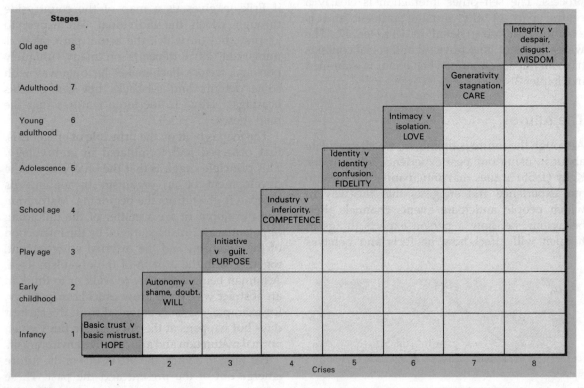

Figure 2.4 Erikson's developmental stages and associated psychosocial crises (adapted from Erikson (1985)).

any positive resolution to a developmental task, he will tend to get stuck at that stage (the technical term being 'fixated'), and his further development will be impaired. Developmental 'repair work' can be done at a later time but, in general, the further on in time this work is done from its optimal stage, the more difficult it is to do. Such work is being done by all of us all of the time quite spontaneously, especially if the human environment matches our needs and is supportive and enabling. Otherwise, such recovering of earlier stages may be done through counselling or psychotherapy.

Implications of the stages

Table 2.2 gives more detail of the implications of each stage. Stages 1 to 4 are childhood, Stage 5 the transition period of adolescence, and Stages 6 to 8 adulthood. It is worth noting that, according to Erikson, half of our development is completed by the end of childhood and a quarter before the normal threshold of memory (about 2–3 years of age). This again emphasises the relative importance of the early years and how much of the foundation of our personality may not be consciously available to us. The last column in Table 2.2 shows perhaps most clearly how the focus of each stage changes through life, and how each is built on the previous one and reaches forward to the next. Successful outcomes of the adult stages, for example, are likely to enable adults, if they become parents, to create a supportive and nurturing environment for the next generation of children. Equally, early deficits in development have a tendency to reappear in the next generation as the cycle repeats itself. A fuller exposition of Stage 6, early adulthood, is given in Box 2.1. This stage has been chosen because it is the one most likely to be personally relevant to the majority of readers of this book.

THE RELATIONSHIP OF THE PSYCHOLOGICAL SELF TO PHYSIOLOGY AND SOCIOLOGY

A theme throughout Erikson's writing is that of the dynamic nature of human processes, which are endlessly interweaving and interacting. This

---

Box 2.1 Early adulthood: intimacy v. isolation

By 'intimacy', Erikson is referring to the drive and willingness that healthy young adults have to share themselves intimately in work, sexuality and friendship with others: 'The intimacy at stake is the capacity to commit oneself to concrete affiliations which call for significant sacrifices and compromises' (Erikson 1985).

In the preceding stage, adolescence, the central issue is establishing an adequate sense of identity. Without this, the intimacy of early adulthood is impossible. This illustrates how the issues of one stage are rooted in those of the previous one.

The opposite of intimacy is isolation. This may be seen as a wish to remain separate and unrecognised, not to relate effectively with a job or friends or sexual partner. Looking back over earlier stages, such feelings may be traced to a sense of identity diffusion in adolescence or to a lack of trust in infancy.

For a young adult to acquire the capacity to give and receive love, 'that mutuality of mature devotion', Erikson suggests that the building blocks from earlier stages – fidelity, competence, purpose, will and hope – need to be adequately in place. Equally, he suggests that the capacity for care in mid-adulthood and for wisdom in old age both rest on the capacity to love in young adulthood. Thus each stage depends on the previous ones and informs those that follow.

---

is true of the eight stages, and it is also true of the three major organising principles in life – **soma**, **psyche** and **ethos** – the content of the first three chapters of this book. Erikson (1985) writes:

A human being's existence depends at every moment on three processes of organisation that must complement each other.

1. The biological process of the hierarchical organisation of organ systems constituting a body (soma).
2. There is the psychic process organising individual experience by ego synthesis (psyche).
3. There is the communal process of the cultural organisation of the interdependence of persons (ethos).

To begin with each of these processes has its own specialised methods of investigation ... In the end, all three approaches are necessary for clarification of any intact human event.

What makes clinical work so instructive is the rule that to approach human behaviour in terms of one of these processes always means to find oneself involved in the others, for each item that proves relevant in one process is seen to give significance to, as it receives meaning from, items in the others.

Table 2.2   Implications of Erikson's eight life stages (Adapted from Erikson 1985)

Stage	Age (approx.)	Task	Favourable outcome	Unfavourable outcome	Lasting accomplishment of successful outcome
1	Infancy (0–1 year)	Basic trust v. mistrust	Feelings of being wanted and loved and cared for. A sense of stability and order in experience – the result of physical and emotional 'mothering'.	Life is chaotic and unconnected. Child likely to be psychologically and possibly physically disabled. Higher infant mortality than usual. Retardation, possibly autism.	Drive and hope
2	Toddler (1–3 years)	Autonomy v. shame and doubt	Learns to stand on own two feet. Feeds self and begins to control bodily functions and use language to meet basic needs. Learns to say and accept 'no' as well as 'yes'. Begins to learn rules of society.	Lack of autonomy, passive dependence on others. Unable to assert own will, resulting in over-obedience. Paradoxically, is unable to accept 'no' and so results in constantly rebellious person-ality, perhaps delinquency.	Self-control and will power
3	Pre-school (about 4–5 years)	Initiative v. guilt	Has developed memory, can go and come back, both in place and time. Starts to learn adult gender roles. More loving, cooperative, secure in family. Good chance of becoming able to make moral choices.	Always wants to be 'in control'. Sense of competition drives individual to be over-competitive. May be always outside the law.	Direction and purpose
4	School (about 6–12 years)	Industry v. inferiority	Learns the basic skills of society – the 'how to's, the 'three Rs'. Learns to feel worthy and competent.	If person fails to learn industry, begins to feel inferior compared with others. If over-learns industry, may become too task-oriented and over-conform to society.	Method and competence
5	Adolescence (age 12 to late teens or early adulthood)	Identity v. role confusion	Sexual maturation and sexual identity. Ponders question 'Who am I?' as distinct from family. Develops social friendships. Tends to reject and be in conflict with family. Begins to discover role in life.	May not achieve an identity separate from family. May not become socially adult or sexually stable.	Devotion and fidelity
6	Early adulthood	Intimacy v. isolation	Learns to share passions, interests, problems with another individual. Also relates to others at work, in community, as well as in family. Achieves stability	Inability to be intimate with others. Becomes fixated at adolescent level, preoccupied with sensation-seeking and self-pleasure. Avoids responsibility and lacks stability.	Affiliation and love
7	Middle adulthood	Generativity v. self-absorption and stagnation	Fosters creativity and growth in others younger than self. Provides leadership, seeks to contribute to community, next generation, world. 'Minds the store'. May be most creative period of life.	Growth limited, remains rooted in past. Becomes 'cog-in-wheel', automated. May experience breakdown of zest for life. Feels life is passing him/her by.	Production and care
8	Old age	Ego integrity v. despair	Recognises and accepts diminishing faculties. Realises and faces own death. Feeling of having lived a 'good enough' life, paving the way for future generations. Dignity of truly 'wise' person.	Reaps bitter fruits of what was sown or not sown earlier. Fears death. An old age of misery, anxiety and despair.	Renunciation and wisdom

Relevance of psychological self to nursing

The concept of 'whole-patient care' so central to the modern philosophy of nursing is derived from the vision of the nurse–patient interaction as an 'intact human event'. A blueprint or map of the whole of human development, on which we can place our own and the patient's situation, gives us a sense of perspective. This allows us to understand what is happening a little better, and to generate ideas in general terms about what the issues might be for our patients, thus being more free to respond to the unique concerns of the individual in front of us.

HOW DO WE MAKE SENSE OF WHAT IS HAPPENING NOW?

Having reviewed the idea of whole lifespan development, let us now consider this second question more closely.

PERCEPTION

When two people interact, their behaviour towards each other depends on the information that they receive through their senses (Fig. 2.5). Human beings do not, however, receive information in the same way as does a tape-recorder or camera. These mechanical devices record everything, without selection or discrimination, in an entirely passive way. They only *record* information; they do not make sense of it. Human perception is far more complex. It is *both* recording *and* making sense – actively selecting, ignoring and interpreting in order to create meaning. It is commonplace to take a photograph of an event and to later see things in it that were

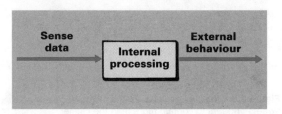

Figure 2.5　From sense data to behaviour.

not noticed at the time, for example reflections in water or the colour of a dress. Similarly, a tape-recording of a conversation often has unwanted sounds in it that were not noticed when it was made.

The figure–ground relationship

The human mind selects from sensory data to construct images that are meaningful. It actively organises information into a focus for attention (figure) set against a general background (ground). For the musician, this may be the sound of one instrument against all others; for a lover, the sight of the loved one in a crowded room. This process of discriminating between figure and ground is a way of reducing the complexity of the perceptual world so that is it manageable and serves our purpose. We can also easily be misled by what we perceive into making inappropriate interpretations of sensory data. Optical illusions show this clearly and hint at our more general capacity to distort evidence and to make mistakes. This central information-processing gives rise both to the richness of our internal world and to our capacity to distort evidence and make mistakes. Sachs (1986) gives fascinating accounts of what can happen to people when these neurological processes go wrong.

Social influences on perception

It is not surprising that the way we perceive the world is strongly affected by social factors. We often force our view of people and events into stereotypes and behave accordingly rather than in response to the new evidence before us. There is a common resistance to testing against external reality; we often prefer our own particular version of what we think or feel or want. Yet we can be strongly affected by what others say or write, even though the content may be blatantly false; hence the severe view taken in law of slander and libel.

Memory, forgetting and attention show similar general properties of being selective, according to the purposes and meaning of what is being attended to, remembered or forgotten. So another question arises: how does the mind do the selecting, interpreting and distorting that creates meaning out of sensory data?

COGNITION

It can come as quite a shock to realise that the visual picture we have of the world – full-size, three-dimensional – is derived from two images, each the size of a thumb-nail, that are thrown onto the retina of each eye by the lens in front. The images are curved, but basically two-dimensional like a camera's image. The brain processes the information from these two images and *constructs* what we see. This construction then becomes a *representation* of the outside world, inside us. The analogy of a map may be helpful once again. The map is not the countryside but it represents it accurately and effectively. The capacity to make these representations (sometimes called mental images, schemata or structures), and internally to compare, contrast and link them, is what is known as cognition. When we see, hear, taste, touch or smell something a second time, we experience re-cognition.

Piaget's developmental stages

Jean Piaget, a Swiss psychologist, was one of the leading investigators into how we come to know the world and change our view of it as we grow up. Like Erikson, he proposed that this cognitive development followed a general pattern for all people. In Piaget's formulation, this pattern was characterised by three main stages from birth to maturity:

- sensorimotor
- intuitive
- operational
  - concrete
  - formal

The sensorimotor stage. In the first stage, a baby gets to know the world by what it experiences through its senses and by what it does *to* the world through its muscle movements, i.e. through action. A young baby uses its mouth to take in food, smile, cry and explore the world around. Older babies, crawling, do not *know* that they cannot go through a closed door; to gain this knowledge, they have to crawl and bump their heads. They can only learn by experiencing the world through the body – by using the senses and by making movements. Hence this stage is called sensorimotor.

The intuitive stage. In the second stage, children know the world in an intuitive way by noticing regularities and seeing the connections between events. Children of primary-school age tend to be over-impressed by appearances, often jumping to conclusions and reversing cause and effect. They have their own logic to work out why things are as they are, which is centred on themselves and their own experience: 'It's dark because it's my bedtime, so the sun goes to bed as well.' When asked to compare a line of sweets with a cluster, as in Figure 2.6, a child at the intuitive stage will say that the line contains more than the cluster, even though the number is the same, because the line *looks* longer. The rule for deciding 'more' and 'less' is not yet fully understood.

The operational stage. In concrete operations, a child in late childhood can think about his own thinking, can understand contradiction and can apply logic to experience: 'It can't be heavier just because it has changed shape.' Learning takes a big stride forward at this stage, when ideas are tested against external reality to see whether or not they make sense. It is now possible for the child to say: 'Just because I think it is so, doesn't make it true.'

In **formal operations** thinking, which may start in adolescence, a person can deal with pure abstractions and hypothetical situations, and can carry out experiments in thought rather than simply in action. This is a long way developmentally from the earliest sensorimotor learning

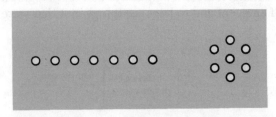

Figure 2.6   Intuitive thinking. To the child, the line of sweets appears to contain more than the cluster.

of a baby, and opens the door to interest in moral and social ideals, grand theoretical designs and adult religion. The sense of the power of such ideas is part of the reason why many adolescents and young adults tend to be so energetic in their criticism of the world around them.

Adaptation and achieving a balance

Although these cognitive capacities change and develop as we mature, they are the result of the same unchanging mental processes operating on experience throughout our lives. The central process is adaptation – the way in which our knowledge and understanding of the world changes under the constant impact of our experience. Adaptation can be broken down into two components: assimilation and accommodation.

Assimilation is the process by which we try to interpret new experience in terms of what we already know. For a young child, for example, a squirrel might be understood as a cat with a big tail. We try to impose our understanding onto the world and make the world fit our view of it.

Accommodation is the process by which we change our mental structures under the impact of new experiences, because the new cannot be understood in terms of the old. Many people report experiences of 'the penny dropping' when they understand something in a new way, often quite suddenly after a painful period of incomprehension: 'I *see* now. I couldn't see what was meant before.' This is a dramatic example of accommodation, which more commonly happens imperceptibly.

Degrees of adaptation. Before we can be fully adapted to the world, our processes of assimilation and accommodation must be in dynamic equilibrium such that we make sense of the world according to what we already know but, if that does not fit, we change and extend our understanding. Few of us are quite so readily adaptable, and we vary, as we shall see later, in our tendency to hold on to the old order or seek out new experiences. Patients who are in hospital or seriously ill for the first time are under considerable pressure to adapt to new circumstances and to change their understanding of themselves. Some

do this better than others. Some regress to an earlier developmental stage, so that their way of thinking is more like that of a child in the intuitive stage than that of an adult who can reason.

It is probably best to assume that, for most people, the immediate response to unexpected change is to resist it. This conservative impulse is very strong. People have been known to prefer death in their familiar home rather than moving away when a predictable disaster such as a volcano or flood threatens them. However, if we change too readily under every pressure from outside, we may lose our sense of continuity, meaning and identity. So a balance between the two processes is the optimal position – another example of the tension between opposites that we somehow need to maintain if we are to remain healthy.

SELF-CONCEPT AND CHANGE

Making sense of the external world is difficult enough, but making sense of the self is another matter. The self is a notoriously slippery and imprecise concept, one which is difficult to define. Carl Rogers, a highly influential American psychologist, placed the self at the centre of his theory. He represents the humanistic school of psychology with its emphasis on human worth and individuality and on the individual's right to determine his or her own actions.

Carl Rogers (1974) suggests that we all create out of our experience of the world a picture of ourselves, with evaluations attached, which is our self. I can get on well with my self, or be in conflict with my self or be 'beside my self', but my relationship to the self is a psychological reality that is unavoidable. Rogers emphasises that each person is the centre of a continually changing world of experience and behaves according to that subjective experience. Thus, to truly understand someone else's behaviour, it is necessary to understand the world *as that person sees it*, from an internal frame of reference, rather than from an external framework. As individual worlds are essentially private, this can only be (partially) achieved by good communication and empathy between those who seek to understand one another (see Ch. 17). Rogers also assumes that human beings have an inner drive to develop themselves in the direction of health, competence and full functioning, when they are free to do so.

The centre, then, of a person's world is the self, and the individual tends to behave in ways that are consistent with his view of the self. Someone who sees himself as inarticulate is not likely to volunteer for public speaking. Someone who has learned that she can do most things she sets her mind to has, by that pattern of thinking, made it more likely that she will succeed in the next task – the self-fulfilling prophecy again. However, life is not always as simple as that.

Self-consistency

If a nurse (assumed in this instance to be female) is receiving information from the world that is in some way inconsistent with her view of herself (e.g. she might define herself as 'helpful' yet be accused of being difficult and obstructive), she has a problem, both cognitive and emotional, which can be coped with in several ways. In Piaget's terms, there is dissonance between how the nurse thought things were and new information; thus, her equilibrium is disturbed. The nurse might adopt one of the following strategies:

1. She can ignore the information completely so that there is nothing to adapt to: 'It went over her head; water off a duck's back', an observer might say.
2. She can take it in but, because of painful dissonance, discount it or discredit the person who said it so that it loses its power to disturb: 'He always says things like that. It's rubbish!'
3. She can experience the dissonance, take the information on board and modify her view of herself accordingly: 'Some people see me as unhelpful and maybe I am sometimes, even though I don't want to be or see myself like that.'

The third strategy is an example of accommodating to new experience whereas (2) shows the nurse maintaining her old view of herself and perhaps distorting the world to suit herself. Adopting (1) is to refuse to acknowledge what is actually happening – the familiar head-in-the-sand technique of coping.

This line of thinking leads us to look at other related mechanisms of the mind that we all use to some extent in coping with and making sense of our everyday lives.

MECHANISMS OF THE MIND

The wide range of theories concerning perception, cognition and the self that have arisen from different fields within psychology illustrate the diversity of approaches that may be taken in answering questions about the way human beings function. In this discussion, however, we will draw upon one approach in particular – the psychodynamic understanding of the person. Four principal concepts, each referring to a different aspect of the interaction between thinking, feeling and behaving, inform the psychodynamic approach. These concepts are:

- unconscious processes
- regression
- transference
- defence.

Unconscious processes

It is commonplace for a person to engage in sport or games, using the body in play. It is perhaps even more common to play with thoughts and feelings in the interior world – imagining, pondering and experimenting. For some people, this mental play is highly creative and a safe haven from the unyielding reality of the outside world. For others it is full of fear, danger and persecution – to be avoided if possible, often by turning away to activity in the outside world. It has a quality different from that of the thinking needed to get things done. The question 'Where would I *really* like to go on holiday?' is quite different from 'Where do I make the bookings for the coach?'. The everyday use of the term 'fantasy' refers to this capacity to consciously imagine and daydream.

Phantasy is also used in a different way by psychodynamic theorists such as Klein (1963) (the spelling denoting this different meaning). These theorists use it to refer to the imaginative activity that is *unconscious* and which underlies *all* our thinking and feeling, rather than just the feelings of which we are aware. They suggest that such phantasy begins very early in childhood and is primarily concerned with bodily processes and relating to others. It becomes more and more symbolic and elaborate as we develop but never loses its primitive roots in infancy. Perhaps you can recall the intense, vivid memories and feelings of childhood – of being abandoned, lost or heroically saved, or of burglars under the bed, for example – which seem to exist independently of whether any of those things actually happened to us. They appear to be products of the mind rather than of direct experience, even though, of course, such events can and do actually happen from time to time. The figures and relationships in fairy tales show something of the intensity and timeless quality of such phantasies.

Klein suggests that our capacity to adapt to the outside world is supported or impaired by such phantasies. When a person is threatened or stressed, especially over a long period of time, adult reality-centred thinking can be weakened such that underlying phantasies become more apparent. A patient may be prey to primitive fears of persecution, which make it almost inevitable that any gesture of help will be viewed with suspicion. Another might interpret quite routine care as evidence of being held in special regard and affection by a nurse. To be aware of these things may help the nurse to understand and be less fearful of some of the more unexpected, even bizarre, thoughts, feelings and behaviour of some patients. It may also, incidentally, help her to understand her own internal world, with all its hopes and fears, alarming as this can be at times. (See the reference to Menzies [1961] later in this chapter.)

Regression

Regression, in general, means reversion to an earlier state or way of functioning. If adults are stressed, it is possible for them to regress to earlier patterns of behaviour that are never entirely outgrown and so remain available for use. Regression may be seen as an attempt by individuals to protect themselves from painful states of mind. It is usually ineffective in doing this because, although one set of anxieties is avoided, it compels people to re-experience other anxieties appropriate to the stage to which they have regressed. Ill patients who are actually helpless and dependent may feel so anxious that they may well regress to a more infantile state, but they are then likely to feel the other anxieties of that stage, such as unrealistic fears of danger or abandonment. If nurses can allow patients to regress into such a dependent state and respect their anxieties without mocking them, they are likely to help them recover more effectively.

In psychotherapy, regression is regarded as a positive process if it allows the patient to return to and complete the developmental work of an earlier stage, i.e. to get beyond fixation and become more free to grow and develop in a way that brings greater satisfaction.

Transference

Transference is the process by which one person relates to another person in present circumstances in ways that are rooted in the past. A nurse, for example, might react to a doctor as if he were her father, perhaps feeling put down or undervalued like she did at home. She may know that the doctor is not at all like her father but nevertheless find herself having 'familiar' feelings when the doctor looks at her. Another nurse may find herself attracted to patients who live in the country because she was most happy when she used to live in the country.

Experience in the past gives us all a readiness to interpret the present not so much in terms of what *is* as what *was*. After reflection, it is often possible to see this quite clearly and to note our transference reactions. A clue is when we almost instantaneously feel strongly about someone or something. Such strong feelings are more likely to be linked to past events than to present ones. Whole patterns of relating to others can be adopted over a long period of time, sometimes a lifetime, which are repetitions of earlier patterns and quite unconscious. This helps to explain why it is notoriously difficult to change human behaviour once a pattern has been established. Such ideas about transference tie in with what was said earlier about Erikson's stages and Piaget's concept of assimilation.

Defence

The previous three mechanisms of the mind may leave the reader impressed by the tendency of human beings to distort what is in front of them. How does anyone manage the real world effectively with all this going on? Paradoxically, it is this rich infusion of the present with the past and with the anticipation of the future that gives us our human capacity for creativity and for civilisation-building.

The human psyche has evolved ways of protecting itself from the feelings of anxiety that inevitably arise from this rich mix of conscious and unconscious feelings. These are called 'mechanisms of defence'. They can be consciously adopted to ward off danger from the outside world (e.g. 'attack is the best form of defence') or unconsciously used to cope with anxiety arising from within. In the latter case, a person may be very uncomfortable about admitting to angry or sexual feelings towards someone else and use the mechanism of denial to protect himself against the conflict these feelings induce.

Such defence mechanisms can have a positive aspect by helping an individual to control and understand his emotional experiences. When defences are 'down', we may feel overwhelmingly vulnerable and be unable to function. However, defence mechanisms also have a negative aspect if they are so strong that they make it difficult for us to act spontaneously or with trust. Thus, potentially rewarding experiences may be inaccessible to the over-defended person.

Regression and denial were two of the defences described by Anna Freud (1936). There are several others also considered in the literature, of which projection and introjection are two.

Projection. This means 'to throw in front of'. It is the mechanism by which an attribute, originally experienced in oneself, is thrown out and located outside oneself, generally in another person: 'I don't dislike *him*. He dislikes *me*.'

Denial and projection here go hand in hand. Violent projective processes probably underlie all bullying, scorn and contempt and can be seen between groups, cultures and nations as well as between individuals. Feelings of persecution are probably strongest in those who would deny feeling aggressive towards others.

Introjection. This process works in the opposite direction to projection. Something is first experienced outside oneself and is taken in as if it were one's own. If someone we love or respect is hurting us, it may be easier to blame ourselves rather than face the distress of confronting the other person: 'It must be my fault that he treats me so badly.' Introjection can act more positively when we bask in the success of someone we know and feel it as our own. If this goes too far, however, it can amount to a form of psychic stealing in which we rob the other person of good things, even 'forgetting' where they came from, and claim them for our own. A student, for example, may so envy the knowledge and wisdom of a teacher that after taking in all that he possibly can, he refuses to acknowledge the teacher's contribution to his development.

Defence mechanisms in nursing

Menzies (1961) studied the ways in which the social system of a hospital was organised to protect the staff from being overwhelmed by the stress and anxiety generated by their jobs. This was originally an investigation into the low morale and high drop-out rate of nurses. Menzies found that there was little acknowledgement of the stress experienced by nurses when patients and relatives projected onto them such feelings as depression, anxiety or disgust at illness. These feelings 'put into' the nurse added to the stress of actually doing the job and responding to patients' needs.

Menzies listed the ways in which the social setting of nursing produced techniques of reducing or dissipating anxiety. She described these defence mechanisms as collusive agreements – often unconscious ones – within the social system of the institution itself. Box 2.2 gives this list as presented by Barber (1989). It can be helpful to nurses to be familiar with these professional

Box 2.2 **Menzies' social defences in nursing practice**

1. Splitting up the nurse–patient relationship
2. Depersonalisation, categorisation and denial of the significance of the individual
3. Detachment and denial of feelings
4. The attempt to eliminate decisions by ritual task performance
5. Reducing the weight of responsibility in decision-making by checks and counter-checks
6. Collusive social redistribution of responsibility and irresponsibility
7. Purposeful obscurity in the formal distribution of responsibility
8. The reduction of the impact of responsibility by delegation to superiors
9. Idealisation and underestimation of development possibilities
10. Avoidance of change

defence mechanisms so that the conflicts and anxieties thus avoided may be confronted in a more realistic way.

CAN WE PREDICT OUR OWN BEHAVIOUR?

This question immediately raises the issue of psychological consistency, i.e. of whether there is *anything* constant about us, given our changing moods and circumstances. The familiar tension between apparent opposites is here again, this time between continuity and change. Children are used to being greeted by fond but distant relatives with a remark such as 'My, how you've changed!' And yet it is clear that they are instantly recognisable.

Some degree of consistency is necessary for life to be tolerable at all. Imagine not being able to predict anything about the behaviour of the people we know. When travelling by bus, train or aircraft, we assume that the physical and mental functioning of those in control is predictable and hence reliable and safe. The fields of personality, intelligence and motivation are three traditional areas in psychology in which the issues of consistency, predictability and individual differences are dominant.

PERSONALITY

This is one of the most controversial and perplexing areas in psychology, and illustrates well the variety of ways of studying the person and the differing theories that result. The idiographic–nomothetic distinction made at the beginning of the chapter helps to select just two approaches to the study of personality from the many available:

- trait theories
- cognitive theories.

A fuller treatment is given in Pervin (1993).

Trait theories

The trait or type approach is a systematic version of our common tendency to describe people we like as 'perceptive' or 'friendly' and those we do not like as 'stupid' or 'cold'. Traits that are considered opposite to each other, such as 'active–passive', are used to define a continuum in terms of which people vary. This variation is tested on large numbers of people with the expectation that a few will score towards the extreme ends of the scale and that most will score in the middle. The idea is to create reliable, objective tests and, on the basis of scores, to predict other aspects of behaviour that may be of interest. Are dominant people good leaders? Is conformity linked to anxiety? The number of traits required to do justice to the rich variations in human personality is a matter of debate.

Eysenck (1967) and Cattell (1965) use a statistical technique called factor analysis to reduce the complexity of large numbers of traits to a few underlying factors. For Eysenck these factors are:

- extraversion–introversion
- neuroticism–stability
- psychoticism–impulse control.

Each element of these three pairs indicates a personality type for Eysenck and is the result of a cluster of traits that go together; for example, an introverted type is likely to be patient, quiet and thoughtful. It is important to remember that most people are not at the extremes of these pairs of traits but are somewhere in the middle. This means, for example, that a balance between introverted and extraverted tendencies is more common than is a heavy bias in one direction.

Eysenck (1967) sought to find a basis for personality within the body. He suggests that any tendency towards neuroticism, for example, is built into the nervous system and is, at least to some extent, genetically determined. His desire to see psychological realities in physical terms indicates his strictly scientific approach to the study of personality and contrasts with other, more subjective, approaches.

Cognitive theories

The cognitive approach may be summed up in the phrase 'As a person thinks, so he is'. We have seen earlier that our view of the world is constructed by ourselves as we interact with it. This more subjective view implies that events do not have meaning in themselves but only in what we make of them.

This focus was explored by Kelly (1955), who believed that how we make sense of things – our construct system – *is* our personality. If I choose to see other people in terms of the construct 'strong–weak', that perception will affect both my behaviour towards them and also my view of myself. Kelly says that the judgement 'strong' about someone does not describe a trait in that person but only how the perceiver sees him. There will always be alternative ways of seeing an individual; thus, a domineering person may be seen as strong by one person and rather pathetic by the next. Kelly takes the view that there is no absolute truth about a human being, but merely attempts by others to make sense of their experience of him or her.

INTELLIGENCE

The concept of intelligence is as familiar to us as the concept of personality, yet it, too, is problematic. Key points that have emerged from a great deal of study and debate concerning the notion of intelligence can be summarised as follows:

1. There is no one definition of intelligence that is agreed by all psychologists, although most would include reference to reasoning power and problem-solving ability. What intelligence actually refers to is therefore as much in the mind of the psychologist as it is in the mind of the subject.

2. Because the word 'intelligence' exists, there is a tendency to think that it refers to something real about a person that can be measured, such as height or weight. This false but very common kind of reasoning is known as 'reification' – the tendency to make real and concrete that which is abstract.

3. Intelligence is assumed to be distributed in the population at large in the same way as height or weight, i.e. according to the normal distribution curve (Fig. 2.7). According to this curve, few people have extremes of high or low intelligence and most are in the middle range. We do not know whether this is true or not. We tend to assume it is and to design tests that confirm this assumption.

4. The reasons for the measured differences in intelligence between individuals have been a source of intense, even violent, debate. In the earlier part of the 20th century, it was assumed that these differences were genetic in origin and hence fixed for life. After the 1950s, environmental factors were emphasised. Nowadays, an interactionist position is generally adopted, which acknowledges the indivisibility of both influences.

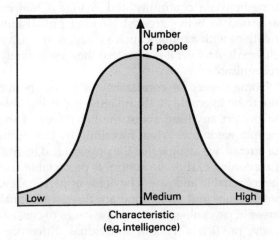

Figure 2.7   The normal distribution curve.

5. Important political and social decisions have been based upon these shifts in emphasis. The most striking has been the way in which children were, up to the 1960s, allocated to different types of school in the public sector depending on their intelligence and 'type of mind', as measured at age 11 and beyond. How children performed at the age of 11 was assumed to be a reliable predictor of their abilities for life. A more egalitarian period followed, which emphasised the importance of keeping opportunities open for all and encouraged the growth of the Comprehensive educational system.

MOTIVATION

Different people are motivated by different things. Some pursue money or prestige, wanting to see a tangible result for their efforts. Others do things for the satisfaction they derive from the activity itself. Most of us do things for mixed motives, so a mixed approach seems appropriate once more in order to do justice to the complexity of human behaviour.

Each theory of motivation tends to focus on one aspect only of this complex subject. Reinforcement theory and Maslow's hierarchy of needs, for example, have contrasting assumptions and are built around very different central concepts.

Reinforcement theory

Skinner (1953), an American experimental psychologist, has shown how animal behaviour can be controlled and 'shaped' by reinforcement, i.e. by the linking of rewards to desired behaviour. This theory of **operant conditioning** (Fig. 2.8) has also been applied to human beings.

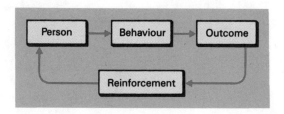

Figure 2.8 Operant conditioning.

In simple terms, if a person is rewarded for a particular behaviour, this behaviour is reinforced and is more likely to be repeated. The relationship between outcome and behaviour can be altered accordingly to a 'schedule of reinforcement', different schedules producing different effects. For example, when a child is learning a new skill in mathematics, a teacher will often tick each correct sum. After the child is more advanced, the teacher may demand a whole page of sums before a tick is given, thus hoping to encourage him to keep on with the task longer without reward and so develop his knowledge and skill. People play slot machines in the knowledge that they *might* be rewarded sometime, and this conviction can sustain very persistent behaviour even in the face of no reward. The whole betting industry is built on this characteristic of human behaviour.

At root, the assumption is that we act the way we do because of the results that are obtained outside of the action itself. This is **extrinsic motivation** and can explain a good deal of simple behaviour. It is inadequate, however, as an explanation of more complex behaviour involving higher cognitive processes.

Maslow's hierarchy of needs

The focus here changes to the concept of 'needs', which by definition are intrinsic to a human being. A need is a state of deficiency in a person that motivates or energises that person to satisfy the need. This is most directly seen with physiological needs. If hungry, I seek food. If tired, I rest. Further needs are psychological and are more open-ended in nature; they are likely to be learned rather than just given, and include, for example the need to develop relationships involving reciprocal affection, or the need for feelings of self-worth. Maslow (1970) suggests that these deficiency needs are hierarchical, in that higher-level needs will be attended to only after lower-level needs are satisfied (Fig. 2.9).

Maslow adds another layer, called growth needs, above the deficiency needs. These needs motivate behaviour that does not result from deficiencies but from our instinctual tendency

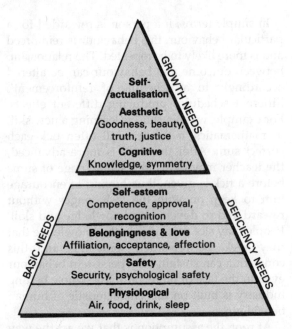

Figure 2.9 Maslow's hierarchy of needs.

towards growth. These growth needs will be attended to only when basic needs are reasonably satisfied. They include aesthetic and cognitive urges associated with virtues such as justice and goodness, and with the pursuit of knowledge, order and beauty. The highest need in Maslow's view is the need for self-actualisation – the unfolding and fulfilment of the self. Like Rogers, Maslow takes an optimistic view of human nature and embraces the humanistic values of what has been called the 'third school' in psychology.

Implications for nursing

Anyone caring for another is likely to have observed that, if that person's basic needs are not met, these unmet needs define the most urgent task for the carer. When these have been satisfied, at least to some extent, other needs become apparent, in an open-ended way. Maslow's hierarchy of needs helps us clarify this experience and can guide nurses' thoughts and actions about their own needs *and* when helping patients. It also endorses what has been said before about how important it is for each patient to be recognised and treated as a unique person by those who are caring for him. Only by close attention to what the patient says and does can the nurse know which of the patient's needs are most urgent at any given time. This interactive process is examined more closely in Chapter 17.

CONCLUSION

Although we started with three basic questions, the pursuit of partial answers has generated more questions, which in turn could generate more. Perhaps the discussion is best left open-ended, for the psychological self is itself open-ended.

This final quotation points to the future in its expression of the way we are beginning to think in the health care professions about how our psychological and physical selves interact:

One of the most exciting and fast-expanding areas in recent years has been the extension of psychological thinking to problems of physical ill-health. What such work obliges us to do is to break down the distinction between mind and body and to become aware that psyche and soma interact in subtle and complex ways. Increasingly it is recognised that psychological factors play some role in the causation of physical disease and that disease, in turn, poses major problems of a psychological nature for the individual. Body changes in ill-health occur in a context of thought, feeling and behaviour from which they cannot be extracted. (Berryman et al 1987)

Summary

We very rarely, unless prompted, stop to consider our psychological selves, yet an understanding of our own development and patterns of thinking and feeling can greatly enhance the care we give our patients, our interaction with colleagues, and our own personal fulfilment.

In this chapter the two main approaches to the science of psychology – idiographic and nomethetic – are considered. A combination of these is likely to give the best balance and the greatest potential for insight into psychology.

To make us what we are, genetic, environmental and cultural factors all contribute, in a continuum of advancement throughout the lifespan, in a progression of stages (according to Erikson 1985).

Having reached the present, we need to make sense of what is happening to us, using the powers of perception and cognition; Piaget's theory of cognitive development gives a framework for this. To use the information gleaned, we have to both assimilate it and accommodate to it, simultaneously adapting and attempting to maintain some degree of self-consistency. The psychodynamic approach to the interaction between thinking, feeling and behaving allows an insight into this area.

Lastly, can we predict our own behaviour? Our underlying personality and motivation would appear to be consistent, but can be influenced by many external factors. Only if our basic needs are met can we move to the next layer of Maslow's hierarchy of needs, and continue the journey towards self-actualisation.

REFERENCES

Barber P 1989 Developing the 'person' of the professional carer. In: Hinchliff S M, Norman S E, Schober J E (eds) Nursing practice and health care. Arnold, London

Berryman J C, Hargreaves D J, Hollin C R, Howells K 1987 Psychology and you. BPS and Methuen, London

Cattell R B 1965 The scientific analysis of personality. Penguin, London.

Erikson E H 1985 The life cycle completed. Norton, New York

Eysenck H J 1967 The biological basis of personality. Thomas, Illinois

Freud A 1936 The ego and the mechanisms of defence. International Universities Press, London

Kelly G 1955 The psychology of personal constructs. Norton, New York

Klein M 1963 Our adult world and its roots in infancy. Pitman, London

Maslow A H 1970 Motivation and personality, 2nd edn. Harper and Row, New York

Menzies I 1961 The functioning of social systems as a defence against anxiety. Tavistock, London

Noonan E 1983 Counselling young people. Methuen, London

Pervin L A 1993 Personality: theory and research, 6th edn. Wiley, New York

Rogers C R 1974 On becoming a person, 4th edn. Constable, London

Sachs O 1986 The man who mistook his wife for a hat. Picador, London

Skinner B F 1953 Science and human behaviour. Macmillan, New York

FURTHER READING

McGhie A 1986 Psychology as applied to nursing, 8th edn. Churchill Livingstone, Edinburgh

Menzies Lyth 1988 Containing anxiety in institutions: selected essays, vol. 1. Free Association Books, London

Niven N 1989 Health psychology. Churchill Livingstone, Edinburgh

Segal J 1985 Phantasy in everyday life. Penguin, Harmondsworth

The sociological self

Tepi Corbett

Individual nursing care requires the nurse to have a knowledge of not only the psychological aspects of her patients, but also the sociological influences determining personal and culturally-related responses. This chapter aims to:

- highlight the relevance of an understanding of sociology
- introduce the structuralist and interpretative approaches to sociology
- explore health as a social construct
- discuss the notion of the sociological self, considering socialisation, roles and role conflicts, and how these impact on nursing practice
- examine the influence of culture on the sociological development of the individual.

INTRODUCTION

Prior to the mid-1980s, the approach to the education of health care professionals was almost entirely based on medical disease. Nursing tended to be task and excessively physical in orientation, despite the fact that official nursing training syllabuses included such topics as 'the social aspects of disease'. It was not until 1979 that legislation brought about a change of emphasis in the pre-registration education of nurses. The concept of holism became the centre of the curriculum.

The significance was that, from then on, nursing students were encouraged to learn how to fulfil not only the physical needs, but also the psychological, social and spiritual needs of patients. In this context, it became necessary to increase and update the knowledge base of the students, particularly in relation to social and behavioural sciences. Although sociology continues to remain a marginal subject, it is now acknowledged that it could act as a humanising factor in the education programme involving:

not just the acquisition of knowledge but the development of a new way of looking at the world – one which calls into question much that we have taken for granted. (Cook 1993)

The physiological and psychological dimensions of the self have been explored in previous chapters. This chapter aims to consider the cultural and social activities that influence 'self' and the fulfilment of human needs during health and illness. It is, however, only an introduction. The references given in the text are there to invite the reader to think sociologically and to develop a three-dimensional 'sociological imagination'. This, as proposed by Giddens (1993), is a creative and enterprising way of looking at social life from an anthropological, historical and future perspective.

SOCIOLOGY IN THE REAL WORLD – THE RELATIONSHIP BETWEEN SOCIOLOGICAL KNOWLEDGE AND COMMON SENSE/LAY KNOWLEDGE

The majority of people are able to be social and survive in social environments because they are aware of the beliefs, values and norms of that society. In other words, their behaviour is embedded in and directed by the way things are in the society in which they live. Social etiquette – the conventional laws of courtesy between the members of the society – could be used as an example here. The reader may well ask 'Is it not just common sense to behave with decorum in Church, attend a formal interview smartly dressed or address a dignitary in a courteous manner?'

Activity 3.1

Reflect on your activities for the last couple of days and choose four different situations in which you found yourself.

- How did you behave in each of the situations?
- If your behaviour was different in the different situations, why do you think this was so?

Individuals generally attempt to behave in accordance with the expectations of the society in which they live. This conduct is largely guided by social determinants, namely the values and norms common to all those raised within a particular culture or belonging to a particular group. Values serve as general guidelines for conduct, as they define what is worth while and worth striving for, or what we might believe to be right or wrong. For example, in Western societies, monogamy – being faithful to a single marriage partner – is considered to be a prominent value, whereas polygamy – allowing a husband or wife to have more than one partner – is dominant in many African cultures. Norms differ from values insofar as they provide specific guides for action indicating what is acceptable and appropriate behaviour in particular situations in a given culture. Differences between cultures can easily be realised through considering, for example, eating habits. In Western societies, it would be considered to be the height of bad manners to allow a loud and prolonged burp to escape at the conclusion of a formal dinner. In contrast, the Bedouin of North Africa regard this as the highest possible compliment to the host. Regardless and because of cultural differences, values and norms make social life predictable and comprehensible (Haralambos 1986).

However, cultural norms and values are generally taken for granted. They become so much part of the members of a society that individuals may be totally unaware of, or indeed deny, the existence of any guidelines for acceptable social behaviour. Instead, their belief may be that it is only natural or common sense that everybody should act in a particular way in a given situation.

Activity 3.2

1. Complete the following sentences:
    I believe that:

    - people live in family units because ...
    - pupils who succeed in school do so because ...
    - teenagers become delinquent because ...
    - the stability of marriage is decreasing because ...

2. Get together with a group of your peers and compare your answers to identify the commonalities and differences of your responses.

3. Suggest reasons for these commonalities and differences.

Having completed the activity, the reader may well have found that 'common sense' beliefs are not so common after all, even in a small group of people. The members of the group will probably have seen the world largely as a mirror of the familiar features of their own lives, in which their private thoughts and feelings predominate. This shows the importance of making explicit the images that individuals may have of society, because appreciating the behaviour of individuals from their individual social viewpoints helps to understand what makes them 'tick'.

Given that social determinants shape and define accepted ways of behaviour for the members of a particular society, it is essential to appreciate that there may be considerable variations not only within different societies, but also within the varied cultures that exist in any one society.

It is particularly important for health care professionals to be able to differentiate between cultural variations of behaviour. This can be illustrated by the fact that, for example, interaction patterns may vary greatly between cultures. Because of cultural 'teachings' in a number of Asian societies, respect for others is portrayed through maintaining a large interpersonal space, averting the eyes and keeping the head low. From this type of behaviour, Americans would imply that the person is distant, submissive or evasive. So, if health care professionals are armed only with 'common sense' knowledge when, for

example, making an assessment of the health status of a patient, they may well come to an erroneous conclusion about the person's behaviour. Thus, although common sense/lay knowledge gives the reader an excellent starting point, sociological knowledge provides a scientific basis that will guide professional decision-making. In fact, Giddens (1992) proposes that a highly illuminating perspective can be achieved through the study of sociology for its:

scope is extremely wide, ranging from the analysis of passing encounters between individuals in the street up to the investigation of global processes. (Giddens 1992)

Every individual, in addition to the physical and psychological component of the self, has a social integrity through which the cultural heritage of his society is safeguarded and passed on to the next generation. As social changes become more rapid and far-reaching, social phenomena that could previously be understood by common sense require a rational and more scientific investigation for us fully to understand how best to care for the individual.

Case example 3.1 illustrates how, for example, a change in the economic status and the nature of the relationships between individuals within a family may directly influence the provision of care. If a nurse is not aware of or has not investigated such change, the care that she delivers may be inappropriate within the context of holistic individualised care.

SOCIOLOGICAL THEORY

STRUCTURALIST AND INTERPRETATIVE APPROACHES TO SOCIOLOGY

It is claimed that reality is socially constructed (Berger & Luckman 1966). How and what sense is made of that construction depends very much on the way in which society is perceived.

In activity 3.3, the reader is presented with two sets of apparently opposite statements. These illustrate two comparative and contrasting

Case example 3.1 Social change

It was the first time that Helen, a third-year student nurse, had been given management responsibility for a group of patients in one of the bays in the ward, under the supervision of an experienced qualified nurse who was her mentor during that clinical placement. The reason for assigning the responsibility to Helen was to give her an opportunity to experience the complexities involved in the provision of holistic and individualised care for a group of patients.

One of Helen's patients was Trevor, a 36-year-old married man who had three young children. He was a happy contented man, despite the fact that he had been made redundant from his job nearly 2 years ago and had not been in paid employment since. His wife was a very attractive woman who had returned to full-time employment a year ago in a large nationwide company where she had worked before and where she now was a well-respected management consultant.

Trevor had been admitted to hospital following an accident in which he had sustained burns to the right side of his body, particularly his arm and leg, and left hand. The latter were comparatively minor, but the former required extensive skin grafts. However, he had fully recovered from his operation and was due to be discharged home in the next couple of days, although he would need care as an outpatient for a considerable time.

Helen had been organising appointments for Trevor that morning. She had remembered to make appointments for him to attend his local health centre for twice weekly dressings, to see the dietician who would explain and advise him on the special dietary needs that had resulted directly from the extensive tissue damage caused by the burns, and to attend the consultant's outpatient clinic in 4 weeks' time.

Although Helen was finding the management responsibilities quite challenging, she had certainly not found it difficult to sort out times for Trevor's appointments as he was not working and could, therefore, attend at any time. Quite pleased with her achievements, Helen proudly went to a review meeting with Joan, her mentor, and felt that she would surely get a 'well-done pat' on her back rather than the usual 'Did you consider . . .?'. This time she had thought of everything. She had not needed prompting but had used her initiative instead and organised all the necessary follow-up care. Or so she thought!

Flustered and red-faced Helan emerged from the seminar room where she had met her mentor. How could she have been so stupid? Now she would have to sort out all those appointments again, as well as organising home-help services. It had never occurred to her that the nature of the roles of the individuals within Trevor's family had reversed. He was a 'house-husband'; he was quite content to look after the children and do all the housework whilst his wife, Vicky, went out to work. They had long since mutually agreed that, because of the better career prospects and job opportunities, Vicky would return to full-time employment, whereas he would take on the responsibility of running the home. It made no difference to him what 'certificated' sickness he had. He still had the children to look after, to take them to and fetch them from school and so on, and would not, therefore, be able to attend at just any time.

Helen had come to realise that change in society is a major component in any change in nursing. For health care workers to be able to provide holistic and individualised care, they must be fully conversant with the elements of current and foreseeable social change.

Activity 3.3

Answer the following questions:

- Does society make man, or man make society?
- Is sociology about man in society, or society in man?

Why do you think you replied in the way in which you did?

approaches to the study of man and society: the structuralist and interpretative approaches.

In the structuralist approach, man is seen to exist and be largely controlled by the economic infrastructure of society. The rules, roles, customs and laws that relate to the structures, systems and institutional frameworks constrain, enable and regulate the existence of man. Although man has a choice of action, a relatively passive role is adopted with the individual being a receiver of and responder to society.

The interpretative approach, in turn, would consider man as an agent who actively changes and manipulates society in face-to-face interactions within all forms of social organisations. Its emphasis lies in the belief that man is the creator of society and the social world.

Although the two approaches appear, on initial evaluation, to be poles apart, they are in reality closely connected and complementary, as they both represent ways of observing the social world, albeit through the use of different conceptual frameworks. These allow for the use of a variety of investigatory approaches and for the adoption of different methods of data collection and data analysis, which, in turn, provides for richer explanations about the social world in which we live. Neither one of the approaches is necessarily more correct than the other.

Bennett (1992) proposes that it is particularly relevant to nursing to have some awareness of the two approaches. This is because, if prospective nurses are familiar with the approaches, they will be helped to understand their future roles within the complexity of the health care system and to appreciate the social and cultural origins of their patients more fully.

The structuralist approach is macrosociological, as its focal point is society as a set of interrelated, interdependent parts or systems. These include the political, economic, educational and medical systems. Within the latter, the actors (nurses and patients) are depersonalised into passive role-receivers, and the structuralist organisation structures, control and adapt social relationships and actions, either in a coercive and divisive or a harmonious and cooperative fashion. The interpretative approach tends to be microsociological, the sociological self being seen to be active in a symbolic world where meanings are constructed and shared rather than externally imposed. The individual negotiates and constructs future roles with others in society. He interprets the culture in which he lives in a unique and distinctive manner, and is active in the construction of meaningful relationships during the process of giving and receiving care.

The interactionist approach is considered to be more relevant and immediate to the work of health care professionals as it concentrates on the microsociological processes, such as the dynamics and relationships within families, whereas the structuralist approach would be to look at family in the context of family patterns that result from, for example, unemployment. As the effectiveness of nursing depends very much upon the formulation and management of interpersonal relationships, knowledge of how the patient feels about being a patient appears more appropriate

than is knowing what percentage of, for example, single parents suffer physical ill-health.

Sociological theories are not always as clear cut as it appears from the above. They are complex and therefore beyond the scope of this chapter, but they all have a common purpose, i.e. investigation that will contribute to a better understanding of social phenomena. Knowledge of sociological theories will provide insight into the theories relating to health care. Indeed, Cox (1979) claims there is a symbiotic relationship between nursing and sociology. The provision of holistic care can be more effectively realised if health care practitioners are able to base their practice on empirical data relating, for example, to changing patterns of disease, dependency and death, and to people's perception of and responses to illness. Both major approaches have their importance, and the skill is in knowing which to use and when.

HEALTH AS A SOCIAL CONSTRUCT

The images of health through the ages have been varied and generally linked to the practice of medicine, and scientific and/or technological developments and beliefs systems. The concept can be presented on a continuum, at the extreme ends of which are biomedical concepts and health as a socially constructed state (Figure 3.1). However, one has not evolved from the other, as can be seen from the history of Ancient Greece, where both concepts are described. They developed in tandem and still exist as such today.

The biomedical concept emerged as a mechanistic perspective. It was based on the belief that to be healthy was to be free from recognisable disease. As the central tenet, the role of the physician was seen as treating disease:

to restore health by correcting any imperfections caused by the accidents of birth and life. (Dubos 1960)

It is this concept that informed the ideology of traditional medical education. The study of the structure and process of disease became a predominant feature in the education of physicians.

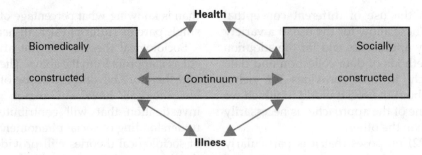

Figure 3.1   Conceptions of health.

This trend still persists today, but social sciences are gaining a stronger hold. However, it appears that the development of medical services, based on the biomedical concepts of surgery, immunological responses to transplants, chemotherapy and the molecular basis of inheritance, are given priority, not only in the provision of sciences, but also in medical education and medical careers (Townsend & Davidson 1982). Indeed, biomedical research predominates in medical research and medical education.

Similarly, nursing and nurse education had a biomedical emphasis until the 1970s. Then, with the emergence of a professional reform movement, 'the new nursing', the focus of nursing moved away from a medical, disease-orientated approach to become more person-centred and individualised. Where the caring role of the nurse had previously centred around the biological functions of the patient, it now began to extend to the psychosocial aspects of the individual and the recognition of the patient as an active participant in, rather than a passive recipient of, care (Corbett 1995). Thus, with the changing emphasis of care, the study of the sociological self has become a predominant feature in the education not only of nurses, but also of other health care professionals, including doctors.

In turn, health as a socially constructed state also had its origins in Ancient Greece. The teachings of the goddess Hygeia advocated that rational social organisation and rational behaviour by an individual were the most important commodities in the promotion and maintenance of health. The World Health Organization (WHO) gave credence to this approach at its foundation at the end of the World War II. WHO, the current authoritative agency on health, included the social perspective as a component of its definition of health. This brought about increased awareness of the need to include social and socioeconomic factors not only within education related to health, but also within the design and provision of health services.

In societies where health and illness present as social categories, health is seen in the context of distribution of illness, epidemiological patterns and class structures of that society. The existence of bacteria, viruses and 'injury' to mind and body are acknowledged. However, the real meanings that are given to them, whilst making sense of them, are social.

Helman (1992) describes how, for example, the presentation of illness and the way in which an individual responds to it are determined by, to a large extent, sociocultural factors. These factors influence which symptoms and signs are perceived as abnormal in a given culture, and shape the physical and emotional changes that occur into a pattern with which the individual sufferer, and people around him, identify. The gap between subjective feelings of altered health status and their social acknowledgement is connected by what Helman calls 'its own language of distress', which also describes 'folk illness'. These

can be 'learnt' in the sense that a child growing in a particular culture learns how to respond to, and express, a range of physical or emotional symptoms, or social stresses, in a culturally patterned way (Helman 1992)

and which are shaped further by cultural and social forces, such as television, newspapers and magazines, and the dominant ideology of the society. It is through this language that the consensus of what constitutes not only illness but also wellness among the members of the culture is expressed. An awareness of this by health care professionals is of paramount importance to enable them to provide culturally sensitive care, as can be illustrated by Case example 3.2.

The concept of health as a social construct is also affirmed by Gomm (1982), who proposes that:

The constitution of health and illness is a socially negotiated process which partakes of prevailing ideologies and world views, and which can be explained sociologically. (Gomm 1982)

As illustrated, there can be varied perceptions of the concept of health between different societies and even in the sub-cultures of a single society. The knowledge, experience and expertise of professionals involved in health care will, in the future, greatly influence the extent or limit to which health and illness are recognised as socially constructed states.

Case example 3.2 The question of healthy eating

In response to the Health of the Nation strategy (Department of Health 1992), a fundholding GP practice in a city in northern England provides opportunities at the health centre for mothers to learn about diet and nutrition. A special meeting is organised once a month at the end of one of the bi-weekly baby clinics. Mothers are invited to bring with them any members of their family who might be interested. The health visitors who usually run the clinics choose a topic that they consider to be particularly pertinent or that has been requested by mothers. Sometimes they deliver the talk themselves; sometimes they invite an expert on the topic. Whatever the case, the health visitors take it in turn to prepare an information sheet on the subject of the talk and make it available for the mothers who were unable to attend.

In a recent practice management meeting, it had been noted that quite a number of, particularly West Indian, babies and children appeared to be overweight. Because of this, and in order to emphasise the importance of healthy eating, it was decided to invite a dietitian from the local hospital to talk about the prevention of obesity.

The event was extremely well attended, perhaps because a few mothers were concerned about their children being teased and bullied at school and being called names such as 'Michelin tyre man'. The talk, and especially the discussion that followed, proved to be very enlightening. The dietitian, Angela, was very charismatic and appeared to have a great deal of insight to the variations that existed in the beliefs and practices about food in different cultural groups. The audience immediately warmed to her, as she did not just tell them not to eat this or that, but seemed to be able to understand the issues that were of concern to individuals, particularly those belonging to ethnic minorities.

Angela explained how food was much more than a source of nutrition: it was a social 'convention'. She found that although all human societies process their food supply in some way, a great many cultural variations exist in terms of what substances are regarded as food and, indeed, how food may be grown, gathered, presented and consumed. Substances that may be acceptable as food in one society or culture may be rigidly forbidden in another. She gave an example of the unacceptability of dogs, cats and mice being used as food in the UK, despite the fact that they may well be edible, and how religious groups have strict taboos about not only the ingestion, but also the handling of certain foods.

In a similar vein, Angela demonstrated through the use of slides how there are variations in what is considered to be healthy and beautiful in different cultures, as had been found by anthropologists studying the physique and body images within different societies. She gave examples of: how wealthy men in some West African cultures send their daughters to 'fattening houses' where they are fed with fatty foods and denied exercise to make them plump and pale, to indicate both wealth and fertility; and of how some West Indian mothers, because malnutrition has been so common in the communities from which they have come, appear to desire to see their offspring as big fat babies, because they believe that a plump, cherub-like baby immediately gives the impression of an affluent family. Angela also explained how scientists had found a great deal of evidence to suggest there to be an extremely strong desire to maintain cultural continuity through the adherence to traditional beliefs and practices relating to food, particularly among immigrant ethnic minority groups. She hastened to add, however, that such things as unemployment, low income, social isolation, long working hours, lack of leisure time and cultural change itself, issues often beyond the control of individuals, also influence health and nutrition.

It was only after this that Angela told her extremely captive audience about the importance of healthy eating and what makes up a healthy diet. The talk had been a great success and, as transpired later, produced a number of positive outcomes, including a reduction in the number of potential 'Michelin tyre men'.

THE EFFECTS OF CULTURE ON HEALTH BELIEFS

Clearly, perceptions of health and illness vary in different cultural and social groups. Health behaviour, like all other behaviour, is determined by the values and beliefs that the members of a society hold. Indeed, Townsend & Davidson (1982) propose that:

the pursuit of health has increasingly been acknowledged to be a social and not merely a technical enterprise.

However, despite health promotion and the wide availability of preventative health programmes (e.g. well-woman clinics), health behaviour varies greatly, even in a single society whose members are endowed with the same cultural heritage. To make sense of this, Abraham & Shanley (1992) propose the use of a health belief model, which lists the four key components of a person's belief about his health (Box 3.1).

Box 3.1 Key components of a health belief model (Adapted from Abraham & Shanley 1992)

The key components are a person's beliefs about:

- how susceptible we are to the illness in question
- the seriousness or severity of the illness
- the potential costs
- the effectiveness of this action in relation to possible alternatives.

If an individual's belief in each of the components were identified, they would act as key informers of whether or not he would, on the appearance of a symptom or a prompt such as media coverage, take some action in relation to his health.

The significance of the above model to the reader is that it would provide a useful tool for assessing and making sense of the patient's health beliefs. Having done this, the nurse could then identify, together with the patient, a plan of action to promote health behaviour, not only in the individual patient, but also in the individual's society. The latter would, in a small way, address some of the inequalities in health identified by Townsend & Davidson (1982).

The section below illustrates how, for example, religious beliefs might influence the health behaviour of an individual.

Illustration: the religious context of patient care

Religious laws touch upon many aspects of daily life and may well influence the way in which an individual perceives health and illness. Religious beliefs frequently affect, for example, such things as family planning, infertility, diet and nutrition. The significance of this to health care professionals is that these beliefs may well influence the provision and delivery of health care. An adherence to religious convictions may be valued much more highly than is the advice of health care practitioners. Conflict may result, particularly when treatment and care is refused on behalf of dependant children. It is important, therefore, that the extent and strength of the individual's beliefs are ascertained to ensure that the patient's spiritual needs are appropriately met.

Family planning and infertility

- Catholic theologians do not approve of the use of 'artificial' contraception, although it is permissible to use the 'rhythm' method.
- Obtaining semen by masturbation for analysis or for artificial insemination is considered 'unnatural' by the Catholic Church and 'wasting of the seed' by orthodox Jews.
- Artificial insemination by the husband (homologous insemination) is allowed only if the semen is already deposited in the vagina, and artificial insemination by donor (heterologous insemination) is forbidden and is considered to be adultery by the Catholic Church.

Diet and nutrition

- In Judaism, all pig products are forbidden, as are fish without fins or scales, and birds of prey. Animals that chew the cud, have cloven hooves and are kosher (ritually slaughtered) may be eaten. Meat and milk products may not be consumed within the same meal.

- In Hinduism, the killing or eating of any animal, particularly the cow, is forbidden. Fish and eggs are only infrequently consumed, but milk and milk products can be eaten because they can be obtained without taking an animal's life.

Medical intervention

- The creed of Christian Scientists proclaims the non-reality of pain and sickness and diseases caused by germs, micro-organisms and viruses. Healing is claimed to be through faith, i.e. spiritual healing, and not through medical intervention.
- Jehovah's witnesses believe that all government institutions are under the control of Satan. They undertake no military service and will not allow medical treatment using any blood derivatives.

Rituals associated with dying

- Among orthodox Jews, there is a precise procedure for mourning. For 7 days following the funeral, the bereaved must remain at home and be visited only by consolers. Recreation and fun are forbidden for a whole year.
- Muslim men are expected to sit with a dying relative to pray and touch the patient. A woman may sit with her dying husband but may not touch him in any way.

EFFECTS OF CULTURE ON HEALTH CARE SYSTEMS

As the continuing development of transport systems and the formation of economic communities bring different cultures close to each other, the goals of health care should be made culturally more sensitive. Health care professionals need to be fully aware of the health beliefs, traditions and practices of different cultural and ethnic groups in the particular society in which they practise.

Lynman (1992) proposes that seeking knowledge of the patient's perspective on health

Activity 3.4

Place yourself in the position of a Polish student, a qualified nurse in his own country, who has come for an orientation programme in your college before being allowed to register as a qualified nurse in this country.

Describe what would you need to do, as his mentor, to ensure that he is competent to deliver culturally sensitive care in this country.

is imperative to be able to provide culturally sensitive care. This is because the patient normally uses his lay 'carers', i.e. family, friends, spouse or partner, for initial advice. Important decisions can thus be made outside the formal health care system in order to solve any problems. These may have great relevance for subsequent health care.

There are cultural variations in terms of the relevance and value of 'scientific' health care. Alternative medicine or therapy has recently gained a much stronger foothold, which is affecting the health beliefs of the society. Methods of healing that were applied centuries ago are becoming prevalent but are not, as yet, contained in the UK's public health care system. This raises concerns about people's health status. Are those with belief in naturopathic health care absenting themselves from 'conventional' care and not accessing alternative care because of the cost?

Health promotion and health education activities need to be conducted with a full awareness of the changing nature of the health culture. Lynman (1992) highlights the imperative to attend to the total context of the client's situation and proposes that:

there is a need for culture-specific information as well as information on a broader conceptual level. (Lynman 1992)

THE SOCIOLOGICAL SELF

The biophysical component of man is frequently, in lay terms, compared to models such as a combustion engine or a battery-driven machine. This comparison may be illustrated by sayings such as 'I need to let off steam' or 'I took laxatives because I needed a good clear out'. Health care professionals enforce the use of these mechanical metaphors further by employing phrases such as 'Your heart isn't pumping as well as it should' or 'You need to recharge your batteries'.

Models are also used in psychology and sociology, although they are theoretical rather than actual representations of man. An analogy is made of observed human behaviour in a psychological or social context and is subsequently used to explain behaviour and/or predict possible future actions. Two such models have been proposed by Abraham & Shanley (1992): a computational model and a dramaturgical model.

The computational model

Information about the events of the world and how one should react to these are stored in an individual. The self – the computer – is programmed. It has a capacity to process information to select the most appropriate response to a given situation within that programme. However, distinct differences exist between the computer and the self. Unlike the computer, in which all permutations are set, human beings are able to add to their programmes. Interactions with different groups in society will modify individuals' behaviour; their beliefs will change and their behaviour will become similar to that of the members of the group. The social self will thus become reprogrammed. The computer, of course, is not able to learn from interactions and cannot voluntarily change the way it is programmed; it functions as an automaton.

There are occasions when a nurse may appear to act like a computer, for example in the event of a cardiac arrest. It may look as if she has been 'programmed' to perform in a certain way because she seems to go onto 'automatic pilot'. She ascertains that cardiac arrest has taken place and instigates resuscitation procedures that she has learnt, and carries on with these until such time as the resuscitation team arrives on the scene and takes over.

Activity 3.5

Reflect on the encounters that you have had with patients whilst you have been on clinical placements.

- Have there been times when your patients appeared to have behaved like computers?
- Why do you think your patients behaved in the way that they did?

Compare your responses with the members of your peer group.

The dramaturgical model

This model cites self within the context of social drama. The individual acts in accordance with an evolving social script:

the way we talk with friends, eye strangers, walk along a crowded street, and much else that we regard as ordinary, taken for granted, indeed natural, are essentially social constructs ... prefabricated by the society, the community, the social class, the occupation or organisation of which we are established or temporary members. (Burns 1992)

Activity 3.6

Imagine yourself to be taking part in a public performance (a play or pantomime). How should you portray yourself in order for the audience to enjoy your performance?

What should you know and how should you perform in order to convey the messages that the creator of the play or performance has intended?

An individual, in order to 'put on' a convincing performance, must be able to convey to 'the audience' the message contained in the script in such a manner as 'the author' intended and the 'audience' understands. The effectiveness of the performance will not only depend on the performer's skill to act, but also on his knowledge of what other roles are being played by the other members of the cast and how tell they are performing. All these aspects will influence the total effect. A positive response from the audience and its ability to identify with the 'plot' will also enhance the quality of the performance.

The direct relevance of this to health care professionals is that the better they understand the requirements and context of the professional roles, the roles played by the members of the multidisciplinary team, the patient's disposition in the context of his or her own biological self, and the purpose of the care, the higher will be the quality of the professional performance. The part of the carer will be 'played' convincingly and with feeling, in the knowledge of what the whole 'performance' is about.

Although the two models of the social self have been explored separately, it is important to acknowledge their complementary nature. This is because:

we must have ready-made guidelines or scripts stored away ... must attend to other's behaviour and ensure that what [they do] will fit into others' representation of the shared situation. (Abraham & Shanley 1992)

An exploration of the theory underpinning social roles within a framework will provide the reader with guidelines for the shared situations to which Abraham & Shanley refer.

SOCIALISATION

Socialisation is a process that preserves the cultural heritage of society and provides a bridge between generations throughout an individual's life cycle. It is most intense in infancy (primary socialisation), the most formative years of an individual's life. Each child is unique, an individual who acquires different values, attitudes and beliefs and develops a personality of his own.

Societies differ widely in their socialisation practices. However, provided that the process proceeds reasonably well, the individual will eventually be able to fulfil his social role functions, making adjustments as he moves along in a changing society.

During primary socialisation, the most important agents of socialisation are contained within the immediate family unit, i.e. the carers of the child with whom the child can form a lasting bond. The importance of maintaining the bond cannot be over-emphasised. For example, when a child is hospitalised, his parent(s) or carers are, whenever possible, encouraged to stay and participate in his care.

The child learns the behaviour characteristics of his parents or carers and also, to a lesser or greater extent, of those in his immediate community. The influence of people other than the family is more important today than previously because of the altered working patterns of women. The peer group, for example, at a day-care centre, begins to assert its influence during what is called the secondary socialisation phase. Other agents of secondary socialisation include schools. Here, alongside the formal curriculum, a hidden curriculum exists whereby the children learn to accept and respond to the teaching staff and their authority. Schools can be extremely influential agents of socialisation for those children who:

escape from the restricting aspects of the social backgrounds from which they come (Giddens 1993)

referring to the under privileged.

The influence of the mass media, particularly the television, as an agent of socialisation is enormous. A great deal of delinquent and deviant behaviour is thought to be caused by uncontrolled exposure to television, especially in terms of violence. However, Giddens (1993) proposes that the mass media has many beneficial effects, as it conveys information to which people would not otherwise have access.

Both primary and secondary socialisation are influenced by a variety of social factors, including social class, agents of socialisation, economic relationships to the community, critical points in the life of an individual, residence patterns and household structures.

Activity 3.7

From your observations of and caring for children, draw conclusions as to how children are socialised into patterns of illness behaviour.

What influences, if any, do:

* ethnic background
* the health of parents
* social class

have on the process?

It is becoming increasingly difficult to determine when primary socialisation ends and secondary socialisation begins because of the changes in family structures, particularly in the employment patterns of parents. Gomm (1982), however, proposes that primary socialisation is about learning the basics, and secondary socialisation is about applying the basics to specific roles, without there being any age divide.

Anticipatory socialisation

Although the major focus of socialisation has been centred on child development, other 'milestones' in an individual's life can be identified as specific socialisation periods. One such period is the anticipated entry into a professional life, which sometimes calls for a shift in the individual's beliefs and values, for example to fulfil entry criteria.

Activity 3.8

How did you prepare yourself for entry into the nursing profession?

How, if at all, did your values and beliefs about society change?

Sometimes, anticipatory socialisation can be problematic and create role strain. This happens if an individual has formed an 'erroneous' impression about, for example, an occupation, and reality does not represent his expectations. No scientific evidence for this exists, as yet, but it is suggested that beliefs, attitudes, values and motives of adults are evolving continuously, although gradually, throughout their working life (Gahagan 1980).

Professional socialisation

Professional socialisation is a continued form of anticipatory or preparatory socialisation. It is about learning shared meanings of the professional culture. Students acquire the intricacies of the role of the nurse and knowledge of the rights, responsibilities, obligations and values of the profession.

Abraham & Shanley (1992) identify that there may be feelings of bewilderment during initial encounters, for example with a hospital, until such time as language becomes shared between professionals:

New ways of talking gradually become new ways of thinking. (Abraham & Shanley 1992)

Socialisation is gradual, but students may find difficulties in adapting to and understanding what is expected of them, and role strain may, potentially, develop.

The reader may well have experienced role strain, adjusting to the different requirements of the role set until such time as he or she has become fully socialised as a member of the professional culture and conformed to its expectations.

However, it is appropriate here to recognise that the structuralist approach to professional socialisation differs from that of the interpretative approach. The former views it as the making of the professional and the acquiring of the professional culture through:

the process of socialisation which reconciles the opposition between the functioning of the social system and the actions of individual members of society. The core values are internalised through this process so that there is a correspondence between the norms and values of the system and the subjective meanings of the actors within. (Bond & Bond 1994)

In accordance with the interpretative view, an individual does not become a professional during the process of preparatory education programme but whilst actually occupying the role and status of a qualified professional and negotiating with individuals and situations that she meets. It is only then that the organisation of the environment begins to influence professional behaviour.

SOCIAL ROLES, MULTIPLE ROLES AND ROLE SETS

The concept of social role refers to a role that is enacted within a group and incorporates appropriate behaviours – role-appropriate behaviour. This behaviour includes the accepted rules and expectations assigned to that role, which denote the functions that an individual undertakes whilst within a particular role. There are kinship roles (mother/son), gender roles (male/female), age roles (child/adult) and occupational roles (doctor/nurse), and they are derived directly from social structures. Although the roles are occupied by individuals, they do not exist in isolation but are complementary. They are intertwined within social systems; for example, parents and child(ren) are in a family, students and teachers are in an education system, and nurses and patients are in a health care system.

As can be seen from Activity 3.9, an individual may have several concurrent roles in his social life, in which he will be expected to behave in a certain way. If an individual has learnt, generally through the process of socialisation, the role-appropriate behaviour, the uncertainty and trauma of social life are minimised because:

Role . . . informs the role bearer of the appropriate dress, duties, talk, obligations, privileges and rights. (Smith 1981)

For example, it is unlikely that a ward manager would go on duty dressed in a jogging suit, address the staff in a manner similar to a sergeant major in the army addressing new recruits during drill practice, be disrespectful towards doctors or patients, or accept personal gratuities from patients or their relatives.

Gahagan (1980) supports this by claiming that there are certain expectations affiliated to social roles in relation to the degree of general

Activity 3.9

Read the account below.

Gary was delighted! After weeks of trying, he had finally managed to get tickets to a rare concert of his favourite pop group. His wife and children found the determination with which he had set about ringing ticket agents and even approaching the 'black market' amusing.

However, Gary's friend and long-standing golf partner, with whom he played in a weekly match, was annoyed. 'Your fanaticism will do you no good if you want to renew your position as a club secretary for next season. Besides, your doctor won't be pleased either. He told you to stop rushing about because of your blood pressure.'

Gary had been sure that he would succeed in the end; he had even cancelled the day out in his business diary so that his secretary could not book any appointments that would prevent him from attending the concert. Gary's mother had been equally convinced of her son's eventual success: 'I knew he would do it; he'll turn heaven and earth to get something that he wants. I am just surprised that he hasn't convinced his next door neighbour to go with him! He'll have to leave home early, though, to travel from Brighton to Glasgow and back in one day.'

Make a list of the different roles that you can identify Gary to have.

How does your list compare with Figure 3.2?

consensus of expectation, the penetration of the role into all the behaviour of an individual, the legal sanctions associated with the roles and, in

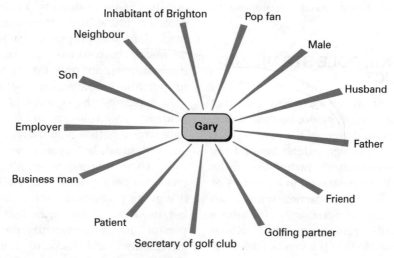

Figure 3.2   An individual's different roles.

the case of professional roles, the code of conduct.

A general consensus is that, for example, the role of the student is to learn. In an education system where the central tenet is adult education, the student may well, on occasions, teach. This might, to a person with a traditional view of education, present some difficulty and result in only marginal consensus about the nature of a teacher–student relationship.

Some roles 'infiltrate' the total behaviour of an individual. A religious leader, for example, is 'required' to be an ardent believer, benevolent and moral in both public and private life. In contrast, no such demands are made of a plumber. As long as he carries out the job safely and to an agreed specification, he can do so dressed in shorts, singing the latest pop song. The role of a plumber makes no demands on the person outside the job.

Role expectations may also be supported by legal sanctions. A parent may be punished by imprisonment for failing to fulfil the physical care needs of his child. If, however, he fails to provide any recreational facilities for the child, no legal punishment will be endorsed. Similarly, a code of conduct, which is one of the hallmarks of a profession, will provide guidelines of behaviour within a professional role. Any deviation from the guidelines, as in the case of nurses, may result in the removal of the 'offending' individual's name from the professional Register, which demands that she ceases to practise in that role.

STEREOTYPING, ROLE STRAIN AND ROLE CONFLICT

The reader may or may not have had a distinct view of the role of a nurse, before becoming one, based on a stereotypical view of the professional. Stereotyping may, however, extend beyond the role itself. The personality characteristics of the role occupants may be portrayed in a positive or negative sense. The latter carries with it an inherent problem, not necessarily for those entering a particular profession, but for those outside it. To illustrate this, the view of a female

Activity 3.10

1. Describe how you saw the role of the nurse before you started your education programme.
2. How do you see the role of the nurse now?
3. If there are differences between (1) and (2), why do you think this is?

nurse as a sex-symbol – as frequently depicted in caricatures and comic films – or of a male as sexually deviant because he has entered a predominantly female occupation, may influence the degree of support that potential recruits to nursing get from their families and friends. Equally, an individual who entered nursing with a romantic notion of a nurse's role consisting solely of 'soothing the fevered brow' may have a problem. The reality, in this instance, does not represent the role expectations and role strain results.

A role function and the role occupant may also present as a mismatch. Generally, an individual is selected for a role because he appears to have the aptitudes and personality to enact the role. If, however, it transpires that the individual and his role partners (fellow workers) do not perceive the role function in the same way, or the individual simply does not have the ability to carry out the function, role strain will result. For example, a student nurse who has chosen a particular branch of nursing may find out during the 'sampling' of the branch in the common foundation programme that she has made an inappropriate choice. Unless the mismatch is rectified, the outcomes will be unfavourable, not only for the student, but also for potential employers and patients.

In exploring the concept of role strain, it is evident that role strain relates to internal antagonism between an individual and one role. An individual, however, generally has multiple roles. There are times when it may be difficult to enact competing roles comfortably. For example, it may be problematic for a patient to combine her usual work role with that of a patient. A person in a powerful position in local government and used to being totally 'self-directing' may find it hard to accept and enact a dependent role. The role conflict that results may be so strong that it may even make the individual discharge herself from hospital against medical advice.

Some role functions may have totally conflicting demands. For example, it is difficult to appreciate the dilemma that a chaplain in the army may have: on one hand, he is employed to preach peace for all; on the other, he is expected to fight a war.

Activity 3.11

Reflect on the concepts of 'role strain' and 'role conflict'.
   Refer back to Activity 3.9. Identify instances when Gary might experience role strain. Explain your reasons in each case.
   Identify any possible conflicting roles and explore these with the members of your peer group.

As can be determined from above, the roles that individuals may have, in both their private and public lives, have a powerful influence on social life. However, a role is frequently more stable than is the role occupant (Groenman et al 1992). It provides guidelines for appropriate behaviour in different circumstances. Individuals tend to have a strong sense of conformity. Sometimes they even conform against their better judgement. For example, it is much easier for students to approach their duties during clinical placement in a task-orientated way – if that is common practice in the area – rather than attempt patient-centred holistic care, which they know to be more beneficial to the patient. It can be very stressful for a new role occupant to differ greatly from customary behaviour, because social pressures exerted by those who control entry into a particular role are very strong. This is particularly relevant in the case of the sick role (Case example 3.3).

THE SICK ROLE

Given that the effectiveness of a social system depends on the effectiveness of the role functions it contains, a text for students engaged in health-

Case example 3.3   Role conflict.
(Reproduced from Bennett 1992)

George, a 72-year-old man recovering from a stroke, had just spent an hour making three of his own cigarettes with one hand. The nursing staff were thrilled to see his achievement, whilst gently and appropriately admonishing him for smoking. George wheeled himself to the day room and was about to light his cigarette when a physiotherapist arrived to take him for his treatment. George refused to move and a row ensued. He was taken for treatment and was later returned in an angry and unrepentant mood by an equally angry physiotherapist. The nurse and the physiotherapist presented a united professional approach to the patient but argued in the ward office about the relative merits of forcing a patient to undergo treatment.

related studies must explore the concepts of 'wellness' and 'sickness'. Being well implies that an individual is able to function appropriately – in the context of his biopsychosocial self – in the roles that he occupies. There are times, however, when an individual may need to withdraw from the obligations and activities that these roles imply. He may be either temporarily or permanently unable to enact his 'normal' roles and assumes, as Parsons (1951) proposes, a sick role in a health system.

Activity 3.12

Given that social roles provide us with guidelines on how to behave in society, how should an individual enact a sick role?

Society does not, however, allow the adoption of a sick role without regulation. It is the physician who:

is involved with the authority to admit and discharge individuals in their passage through the sick role. (Mann 1983)

In doing so, the physician keeps a social and emotional distance and deals with each sick role occupant on equal terms. In return, the sick individual is exempt from his normal role obligations and is not held responsible for his own condition. This is, however, conditional. The individual is expected not to use sickness for gainful purposes, either in terms of using the system fraudulently or of prolonging the period of sickness. He is also expected to seek and act on the advice of qualified professionals. The above forms the basis of what could be termed a contract between the physician or nurse and the patient in the sick role. There may, however, be varying levels of lack of role compliance on behalf of the patient, particularly if the advice given by the professional does not coincide with the patient's wishes and expectations.

Activity 3.13

Many conditions, such as sexually transmitted and smoking-related diseases, are morally 'loaded'.
  How do you think this moral perspective may affect:

* the sick role
* the interaction between the doctor and the potential sick role occupant
* the relationship between the nurse and the potential sick role occupant.

Attempt to substantiate your conclusions with evidence from the media (television, radio and newspapers).

Parsons (1951), acknowledging that becoming ill is a natural event, categorises sick role behaviour as deviant. This deviance, however, does not necessarily contain negative aspects. The enactment of the sick role, providing it adheres to the contract previously mentioned, will improve the functioning of social systems. This is because the health system is designed, ideally, for the purposes of optimising the health status of the nation as a whole. The latter, however, begs the question that the reader may wish to explore: how forceful is medicine as an agent of social control?

Whatever the response to the question in Activity 3.14 may be, each member of society has a unique view relating to the concepts of health and sickness. This view will be an integral

Activity 3.14

Explore the following with the members of your peer group:

* How forceful is medicine as an agent of social control?

part of the cultural beliefs and values of the individual in the context of the society in which he lives.

George's experience in the sick role (see Case example 3.3) was unhappy. He had obviously achieved a great deal by rolling a cigarette, despite the fact that he could use only one hand. However, the structural constraints imposed on him almost negated not only his positive experience, but also the experience of the individuals enacting the professional roles. The adoption of a more interpretative approach, whereby George, the nurse and the physiotherapist would take a negotiating approach to designing the treatment schedule for George, would have made it a much happier and a more satisfactory situation for everybody within the context of their respective roles.

CULTURE

It is likely that the reader will have come up with two distinctive definitions of the word culture.

Activity 3.15

How would you define the word 'culture'?

Most people use the word in the context of art, literature or music. The actions that would be undertaken in the context of, for example, art culture used to be considered rather sophisticated and available only for the 'élite' – largely middle-class intellectuals. Media coverage, however, has changed all that, and all members of the society now have access to this kind of 'culture'.

Sociologists, whilst recognising the above, have extended the use of the term culture to embrace:

the values the members of a given group hold, the norms they follow and the material goods that they create. (Giddens 1993)

Indeed, Martin and Belcher (1986) consider culture to be a philosophy of life and death in society. It contains the human heritage of a society in the form of rules, values and beliefs of that society. These are passed to the next generation during the process of socialisation. Individuals learn to 'act' in accordance with role-appropriate behaviour in human practices such as child-rearing, marriage, dress, work and religion. They learn values in terms of what is right and wrong in their culture and beliefs about the world and the nature of society.

Cultural heritage is not about the physical environment, but about the way in which the environment is used, or indeed abused, as highlighted by, for example, Greenpeace issues such as anti-pollution and the slaughtering of whales. Nor is cultural heritage about such things as genetically determined characteristics, such as skin colour. However, it *is* about the way in which the members of a group sharing the same skin colour behave.

Culture is pervasive at all levels of human functioning in society. Because of its profound effects, there is a tendency to assume that the culture that an individual 'owns' is the best one. This is not so. For example, monogamy is the natural form of marriage in Western industrial societies, and polygamy is, in the main, frowned upon and against the law. In some societies, for example in a number of tribal societies of Africa, the only accepted form of marriage is polygamy. The polygamous society would struggle to exist within a monogamous structure. Gender-related issues, such as the role of women in politics, education, religion and employment, are, to a large degree, culturally 'informed'. Ongoing, and sometimes very fierce, debates under the banner of actual and proposed legislation relating to equal opportunities are taking place worldwide. Such issues as paternity leave have a direct relevance to marriage and family patterns in society, and will in the future become part of the cultural heritage.

There is universal recognition of the fact that food and water must be ingested to meet biological needs. However, there are great cultural diversities in terms of 'what' and 'how'. Food that is acceptable, and even a delicacy, in one culture may be considered totally inedible in another. For example, feelings of hunger generally produce images of food. These images, frequently 'informed' by religious beliefs and practices, have variations from, for example, thick beef steaks cooked to a crisp, to raw fish.

Variations exist not only between different cultures, but also within the sub-cultures of a dominant culture. In modern Britain, many sub-cultures – Italian, Pakistani and Chinese for example – live side by side. This cultural diversity, predominant in industrialised societies, presents its own challenges. Children within the sub-cultures are exposed to the influence of norms, beliefs and values beyond their 'own' culture, and may face difficulties in, for example, settling in at school or accepting the practices relating to courtship and marriage. Their 'own' cultures make demands on them in terms of their dress and their gender roles that may result in what their parents would identify as culturally deviant behaviour.

Activity 3.16

Identify the different sub-cultures that exist in the community in which you live.

Taking each sub-culture in turn, identify the 'idiosyncracies' that you believe them to have in terms of:

- family structure
- gender-related behaviour
- child-rearing practices
- nutrition.

Compare your findings with the members of your peer group.

The text so far has concentrated on cultural diversity, but there are a number of cultural universals that are to be found in all human societies. All people have a language by which they communicate; it is the specific language that differs. Each culture has some form of family and marriage system, religious rituals and medicine, which are based either on scientific methods or on the supernatural. There is universal recognition of the importance of hospitality, be it expressed by offering food and drink to guests or – as in some Eskimo groups – by lending the wife for the night to keep a visitor warm. Whatever the diversities or universals, the individual's total view of the world is, all in all, culturally determined:

whether the earth is considered to be round or flat, at the centre of the universe or not, whether the cosmos is believed to be inhabited by one deity or many, by ghosts, demons or ancestral spirits is all determined by culture. (Winefield & Peay 1980)

Summary

It is only since the 1980s that the importance of a structured understanding of the sociological self – as opposed to an assumed common sense approach – has been realised, to enable the provision of truly individualised patient care. This is especially relevant in a multicultural society, such as that of the UK, so that cultural differences in practice can be recognised and, as far as possible, incorporated into the plan of care. Changes in social status imposed by, for example, parenthood or unemployment will also influence the needs of patients coming into contact with the health care services.

The main approaches to sociology – structuralist and interpretative – appear to be opposite ends of a spectrum, but are in fact complementary; their combined use allows a variety of research techniques and methods of application to nursing care. Also important to study is the notion of health as a social construct, which helps in the understanding of an individual's response to illness and health care.

Man is a social, socialised and culturally-influenced being, and his (and his carers') sociological self cannot be separated from his physiological and psychological characteristics if health care is to be truly holistic.

REFERENCES

Abraham C, Shanley E 1992 Social psychology for nurses. Understanding interaction in health care. Edward Arnold, London

Bennet K R 1992 The sociological self. In: Kenworthy N, Snowley G, Gilling C (eds) Common foundation studies in nursing. Churchill Livingstone, Edinburgh, pp 59–74

Berger P L, Luckman T 1966 The social construction of reality: a treatise in the sociology of knowledge. Doubleday, New York

Bond J, Bond S 1994 Sociology and health care, an introduction for nurses and other health care professionals, 2nd edn. Churchill Livingstone, Edinburgh

Burns T 1992 Ervin Goffman. Routledge, London

Cooke H 1993 Why teach sociology? Nurse Education Today 13: 210–216

Corbett T M 1995 The nurse as a professional carer. In: Ellis R B, Gates R J, Kenworthy N (eds) Interpersonal communication in nursing. Churchill Livingstone, Edinburgh

Cox C 1979 Who cares? Nursing and sociology: the development of a symbiotic relationship. Journal of Advanced Nursing 4: 237–252

Department of Health 1992 Health of the Nation – a strategy for health in England. Cmnd 1986. HMSO, London

Dubos R 1960 Mirage and health. Allen & Unwin, London

Gahagan J 1980 The foundations of social behaviour. In: Radford J, Govier E (eds) A textbook of psychology. Sheldon Press, London, pp 577–601

Giddens A 1993 Sociology, 2nd edn. Polity Press, Cambridge

Gomm R 1982 Health as a social product. In: Gomm R, McNeill P (eds) Handbook for sociology teachers. Heinemann Educational, London, pp 86–92

Groenman N H, Slevin O D'A, Brickenham M A 1992 Social and behavioural sciences for nurses. Campion Press, Edinburgh

Haralambos M (ed.) 1986 Sociology a new approach, 2nd edn. Causeway Press, Ormskirk

Helman C G 1992 Culture, health and illness, 2nd edn. Butterworth Heinemann, Oxford

Lynman M J 1992 Towards a goal of providing culturally sensitive care: principles upon which to build nursing curricula. Journal of Advanced Nursing 17: 149–157

Mann M 1983 The Macmillan student encyclopaedia of sociology. Macmillan, London

Martin B, Belcher J 1986 Influence of cultural background on nurses' attitudes and care of the oncology patient. Cancer Nursing 9(5): 230–237

Parsons T 1951 The social system. Routledge & Kegan Paul, London

Smith J P 1981 Sociology and nursing, 2nd edn. Churchill Livingstone, Edinburgh

Townsend P, Davidson N 1982 Inequalities in health: the Black report. Penguin, Harmondsworth

Winefield H R, Peay M Y 1980 Behavioural science in medicine. George Allen & Unwin, London

FURTHER READING

Calvert S, Calvert P 1992 Sociology today. Harvester Wheatsheaf, London (Useful text for those students who have not read sociology before. Concepts and problems are explored in the context of major changes in British society in the 1980s. Up-to-date research evidence is used to augment issues. Also contains very useful references for further reading.)

Giddens A 1993 Sociology, 2nd edn. Polity Press, Cambridge (A must for all discerning students because of its compulsiveness, lucidity and liveliness. Provides good comparative studies, both inter- and cross-culturally. Reader-friendly.)

Leathard A 1990 Health care provision. Past present and future. Chapman & Hall, London (Up-to-date book on the developments in the NHS. The training of various professional groups in the health and welfare services is put into context. Excellent for its succinctness.)

Lynan J 1992 Towards the goal of providing culturally sensitive care: principles upon which to build nursing curricula. Journal of Advanced Nursing 17: 149–157 (An insightful account of cultural influences on health care and particularly nursing care, with special emphasis on communication.)

Robinson J, Gray A, Elkan R (eds) 1992 Policy issues in nursing. Open University Press, Buckingham (An analysis of contemporary issues in nursing approached through policy studies in history, sociology, economics and management. Provides useful references for further study.)

Stress and the individual

Margaret Clarke

'Stress' is a term readily heard and spoken in today's Western society, but what is it and how does it affect the nurse, both in terms of her caring for patients and with respect to her own health? In exploring these issues, this chapter aims to:

- investigate the definition of stress
- compare models for understanding stress
- describe methods of coping with external demands
- discuss the potential role of stress in selected illnesses, referring to some known research methods and studies
- consider how the nurse can help to alleviate patient and personal stress, emphasising information-giving and stress-reducing strategies.

A recent newspaper article (Radford 1994) reported ways in which British white collar workers cope with the 'worst levels of stress in Europe'. It went on to state that stress and stress-related illness costs the nation 90 million working days and £13 billion in absenteeism each year.

The article highlights issues that will be discussed in this chapter. First of all, what is stress? Within that same newspaper article there was a statement that British white collar workers have the lowest 'feel-good' factor in Europe. Does the report suggest that stress is the opposite of 'feeling good'? This chapter considers the different ways in which the term 'stress' is used and the different meanings that people give to it. Second, the article implies a link between stress and illness, which is an important consideration for nurses. Third, there is a clear implication that stress can be measured, so that one can compare one group of workers with another. Finally, the issue of coping with stress was touched upon in the newspaper report, since it went on to list methods that the workers said they used to cope with stress. These are not the only issues that will be discussed in this chapter, but the newspaper piece shows very well how stress has not only become a part of our everyday concerns, but has become 'newsworthy' as well. It is crucial to understand clearly what is meant by the term 'stress', as well as being able to infer how other people define it from the way in which they use the term.

DEFINITIONS OF STRESS

In science, the term 'stress' means any change within a system induced by force. Physicists and engineers define stress as the force per unit area that will distort an object. Physiologists believe that stress is something that disturbs the physical or chemical balance (homeostasis; see Ch. 1) within an organism. Psychologists employ the term to denote emotional tensions that arise from psychological demands. Although the word is most commonly used by the public in this last sense, both the physiological and the psychological aspects of stress must be considered in order for the concept to be fully understood. Even though stress may arise from psychological demands, it prompts a physiological response.

Although the term 'stress' normally has negative connotations, not all stress is painful. Most readers will be able to describe the pleasure associated with some kind of stressful activity. Why do people sky-dive, hang-glide, climb Mount Everest or make love? All of these activities produce stress, yet they are rarely described as stressors.

Probably the simplest definition of stress is that given by Hans Selye (1976) – 'the wear and

Activity 4.1

1. Make a list of about 10 stressful activities in your life at the moment. Try to include some that produce pleasurable responses.
2. For each, list the obvious changes that these activities cause in you.
3. Discuss your lists with a colleague to see if there are any shared experiences and responses.

tear caused by life' – but this definition implies that it is impossible to have a completely stress-free life, in fact, complete freedom from stress means death. Selye was intent upon clarifying the meaning of stress. Prior to his writing, the word was not used in medicine or nursing. His research led him to the discovery of physical responses to all kinds of damage, including psychological injury. His work and his model of stress are discussed later in this chapter, as are other ways of looking at stress.

MODELS OF STRESS

Bailey & Clarke (1989) describe three main approaches to understanding stress. They are:

- the stimulus-based model
- the response-based model
- the transactional model.

A brief examination of these approaches will help to clarify how different people use the word 'stress' and may help the student nurse to choose the model that will be most helpful to her in patient care. Most professionals today find the transactional model most useful, but, since it has developed from the other two, it is also important to understand the earlier models.

THE STIMULUS-BASED MODEL

This model describes 'stresses' as the external or environmental factors (stimuli) that provoke a response, or series of responses, in the individual. These responses are known as 'strains' (Fig. 4.1). The model played an important role in stimulating research that furthered the understanding of

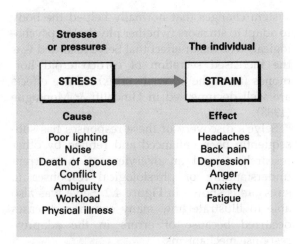

Figure 4.1 The stimulus-based model of stress. (After Bailey & Clarke 1989.)

stress and the conditions under which it occurs. It also led to newer and better definitions, which, in their turn, stimulated research. The initial research into stress as a stimulus involved studying what kinds of stress caused strain, and what was the nature of the strain that occurred.

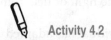

Activity 4.2

Take a moment to write down a list of events that you think could be stimuli causing strain. Then use the list to see whether or not any of the items on it correspond to those stimuli that have been researched.

A commonly listed stressor is loud and continuous noise. This, together with very high or very low environmental temperatures, has been investigated as a stimulus for stress. Other stimuli are poor lighting, conflict, ambiguity, excessive load and the death of a spouse. Similarly, the responses, or strain, have also been investigated. These include headaches, back pain, depression, anger, anxiety and fatigue.

The stimulus-based model is attractive because it is simple. Unfortunately, it is too simple. With such a model, the stronger the stimulus, for example noise, and the longer it continues, the worse the strain. Similarly, the effect of a stimulus of the same kind, duration and level of intensity would be the same every time it occurred, and

the same for every individual. However, the evidence is that things are not this simple. Macpherson (1974), reviewing the literature on thermal discomfort, came to the conclusion that what were intolerable conditions for some people induced only mild discomfort in others. He also came to the conclusion that something that causes great distress on one occasion may cause none at all later. For example, the loud noise of a road drill outside when a student is trying to listen to an important lecture is likely to have a different effect from the noise of a disco, although the noise levels may be similar.

What is wrong with the stimulus model of stress is that it takes no account of adaptation, which is the process by which individuals 'accommodate' to their environment. This accommodation happens within the sense organs, which, when exposed to a constant level of stimulus, stop responding to the extent they did initially, and may even stop responding altogether. Psychologists also talk about adaptation, as meaning the way in which perception and interpretation of the world change with experience. In addition to this problem, the model takes no account of individual differences, nor does it account for motivation, since this is a factor that will alter quite considerably how people respond to adverse conditions. Furthermore, there is no recognition of the meaning that events have for people. The meaning that a jet plane noise has for the person whose relative has been killed in an air crash may be very different from the meaning for someone excited about going on holiday.

There is another major stumbling block with this model. In any stimulus–response model, the greater the stimulus, the greater the response, and, conversely, the less the stimulus, the smaller the response. This simple relationship breaks down completely when considering the effect of complete absence of stimuli upon human beings. Lack of stimulation is known to be a situation that is extremely stressful: it is an ingredient of brainwashing. Nurses need to be aware of such deleterious effects, since patients may be exposed to environments that are very impoverished in terms of stimuli.

In summary, the stress–strain explanation has produced some useful information, but the model is not entirely helpful, because it fails to recognise all the factors involved in stress. In particular it fails to take account of adaptation and individual differences.

THE RESPONSE-BASED MODEL

This model is one in which the word 'stress' is used to describe the changes that take place within an individual in response to damaging or potentially damaging external or internal demands on the body. Stress is what happens as a result of provocation of some kind. The provocation is, therefore, the stressor: that which causes stress.

Selye pioneered the response-based model in the 1930s. His powers of observation prompted him to ask questions and to seek explanations for oddities that others took for granted. Whilst still a medical student, he wondered why sick people all seemed to exhibit some common characteristics or symptoms, even when they had distinctly different illnesses. He wanted to learn more about this phenomenon and was amazed to discover that no one had ever investigated it. His advisers laughed at his idea of researching the 'general syndrome of disease'. Selye became an excellent endocrinologist and eventually managed to fulfil his wish to research the 'disease syndrome' (those common symptoms that all ill people demonstrate) through his studies of the endocrine system. He discovered physiological changes that occurred in response to physical and psychological damage and eventually called these changes stress, or the stress syndrome.

General adaptation syndrome

Selye called the body's set of physical responses to stressors the general adaptation syndrome (GAS), because it was the same whether the cause was a physical one (such as infection, haemorrhage or burns) or a psychological one (such as bereavement, occupational problems or loneliness). Selye's definition of stress was 'the non-specific response of the body to any demand'. This response was a set of endocrine and nervous system changes that normally helped the body to adapt to stressors (whether physical or psychological). The major effect that Selye recorded was the increased secretion of corticosteroid hormones (from the adrenal cortex), whose effects are well documented in Hinchliff & Montague (1988).

Selye's discovery of these responses has subsequently been enhanced and refined by other researchers, and an overview of the current understanding of physiological responses to stressors is shown in Figure 4.2. Selye was also able to illustrate how many common diseases occurred because of errors in the adaptive response mechanisms.

The phases of the GAS

Selye described the GAS as a system that operates in three phases (Fig. 4.3). Each phase has certain characteristics, as follows:

- Alarm phase: palpitations, tachycardia and tremors. The individual is galvanising bodily resources to maintain life, to fight or flee from danger.
- Resistance phase: the individual has adapted to the stressor. Symptoms of the alarm reaction diminish or disappear, but the capacity to cope with further stressors is diminished.
- Exhaustion phase: symptoms reappear because stressors continue to increase, or because new stressors make demands with which the body cannot deal successfully. Adaptation is no longer present and death may occur.

Some of the physical symptoms of the alarm phase may be well known to the reader. They are due to the action of the sympathetic nervous system and the release of the hormones adrenaline and noradrenaline from the adrenal medulla. Selye built on the work of Cannon (1932) who had described the important role of these hormones in what is known as the fight–flight mechanism. Selye's own work did, however, reveal the importance of the glucocorticoid hormones (from the adrenal cortex) in stress. The effects of these two groups of hormones are

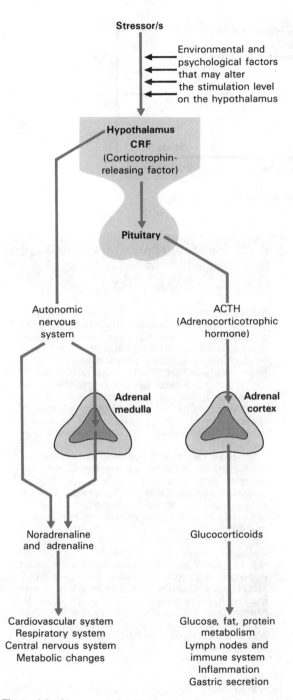

Figure 4.2 Nervous and endocrine responses to stressors.

Table 4.1 Main actions of adrenaline and noradrenaline (the catecholamines)

Organ/system	Effect
Heart	Increased cardiac output
Blood vessels	Dilatation of arterioles supplying skeletal muscle Constriction of arterioles supplying gut and skin
Respiratory system	Increased breathing rate Bronchodilation
Nervous system	Increased arousal and tensing of muscles
Eyes	Pupil dilation
Metabolic effects	Glycogen breakdown to form glucose for energy production Fat breakdown to release fatty acids for energy production

Note: These effects occur rapidly in response to stressors and can be short-lived.

Table 4.2 Main actions of the glucocorticoids

Function	Effect
Carbohydrate metabolism and fat	Inhibits glucose intake in tissues, except for brain and heart, thus increasing blood glucose levels Stimulates glucose production from stored glycogen, proteins and fats Enhances the effects of adrenaline, noradrenaline and glucagon in glucose production from stores
Protein metabolism	Breaks down protein molecules Depresses protein synthesis (including immunoglobulins) Deaminates; increases urea production
Immune system	Decreases mass of all lymphatic tissues Decreases numbers of circulating lymphocytes and other white blood cells
Inflammatory response	Reduces inflammation
Other functions	May enhance learning Enhances urinary excretion Promotes gastric secretion and the development of peptic ulcers

Note: The effect of the glucocorticoids is slower and longer lasting than that of the catecholamines.

shown in Tables 4.1 and 4.2. It must be remembered that in stress they are released together and therefore strengthen one another's actions.

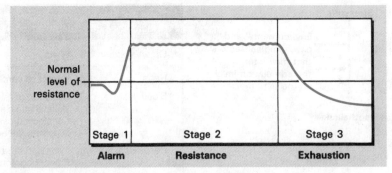

Figure 4.3 The three phases of the general adaptation syndrome. (After Selye 1976.)

In Selye's model of stress, the main point of the response is to enable the body to adapt, i.e. to restore homeostasis, at the earliest opportunity. Selye's further work showed how optimum levels of stress hormones enable the body to adapt to extra demands, whereas high and continuing levels of these substances can lead to increased vulnerability to disease. Take a moment to think about the stressors that white collar workers encounter in the workplace. How helpful are the physiological responses that occur, continuously, during the alarm phase of the GAS? This is an important point to consider when thinking about the relationship between stress and illness. Selye's model has particular application in nursing, as patients and relatives are likely to display one or more of the signs of the stress response.

Limitations of the response-based model

Some writers believe that the response-based model is limited. Whilst they accept that the stress process consists of many fundamental physiological changes, the response model of stress still presents man as a passive being reacting to a hostile environment (Bailey & Clarke 1989). In fact, in his writings, Selye acknowledged that factors other than purely physiological ones were obviously influential in the stress response and its subsequent development (Box 4.1).

THE TRANSACTIONAL MODEL

The transactional model owes much to the work of one particularly influential researcher, Richard Lazarus, who, like Selye, has devoted many

---

Box 4.1 Hans Selye's broader view of stress (Reproduced with kind permission from Selye 1976)

'We must differentiate within the general concept of stress between the unpleasant or harmful variety called *distress* (from the Latin dis = bad as in dissonance, disagreement) and *eustress* (from the Greek eu = good, as in euphoria). During eustress and distress the body undergoes virtually the same nonspecific responses to the various positive or negative stimuli acting upon it. However, the fact that eustress causes much less damage than distress graphically demonstrates that it is 'how you take it' that determines, ultimately, whether you can adapt successfully to change.

It may be said without hesitation that for man the most important stressors are emotional, especially those causing distress. Naturally, purely physical demands upon the tissues of our body, such as a wound healing, restoration of lost blood, fighting of infections or poisonings can also become of paramount importance. Yet these are far less commonly met in normal life than the emotional stimuli with which we are almost constantly faced; besides, even somatic reactions affect us largely because of the nervous responses (fear, pain, frustration) which they evoke. This is probably because among all living beings, man has the most complex brain and is the most dependent upon it. Thus, it is especially true that, in our life events, the stressor effects depend *not so much upon what we do or what happens to us but on the way we take it.*'

---

years to work in the field of stress. Lazarus's first publication was in 1966, and he has elaborated and developed his concept since that time.

The transactional model takes into account that the human being is a thinking being with memory of past events, the ability to predict (even if very inaccurately) the future, and also the ability to try to influence events, rather than passively responding to them. The fact that human beings also respond with emotions was implicit in the response-based model discussed above. Individual differences are taken account of in the transactional model, since the past history of each individual will be different, and each individual may interpret situations differently, as well as having an individual style of coping with events.

The term 'transactional' comes from the central component of the model, the concept that individuals engage in transactions with their environment. That is to say, they in some way adjust the environment and make it different from what it was before. This means that the individual has a tool by which he can prevent or ameliorate stressors. Another term that is associated with the transactional model is 'interactional'. This signifies that there is interaction between the individual and the environment: the person adapts to the environment, but also adjusts the environment, so the process is not just one way. The transactional model shifts our view of man from one who responds to the environment to one who shapes it. Far from merely responding to stimuli, the person is responsible for creating many of the stimuli on which he must act.

Coping

Lazarus does not, however, use the term 'stressor', but instead writes about demands made on the individual by the environment. Sometimes other terms, such as 'threat', 'loss', 'harm' or 'challenge', are used instead of 'demand'. Another major concept is that of coping, which can be defined as the efforts made by the individual to meet the demands exerted by the environment. Successful coping can be defined in terms of the outcome, i.e. that the individual manages to keep stress levels within an optimum range for himself.

An important aspect of the transactional model is that Lazarus introduces the idea of appraisal. First of all, the individual appraises the threat and its potential for harm. This is termed primary appraisal. Following this comes secondary appraisal, which is the estimation the individual makes of his capacity for coping. Finally comes reappraisal, which is the assessment of the effec-

tiveness of coping; i.e. it is a reassessment of the environmental potential for harm. Like any explanation, this is an oversimplification, since it has made the process appear to be isolated and clearly defined, with a beginning and an end. In practice, 'the individual should be seen as a dynamic system attempting to control levels of threat and demand to which he or she is exposed by effective coping' (Bailey & Clarke 1989). But where is stress in all of this? It can be defined as occurring when there is an imbalance between the demand made on the individual and his ability to cope.

Figure 4.4 provides a summary of the transactional model.

The transactional model in health care

There are clearly differences between the transactional model of stress and the others considered above. What are the benefits of this model for health professionals? First, it makes clear statements about individual differences. This is useful for health professionals since it directs attention to the fact that patients and clients are individuals who need to be individually assessed. It helps in understanding why one person may find a visit to a dentist terrifying, whilst another treats it as just routine. Furthermore, the work of Lazarus and others shows not only that the way in which people interpret things may be very individualistic, but also that they can be assisted to see things differently by giving them information. This helps to explain the vast amount of research that has shown that most people can cope better with surgery if they are given good information prior to operation. However, the most important aspect of the model is that it has shown that people can be helped to cope with situations that they perceive as threatening or demanding.

Methods of coping

Lazarus (e.g. Lazarus & Launier 1978) has carried out a great deal of work that has investigated coping. He argues that there are two types of coping: problem-focused coping and emotion-focused coping.

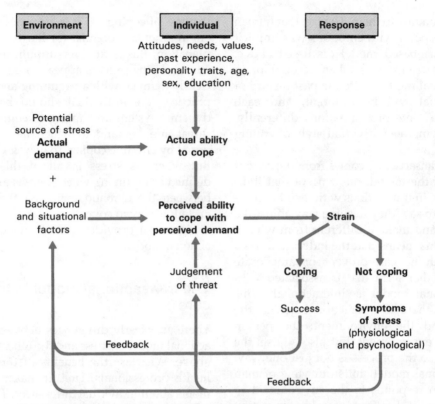

Figure 4.4   A transactional model of stress. (After Sutherland & Cooper 1990.)

Problem-focused coping

Many situations that challenge, or make demands on, individuals do so because they present people with problems. Problem-focused coping attempts to deal with these. For example, a nurse at work who is suddenly confronted with two patients arriving at the ward door for admission at an identical moment whilst she is already very busy has great demands placed on her. One problem-focused method of coping would be to seek help. Another would be to establish priority between the competing demands. Which patient needs the most urgent attention? The other is politely asked to wait. By coping effectively, the nurse avoids the stress that might otherwise occur.

Emotion-focused coping

However, there are many challenging and demanding situations that either are not amenable to problem-solving or that are so complex that other forms of coping, for example emotion-focused coping, are also needed.

In discussing the response definition of stress, the action of the autonomic nervous system was mentioned. A description was given in Table 4.1 of the increase in pulse rate and blood pressure and the tensing of muscles that occur when the sympathetic nervous system is active. Figure 4.2 also shows how psychological factors, such as fear and anxiety, bring about physiological responses to problems and stressors; when these become excessive, the ability to cope with the challenge may be impaired.

Emotion-focused coping includes a range of methods that help to reduce high levels of fear and anxiety and their accompanying effects. This then conserves energy to deal more effectively with the problem at hand. Methods of emotion-focused coping include deep breathing and relaxation, which counteract the effects of the catecholamines.

As stated above, not all challenges or demands can be coped with by problem-solving techniques. Some of the most demanding situations come into this category; for example that facing the individual who is bereaved by the loss of a close relative. There is no way that coping can make good the loss. Instead, emotion-focused coping may help by reducing or ameliorating some of the mental anguish and physical symptoms experienced. This may help the individual in the short term and also provide time in which to come to terms with the loss.

For some people, taking alcohol or tranquillisers is an emotion-focused method of coping. Whilst these substances may indeed help with emotions in the short term, they may themselves unfortunately cause health problems in the long term if a dependency develops.

Denial and coping

Another coping method that can help people with severe demands is changing the way of perceiving or interpreting the demand. Included here are ego defence mechanisms, as described by Freud (1946), including the process of denial. In using denial, the individual acts as if the loss or demand no longer exists. It should be noted that this is not just a simple matter of putting the issue mentally aside and concentrating on something else instead. It is an unconscious process: the knowledge of the loss is just not available to the individual's conscious self.

It was believed that this was a mentally unhealthy response, which later caused difficulty. Indeed, the basis of much of Freud's work was to recover memories of incidents in the individual's childhood that had been denied and were causing problems in adult life. However, Lazarus (1979) has argued that, at least in conditions of excessive physical trauma or disease (e.g. spinal cord injury), denial buys the sufferer time. When the individual has recovered his physical reserves, he is better able to face the problems of his new life.

An interesting study by Gyllensköld (1982) showed the process of denial in operation. Her background was in clinical psychology, and she carried out a series of fairly long interviews with a group of 22 women newly diagnosed as having cancer of the breast. These interviews continued for a period of about a year, during which time the women were both coming to terms with the diagnosis, and also undergoing and coping with treatment. Gyllensköld reported the women using denial and other defence mechanisms during the course of the interviews. What was particularly interesting was the lability of these coping methods. One moment the individual was using, for example, denial or projection, the next she was not and was fully in touch with reality.

Intellectualisation and coping

Another defence mechanism, first described by Lazarus (1976), that is of particular relevance to nurses is the process of intellectualisation. Here the individual treats an emotion-laden problem as if it were simply an intellectual problem to be solved dispassionately. This was first described in relation to medical students, but nurses also use this strategy, occasionally in relation to patients.

Challenging beliefs

Whilst the use of defence mechanisms can be seen as a passive method of coping that is not under the individual's control, other methods of coping are under control, and can be taught or used by nurses or therapists as a coping strategy. These methods can be classified as involving a change in beliefs. For example, it is possible for an individual, when faced with a threatening situation, to learn to say to themselves such things as 'Now I am calm. I am going to assess this situation calmly and deal with it', or 'I know I can cope, there is nothing to be afraid of'. Combined with deep breathing, such methods can be a very successful way of coping with frightening situations. Firemen and policemen, for example, frequently have to act when under great threat; occasionally, so do nurses.

Some of the ways in which nurses can help people to come to terms with illness or an operation also involve changing the ways in which the individual sees the threat. This involves helping the person to see things in a more realistic light, since reality is frequently less frightening than is the image.

Support groups

Patient support groups are groups of people who have a common health problem and who provide support to one another in coping. A group like this not only inspires a newly diagnosed patient in living with the disease, but can also give practical advice that will help with the day-to-day management of such a chronic illness.

Social support in general is frequently important in helping individuals to cope when they are faced with great challenges. Definitions of social support are somewhat cumbersome, but its function has been described. Cobb (1976) has suggested that the recipient of support feels cared for, esteemed and valued and belongs in a mutually helpful network. Such support can derive from a variety of sources, for example a spouse, parent, friend or work colleague (Callahan & Morrisey 1993). For nurses, given the emotional content of their role, having such social support may make the difference for them between coping and not coping.

Coping and control

Bailey & Clarke (1989) have defined coping as 'any activity by the person which changes his perceived relationship with his environment (internal or external) to the point where he no longer regards it as threatening, *whilst the attainment of personal control is the outcome of successful coping'* (italics added). They go on to argue that individuals who feel a sense of effective control over events also have a sense of self-esteem, believe in their ability to influence events and have a sense of autonomy. This may go some way to explaining those people who apparently thrive on pursuing dangerous careers or hobbies, such as racing drivers and mountain climbers. Bailey

& Clarke (1989) suggest that the greater the threat, the greater the self-esteem, if and when personal control is gained. That is to say that effective coping at a very high level of demand is rewarding to the individual achieving it.

Antonovsky (1979) suggested a related phenomenon, 'psychological coherence', which develops from a consciousness of increased mastery over threat. This is not simply a sense that one has coped well on a particular occasion but a psychological shift in the individual's view of himself. Antonovsky described a sense of coherence as arising from the individuals having a dynamic, pervasive and long-standing feeling not only that the internal and external environment is predictable, but also that there is a strong chance that things will work out as well as expected.

There are three components to a sense of coherence (Antonovsky 1979, 1987): comprehensibility, manageability and meaningfulness. Comprehensibility occurs when the information represented by the stimulus is perceived as structured and clear; there is a logic to the situation. Manageability is 'the extent to which people perceive that resources are at their disposal that are adequate to meet the demands' (Antonovsky 1984). This does not mean that these resources have to be under direct personal control; they may be controlled by others in a way that is likely to be effective. Meaningfulness denotes emotional investment in life. The individual has a sense that there are important areas in life, which, although very challenging, are well worth the emotional effort and time needed to cope.

Emotional coping and health care

Antonovsky's views are frequently considered important within the health care professions (see, for example, Sullivan 1993), since he identifies a relationship between psychological coherence and health. His model is called a salutogenic model. Sullivan considers that psychological coherence acts as a buffer against stress. Seligman (1975) has suggested that people experience a sense of helplessness when their efforts to achieve

Box 4.2 Potentially demanding elements in the role of a hospital staff nurse

Unpredictable workload

Patient admissions are controlled by medical staff and contracts with purchasers. It is this element that makes a great difference to the workload.

Conflicting demands made upon the role of staff nurse

Patients, relatives, senior nurses, student nurses, medical staff and therapists, for example, may all expect the staff nurse to play a slightly different role.

Potential for having to work beyond the level of competence

During staff shortages owing to sickness, a staff nurse may have to take responsibility for which she is not yet ready.

Feelings of not being completely informed

Communicating with patients and relatives can sometimes be difficult as the staff nurse may not know what they have been told by others, for example medical staff.

Time pressures

This can lead to cutting corners and dissatisfaction with the quality of care given. It can result in the nurse feeling conflict between the ideals she holds and the reality of what is possible.

Possible lack of feedback on performance

Senior staff may not give frequent feedback upon the nurse's work.

Acting as a mentor, supervisor or assessor to student nurses

This can lead to feelings of pressure and inadequacy if the staff nurse is pressed for time or believes that the student is more knowledgeable.

Personal pressures

The staff nurse has a private life outside the workplace, which can impose its own demands. For example, a female nurse may be the breadwinner within a relationship.

---

personal control have no effect that they can perceive. Those who experience a sense of helplessness are more likely to become depressed and anxious than are those who experience a sense of personal control. Burnout seems to be a related phenomenon, although it is specifically job-related and occurs when work creates such frustration of goals that the efforts made have no effect on outcomes. It is associated with low self-esteem, and has been described particularly in those professions, such as teaching, social work, nursing and medicine, that are concerned with the welfare of others. There is usually a greater degree of emotional exhaustion.

This can be related to occupational stress. In Box 4.2, those elements of a hospital staff nurse's role that could be particularly stressful are picked out. In contrast, in Box 4.3, the stressful elements of being made redundant are listed. These are not, by any means, exhaustive lists. It must also be remembered that people are individual, both in the way they perceive events and in the way in which they cope. Interestingly, given that anxiety and stress are linked, several studies of nursing have shown satisfaction and anxiety to

Box 4.3 Demands made when a person has been made redundant

Loss of self-esteem

Feelings of loss of control

The person was unable to influence the decision that he or she be made redundant.

Loss of role

Think how much of the week is taken up at work, where we take on a role that is different from that at home.

Loss of structure to the weekly routine

Threat owing to reduced income

Threat of losing the home

The person may be unable to keep up mortgage payments.

Anxiety about getting another job

---

be positively linked. This shows that whilst nursing may be very demanding, it is also a very satisfying profession (Bailey 1985, 1986).

STRESS, COPING, HEALTH AND ILLNESS

In the newspaper article mentioned at the beginning of this chapter, a link was suggested between stress and illness. How might the possibility of such a link be researched?

Activity 4.3

How would you set about investigating the relationship between stress and illness? Write down some of your own ideas, then discuss them with student colleagues or other friends. What ideas did you have?

Retrospective research into stress-related disease

One approach to research is to identify a group of people with a disease that is thought to be stress-related (e.g. duodenal ulcer) and to ask them about the stress they experienced in the period of time before the onset of the illness. A control group who have not developed the illness are also asked about the stress they experienced during the same period of time. The two groups are then compared.

Activity 4.4

Discuss with colleagues or friends the question 'How may illness affect an individual's recall of recent events and memory in general?' Think about your own experiences, as well as considering what others might remember. Make a list of your collective views.

There are, however, problems with this approach. First, there is the issue of memory, which may be selective: remembering major events is easier than remembering all the minor irritations that, nevertheless, accumulate. A further problem is that memory may be affected by the influence of the current situation. An ill person may be trying to make sense of the question 'Why me?' and be reflecting on negative events before the research takes place. Third, the stress reported by one individual may not be of the same order as the stress reported by another. Finally, even if one could categorically state that those with, for example, duodenal ulcer experienced more stress in the run up to the onset of illness than had the control group, this does not necessarily mean that the stress caused the illness.

Clearly, this type of study design contains many pitfalls in establishing an unequivocal cause and effect relationship between stress and illness. On the other hand, retrospective studies may be used to give researchers leads that can then be followed up with more rigorously designed studies.

Prospective research

In prospective research, the researcher follows up a group of people over a long period of time, recording stressful events as they happen. The illnesses of individuals from the group are then recorded and related to the levels of stress experienced. Differences between the experienced stress levels of this sub-group would be contrasted with the experienced stress levels of those who did not develop any illness. Whilst such a study is more rigorous than is the retrospective study, it is not without its own problems. It is not easy to maintain contact with a group of individuals over a long period of time, and comparisons of the stress experienced by different subjects is difficult because of the subjective nature of stress. In practice, what has been done in prospective studies is to record major life events and other objective circumstances, rather than experienced stress. This is more reliable in terms of measurement, but is only a proxy for stress, since not everyone responds in the same way to major life events.

Major life event stressors

A programme of research that systematically investigated the effect of major life events was carried out by Holmes & Rahe (1967). First of all they identified a series of major and minor events that are common in the lives of those in Western society, for example getting married, suffering bereavement, getting a parking ticket and going on holiday. Next, a group of people were asked to rate these events in terms of 'severity' of the need for readjustment. Having obtained these results, they were then converted into rather arbitrary 'life change units', the death of a spouse being given the arbitrary maximum value of 100 and all the other events being related to this. This formed a scale called the Social Readjustment Scale. The scale was then used to compare individuals' scores, in terms of events needing readjustment over a period of time. It has been used in both retrospective and prospective studies. There have been criticisms of the scale, both because it incorporates positive and negative events, for example getting married and getting divorced, in the same scale, and because it simply tots up scores without taking into account how the person feels about the event. Evidence from this type of study has been suggestive of a link between stressful life events and the onset of illness, but it cannot be regarded as completely unequivocal (Box 4.4).

Box 4.4 Examples of life stress events

Death of spouse
Death of close family member or friend
Major personal illness or injury
Marriage
Moving house
Marital separation/divorce
New baby
Loss of job
Parent(s) coming to stay permanently
Major change in financial status
Sexual problems
New job
Retirement
Minor violations of the law

All of these events represent a change in lifestyle. Generally, the bigger the change, the more stressful it is, even if it is a change for the better. Not all individuals will have the same response level to these events.

DISEASES RESULTING FROM STRESS

Apart from studies using the Social Readjustment Scale, which treat events in terms of scores and also treat different illnesses as equivalent, there have been studies that look at the relationship between more differentiated events and specific illnesses. For example, some research has looked at the relationship between the incidence and onset of coronary heart disease and the way in which an individual typically reacts to stressful events. A coronary-prone, or type A, personality has thus been described. This is the person who typically drives himself hard, seems to be constantly under pressure of time, is competitive and may show hostility to others (Rosenman & Friedman 1974). Other studies, which have investigated people who develop cancer, suggest that individuals who have difficulty in expressing their emotions are more susceptible to cancer. Furthermore, those who respond to the disease with helplessness have a less favourable outcome of the disease, and those who fight the disease aggressively have a more favourable outcome (Pettingale et al 1985, Bailey & Clarke 1989). The studies quoted above have investigated, somewhat globally, the relationship between illness and stress. However, it is also worth remembering the physiology of stress, as elucidated by Selye, and relating this to both the onset and the course of the illness.

The damaging effects of stress

Whatever the stressor, and whichever model of stress is chosen to aid the management of stress, there are common signs and reactions of which it is important for nurses to be aware.

Immediate physical responses

Easily measurable and widely accepted and reliable indicators of stress are:

- a rise in the blood level of adrenaline
- a rise in the blood level of corticosteroids
- a rise in blood pressure
- a rise in sweat secretion.

Recognisable acute changes

These are variable, but most people can recognise several of the acute stress response symptoms listed in Box 4.5. Any one of these changes may occur in an individual who is 'distressed'. Fortunately, the timespan of the clinically measurable

Box 4.5 General stress response symptoms

General irritability
Pounding of the heart
Dryness of the throat and mouth
Impulsive behaviour
The urge to cry or run and hide
Poor concentration
Feelings of weakness and/or dizziness
Becoming easily fatigued
Anxiety, but concerning nothing in particular
Tension/alertness: being 'keyed up'
Trembling or nervous twitching
Being easily startled
Giggling; nervous laughter
Stuttering or other speech defects

Grinding of the teeth
Poor sleep patterns/insomnia
Being fidgety
Frequent urination
Diarrhoea, feeling sick or vomiting
Migraine headaches
Pain in the neck or lower back
Loss of appetite
Increased smoking
Increased alcohol consumption
Other drug use
Nightmares
Accident-proneness

response or the self-observed response is often relatively short, and it is therefore unlikely to lead to a long-standing, debilitating illness. However, modern life – with its rapid pace, variety of activity and mounting pace of change – appears to be provoking longer periods of stress, with resultant illnesses.

Diseases resulting from stress

Stress-induced illness remains a controversial subject among health care professionals, but most writers on the topic believe that enough is now known about causal pathways (e.g. endocrine changes and changes to the immune response) for stress-related illness not to be ignored. Box 4.6 lists widely accepted and researched disorders that *may* have stress as an underlying cause (although this does not mean that stress is their only possible cause).

Stress and hypertension

Some links have been clearly established through research. One of the major effects of both sympathetic nervous system stimulation and catecholamine release (see Table 4.1) is an increase in blood pressure. Should the hormone levels be exceptionally high, and should this state last for a length of time, hypertension can become chronic. It is worth noting that untreated persistent hypertension increases the probability of both stroke and coronary heart disease. Myo-

Box 4.6 Some illnesses generally accepted to be stress-related

- Cardiovascular disease (angina, myocardial infarction) precipitated by hypertension and high blood cholesterol
- Gastrointestinal disorders (duodenal and gastric ulcers)
- Diabetes mellitus
- Hayfever (immune response abnormalities)
- Eczema and other atopic skin disease (immune response abnormalities)
- Eclampsia and renal disease, secondary to hypertension
- Rheumatoid diseases (immune response abnormalities)
- Cancer (this is a massive subject, comprising a great variety of disorders, and is widely researched)
- Multiple sclerosis, myasthenia gravis, rheumatoid arthritis (all thought to be autoimmune disorders, which may be stress-related)
- Mental illness (ranging from anxiety to some severe conditions arising from over-compensation in coping with initial stress, e.g. unacceptable sexual behaviour)

cardial infarction and stroke are extremely serious and cause not only premature death, but also high levels of morbidity.

Stress and diabetes

The effect of synchronous high levels of catecholamines and cortico-steroids is to bring about the conversion of glycogen and amino acids to glucose. There is speculation that a prolongation of this response could lead to diabetes mellitus if pancreatic capacity for insulin production were insufficient. Similarly, the accompanying altered fat metabolism is believed to increase cholesterol levels. Prolonged high cholesterol levels have also been linked to an increased likelihood of coronary heart disease. Research in which cholesterol levels have been monitored over time, which has included periods of increased stress, has shown raised cholesterol levels associated with the times of increased stress (Clarke et al 1975). This relationship was confirmed in a study by Tucker et al (1987), who concluded, however, that 'when it comes to serum cholesterol levels, the perceptions people have of their problems play a more significant role than the problems themselves'. This latter finding confirms the importance of transactional views of stress.

Stress and reduced immunity

High levels of circulating corticosteroids are known to be associated with changes in immunity (Boore 1988). They have the effect of depressing the number of circulating antibodies and the number of eosinophils, and of suppressing the inflammatory response. This increases the susceptibility of the individual to infection. It also reduces fibrosis, a process important in wound healing. A wound increases the chances of organisms entering and makes both the immune response and the healing process important. This obviously has significance for patients undergoing major operations. It has been suggested, again with less firm evidence, that there is a reduction in immune defences mediated by the stress associated with the onset of cancer.

Stress and peptic ulcers

Another effect of high levels of circulating corticosteroids is an increase in the secretion of both hydrochloric acid and pepsinogen in the stomach. In turn, these two factors lead to a higher probability that peptic ulceration will occur, which has been induced experimentally by subjecting animals to stress. Stress-related peptic ulcers associated with, burns for example, are now preventable using histamine blockade as a regular part of the care programme.

Whilst there is little unequivocal evidence for the link between stress and illness, there is much suggestive work, and there are also physiological facts, to support such a hypothesis.

STRESS AND COPING AND THE APPLICATION TO HEALTH CARE

Regardless of whether or not stress causes illness, there is little doubt that being ill acts as a stressor, which is exacerbated by having to go into hospital for investigation and treatment. There are many issues here. Being ill creates many uncertainties, those of diagnosis, prognosis, treatment, disruption of family life and responsibilities, and the consequences of the illness even if a full recovery is made. The treatment may, in itself, act as a stressor, frequently of a physical nature. For example, having a major operation involves loss of blood and physical trauma to tissues, and, if a general anaesthetic is used, a period of starvation leads to the depletion of endogenous energy stores. Pain is also a very powerful stressor.

The role of the nurse with distressed patients

Since one of the major problems for patients, and also for their partners, parents, children and friends, is uncertainty, one way of helping is to give patients accurate and timely information. A good deal of research by nurses and others has shown the value of this (Mathews & Ridgeway 1984). It not only helps patients to feel a greater sense of personal control, but actually also increases the speed with which they get better. Therefore it is common practice to produce leaflets and information pamphlets that can be sent to patients before they come to hospital.

The importance of information

Information leaflets are clearly worthy attempts to help people to cope with the experience of illness and going into hospital, but this may be an inadequate approach to meeting patient needs. To keep patients fully informed, the aim should be a continuous and individual strategy. A person's information needs should be assessed and the results of the assessment used to identify the best way to give the information. Individual interaction allows the nurse to assess whether the patient understands the information. It also allows the patient to ask questions to reflect his or her individual concerns. Using written information and individual interaction together is a good approach, since written information means that the person has a record that can be referred to and does not rely on memory. This is important because Ley & Spelman (1967) have shown that memorising and retaining information may be reduced by anxiety and stress.

Knowing what is going to happen before it happens allows the individual to anticipate events and to prepare coping strategies. It also converts an unknown, strange, event into a more predictable one. Research has shown that most individuals cope better if the information that they receive is specially tailored to their needs and allows them to anticipate how things will affect them personally. In relation to procedures that they undergo, for example, it is useful if the person has been told the points at which discomfort or pain will be experienced, and also the nature of the discomfort and pain. (Johnson 1973). It is also beneficial if he has been told how to help, for example, by adopting a good position, keeping still at crucial moments, using deep breathing and so on.

When health professionals give information to clients or patients, they frequently give it from the professional's, rather than the client's, point of view. They say what they are going to do, rather than what the patient's experience will be. Whilst better than nothing, this type of information does not really meet the client's needs, which may be one reason why patient support groups are successful – they are able to speak from the patient's point of view.

One of the advantages of the transactional view of stress is that it allows for individual differences. Using such a model as a theoretical framework for research, it has been found that not all individuals wish to be given information. Some prefer to take a passive role and leave it to the doctors and nurses, so it is important that information is not forced upon them.

The stress of loss

Unfortunately, the course of some illness is itself uncertain, and health professionals are then unable to give precise information about the future. Sometimes the prognosis is very poor, in which case knowing the truth and reality of the situation becomes in itself a major negative event.

One of the major stressors is loss or anticipation of loss, and this has great significance in health care. Losses include bereavement, a major change in body image through the actual loss of a part of the body or a loss of its function and knowing that one is dying.

The process of adjustment to such losses has been described in the literature (Kubler-Ross 1969, Parkes 1975, Worden 1983, Roberts 1986). The descriptions have much in common, even though the terminology may be different. Elizabeth Kubler-Ross was one of the first to describe the process that she identified as a series of stages (see Ch. 19).

STRATEGIES FOR COPING WITH STRESS

Earlier in this chapter some of the demands that might be experienced by a hospital staff nurse were listed. Student nurses may also be subject to such demands during periods of clinical practice (Box 4.7), but there are other demands imposed simply as the result of being a student. It is important to develop personal coping strategies and then teach them to others, both colleagues and patients.

Seeing things differently

One purpose of education is to allow students to benefit from the experience and knowledge of others. Learning theory may be a 'drag', but theory can be used to help a greater understanding of situations that are encountered. Knowing that anger is a normal response to loss and that a patient can displace that anger onto health care professionals can help the nurse to cope, since one can put it into perspective rather than believing that the angry person has 'got it in for you' personally.

A particularly useful shift of perception is understanding role theory (see Ch. 3), since this provides a tool for interpreting behaviour that might otherwise appear out of character. For example, a particular student is well supported in his studies by a tutor who, he believes, respects and likes him. However, the student fails an examination and embarks upon an appeal. To his astonishment, the tutor appears to be on the college's side, rather than his. This can be understood in terms of role theory. The tutor has the role of being a member of staff of the college during the hearing, and, for the time being, this role takes precedence over that of tutor. Understanding this helps in coping later when, once again, the student needs the help of the tutor.

Being assertive

Assertion can be defined as expressing one's own point of view, or stating one's own needs whilst still respecting other's views and needs. Being non-assertive is defined as denying one's own needs in order to allow someone else's needs to be satisfied. Assertion should be differentiated from aggression, which is seeking to dominate or to get one's own way at the expense of others.

Nursing is still a predominantly female profession, and many women still find it difficult to assert themselves. If this happens, a nurse many feel threatened and her self-esteem challenged, perhaps because of feeling unfairly treated, or because another's needs have been given greater priority. Being assertive can counteract this and is a way of coping with stress. In recognition of this, many colleges of nursing and midwifery offer their students assertiveness training.

Relaxation techniques

Relaxation is often regarded as helpful in psychological stress. There are a number of relaxation methods. Here, there will be only a brief description of the most common. Again they are techniques that need practical or experiential learning. It is well worth experiencing at least one of these personally, since they can be useful for patients. Whilst it might not be appropriate for the nurse to teach patients herself, it is helpful to know what is involved so that she can be supportive.

Meditation

One of the best known relaxation methods is meditation. It involves a mental exercise that also affects the body's physiology. The purpose is to gain control over attention, so that the practitioner of meditation can choose what to focus attention on, rather than attention being subject to unpredictable events. This not only gives the individual a feeling of control, but can also be used to cut out obsessive thoughts. These can be a distressing feature of stress, in relation to, not only major life events, but also some of life's minor but repetitive 'hassles'.

There are many different ways of meditating, most of which involve focusing the attention on an object, be it imaginary or real. Deep breathing is also involved. Research has shown that meditation slows the heart and respiratory rates and decreases muscular tension, as well as inducing alpha waves in the brain. The technique can also increase the blood flow to the periphery such as the fingers and toes.

Figure 4.2 shows how 'higher' activities in the cerebral cortex, such as concentration and attention on a particular objective, may alter the activity of the hypothalamus, which can, in turn, affect the activities of the autonomic nervous and endocrine systems.

Autogenic training

This is a relaxation technique that uses a protocol to bring about a general feeling of bodily warmth and heaviness in the limbs and torso. In contrast to meditation, the induction of bodily relaxation can bring about relaxation of the mind. Physiologically, the effects are similar to those identified in the section on meditation. Autogenic training can be used to help in specific diseases, such as Raynaud's disease, migraine and even hypertension.

Progressive relaxation

In this method, people are taught to contract and then relax groups of muscles so that they can become aware of the difference. Earlier in this chapter, the effects of prolonged tension in muscles was mentioned. If one can recognise when this is happening and deliberately relax, some of the negative effects of stress can be diminished. This method is also said to relax the mind as well as the body, but it does not, apparently, affect the alpha rhythms of the brain, unlike the methods discussed above.

REFERENCES

Antonovsky A 1979 Health, stress and coping. Jossey-Bass, San Francisco

Antonovsky A 1984 The sense of coherence as a determinant of health. In: Matarazzo J D (ed.) Behavioral health: a handbook of health enhancement and disease prevention. J Wiley, New York, pp 114–129

Antonovsky A 1987 Unravelling the mystery of health. Jossey-Bass, San Francisco

Bailey R 1985 Antogenic regulation training. Sickness absence, personal problems, time, and the emotional-physical stress of student nurses in general training. Thesis submitted for degree of PhD, University of Hull

Bailey R 1986 Coping with stress in caring. Blackwell Scientific, Oxford

Bailey R, Clarke M 1989. Stress and coping in nursing. Chapman & Hall, London

Boore J 1988 Endocrine function. In: Hinchliff S, Montague S (eds) Physiology for nursing practice. Baillière Tindall, London, pp 190–198

Callahan P, Morrisey J 1993 Social support and health: a review. Journal of Advanced Nursing 18: 203–210

Clark N, Arnold E, Foulds E 1975 Serum urate and cholesterol levels in air force Academy cadets. Aviation and Space Environmental Medicine 46: 1044–1048

Cobb S 1976 Social support as a moderator of life stress. Psychosomatic Medicine 38: 300–314

Freud A 1946 The ego and mechanisms of defence. Hogarth Press, London

Gyllensköld K 1982 Breast cancer; the psychological effects of the disease and its treatment (translated by Patricia Crampton). Tavistock Publications, London

Hinchliffe S, Montague S 1988 Physiology for nursing practice. Baillière Tindall, London

Holmes T H, Rahe R 1967 The social readjustment rating scale. Journal of Psychosomatic Research 11: 213–218

Johnson J E 1973 Effects of accurate expectations about sensations on the sensory and distress components of pain. Journal of Personality and Social Psychology 27: 499–504

Kubler-Ross E 1969 On death and dying. Macmillan, New York

Summary

Life today has become extremely complex, and all of us feel that we ourselves are affected by stress and that we can recognise its effects on others. But what is stress? The definition of stress to some extent depends on whether one is considering physiological or psychological parameters, and is complicated by the fact that stress may be pleasurable as well as damaging.

Various models have been suggested as a framework for studying stress – stimulus-based, response-based and transactional – the latter probably being the most useful in the health care setting. It recognises that the individual interacts with past and present individual influences, adapting to and adjusting his environment. The action of a person to meet environmental demands is described as 'coping'. Many strategies are employed to

help an individual to cope, some of which are described in this chapter.

As a result of the investigation of major life events and illness, stress is believed to be important in the aetiology or exacerbation of many diseases, several of which are discussed in the text. The nurse has an important role in preventing and alleviating as much of the patient's stress as possible, for example by giving information and by suggesting stress-reducing strategies.

Today's NHS is subject to change after change; political and personal powerlessness is also being felt throughout the economic sector and even in the home. Thus the nurse must be aware of the areas in which she, too, is at risk of stress: a nurse suffering stress will be less able to help a patient in the same position.

Lazarus R S 1966 Psychological stress and the coping process. McGraw Hill, New York

Lazarus R S 1976 Patterns of adjustment. McGraw Hill, New York

Lazarus R S 1979 Positive denial: the case for not facing reality. Psychology Today (Nov): 44–60

Lazarus R S, Launier R 1978 Stress related transactions between person and environment. In: Pervin M, Lewis M (eds) Perspectives in interactional psychology. Plenum Press, New York, pp 287–327

Ley P, Spelman M 1967 Communicating with the patient. Staples Press, St Albans

Mathews A, Ridgeway V 1984 Psychological preparation for surgery. In: Steptoe A, Mathews A (eds) Health care and human behaviour. Academic Press, London

Parkes C M 1975 Bereavement; studies of grief in adult life. International Universities Press, New York

Pettingale K W, Morris T, Greer S 1985 Mental attitude in cancer; an additional prognostic factor. Lancet i: 750–753

Radford T 1994 White collar workers turn to chocolate, tea, coffee, alcohol and smoking to cope with worst level of stress in Europe. The Guardian, 14 November

Roberts S L 1986 Behavioural concepts and the critically ill patient, 2nd edn. Appleton Century Crofts, Norwalk, CT

Rosenman R H, Friedman M 1974 Neurogenic factors in pathogenesis of coronary heart disease. Medical Clinics of North America 58: 269–279

Seligman M 1975 Helplessness: on depression, development and death. W H Freeman, San Francisco

Selye M D 1976 The stress of life. McGraw Hill, New York

Sullivan G C 1993 Towards clarification of convergent concepts: sense of coherence, will to meaning, locus of control, learned helplessness and hardiness. Journal of Advanced Nursing 18: 1772–1778

Tucker A, Cole G E, Friedman G M 1987 Stress and serum cholesterol: a study of 7000 adult males. Health Values 11: 34–39

Worden J W 1983 Grief counselling and grief therapy. Tavistock Publications, London

Pain

Christopher J Goodall

CHAPTER CONTENTS

Pain is a component of many different
illnesses. The aims of this chapter are to:

- examine the individual nature of the pain
  experience
- outline the physiology and modulation of
  pain
- study the clinical features and assessment of
  pain
- discuss pharmacological and non-
  pharmacological methods of pain relief, and
  their evaluation.

THE INDIVIDUAL NATURE OF PAIN

'Will it hurt?' is the question almost everyone asks when facing a medical procedure, from a filling at the dentist to major surgery. One of the most demanding experiences in nursing is caring for patients who are in pain, maybe the acute severe pain of appendicitis or the chronic grinding daily pain of arthritis. Nurses need to assess those patients carefully, plan and carry out their care sensitively, and evaluate that care fully. They will want, above all, to empathise with their patients, to be with them and to show that they care.

Pain presents a tremendous challenge to nurses. While it is very satisfying for a nurse to reach out to a patient in pain, to try to understand his suffering and to show that she understands, the personal nature of the pain experience prevents her from fully empathising. Words are inadequate to explain one's pain, although people in pain often use highly descriptive words, such as burning, crushing or stabbing.

Activity 5.1

Within your group of nursing students, there will be many past experiences of pain. One person may have suffered from migraine, another from toothache and a third from appendicitis. It is useful to talk about these personal experiences of pain with your colleagues. Try to explain, as fully as you can, what your pain was like. When it is the turn of the others, listen to them carefully. Can you really grasp the intensity and quality of *their* pain?

Group discussions may reveal that people have not only very individual experiences of pain, but also differing attitudes to it, often based on previous experiences. They may face a dental appointment for a filling with equanimity, because their past experience of that dentist has taught them to trust her. Others, however, may feel apprehensive, even fearful, about dental treatment, because of a previous traumatic encounter.

Pain is personal. It is an individual experience to which people react in an individual manner, their reactions being based on individual life histories. The key to the effective treatment of pain, therefore, is to assess the patient fully and carefully, and to act on what he says about his pain. In other words, nurses should treat each person as the 'expert' in his own symptoms, including pain: he knows better than any nurse or doctor what he is feeling. In individualised nursing care, there is no place for the issuing of pain killers during a routine 'drugs round'. This is an excellent method of ensuring that patients must wait, in pain, for the nurses' convenience and set routine. Nor is it a mark of individualised care to decide that Mr Jones, being 3 days post-operation, has no further need of injections of a strong analgesia (or pain killer) but can now make do with less potent tablets. Mr Jones, being an individual, may not fall in with such ward routines and expectations. He may actually *need* a further injection.

This chapter examines not only the physiological nature of this important life experience called pain, but also the psychological factors that play a part in that experience. It also considers, briefly, the various responses to or treatments of pain that are now available. A chapter of this length can only provide an introduction to this fascinating and vital subject; consequently, there is a list of further reading at the end.

PHYSIOLOGY OF PAIN

NERVE ENDINGS

Everyone knows that it hurts to prick a finger with a needle or to touch a hot oven with a hand; these are very common examples of causes of pain. A patient following an abdominal operation may also experience pain if his gut distends with trapped gas. A person with an arthritic knee joint feels pain, especially if her leg is suddenly jolted. In each of these cases, the starting point of the pain is the stimulation of nerve endings – in the skin, the gut or the joints respectively.

Nerve endings within the skin can be stimulated by various factors, including temperature and pressure. Putting one's foot into a warm bath may be a pleasant sensation, but if the water temperature is too high, the experience is that of pain. Free nerve endings in the skin that respond to harmful or *noxious* stimuli are called *nociceptors*. The skin is very well supplied by such nerve endings, in order to warn a person of harmful or potentially harmful stimuli. In this situation, nociceptors play a major role as information-gatherers.

Skin that is cut or pierced, for example by a scalpel or needle, also produces the sensation of pain (unless either the skin or the whole patient is anaesthetised). However, the intestine, if cut during surgery, responds to neither the action of the scalpel nor the burning of diathermy (a method of heat-sealing severed blood vessels during an operation). Instead, nerve endings in the gut wall that respond to stretch are stimulated if, post-operatively, there is a build up of gas within the intestine. This explains the pain experienced as 'wind' by patients 2 or 3 days after their abdominal operation (see Case example 5.7).

Question 5.1

Can you think of another hollow organ that, when over-extended, will cause pain?

Brain tissue, when incised, also does not cause pain, so a brain operation might be possible without an anaesthetic. However, the skin covering the skull and the meninges within the skull (the membranes covering the brain itself) would give rise to pain if cut, so would need to be anaesthetised.

(One answer to Question 5.1, incidentally, is the bladder. Some patients develop urinary retention, which means that they cannot pass urine. The bladder fills more and more, and the bladder wall stretches to accommodate the increasing volume of urine, thus stimulating stretch receptors within the wall. This explains why urinary retention can be so painful and should be treated swiftly – see Case example 5.3, below.)

NERVOUS PATHWAYS TO THE BRAIN

For a noxious stimulus to be perceived as pain, nerve impulses must travel from the stimulated nerve endings to the brain. There are different pathways followed by nerve impulses, which give rise to the sensation of pain of differing qualities. Case example 5.1 illustrates two types of pain.

Case example 5.1

Mrs Edwards is having a blood test in the outpatients department. She is well used to these, so is not particularly bothered by the test. As the needle pierces her skin just above the vein, she feels a sharp, pricking sensation, which is very clearly localised. This sensation rapidly passes off, however, and is replaced by a duller pain, somewhat harder to pinpoint to one particular area. This ache continues even after the needle is withdrawn. The technician hands Mrs Edwards a cotton wool swab to press on the puncture site in order to stop any bleeding, and applying this pressure seems to help to relieve the pain.

Physiologists distinguish between *fast pain* and *slow pain*. Each sensation has different receptors, nerve pathways within the spinal cord and pathways to the brain.

Fast pain (that initial sharp pain Mrs Edwards felt as the needle entered her skin) occurs when certain nociceptors are stimulated. These receptors are served by small-diameter myelinated fibres (Aδ fibres), which travel to the spinal cord, where they synapse (see Ch. 1 for details of nervous tissue anatomy and physiology).

From the synapses in the spinal cord, fibres cross to the opposite side of the body and carry impulses up to the brain stem, the thalamus and the cerebral cortex. Such nerve tracts are named according to their source and destination; hence, spinothalamic tracts convey nerve impulses from the spine to the thalamus.

Fast pain is usually sharp and can be well pinpointed or localised.

Slow pain (the dull ache following the needle insertion) occurs with the stimulation of polymodal nociceptors by certain substances, such as bradykinin and prostaglandins, released from damaged cells. On being stimulated, these nerve endings send impulses along much finer, non-myelinated nerve fibres (C fibres) to the spinal cord, where they synapse with other fibres. Nerve signals then cross to the opposite side of the body and travel to the reticular formation within the brain stem (these nerve tracts thus being known as spinoreticular tracts). From here, impulses travel to the hypothalamus, thalamus and cerebral cortex.

Slow pain is more difficult to localise than is fast pain. Consequently, Mrs Edwards would experience the later, duller ache in a somewhat wider area of her arm than the initial sharp, highly localised fast pain.

Fast pain and slow pain pathways are shown diagrammatically in Figure 5.1.

It should be noted that the dull ache of an arthritic joint is caused by the release from damaged tissue cells of substances such as prostaglandins. There are certain drugs available that help reduce the pain of arthritis by blocking this production; these are known as anti-prostaglandins.

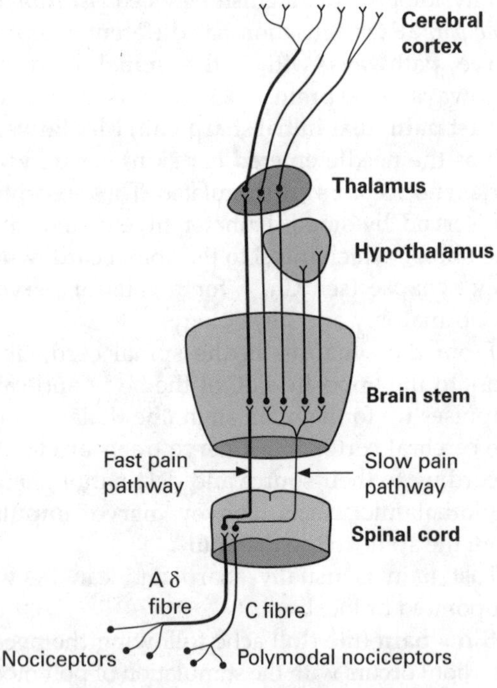

AREAS OF THE BRAIN INVOLVED IN PAIN SENSATION

Nerve impulses reach the cerebral cortex after travelling via different routes, as described above. Impulses reaching the thalamus give rise to a generalised sensation of ill-defined pain (for example in a leg or arm). It is the somatosensory cortex that pinpoints the source of the pain, as it does with sensations other than pain. The thalamus acts as a relay station, passing on the nerve signal to its higher command centre.

Nerve impulses reaching the reticular formation are similarly relayed, but within the reticular formation itself, these nerve impulses activate adjacent nerve cells. In this way, more areas of the brain are activated, so the source of the pain signals cannot be exactly localised. Because slow pain messages are sent via the spinal cord to the reticular formation, this type of pain is not well localised.

REFERRED PAIN

Nurses on coronary care units (CCUs) know that the pain associated with a myocardial infarction (heart attack) is not only experienced in the centre of the chest, but also seems to travel down the left arm to the fingers of the left hand, and up into the left jaw. This is an example of **referred pain**. Knowledge of the physiology of pain helps to understand this phenomenon.

Nerve fibres travelling from internal organs, such as the heart, enter the spinal cord via the dorsal horn of grey matter ('dorsal' referring to the posterior area of the spinal cord). Other nerve fibres from the skin also enter the spinal cord in the immediate vicinity. Within the dorsal horn, intermediate neurones link these 'afferent' (or incoming) nerve fibres, and in this way the brain is deceived into interpreting the pain impulses as coming from the skin of the left arm rather than, or as well as, from the heart muscle.

Referred pain can be felt in peripheral structures some way distant from the actual source of the

Figure 5.1   Fast and slow pain pathways.

pain. A patient with an inflamed gallbladder often feels only generalised upper abdominal pain, as well as pain very closely localised to the tip of the right shoulder. Referred pain has an important role in arriving at an accurate diagnosis, and suggests how important it is for the admitting nurse to listen carefully to the patient's description of his pain.

PHANTOM LIMB PAIN

When a leg is amputated, the nerve pathways above the level of the operation remain intact, as do the brain areas served by those nerves. It is often the case that a patient experiences severe pain in his amputated limb – in a leg that is no longer there. Such pain can be very difficult to treat, but it is important for the nurse to show that she believes the patient's pain is *real* and not imaginary. Phantom limb pain causes real suffering for the patient. It also shows that pain is a sensation, rather than just the stimulation of nerve endings.

ENDOGENOUS PAIN KILLERS

Most people have heard of cases in which a soldier in the heat of battle receives a serious wound but remains unaware of it until the excitement abates. In such a case, severe tissue damage does not seem to give rise to the expected warning signal of pain. There are several possible reasons for this, one of which involves the nervous system's own natural opioids or pain killers.

Morphine, one of the products of opium, has long been known as a highly effective analgesic or pain killer. However, only as recently as the 1970s was the discovery made that morphine acted by joining with certain receptors in different parts of the nervous system, including the brain stem and spinal cord.

The presence of these 'opioid receptors' within the nervous system suggested to physiologists that there must be one or more naturally occurring (endogenous) analgesics that would 'fit' these receptors – it is unlikely that the human body would contain opioid receptors that had no function but to wait around until the human race developed drugs to fit them!

It was discovered that cells within the brain and spinal cord secreted substances that joined with these receptors, thus inhibiting the transmission of nerve impulses at synapses. In this way, they acted like the opiate drugs, morphine and diamorphine. These endogenous (built-in) opioids consist of three main groups:

- endorphins
- enkephalins
- dynorphins.

These block (or inhibit) the passage of nerve impulses by attaching to pre-synaptic receptors of $A\delta$ and C nerve fibres. It is suggested that they work by blocking calcium channels within nerve terminal membranes (Guyton 1991). Once these calcium channels are blocked, the nerve terminal membrane cannot secrete the neurotransmitter required to ensure the passage of a nerve impulse from one neurone to the next thus blocking the transmission of pain.

The endogenous opioids are especially secreted when the body is undergoing stress, for example during an athletic event. When one rubs the skin over a bumped elbow, the pain experienced diminishes, partly because the stimulation of nerve receptors in the skin brings about secretion of endogenous opioids from within the pain pathways. These then block or diminish the transmission of pain signals up to the brain (Guyton 1991). The next section, however, gives an alternative explanation of this phenomenon.

It is thought that acupuncture has its analgesic effects also by stimulating the secretion of the endogenous opioids.

THE 'GATE THEORY' OF PAIN MODULATION

The effects of rubbing an injured area play an important part in the 'gate' theory of pain modulation, which is here described in very simple terms (Case example 5.2).

This profile illustrates that there is much more to pain relief than just drugs, as this staff nurse realised. Figures 5.2 A–C explain, using a series of simple, highly figurative, diagrams, how such nursing measures might be helping Miss Philips.

Case example 5.2

Miss Philips is awakened every night by the pain in her foot. She has long been a cigarette smoker, and now, as a complication of this, she has gangrene in the toes of her left foot. She is currently in hospital awaiting an operation to remove the foot. Last night, she asked the nurse for some pain killers, which were only partially effective.

Tonight, there is a different nurse on duty, who brings her not only two tablets but a cup of tea. The nurse then sits down by Miss Philips and they talk about their families and the holidays they have enjoyed.

'Will you rub that awful leg for me?', asks Miss Philips, and the staff nurse gently massages the left leg as the two of them converse.

After half an hour, Miss Philips is feeling drowsy and thinks she will try to get off to sleep once again. 'You know, my foot feels so much better now. Pity you aren't on duty every night.'

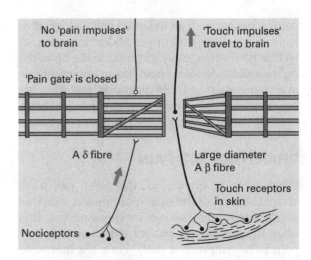

Figure 5.2B   (Highly figurative.) Nerve impulses from touch receptors in the skin pass through the spinal cord and ascend to the brain, but the spinal 'gate' is closed to the impulses from the nociceptors, and the person feels no pain.

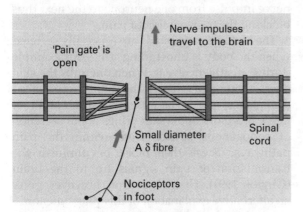

Figure 5.2A   The 'gate' is open to nerve impulses from nociceptors, and the person feels pain.

The nociceptors in Miss Philips' foot are stimulated by ischaemia (lack of oxygenated blood, in the same way as ischaemia causes the pain of myocardial infarction). Figure 5.2A shows a small diameter Aδ nerve fibre travelling from the nociceptors to the spinal cord. Here it synapses with another neurone, which then passes up the cord towards the brain. The figure shows, in a highly diagrammatic form, how a 'gate' in the spinal cord is open to allow pain impulses through.

Figure 5.2B shows what happens when the skin is gently massaged (as, for example, by the

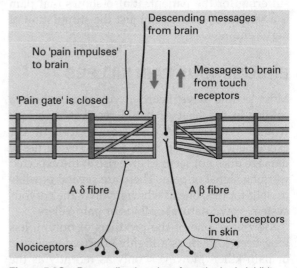

Figure 5.2C   Descending impulses from the brain inhibit the transmission of pain impulses in the spinal cord; the pain 'gate' is closed, and the person feels no pain.

nurse in Case example 5.2). Rubbing stimulates sensory receptors in the skin and sends nerve impulses along large diameter myelinated Aβ fibres to the spinal cord, and thence to the brain. Impulses travel faster along these Aβ fibres than along the smaller diameter Aδ fibres. Again in very diagrammatic form, Figure 5.2B shows how the arrival of these touch-instigated nerve impulses at the spinal cord opens a gate for their own passage up the cord to the brain, but *shuts* the gate to the passage of the slower pain impulses.

In very non-physiological language, rubbing the skin over an affected area keeps the brain 'busy' and stops it being too bothered about impulses arising from the source of the pain. Similarly, in Case example 5.1, Mrs Edwards relieved the pain following her blood test by pressing with a swab on the needle site. This pressure sends nerve impulses along Aβ fibres, thus closing the spinal cord gate to pain impulses.

Question 5.2

What other physiological function is served by the application of pressure to the puncture site?

There is a further factor that reduces (inhibits) the transmission of impulses from the nociceptors through the spinal cord, and hence shuts the gate on those impulses. In Case example 5.2, the nurse chatted with Miss Philips, as well as giving her two pain killers. That conversation will have helped reduce the patient's anxiety.

Messages travelling *down* the cord from the brain, which arise from the person's sense of well-being, help to shut the spinal cord gate against the pain impulses by inhibiting the transmission of nerve impulses from the Aδ fibres across its synapse in the cord. Figure 5.2C shows how these descending messages help to shut the gate.

The gate theory of pain control was first proposed by Melzack & Wall in 1965, and has been modified by them since then. Their theory helps to explain why simple measures such as rubbing a painful elbow reduce the pain felt, and also how there is a strong psychological input to one's experience of pain. Giving Miss Philips two tablets had some effect on her pain, but combining those tablets with company, conversation and a cup of tea eased her pain much more effectively. This is an example of nursing care using a knowledge of physiology and psychology.

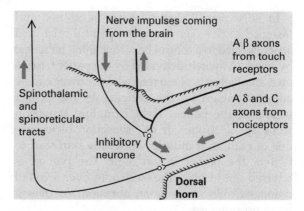

Figure 5.3 'Pain messages' along the spinothalamic and spinoreticular tracts can be inhibited by activity in larger diameter Aβ fibres from touch receptors and descending messages from the brain. Both of these excite the inhibitory interneurone seen in the figure. (Adapted from Rutishauser 1994.)

In summary, the nervous system not only receives and responds to pain-causing stimuli, but also *modulates* the incoming nerve signals and thus the experience of pain. This modulation occurs in the brain and within the spinal cord.

Having studied the highly diagrammatic figures used to help explain the gate theory of pain control, it should now be easier to understand a more conventional diagram, as in Figure 5.3.

TRANSCUTANEOUS ELECTRICAL NERVE STIMULATION (TENS)

Although this is a form of treatment for specific types of pain, it is worth considering here because it helps to explain both the gate theory of pain modulation and the function of endogenous opioids. TENS can be used for pain that has already been diagnosed, such as that of an arthritic joint. It is not used for pain that has not been investigated and identified.

Question 5.3

Why do you think it is so important to make an accurate diagnosis of the cause of a person's pain before starting pain control therapies?

In TENS, small electrodes are moistened and fastened to the skin above the painful area, and are connected to a control box (containing batteries) by wires. A switch, activated by the patient, turns on a small electrical current whose power can be adjusted, again by the patient. As the power increases, the patient feels a tingling sensation from the electrodes. If this sensation turns into one of pain, or if muscles under the skin start to twitch, the power is too high. The patient is advised not to place the electrodes over areas of damaged skin (such as an abrasion) or over a bony prominence.

TENS reduces the patient's sensation of pain by sending nerve impulses along Aβ myelinated fibres, thus closing the spinal gate to pain impulses. It also causes the secretion of endogenous opioids, discussed above. Thus, even after the current is switched off, the analgesic effect can continue for many hours.

An important feature of TENS therapy is that it is *under the patient's own control*. Consequently, the patient feels as if she is contributing positively to the control of her own pain, rather than simply enduring it. Furthermore, TENS avoids the side-effects of drugs. There are few problems in using TENS, providing the instructions are followed carefully. Some patients with decreased manual dexterity find it difficult, and sometimes impossible, to fix the electrodes without help.

CLINICAL FEATURES OF PAIN

It is important for nurses to observe a patient for any signs associated with pain. Patients' verbalisation of their pain is an important diagnostic aid, and the words patients choose to describe their pain can help the doctor to form an accurate diagnosis.

However, some patients are unable to verbalise their pain, while others may choose not to. A young man with a severe learning disability may not know the words to use to tell nurses he has pain. An elderly woman following a stroke may be unconscious, yet still be aware of pain and discomfort. A road traffic accident victim,

following a head injury, may be artificially ventilated in the intensive care unit and thus unable to speak for himself. A very young child will show signs of distress, but cannot use words to describe his pain. All these patients will be unable to talk about their pain to the nurses caring for them. Instead, the nurses will have to judge their patients' pain from their behaviour and other clinical pointers.

Some patients may even refuse to admit to having pain (which they perceive as a sign of weakness) or find it difficult to 'bother the nurses' with their pain.

Case example 5.3 illustrates the possible clinical features that the nurse may observe in a patient with pain.

Case example 5.3

Mr Johnson has had an operation to remove an enlarged prostate gland. Two days afterwards, he is sitting out of bed and taking oral fluids well. There is a catheter in his bladder to drain urine, as well as blood and blood clots that formed following the operation.

When Michael, the student nurse, goes to Mr Johnson with his mid-morning drink, he notices that the patient's face is twisted and grimacing. Neither is Mr Johnson sitting still, but is shifting his position in the chair as if in great discomfort. Michael asks what the matter is, and Mr Johnson tells him of a bad pain in his lower abdomen. The nurse takes the patient's pulse and blood pressure, and finds them both somewhat raised.

When Michael hurriedly fetches the staff nurse, she sees that no urine is draining down the clear plastic tubing from the catheter – it is blocked by a blood clot. By squeezing the tubing towards the urine collection bag, the clot is freed and urine drains again. Mr Johnson's pain swiftly disappears.

Most of the clinical features described here are easy to understand. Moderate pain tends to raise the blood pressure and pulse. The patient is often disturbed and unable to sit still, tossing and turning in bed or in his chair, and having interrupted sleep at night. His facial expression is sometimes distorted by pain, and if he is conscious, he may vocalise about his pain.

There are two important features of the nurses' actions in this profile. First, on seeing that his patient was in pain, the student nurse acted promptly. He treated the situation as an emergency and fetched help. Second, the staff nurse's actions followed a swift yet informed nursing assessment, based on her knowledge of her patient and his operation. The answer to Mr Johnson's pain was not, in this instance, tablets or an injection: neither of these would have unblocked his catheter. The action required was to 'milk' the catheter tubing, thus releasing the blockage that the staff nurse knew, through observation and experience, was there.

The vocabulary of pain

Case example 5.4

Dr Adams is called out to one of his patients who is complaining of 'crushing' pain in the middle of her chest. The lady's daughter is with her, and tells the doctor that her mother also has pain 'like toothache' in the left side of her jaw.

When he arrives at the house, Dr Adams sees Mrs Fewster lying flat on the sofa. Her face is very pale, almost grey in colour, and although it is pouring with sweat, her skin feels cold. She is moaning slightly and seems to be barely conscious.

The doctor takes her pulse and finds that it is very rapid, uneven and feeble. Her blood pressure, which is usually about 140/80 mmHg, is now scarcely audible through his stethoscope. He judges it to be 70/40 mmHg.

He asks Mrs Fewster how she feels; she can barely open her eyes. 'I'm scared stiff, doctor,' she murmurs.

There are clearly some differences between Mrs Fewster's pain and Mr Johnson's. The pain of a heart attack is very severe indeed, and the patient is often terrified. Fear is, in fact, one of the clinical features associated with a heart attack, whereas, by contrast, the usual daily pain of an arthritic knee joint, for example, does not tend to scare the patient. Mrs Fewster's blood pressure is extremely low, rather than raised, as would be likely to occur with moderate pain.

The words a patient might use about his heart pain are commonly 'crushing', 'like a tight band round my chest' and 'like a vice'. Such words are very significant. With appendicitis, a patient might describe it as 'burning', 'stabbing' or 'like a knife'. The chronic pain of arthritis is often described as 'aching', 'gnawing' and 'nagging'.

Different pains have their own vocabulary. The words commonly used tend to emphasise the *intensity* of the pain perceived by the patient. Other words are based on the *affective* nature of the pain – frightening, irritating, annoying (Melzack & Wall 1988).

Severe pain is often associated with feelings of nausea, so words like 'sickening' are also used by patients. Because of this, drug regimens for pain relief often also include an anti-emetic.

Words used by the patient to describe his pain should be recorded accurately by the assessing nurse. They may help to pinpoint his diagnosis and can also help to determine whether or not treatment with certain pain-killing drugs is working. If a patient claims that his pain is 'absolutely terrible' before he takes the prescribed tablets, and an hour after swallowing them says his pain is 'not too bad now', the nurse will know, albeit somewhat vaguely, that the drugs have worked. The trouble with such descriptions is that, in the realm of pain control, they are somewhat inexact. Understanding this is important when considering methods of assessing a patient's pain and evaluating the effectiveness of analgesics and other therapies.

ASSESSING A PATIENT'S PAIN

In order to treat a patient's pain on an individual basis, rather than as a care routine, nurses have an important role in fully assessing their patients both on admission and throughout their stay in hospital, or during a period of care in the community.

Pain assessment tools

Figures 5.4A and B show two related pain assessment tools. These scales are usually printed on small pieces of card or plastic. They are highly effective if correctly used and if the appropriate tool is used for each individual patient.

Figure 5.4A shows a visual analogue scale (VAS), which consists of a vertical or horizontal line with a brief pain desciptor at either end. The

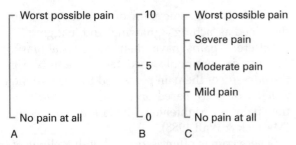

Figure 5.4 (A) Visual analogue scale (VAS). (B) Numerical rating scale (NRS). (C) A simple 5-point verbal descriptor pain scale (VDS).

patient is asked to mark on the scale the point that represents the pain he is currently experiencing. The nurse then measures the distance from the bottom of the scale, for comparison with further readings (for example after the administration of pain-killing drugs).

The numerical rating scale (NRS) shown in Figure 5.4B is similar to the VAS, but has numbers instead of pain desciptors. NRSs can vary slightly; some have simply 0 at the lower end and 10 at the upper, while another may have the full scale, from 0 to 10.

Both the VAS and the NRS are difficult for patients with poor vision to use. Also, for the scale to be effective, the patient has to be capable of representing his pain experience on it, which is not possible for all patients. A patient may see no connection between his 'horrible pain' and the number '8' on the scale in front of him.

Figure 5.4C shows a somewhat different assessment tool – the verbal descriptor scale (VDS). This consists of a vertical or horizontal line with descriptors at regular intervals along it. Some writers claim this is more popular with elderly patients (Raiman 1986), but there are several problems with it. First, the VDS is less sensitive than are the other scales shown, because the patient cannot pick a spot *between* two descriptors. In this respect, slight changes in the pain experience (for example, following analgesia) cannot easily be demonstrated. Some patients, too, may misunderstand some of the descriptors, whilst others may disagree with the order in which some of the descriptors appear on the scale. Those with learning difficulties, and with certain mental health problems, may have difficulty

dealing with a range of verbal descriptors. VDSs can be of different complexity, some with 10 levels, others with only five (as in Figure 5.4C). The simpler, shorter verbal scales tend to be the least sensitive.

Children and babies in pain

Assessing a child's pain presents particular problems for nurses and doctors, both in hospital and in the home. Whilst a young teenager may be able to use appropriate pain vocabulary, and to fill in an assessment tool, a child of 4 or 5 years old will not. A parent may be able to spot signs of generalised distress – the child may be crying and red-faced, unable to stay still and holding his fists clenched tightly. However, another child may be pale-faced, silent and lying absolutely still.

Pain assessment tools have been devised that help the child to communicate his pain. Some use printed faces: some smiling and happy, others frowning. The child is asked to point to the face whose expression seems closest to that of his own feelings. Other simple drawings represent the shape of the body, and the child is encouraged to point to which part hurts him. Appropriate language must be used: 'Does your tummy hurt you?', rather than 'Do you have abdominal pain?'

These drawings cannot be used with babies. Assessing the pain experienced by a baby is very difficult, although it is easier to observe generalised distress in a very young child or baby. Some Canadian research has focused on the facial expression and the pattern of crying in babies during certain invasive and non-invasive procedures, including intramuscular injections. A common response to the injection was squeezing the eyes tightly shut and opening the mouth. Some changes in the quality of the babies' crying were also observed (Grunau et al 1990).

Martikainen & Heinonen (1990) state that newly-born babies – even those born prematurely – require analgesia if undergoing surgery, even though it is very difficult to judge the quantity and quality of pain experienced. They stress the importance of carefully calculating appropriate drug doses for each individual baby, and observing for side-effects, to which such tiny babies are particularly susceptible.

Caring for the young child in pain, and for his distressed parents, is a highly specialised and demanding area of nursing, requiring its own specialised training.

FACTORS AFFECTING THE PAIN EXPERIENCE

It is tempting to assume that the degree of pain experienced relates exactly to the strength of the pain-causing stimulus. This would suggest that a 'major' operation, for example, is more painful than a 'minor' one. However, the experience of pain depends on far more than its initiating event.

Past experience of pain

A person's past experience of pain affects the way in which he reacts to potentially painful situations. Case examples 5.5 and 5.6 demonstrate this.

Case example 5.5

After walking half a mile, two elderly friends, Janet and Doris, admit to feeling moderate pain in their hip joints. For Janet, this is a new situation. She has not experienced such pain before, so she is very worried by it. The worry causes the pain experience itself to worsen. Doris, by contrast, has long had an arthritic hip, so she is almost dismissive about her hip pain. She is certainly not worried by it – she knows what is causing it.

Case example 5.6

After using the same dentist for 10 years, David has no doubts about attending for a tooth filling. He knows the dentist will explain every step of the proceedings and that, from past experience, it will hurt very little. Harry, on the other hand, does not really trust his dentist. The last filling he had was rather painful. On going to the dentist this time, Harry is tense and anxious, almost ready to feel pain as soon as he hears the sound of the drill.

Understanding the cause of pain

The degree of perceived pain is affected by not only the past experience of pain, but also knowledge of the *cause* of the pain. A pain whose cause is known tends not to give rise to as much anxiety as does a pain that is new to the sufferer. In addition, anxiety tends to increase the pain experience itself (Case example 5.7 and Activity 5.2).

Case example 5.7

Roger is in hospital, having had his appendix out 3 days previously. He is looking forward to going home to his wife and children, but this evening he feels a new sort of pain in his abdomen. His abdomen feels 'tight', and it seems to be pulling on his clips. Has something gone wrong inside? Is he bleeding from the operation site, and no-one knows about it? He becomes very agitated and calls the nurse. He is far from soothed when she tells Roger his pain is 'only wind'.

This patient needs information, rather than platitudes, to help him to deal with his pain. Until he receives such information, he is prey to all sorts of terrible imaginings – so, of course, his pain worsens (Activity 5.2).

Activity 5.2

How would you have handled Roger's worries? Discuss with your colleagues what your actions might have been, then read the following passage. Do not bother too much about the medical details of Roger's pain or your response to it, since you may not yet have enough information from your course to help you. Concentrate instead on the way in which you would *respond* to this very anxious patient.

The nurse did not handle Roger's question well, and further explanation is needed. Gas is building up within his bowel because the intestinal contents have temporarily stopped moving onwards, owing to the operation. The nurse should say that this is quite normal following an abdominal operation. The technical term is 'paralytic ileus', but it is not helpful to use it at this stage, nor should she use the dismissive phrase 'only wind'. Following an accurate explanation, Roger is likely to be further reassured by the nurse checking his pulse and blood pressure. He now realises that someone is taking his worries seriously, and the pain will probably be considerably alleviated.

Hayward's (1975) research showed how *pre*-operative information on a patient's condition could help his *post*-operative recovery. A patient who understood what his operation was for, what equipment there might be (such as a drip or catheter) when he came round from the anaesthetic, and what sort of discomfort there might be afterwards, tended to require less post-operative analgesia than did someone given no such information.

It is important to note that Hayward wrote about information, rather than vague reassurances. 'Don't worry, you'll be all right' tends not to provide much comfort to a patient awaiting operation. By contrast, the explanation in Case example 5.8 given by a nurse to a young man with appendicitis provides both information and reassurance.

Case example 5.8

'I'll be taking you down to theatre when the trolley arrives. I'll stay with you while they give you the anaesthetic – no, it's not a mask over your face, just an injection in the back of your hand. You'll go off to sleep really quickly and smoothly. When you wake up, there'll be some theatre nurses looking after you. Don't worry about their odd uniform; they always wear those blue caps down there. When you come back to this ward, I'll be looking after you again. You may have a drip tube in your arm, just to give you some fluid. Your wound may be a bit sore, but we can give you an injection that'll get rid of any pain.'

Here there is both reassurance and useful information. The patient has both the comfort of human company (and therefore some distraction from his situation) and warnings, in language he can understand, about what to expect. He is not patronised. He is told the truth – there *will* be some soreness after the operation – but he is also told what the nurses can do about that.

Culture

Not only does present mood – anxiety or calm, depression or happiness – make a difference to

the amount of pain experienced, but also the culture from which people derive influences their attitude towards pain and how to respond to it. Melzack & Wall (1988) give some hair-raising examples of rituals in Indian villages that seem to be unbearably painful, but which the participants endure without any apparent sign of pain. In some parts of the world, religious enthusiasts 'celebrate' Easter by having themselves crucified – actually nailed to a cross. It is not known whether they feel pain during this procedure, but they do not appear to give any sign of suffering.

People from some cultures are said to respond very vocally to pain, crying and sobbing with much verbalisation. They are not cowards, but are simply carrying out their culturally in-fluenced response to pain. By contrast, the typical British response to pain is that of the 'stiff upper lip': the patient tends to keep to himself any signs of distress. (However, the reputation for silent suf-fering among the British is not always deserved. The author has witnessed a very large rugby player with a dislocated shoulder cry un-restrainedly at the sight of an approaching needle.)

Alcohol and other drugs

A further factor affecting the amount of pain felt, and the response to it, is the influence of alcohol and other drugs. A driver who is very drunk may be cut from the wreckage of a car without requiring any pain-killing drugs from the paramedics. Similarly, heroin users may damage themselves by falling or leaning against a hot radiator without being aware of it. Heroin is not only a sedative, but also a powerful analgesic. As diamorphine, it is used widely in the medical treatment of severe pain.

Other drugs, such as cannabis or even legally prescribed sleeping tablets, can diminish a person's awareness of his surroundings, including those that are dangerous. It is all too easy for a wrist to be fractured when the arm bangs against furniture, or for the buttocks to be severely burned when a person sits on a hot radiator. The drugs that have been taken lead to diminished awareness of pain.

Inability to perceive pain

Some children are born with a nervous system that fails to provide them with the warning power of pain (congenital analgesia). Such children, during the natural rough and tumble of growing up, often sustain severe damage to their limbs, including fractures. Parents and schoolteachers have to observe these children very carefully in order to spot limb deformities – pointers to possible fractures. Cases of congenital analgesia are, fortunately, rare (Melzack & Wall 1988).

Much more common in modern society, with road accidents and other traumatic incidents, is the person with a fractured spine. Below the level of the fracture, neuronal communication is lost, the person being unable both to receive sensory information from the lower limbs and to send out motor instructions.

Activity 5.3 illustrates how tissue damage may occur without the person knowing, and how pain and discomfort can be important warnings.

Activity 5.3

Andy is 18 years old, and, following a car accident in which his spine was broken, he is a wheelchair user. He has no feeling at all from his waist down, nor has he any muscular control over his legs. As if to compensate, his arms and shoulders are now very powerful, and he plays wheelchair basketball whenever he can.

He has been warned about the possibility of pressure sores. The problem for Andy is that, being paralysed, he cannot feel when these areas are becoming sore, and he therefore does not automatically shift position to get comfortable.

Discuss with your colleagues what you might advise Andy to do. If he were a patient in your care, what nursing measures would reduce the risk of his developing pressure sores?

THE PHARMACOLOGY OF PAIN RELIEF

This section contains a description of a few of the drugs that are available for the treatment of pain. More information will be found in textbooks on pharmacology (e.g. Hopkins 1992). It is at present principally the responsibility of doctors to prescribe pain killers (and other drugs), although nurse prescribing is gradually being introduced. The role of the nurse regarding the use of analgesics is that of carrying out an initial patient assessment, safely administering the prescribed drug at the correct time, and observing its effect and any possible side-effects. If a prescribed drug fails to reduce a patient's pain, it is the nurse's responsibility to inform the doctor and to press for the prescription to be altered.

The analgesics described here are grouped according to their comparative strengths. Many of the milder analgesics are available for sale without a medical prescription.

ANALGESICS FOR MILD PAIN

The most common drugs used for pain such as headache, toothache and period pains (menorrhagia) are aspirin and paracetamol. Both may be bought without a prescription, but this does *not* mean that they are without side-effects.

Aspirin

Aspirin is one of a large group of non-steroidal anti-inflammatory drugs (NSAIDs) that were mentioned earlier in this chapter. Prostaglandins, released by damaged cells, are substances that cause pain and promote inflammation. It is joint inflammation in rheumatoid arthritis that causes the main clinical features of pain and stiffness. Aspirin, like the other NSAIDs, blocks or reduces the production of prostaglandins, thus helping to reduce both inflammation and pain. For useful discussions on both prostaglandins and NSAIDs, see Trounce (1994, pp. 105, 183) and Hopkins (1992, pp. 360–361, 355–356).

Adult dose. One or two (300 mg) tablets every 4 hours. The maximum adult daily dose is 12 tablets. The tablets should be taken just after food. For people who have difficulties swallowing large tablets, aspirin can also be taken dissolved in water.

Side-effects. These include gastric pain caused by irritation of the lining of the stomach.

Sometimes a blood vessel can be eroded in the lining of the gastrointestinal tract and the patient can either vomit blood (**haematemasis**) or pass blood from the rectum (**melaena**).

Activity 5.4

Can you discover why aspirin, even in low doses, is no longer normally given to children under the age of 12? You will need to consult textbooks of pharmacology or perhaps paediatric nursing.

Paracetamol

Adult dose. One or two (500 mg) tablets every 6 hours. The maximum adult daily dose is 8 tablets. Like aspirin, paracetamol can be obtained in soluble form.

Side-effects. Unwanted effects are fewer in number than for aspirin, in that paracetamol does not cause gastrointestinal irritation. The maximum daily dose of 8 tablets should *never* be exceded because of the danger of liver damage, which, although treatable if caught in time, may be irreversible. Prolonged daily intake of paracetamol, even at the correct dosage, may lead to kidney damage (analgesic nephropathy).

For the treatment of paracetamol poisoning, see Hopkins (1992, p. 512).

Box 5.1   Look after yourself

Nurses are just as susceptible to headaches and muscular pains as are the rest of the population, perhaps more so because of the strenuous and stressful nature of their work. It is worth emphasising here the very real danger of taking too many paracetamol tablets. This is important because paracetamol is so easily available – even in supermarkets – and because this drug can be 'hidden' within a proprietary name label. For example, some medicines for colds and influenza contain a mixture of drugs, including paracetamol.

As a broad rule, it is preferable to buy a single named drug, so that you can be sure what and *how much* you are taking. Another rule is, if your headache or period pain is not relieved by the correct dosage of a particular analgesic, you need a different drug, rather than more of the same. In such an event you need the advice of your doctor.

ANALGESICS FOR MODERATE PAIN

The pain experienced following a fracture, or convalescing after an operation, is often treated with these drugs.

Co-proxamol

Adult dose. One or two tablets every 6 hours. The maximum adult daily dose is 8 tablets. Each tablet contains a mixture of two drugs:

- paracetamol 325 mg
- dextropropoxyphene 32.5 mg.

Side-effects. One danger of overdosage is clearly that of taking too much paracetamol, so the daily dose of 8 tablets should not be exceeded. Other side-effects include nausea and constipation. If taken in excess, the dextropropoxyphene component may cause respiratory depression. These tablets should not be taken with alcohol.

Dihydrocodeine

Adult dose. One or two (30 mg) tablets every 6 or 8 hours after food. The maximum daily dose is 120–180 mg.

This drug is more powerful than its relative, codeine, and like codeine, which can be found in some cough mixtures, it can help to suppress a cough. It is used for chronic pain when it is not considered advisable to prescribe a stronger narcotic, such as morphine. Even so, both codeine and dihydrocodeine are derived from opium, as is morphine.

Side-effects include drowsiness and constipation. To help prevent the latter, the patient is advised to take the drug after meals.

ANALGESICS FOR SEVERE PAIN

The drugs described here are used for the treatment of severe cancer pain, immediately following surgery and for the severe pain of a heart attack. They can be given orally but are more often given by injection, into either the muscle (intramuscular) or the vein (intravenous).

Morphine

Adult dose. Following surgery, an intramuscular injection of 10 mg morphine may be given, repeated every 6 hours. Patients usually no longer need such a strong pain killer after approximately the second or third post-operative day (although there are individual differences).

Morphine can be given orally, one useful form of which is as a slow-release tablet, MST Continus. These tablets, which are given twice a day to patients with cancer, are provided in strengths rising from 10 mg to 200 mg. Such doses give some idea of how doctors can gradually increase the amount of morphine their patients require over a period of time. A patient with cancer may be started on MST Continus 10 mg twice daily, but over 3 months, this could be increased in stages to MST Continus 60 mg twice a day, and subsequently even higher.

Side-effects. Morphine has many side-effects. One of these, euphoria, is useful, in that the patient feels relaxed and happy despite his diagnosis of cancer. Other side-effects, such as nausea and vomiting, can be severe. An anti-emetic is often given with morphine, especially when the patient is receiving high doses of the opiate. Some patients suffer hallucinations under morphine that are frightening and distressing, and can lead to confusion. In such an event, the nurse needs to stay with the patient, explaining what is happening, and preventing him from wandering or falling. Like other powerful analgesics, morphine can reduce the respiration rate, sometimes severely.

Diamorphine

Adult dose. For a patient in severe pain following a heart attack, 5 mg diamorphine may be given by slow intravenous injection. This drug is not usually given for post-operative pain relief, being most often prescribed for heart attack patients and those in the terminal stages of cancer. As for morphine, the dosage of diamorphine may be considerably increased with the passage of time.

Since patients with cancer often lose much body weight, it is inadvisable to give intramuscular injections, since this can lead to the needle hitting the bone. Diamorphine can be given in mixtures, sometimes with sherry disguising its bitter taste.

Side-effects. The side-effects of diamorphine are similar to those of morphine. Anti-emetics can be given to reduce the incidence of nausea and vomiting. Hallucinations are possible, as is a reduction in the patient's respiration rate.

Diamorphine is even more addictive than morphine, because of the euphoria it causes. However, the risk of addiction is slight when the drug is prescribed for its pain-killing (rather than mood-enhancing) powers. Doctors should not hesitate to prescribe an adequate dosage of diamorphine for someone dying of cancer. In most cases of terminal cancer, pain, as well as the other distressing symptoms, *can* be controlled. In this respect, the hospice movement in Britain has led the way in educating nurses and doctors about the importance of adequate pain relief. Similarly, Macmillan and Marie Curie nurses provide important advice for GPs about pain relief, as well as much needed support and care for the patients themselves and their relatives.

ADDITIONAL DRUG TREATMENTS FOR PATIENTS IN PAIN

The role of anti-emetics has already been noted in reducing the incidence of nausea as a side-effect of, for example, morphine. Nausea may be as miserable a symptom for some patients as is their pain, and, for the postoperative patient, vomiting may cause strain on surgical clips or sutures, thus leading to more pain. There are other drugs besides anti-emetics that may be prescribed for patients in pain.

Night sedation, for example, (as well as other important nursing measures) may help patients to achieve a good sleep. This is particularly important because pain can seem far worse at night (see Case example 5.2, above). Although many analgesics cause drowsiness, which may be sufficient to help the patient sleep, a sedative such as nitrazepam may be prescribed as well.

A related drug, diazepam, is widely prescribed to help reduce anxiety, and it, too, may have a role in effective treatment of the patient in pain.

Its property as a muscle relaxant can also be useful in some cases of back pain, where spasm in the muscles around the spine can lead to severe pain. Diazepam can cause confusion, especially in elderly people, and should be prescribed for only a limited time as it can cause dependence.

The anti-depressant drug amitriptyline can also play a part in the treatment of chronic pain, not only by lifting the patient's natural depression. First of all, amitriptyline causes drowsiness, so may help the patient to sleep. (Some patients, who wish to remain fully alert during the day, may be prescribed the total daily dose of the drug at night time.) Second, when given with analgesics, amitriptyline tends to *potentiate* these pain killers, i.e. they seem to work more effectively, which will again benefit the patient with chronic pain. The effective dose for a younger adult may be 75 mg or 100 mg, but an elderly person may require only 50 mg. The most serious side-effect is that of cardiac arrhythmias. A person who has taken an overdose of amitriptyline may need to be nursed on a coronary care or intensive care unit, where cardiac monitoring facilities (and nurses trained to use them) are available.

INDIVIDUALISING DRUG THERAPIES

On reading the above lists of drugs with their usual daily dosages, it is easy to regard drug prescribing as a somewhat automatic procedure. The truth is far different, because patients require drugs that are prescribed with their individual needs in mind. This is illustrated by Case example 5.9.

In this example, Mr Roberts' individual needs are being met. They are assessed by two well-trained professionals, and new treatment is agreed with the patient. Finally, the changed drug therapy is evaluated for its effectiveness. This profile also illustrates one of the vital roles of the nurse in the community: maintaining contact with patients in their own homes, ready to enlist the help of the GP when it is needed.

THE PLACEBO EFFECT

Sometimes a patient's pain can be reduced by the use of a 'dummy' tablet, one that contains no

Case example 5.9

Mr Roberts is a 68-year-old widower who, for 6 years, has been battling against lung cancer. He is now in the final stages of the disease. His GP has prescribed MST Continus 60 mg twice a day, having gradually increased the dosage from an original daily dose of 20 mg. Because Mr Roberts experiences considerable nausea, his doctor has also prescribed prochlorperazine 5 mg three times a day. Mr Roberts takes the first of these with his early morning cup of tea, 1 hour before breakfast.

The district nurse, on her regular visit every fortnight, notices that Mr Roberts' pain is not well controlled. His face is drawn and pale, and he shifts uneasily in his chair. She also thinks that she can notice signs of depression. She asks the GP to pay Mr Roberts a visit.

The doctor agrees with the district nurse. He judges that Mr Roberts' morphine dosage is probably at the right level, but he prescribes co-proxamol, two tablets, at 10 am, 4 pm and 10 pm. Although a milder pain killer than morphine, this drug will 'top up' Mr Roberts' pain relief in between his doses of MST Continus. The doctor also prescribes the anti-depressant amitriptyline, 50 mg at night. This has a sedative effect, so may also help Mr Roberts to sleep.

Finally, the GP asks the district nurse to visit Mr Roberts each week to evaluate this change in drug therapy.

analgesic drug at all. Such treatment is used only very sparingly. The patient may be someone who complains of pain, but, despite every possible medical test, no cause for the pain can be found. The doctor hesitates to prescribe the strong (and possibly addictive) pain killers that the patient seems to require, so a placebo (the Latin for 'I shall please') is given. The tablet consists of inactive substances that will do the patient no harm. The patient, believing that he is receiving real analgesia, experiences a lessening of his pain.

A patient's account of his pain should always be believed: his pain is real to him. Nurses and doctors should at all costs avoid being judgemental about the people who seek their help. Consequently, patients who complain of pain should be thoroughly investigated, and placebos used only as a last resort. It could well be argued that a person who claims to have pain without there being an apparent physical cause is in need of nursing and medical care as much as the patient

Question 5.4

Why do you think a placebo has the effect of reducing a person's pain? Base your reasons on your knowledge of both the physiology of pain and its cultural aspects?

with, for example, an arthritic joint: both people have pain that is real to them.

Placebo tablets are used in some drug trials, whereby one group of patients receives the drug (not necessarily an analgesic) being tested and the other group receives dummy tablets, manufactured to look exactly like the real ones. Neither the patients nor the doctors participating in the trial know which tablets are real and which are placebos.

PATIENT-CONTROLLED ANALGESIA

Intramuscular injections can be frightening for some patients, and for the cancer patient who has lost a lot of weight, they can also be painful. They additionally lead to surges in blood levels of the drug being injected (within about 1 hour of the injection), followed by periods when the blood level falls to lower than that required to have a therapeutic effect. This means that a post-operative patient written up for morphine 10 mg every 6 hours, may have to wait – in pain – until it is time for his next injection, which is clearly unsatisfactory.

A relatively new method of delivering analgesia uses an electronically controlled syringe pump. The syringe contains a diluted, known amount of the drug prescribed, and the pump is set to deliver a predetermined amount of the drug every time the patient presses the control button. The drug is delivered via an intravenous cannula, so that it has an almost instantaneous effect.

An important feature of this method is that there is no ebb and flow of the drug's blood level, which instead remains almost constant if the pump is used correctly. Furthermore, the patient does not have to wait for a nurse to bring him an injection – the drug delivery is under his own control. The pump has a safety device to ensure that it does not deliver more than a certain

amount of the drug (i.e. beyond the amount that might cause respiratory depression). If the patient presses the control button too often, the pump will not deliver a further bolus of the drug, although it may make a sound or cause a light to flash, which suggests to the patient that it is doing so. In this way, the pump provides both analgesia and placebo.

ADDITIONAL PAIN-RELIEVING STRATEGIES

Drugs have a vital role in the reduction of both acute and chronic pain. They are, however, not the only weapon to be employed against the distressing experience of pain. A brief overview of some of these additional methods is given below.

POSITIONING, REST AND SLEEP

For many patients in hospital, pain seems worse at night. Night is the time when imaginings are darker and when time drags. The nurse in Case example 5.2 (above) realised this, and, instead of simply handing her patient two tablets for her pain, she took time to sit and talk with her.

The nurse may well have helped her patient further by changing the position of the pillows and smoothing the bottom sheet to get rid of wrinkles. When Miss Philips got back into bed after her cup of tea, the nurse could have gently pressed a pillow against her back to give support. How simple all these measures are. There is nothing here that is complicated, nothing at the vanguard of medical innovation, yet these are all effective measures that the nurse can adopt on her own initiative.

Achieving sleep is difficult in a hospital ward because of all the activity, the need for a certain amount of light and, above all, the noise. Nurses on night duty have a responsibility to ensure that noise is reduced as much as possible, so that their patients can enjoy an uninterrupted night's sleep. Sleep and rest enable the patient to be free of anxieties, to gain strength to help healing and fight disease. During sleep, pain is forgotten.

RUBBING AND MASSAGE

On banging an elbow or knee, it is almost an automatic response to rub the affected part in order to reduce the pain; and the gate theory of pain, outlined above, helps to explain how this may work. Massage is qualitatively somewhat different from rubbing, since the former term is usually reserved for manipulation of the skin and underlying tissues according to a pattern established by training. Courses in therapeutic massage are available; such courses teach methods of handling the person safely, having regard to his underlying disease process. Massage can involve both lightly stroking the skin and applying firm pressure to the underlying muscle.

A factor common to both rubbing and massage, as applied to the patient by another person, is physical contact. To be massaged by someone in order to reduce pain is to know that someone else cares and is actively doing something about the pain.

DIVERSION AND MEDITATION

Sometimes, one's mind can be taken off pain by some external factor – conversation, the television or radio, or an interesting book. Even just simple human company can be effective. Many people find ward life in hospitals, or being ill in bed at home, very boring, and when this is the case, the patient has little to do but dwell on his pain and other symptoms.

Having a nurse take an interest in him by listening to his anxieties and questions, or by chatting about families, holidays or cars – anything that interests the patient – can help to alter his mind's focus of attention. As his interest in the subject being discussed grows, so his pain experience diminishes.

Diversion is a useful form of therapy, but it is not the first line of defence against acute pain. Someone in extreme pain from appendicitis needs something more effective than watching a soap opera on the television. One useful feature of diversional therapy, however, is that it is something that the patient's relatives can carry out. Relatives often feel helpless at the bedside of a loved one in pain. If the nurse encourages them to fill the person's time with conversation (while allowing the patient to rest if he needs to), they will feel of more use in such a stressful situation.

Those people who regularly practise meditation often find that it helps them 'step back' from painful experiences. Meditation, whether or not of a religious nature, allows someone to calm the mind, to empty it of unwanted thoughts and to relax deeply.

Meditation is not a technique that can be turned to when a person suddenly experiences pain unless he has previously practised it. Meditation is usually carried out two or three times a day, in a quiet spot of the home, and usually before meals. It can be silent, or accompanied by a regular, soft chanting, with the meditator concentrating on his breathing. It can be, to the onlooker, embarrassing and pointless, but its practitioners claim that the sense of well-being it invokes benefits them tremendously. If they are faced with pain, they are able effectively to distance themselves from it.

HEAT, COLD AND OINTMENTS

People suffering from some forms of arthritis sometimes find that heat, applied in the form of a hot water bottle (making certain its temperature is not too high) or an electric heat pad, can be very soothing to their joints.

Some ointments, rubbed into the skin above the painful joint, provide the sensation of warmth by causing dilation of local blood vessels, which may be demonstrated by the overlying skin turning pink or red.

Although the feeling of warmth can be very soothing, how it actually reduces pain is not entirely clear. If blood flow to the affected area is increased, it may be that blood cells are brought in greater numbers to areas of tissue damage, thus hastening repair (Melzack & Wall 1988). Another explanation makes use of the gate theory of pain modulation. Heat stimulates sensory nerve receptors, sending messages to the spinal cord that shut the 'gate' against other sensory messages from pain receptors.

By contrast, cold packs (consisting of ice chips wrapped in gauze or towelling, or a plastic pack of special gel that has been chilled in a refrigerator) can reduce the inflammation accompanying certain sports injuries, such as sprains. Muscle spasm, too, may be reduced by the application of an ice pack. As first aid immediately following a burn or scald, copious amounts of cold water poured over the affected area will reduce both the pain and further tissue damage.

Some NSAIDs, such as piroxicam, are available as gels or creams, as well as oral preparations. The gel is rubbed well into the skin over the painful joint, and the pain is decreased by the drug's anti-inflammatory action.

INFORMATION TECHNOLOGY AND THE TREATMENT OF PAIN

Computers are now commonplace on wards, in GP's surgeries and in high street pharmacies. They are highly effective at storing information on both patients and drugs. For example, when a patient takes a prescription to his usual pharmacist, she enters details of the newly prescribed drug on her computer. A warning signal appears: the computer has discovered that this new drug is incompatible with a drug the patient was pre-scribed a month ago and which he is still taking. The pharmacist will not have remembered that earlier drug, and the GP is perhaps not abreast of the daily advances in pharmacology and does not realise that he is prescribing an incompatible drug. The computer, however, is able to sift rapidly through its memory and produce a warning.

In another situation, an elderly patient complains to his GP about pain in her wrist. Medical examination suggests she has rheumatoid arthritis, and the GP prescribes an NSAID. The doctor enters this on the surgery computer, which then warns him that this patient has a history of duodenal ulcers; it would be dangerous for a patient with this past medical history to take NSAIDs.

The GP is new to the practice and does not know the patient, and the patient sees no reason

to mention that, 10 years ago, she had an ulcer, since she can see no connection between ulcers and a painful wrist. The computer, however, sees a connection where the patient did not, and warns the GP.

In both these examples, the computer's ability to store massive amounts of information, and to sift through it rapidly, proves to be invaluable in the safe and effective care of patients, including those in pain.

EVALUATING PAIN THERAPIES

Once the patient in pain has been assessed, and various treatments have been planned and implemented, these need to be evaluated for their effectiveness in helping to relieve the pain of that particular individual (Case example 5.10).

Case example 5.10

Mr Harris, an elderly widower with rheumatoid arthritis, is being assessed by a district nurse prior to changing his analgesia. The tablets he has been taking until now have not been very effective, and the GP has prescribed a new drug. After discussing how his pain seems to be affecting his daily life, the nurse shows Mr Harris various pain scales, and he chooses a 10-point verbal descriptor scale as the one he understands best. He points to the fourth descriptor – Moderate and uncom-fortable pain – as being the most appropriate for him at present.

The nurse explains when, and how often, his new tablets should be taken (just after his breakfast and evening meal), and tells Mr Harris she will call again in a fortnight to see how he is getting on. 'Telephone me,' she advises him, 'if you get any indigestion-type pains.'

Here, the patient is not simply given the new tablets and expected to get on with things. The nurse intends to *evaluate* how effective the drugs are at helping her patient's discomfort. Both patient and nurse are happy when, at the next visit, Mr Harris points to the second mark on the verbal descriptor scale: 'Very mild pain'.

Figure 5.5 shows an Assessment→Action→ Evaluation cycle that the district nurse follows

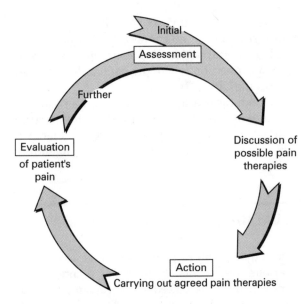

Figure 5.5   An Assessment→Action→Evaluation cycle of pain therapies.

for Mr Harris and which could be used for any patient in chronic pain. The cycle could just as well suit someone in hospital recovering from an operation. Note how the cycle comes round again to Assessment, but this time to a point at which the drug therapy may be either adjusted or left as it is.

Patient assessment is not a one-off event, performed when the patient is first admitted to a ward or seen at home by a district nurse, but a continuing process, as Figure 5.5 demonstrates.

Activity 5.5

With a group of your colleagues, devise a brief profile for a patient recovering from an orthopaedic operation, and show how her care fits the Assessment→Action→ Evaluation cycle. You may find that your cycle occurs within a much shorter period of time than did that for Mr Harris, but you will be sure that it is still appropriate.

Summary

Pain is much more than simply the result of an initiating stimulus; it is an experience with cultural, social, familial and psychological components. The key to effective control of pain is thus a full and individualised assessment of the patient.

Pain arises from the stimulation of nerve endings. Nerve impulses travel along neural pathways to the brain, where the pattern of impulses is interpreted, and pain assigned its characteristics. The 'gate theory' of pain can be used to explain how various external and internal factors help to dimish the sensation of pain.

The starting point for the assessment of pain is the patient's description and the nurse's observations, the latter being of even greater significance when the patient is for some reason unable to communicate the level of his pain.

Analgesics of various types and strengths have a major part to play in the overall management of pain, but other drugs, such as sedatives, anti-emetics and antidepressants, may also be employed. Additional strategies, such as ensuring adequate sleep, massage, diversion and information-giving, may contribute to the lessening of pain. Any treatment method must be evaluated, leading again to assessment and further intervention.

Nursing the patient in pain is very challenging, but perhaps nothing can be more satisfying for the nurse than to see her patient's pain well controlled.

REFERENCES

Grunau R V, Johnston C C, Craig K D 1990 Neonatal facial and cry responses to invasive and non-invasive procedures. Pain 42(3): 295–305
Guyton A 1991 Textbook of medical physiology, 8th edn. W B Saunders, Philadelphia
Hayward J 1975 Information – a prescription against pain. RCN, London
Hopkins S J 1992 Drugs and pharmacology for nurses, 11th edn. Churchill Livingstone, Edinburgh
Martikainen A, Heinonen K 1990 Pain management in new-born infants. Nordisk Medicin 105(5): 144–145 (paper written in Swedish, abstract published in English)
Melzack R, Wall P 1965 Pain mechanisms: a new theory. Science 150: 971–979
Melzack R, Wall P 1988 The challenge of pain, 2nd edn. Penguin Books, Harmondsworth

Raiman J 1986 Towards understanding pain, and planning for relief. Nursing, 3rd Series (11): 411–413, 418–423

Rutishauser S 1994 Physiology and anatomy: a basis for nursing and health care. Churchill Livingstone, Edinburgh

Trounce J 1994 Clinical pharmacology for nurses, 14th edn. Churchill Livingstone, Edinburgh

FURTHER READING

Hopkins S 1992 Drugs and pharmacology for nurses, 11th edn. Churchill Livingstone, Edinburgh (An established text well suiting the needs of today's nurses. It is not just a list of drugs; there are also useful discussions of drugs-related legislation, the nurse's role and the treatment of poisoning by medicines. Highly recommended.)

Melzack R, Wall P 1988 The challenge of pain, 2nd edn. Penguin Books, Harmondsworth (Fascinating, especially the earlier chapters. The physiology of pain is described in great detail, but the whole book is eminently readable.)

Pentrell J M, Wolf A R 1992 Pain in children. British Journal of Hospital Medicine 47(4): 289–293 (A review of the literature, concerning the principal differences – in physiology and pain relief – between babies and children.)

Rutishauser S 1994 Physiology and anatomy: a basis for nursing and health care. Churchill Livingstone, Edinburgh (An excellent new textbook. Clearly written, well illustrated, with just the right amount of detail for nursing students.)

Sparshott M 1993 Managing pain in children: special care for special babies. Nursing Standard 7(25): suppl.

2

Concepts of health

Nursing is as much concerned with the promotion of health as it is with the care and treatment of illness.

This section of the book considers the health–illness continuum, emphasising health education and preventive measures before examining disease patterns and describing how the National Health Service is organised to meet the needs of the general public in both hospital and community environments.

6 Normal health

Diana Forster

An understanding of the concept of 'health' is of vital importance before the whole state of a person, including 'ill-health', can be approached. This chapter aims to:

- explore what comprises 'health' for different people
- outline the reductionist and holistic approaches to health, and examine the disease and positive health models
- consider inequalities in health
- identify the wider social and environmental factors affecting health
- discuss the nurse's influence in the achievement of a healthy lifestyle.

WHAT IS HEALTH?

This question is personally relevant to nurses themselves, and to their work in helping people to maintain as high a quality of life as possible. A variety of approaches towards answering the question will be considered, ranging from individual to community-wide perspectives.

Activity 6.1

Consider the following questions, alone or with colleagues, to begin clarifying your own views about health:

- What does a healthy person look like?
- What personality traits does a healthy person have?
- What kind of activities does a healthy person take part in?
- Are you healthy?
- What would you have to change to make you more healthy?
- Who is the healthiest person you know?
- What is it about them that makes them healthier than you?
- Is health the same as, or different from, well-being?
- What are physical health, social health and mental well-being?
- How can you assess whether or not someone has health? (McBean 1992).

DEFINING HEALTH

How can health be defined? It is commonly thought of as a state of feeling well and not being ill, but health and sickness are not entirely separate concepts – they overlap. There are degrees of wellness and illness. Antonovsky (1987) suggests that we are all terminal cases, and as long as there is a breath of life in us, we are all in some measure healthy. He proposes that the focus of health should be upon enabling people to stay well, rather than concentrating on causes of illness.

This positive view may be used to define health as a state of physical, mental and social well-being – not simply the absence of injury or disease – that varies over time along a continuum. A high level of wellness is at one end of this continuum, with disease or illness and its characteristic signs, symptoms or disabilities at the other. Our position along the continuum varies, but there is no clear demarcation between health and ill-health. Blood pressure, for instance, may be described as low, normal or high, but the degrees merge into each other and the appropriate point at which treatment is necessary may be difficult to determine. Similarly, senile dementia is widely regarded as

a distinct entity, and much research effort goes into the search for its causes. However, studies of cognitive function in elderly people show that 'normality' merges imperceptibly into 'dementia', progressively affecting a minority of this age group. The identification of early dementia is a notoriously difficult clinical area, and diagnostic criteria differ widely.

A large proportion of people rate their health as 'good' or 'fairly good' in spite of suffering from some form of chronic disease or disability. People with impairments move along the health continuum, sometimes feeling at their peak of health and on other occasions feeling less so. One study in which older women were interviewed found that health problems were often played down. The women would typically say, 'Oh I'm fine in myself, it's just this ... stiff knee/high blood pressure/trouble with my waterworks ...' (Bernard & Meade 1993). Health was therefore being assessed not just in terms of the presence or absence of disease, or in terms of function; the women felt well in spite of their illness or disability. We therefore need to understand what people themselves mean when they discuss 'health'.

A woman may feel well and be unaware of a developing breast malignancy, or a man may describe himself as being 'on top of the world' but have an undiagnosed heart defect. It is also possible for people who are terminally ill to experience a sense of well-being; their bodies may be diseased, but they are at peace with themselves and are well adjusted to the ending of their lives. Nurses working in hospices or caring for terminally ill people at home may be familiar with such examples. Woods & Edwards (1989) comment that 'it is not a contradiction to refer to a healthy attitude towards illness or death'.

Blaxter (1990) also reports studies that show that health can be defined as co-existing with quite severe disease or incapacity. Her examples include the case of a Scottish woman who said of her husband that 'he had a lung taken out but he was "aye" healthy enough'. In another study, a daughter reported that her mother 'had been an active woman before [her illness] with no previous restriction apart from general old age, loss of sight in one eye and loss of memory. The doctor said at the inquest she was a very fit woman for her age.' Another woman, aged 79 and disabled by arthritis, is also reported as saying, 'To be well in health means I feel I can do others a good turn if they need help.'

Consider being in a clinical situation with an elderly arthritic woman, wondering how she must feel, being old and suffering from a chronic disability. When asked, 'How are you today, Mrs Jones?' her answer might be surprising. The fact that Mrs Jones has felt well enough to make the journey to the surgery to pick up her repeat prescription and is now on her way to the day centre may cause her to reply with genuine pleasure, 'I feel very well, thank you, dear.'

Equally, someone apparently fit and healthy, prosperous and untroubled by the cares of poverty and poor housing might respond in a very different way. Relationship problems may be the cause of a very real depression or a feeling of purposelessness and futility in life. Conceptions of health can vary widely even within the same person, according to a variety of factors, sometimes emanating from within and sometimes due to external causes.

LIFE EXPECTANCY AND HEALTH

The number of years that people can expect to live is a good overall indicator of the health of a nation. All four countries in the UK have produced health strategies to address the major causes of premature death and preventable illness. The specific priorities and targets vary between the different countries, although they all include circulatory diseases, accidents and certain cancers, with their associated risk factors such as smoking (see Ch. 9). The average lifespan in the UK is increasing by an average of 2 years every decade. According to projected mortality rates, a boy born in 1996 can expect to live until he is 74, while a girl can expect to live until she is nearly 80 (Central Statistical Office 1995). Does this mean that we are becoming part of a healthier nation? Averages such as these, however, hide the inequalities in health and

health choices of which nurses need to be aware and which are a recurring theme in this chapter.

APPROACHES TO HEALTH

Cmich (1984) identifies two basic approaches in 20th-century Western thought. One is reductionism, which, in health care, regards the organism as a collection of components that are considered separately – for example, the body is reviewed as a system of different parts. The other approach is holism, which, in health care, leads to a focus on growth, well-being and self-actualisation.

Holistic health

Attempting to understand the web of influences upon someone's health and well-being involves taking a 'holistic' approach. The term comes from the Greek 'holos', meaning 'whole'. The holistic health approach incorporates a belief in a person's responsibility for his own life, a willingness to cooperate with others, and an emphasis on developing meaningful relationships and a positive outlook on life.

Nurses applying the holistic approach to health care place emphasis on the whole person, taking into account each one's physical, emotional, intellectual, spiritual and sociocultural background. The nurse's focus is on prevention and well-being, and on helping individuals to take responsibility for their own health, although people have more choice and control over some factors affecting their health than others.

Lifestyle

Lifestyle factors include the way or style in which people live their lives:

- what they eat or drink
- whether they smoke
- how much exercise they take
- what risks they take, for instance in relation to drug misuse or safe sexual practices.

Smoking is the greatest cause of preventable death in the UK, with about one in six deaths being attributed to its links with such diseases as lung cancer, respiratory disease and heart disease. Many factors affecting health, for example the quality of the air people breathe, the pressures of the educational system and the state of the roads, are outside the individual's immediate control. However, research suggests that choices about health-related behaviour, such as smoking, are also heavily influenced by people's living conditions. Although the proportion of people who smoke cigarettes has continued to decline in all social groups, the decline has been more marked in non-manual than in manual social groups, so the difference between groups has become greater, thus increasing inequalities in health. Graham (1993) found that women in manual households in her study smoked in order to cope with the demands of their everyday domestic and caring responsibilities, even though they knew and understood the possible threats to their health.

Components of holistic health

The holistic approach to health therefore encompasses a range of dimensions, which may be identified as:

- societal
- environmental
- spiritual
- physical
- mental
- sensual
- social
- sexual.

It thus relates to a wide range of human capacities and qualities.

Cmich (1984) proposes 12 components of the holistic health approach, based upon her detailed analysis of relevant literature:

1. An individual's body, mind and spirit are interrelated and inseparable, functioning as an integrated whole.

2. The spiritual dimension of human beings, in which individuals search for meaning and purpose in their lives, is relevant to all aspects of health and disease.

3. Wellness, as a way of life that is unique for each person, reflects an attitude emphasising well-being and the enjoyment of the highest level of health possible, rather than the absence of disease.

4. Health is an ongoing process, reflecting continuous change as the individual develops throughout the lifecycle.

5. Health and wholeness involve harmony between the person, society and the environment.

6. Self-awareness involves developing knowledge of one's own inner thoughts, motivations and needs.

7. Human beings have the capacity to influence healing in themselves naturally, in both mind and body.

8. Health and illness are psychosomatic, in that both mind and body are involved in all levels of illness and wellness, as mind and body interact.

9. Individuals have the responsibility to be accountable for their own health and well-being, and for their own health behaviour.

10. Each person is not a passive victim if disease develops, but is a responsible participant in illness as well as health.

11. The health professional and patient are partners who share responsibility for the fight against illness and for the healing process.

12. A multidimensional approach is acknowledged in holistic health, including an investigation of alternative healing systems, such as acupuncture, yoga, meditation and biofeedback.

FITNESS

An important aspect of the concept of health is that of 'fitness'. Downie (1990) comments that fitness in its most obvious sense refers to the state of a person's heart and lungs. A fit person, in this sense, can climb stairs or run for a bus without being too out of breath, while an extremely high level of fitness is needed by top athletes to perform well at their sport. Downie (1990) considers fitness under the 'four Ss' of:

- strength
- stamina
- suppleness
- skills.

People who have sufficient of these 'four Ss' to carry out their normal, everyday activities and tasks without undue physical discomfort (such as muscle aches) will probably view themselves as fit (Box 6.1).

Box 6.1 **Effects of exercise upon physical and mental well-being**

Exercise:

- helps people to feel good about themselves because they look healthier and therefore more attractive
- improves the efficiency of the circulatory system and therefore reduces fatigue
- improves appetite and digestion
- helps relaxation by providing an outlet for tension and frustration
- improves sleep patterns
- helps to prevent physical illnesses, such as heart disease and osteoporosis
- increases self-esteem.

Personal fitness targets are likely to vary throughout a person's life in relation to age, disability, etc. Athletes, dancers and sports enthusiasts may seek to develop their optimum fitness, maximising the efficiency and effectiveness of the body as though it were a machine. In this mechanistic view, the heart is viewed as a pump, the lungs as gas exchangers and the muscles as sources of power.

Fitness and mental health

The concept of fitness can be applied to mental as well as physical health. The generally-held view that exercise makes people feel good mentally as well as physically is probably true:

- Exercise results in significant improvement in measures of self-confidence and self-esteem.
- Exercise has an anti-depressant effect, which has been demonstrated among mildly or moderately depressed people in both hospital and community-based populations.
- There is an association between exercise and anxiety reduction.
- Exercise can reduce the immediate physiological response to stress.

The anti-depressant and anti-anxiety effects of exercise are biologically plausible. For example, research in brain chemistry suggests that one of the immediate effects of exercise may be an increase in the brain levels of endorphins, substances whose effects are that of an intrinsic heroin-like substance.

Farrell (1991) describes a mentally healthy person as one who can solve problems in a mature way and who can deal with crises, possibly within the framework of supportive family and social networks. Mental health throughout life is a matter of getting to know oneself and understanding one's own needs, achieving what is possible and coming to terms with what cannot be achieved. Learning to recognise what makes one feel stressed and how to cope with stress is an essential part of a mental health self-care regimen (see Ch. 4).

Aggleton (1990) points out the complexity of defining health and fitness. Some people may be healthy according to some criteria but not according to others. Aggleton cites several examples, which may serve as an exercise to help the reader clarify his or her views of health (Activity 6.2).

Activity 6.2

Consider the following cases. Are they healthy or not:

- A sports enthusiast who is highly skilled in his favourite team sport but consumes 5 pints of lager after every match.
- A well-adjusted, happy and outward-looking chef who happens to weigh 17 stone.
- A well-liked and reasonably content teacher who smokes 30 cigarettes a day in order to cope with her job.
- A sociable young woman who is described as the life and soul of the party, but who cries herself to sleep every night.

INEQUALITIES IN HEALTH

A lifestyle based upon a holistic approach to health therefore helps people to become responsible for influencing their own health and well-being, and to be sensitive to factors affecting them. Such factors include nutrition, physical fitness, stress management and environmental conditions. However, as has already been considered, to maintain health and avoid being physically or mentally ill, people need to live in a healthy environment and have access to a range of goods and services of sufficient quantity and quality (Doyal & Gough 1991). Inequalities in health, are however, still widening: a recent report demonstrates the shorter expectation of life for people who face multiple disadvantage (Acheson 1995). Inequalities exist in relation to:

- social class
- race
- gender
- older age
- disability
- region and locality
- access to services
- health outcomes.

Mortality rates for stroke, for example, are generally higher in the north of England than in the south, in social class V than social class I, and in those born in the Caribbean and African Commonwealth and Indian sub-contintent, than they are among those born in England and Wales (Department of Health 1994).

Seedhouse (1988) speaks of the world of health care as being in a state of crisis:

The turmoil which surrounds the health professions has swelled because of conceptual confusion. The meaning of the world 'health' has again come under close scrutiny, and it has become clear that the notions of 'health' and 'human value', are inseparable ... The members of the disciplines have begun to ask searching questions about the rationale of a health service, about what a health service should truly be for, and about the relationship between ethics and health care. The conclusions that are dawning have massive implications for the whole organisation and structure of health care.

He suggests that health professionals should address the central needs of their clients, in an egalitarian way. He considers that full health can never be achieved in a system that allows inequalities such that some people's material needs are fulfilled whilst other people lack shelter and food, or have a very limited general education and see little purpose in life. Seedhouse (1986) also argues that health is made up of a number of factors that help people to achieve their maximum personal potential. These factors, or foundations for achievement, include the basic necessities of life, such as food, water and shelter, as well as access to information and the necessary skills to make sense of such information and use it appropriately.

As we have seen, there are many social and environmental factors affecting health over which a person may have little or no control. While some environmental factors, for example air and water pollution, may affect everyone, some social factors, such as low income, poor housing or the inability to afford a car, will affect certain groups of people far more than others. Making healthy choices is therefore easier for some, empowering them to take greater care of their own health and well-being.

Reducing inequalities in health experiences and opportunities is a central principle of health promotion, discussed in Chapter 7.

FOLKLORE

Many lay beliefs pertaining to health are encapsulated in folklore. Sayings such as 'An apple a day keeps the doctor away' are well known. Often, we grow up with many such notions and barely notice that they have become part of our own belief system (Activity 6.3).

Activity 6.3

1. Draw up a list of as many different health-related sayings and beliefs as you can think of.
2. Identify those which you grew up with.
3. If you are able, note the origin or source of such sayings.

INFLUENCE OF THE MEDIA ON PERCEPTIONS OF HEALTH

In all its forms, the media is an important and influential source of persuasion. It provides responses to change, and is itself an agent of change. Many advertisements and TV dramas shape attitudes and expectations; they may present desirable situations, but they undoubtedly also leave many people feeling less than adequate. They certainly have considerable influence on images of health and help to shape the norms to which many individuals aspire. It may be useful for the reader to pause and reflect upon the ethics of such practices and on the power and influence of the media in all its forms, especially as this pertains to health (Activity 6.4).

Activity 6.4

Divide a page into three columns.
  In column one, list five items you have recently purchased that you had seen advertised.
  In column two, note the advertising medium you most associated with each product.
  In column three, state whether or not the fact that you had seen this item advertised had any bearing on your decision to buy. Think carefully about this.
  In pairs or small groups, discuss your findings. Note any shared observations about the pressures to buy.

Problems can arise when influences, particularly commercial ones, play a disproportionate part in shaping feelings about what constitutes good health and what can be done towards its achievement. Such messages leave people feeling inadequate and, worse still, may cause them to seek endlessly for an impossible dream or, indeed, give up striving for goals altogether.

Media influences, whether from the press, posters, television or radio are considerable and, to some extent, pernicious, since the messages conveyed can impinge upon consciousness at many different levels, even without being deliberately subliminal. Pausing to consider the implications for health of media persuasion may enable the individual to measure personal health beliefs against what is considered 'normal'. Does 'normal health' equate with the 'desirable' images of health generally portrayed by the media? How realistic are the demands and pressures put upon the individual to achieve this supposedly desirable health status? Are some of the values associated with the desired level of health represented in the media

questionable? Are the norms of health that are assumed to be ideal equally appropriate for everyone?

THE NURSE AS ROLE MODEL

Clarke (1991) discusses the pressure upon nurses to conform to a certain 'healthy' lifestyle image in order to maintain a degree of credibility with patients. She considers how far a nurse should be prepared to change her lifestyle so that she may faithfully reflect her professional teachings. Clarke presents the example of a 125 kg (20 stone) nurse who has nicotine-stained fingers and halitosis and who gets breathless going upstairs in the lift. Should she modify her lifestyle?

Parsons (1979) defines health as 'the state of optimum capacity of an individual for the effective performance of the roles and tasks for which (s)he has been socialized.' This approach emphasises the capacity of a person to fit in with society's norms and expectations, and could be applied to nurses working in professional health care, who are often expected to provide role models for health. Question 6.1 invites the reader to consider his or her own health as a nurse.

Question 6.1

Do you feel tired all the time?
Do you feel you can't cope, and that things get on top of you?
Do you feel at your peak?
Do you smoke?
Do you need to lose weight?
Do you think you drink too much?
Do you need to take more exercise?
Are you over-using drugs, medicinal or otherwise?

Horne (1990) suggests that nurses should take a good look at their own lifestyles and assess how healthy they really are. She invites nurses to define their own health profiles and set health goals, perhaps with friends or colleagues, for 6 months ahead. However, she warns that nurses should remember their mental health in this exercise and not be too tough on themselves.

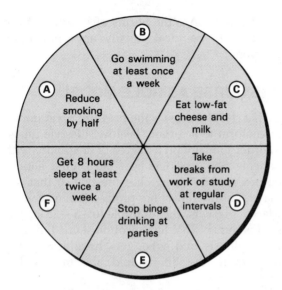

Figure 6.1 Goals for lifestyle changes.

Figure 6.1 gives examples of lifestyle change goals that might be set.

SOCIAL WELL-BEING

Emotional and social health may be considered in terms of:

- feelings
- emotions
- interests
- motivations
- attitudes
- values.

All of these elements change and mature over a person's lifetime.

Social well-being refers to the skills and other abilities that enable us to form friendships and relate to others. 'Lifeskills' are used to help us in the many kinds of contact that occur as part of ordinary social life, for example (Hopson & Scally 1980):

- effective communication
- making and managing relationships
- managing conflict
- being assertive
- working in groups
- influencing others

- managing stress
- coping with life changes.

Individuals engage in transactions with the broader environment in accomplishing the developmental tasks appropriate to each life stage. The social approach defines social health according to whether or not the person is fulfilling expected cultural norms and social functions.

Downie (1990) discusses another dimension of social well-being, viewing the concept as a characteristic of society itself, as distinct from the individuals who make up that society. This approach focuses not upon individual people but upon the structure of society, which includes:

- institutions
- practices
- customs
- political arrangements
- social class relationships.

MODELS OF HEALTH

The disease model of health

This is a negative model of health in which health is viewed as the polar opposite of disease. Disease is usually understood as the presence of some pathology or abnormality in a part of the body. Bacteria and viruses cause many diseases, whilst other diseases, such as cancer, are caused by less easily identified sources. However, diseases may be present without causing any anxiety, distress or symptoms. It may be some time before an abormality or disturbance in the body's functioning becomes apparent to the sufferer. Conversely, people can experience pain or discomfort, but doctors may be unable to identify any cause or underlying pathology. Aggleton (1990) emphasises the distinction between abnormalities that signal disease and the feelings people have about themselves. Someone is said to be ill when he feels pain or discomfort, although disease may or may not be present.

The concept of disease as being the opposite of health is useful as a biomedical model that lends itself to measuring, detecting and recording disease processes in the patient. It is possible reliably to compare different people's health, and to assume that a person who has no trace of detected disease is healthy. However, there are many drawbacks to the biomedical model of health, which emphasises the negative rather than the positive aspects of health that the World Health Organization (1946) definition, quoted below, attempts to highlight.

Positive health

The idea of positive health has, for some decades, featured in published reports, beginning with the definition found in the preamble to the Constitution of the World Health Organization (WHO): 'Health is a state of complete physical, mental and social well-being, and not merely the absence of disease or infirmity' (World Health Organization 1946). This is similar to the definitions already discussed, and it is now quite old and well known. One of the problems with the WHO definition is that it assumes there is one particular state that equates with being healthy; it does not consider the continuum discussed above. Although limited in scope, the idea contained within the WHO statement is, however, an important one. It attempts to move thinking away from solely physical aspects of health – the biomedical approach. The biomedical approach is limited to considering the disease process itself and its diagnosis, management and treatment; it does not go on to consider, for instance, the health of the individual once the disease process has been eliminated or found to be absent. In contrast, the WHO definition does, however, introduce mental and social dimensions and consideration of well-being. It therefore extends ideas about health to include the whole person, rather than just the physical problem the person may be suffering from, leading to a more holistic approach to health, including the influences of society, environment and culture discussed above.

A WIDER APPROACH

'A blend of today's reality and tomorrow's dreams' was the vision created by the 32 Member States of the WHO European Region in 1984 when they adopted the first set of European targets for health. These targets, now reviewed and updated over a decade, express a commitment by Member States to achieve health for all by the year 2000 (World Health Organization 1993). The health outcomes woven into the targets have four themes relating to one another:

1. Ensuring equity in health – by reducing gaps in health status between countries and between groups within countries.
2. Adding life to years – by helping people to achieve and use their full physical, mental and social potential.
3. Adding health to life – by reducing disease and disability.
4. Adding years to life – by increasing life expectancy.

These targets reflect the blueprint for a new health care system that was laid out at the International Conference of Alma Ata (World Health Organization 1978). This conference recognised the need for change and development, identified by many health practitioners, and introduced the primary health care approach to promoting health for all (see Ch. 7).

Primary health care

The term 'primary health care' (PHC) is sometimes thought to mean care at the margins of health services where they come into contact with communities. It then becomes confused with primary medical care or simple curative services, perhaps with the addition of preventive measures such as immunisation programmes. However, the PHC envisaged at Alma Ata is much more than an addition to existing health services, much more than primary medical care. It is a reorientation of all health services towards the needs of communities, both local and national. The vision of PHC presented by Alma Ata challenged many existing ways of thinking and practice in health services throughout the world.

Traditionally, in health care, the hospital has been one category, and everything outside the hospital has been viewed as the community. In the PHC approach, the hospital is regarded as part of the community setting, and the context of people's lives and the wider environment are recognised as having a major impact on the health of people and nations. Inequalities and difficulties with making healthy choices, as we have seen, underpin many aspects of health. 'Nurses witness daily the effects of poverty and the wider environment on the health of individuals and families' and 'nurses have much to contribute to the public health movement' (Royal College of Nursing 1994a).

A HEALTH AND LIFESTYLE SURVEY

A national survey of men and women aged 18 years and over in England, Scotland and Wales was carried out in 1984/85, achieving a random sample size of 9003. Participants were asked in great detail about their health and their lifestyles. Certain aspects of fitness were measured, and participants were invited to express their opinions and attitudes towards health and health-related behaviour (Blaxter 1990). Thus, physiological measurements and verbal reports were obtained.

The information was collected at two home visits. The first of these was carried out by an interviewer who elicited information about:

- personal and family circumstances
- self-reported health
- health attitudes and beliefs
- health-related behaviour, including detailed questioning on diet, exercise, smoking and alcohol consumption.

The second visit was made by a nurse who carried out physiological measurements, including height, weight, girth, blood pressure, pulse rate and respiratory function.

The broad conclusion reached at the end of the analysis of the findings was that circumstances carry rather more weight as determinants of health than do healthy or unhealthy behaviours. All four behaviours studied, particularly smoking, were found to be relevant to health, but they had most effect when the

environment was good. Blaxter (1990) confirms, therefore, that health is affected by general lifestyle, which is in turn related to economic or occupational position. It is only in more favourable circumstances that there is room for improvement by adopting better health-related habits. Health, in all its dimensions, was once again found to be associated with:

- social class
- income
- personal living circumstances
- the wider environment.

The avoidance of behavioural risk factors was found to be protective to only a small degree when aspects of lifestyle not under people's direct control were unhealthy. These findings have important implications for health promotion and health education, and are discussed in Chapter 7.

Normal health, as Blaxter (1990) points out, can accommodate a certain level of symptoms or complaints. To have no symptoms or complaints at all could be described as super-health and is highly extraordinary, occurring only in a small minority of people.

THE BIOPSYCHOSOCIAL PERSPECTIVE

We have already seen that when 'the person' is added to the biomedical model, discussed earlier, a broader picture of health and illness emerges. This is the biopsychosocial perspective, which considers the interplay between the biological, psychological and social aspects of a person's life, fitting in with the holistic model of health.

Biological factors

The biological dimension of the person includes genetic characteristics and physiological functioning, for example with regard to whether the body:

- has structural defects, for example brain damage or a heart defect
- can respond effectively in protecting itself by fighting infection

- sometimes over-reacts in the protective function, such as when allergic reactions to pollen or dust are produced.

As discussed in Chapter 1, the body is made up of a complex system of organs, consisting of tissues that are, in turn, made up of cells. The efficient, effective and healthy functioning of the body's systems depends on the way each of its components operates individually and interacts with others.

Psychological factors

Anyone who has developed influenza, has sprained an ankle or has had severe toothache knows how much psychological damage these possibly minor conditions can cause. The more serious the physical disorder, the greater the likelihood is that it will significantly affect a person's thoughts and feelings. These psychological changes in turn affect the person's physical condition, compounding the ill-health. Research also shows that ill people who overcome their negative thoughts and feelings can speed their recovery (Sarafino 1994).

Psychological factors include behaviour and mental processes such as:

1. cognition
2. emotion
3. motivation.

Cognition plays an important role in health and illness because it includes the processes of:

- perceiving
- learning
- remembering
- thinking
- interpreting
- believing
- problem-solving.

The questions and activities given earlier in the chapter may have helped the reader to explore some of these cognitive factors and how they affect health behaviour.

Emotions are subjective feelings that affect thoughts, behaviour and physiology. Pleasant emotions, such as joy and affection, are con- sidered positive, while others, such as anger, fear and sadness, are negative. Research suggests that people whose emotions are relatively positive are less disease-prone and are likely to recover more quickly from illness than are those whose emotions tend to be negative (Sarafino 1994). Chapter 2 explores the role of personality in health and illness.

Motivation is the psychological factor used to explain why people behave in certain ways. Exercise helps people to look and feel more healthy and attractive, but, in order to begin exercising, they need strong motivation. Motivation provides the necessary drive to enable someone to stick with a programme of exercise or dietary modification. It may come from within or derive from external factors. For instance, parents may become motivated to stop smoking if their children have become aware of the health implications of smoking and try to persuade their parents to quit. (Motivation is discussed in greater detail in Chapter 2.)

Social factors

People live in a social world, interacting with family, friends, co-workers and other members of the community. The social world of the individual is, however, larger than just the people with whom direct contact is made. All people are part of the social system and function at various levels, including:

- community
- culture
- society
- nation.

These social spheres are interrelated, and each individual's health is related to all levels. The society we live in affects the health of individuals, for example by establishing certain health values, including the belief that it is good to be fit and healthy.

The closest social relationships for most people occur within the family. Children learn many health-related behaviours, attitudes and beliefs from parents, brothers and sisters. The influence of community, culture and society on health gradually develops as the child grows, enlarging his or her circle of friends and interacting with more and more people.

The role of biological, psychological and social factors in health and illness are therefore apparent in many aspects, but the interaction between these components is a more complex issue.

THE ENVIRONMENT

To enable people to become all that they are capable of being, many aspects of a healthy environment need to be considered. The effects of several of these aspects upon health will now be discussed, namely:

- housing and health
- social class and health
- ethnicity and culture in health
- work, unemployment and health.

HOUSING AND HEALTH

A close association between poor living conditions and ill-health has been generally accepted for more than 100 years (see Ch. 8). Housing tenure (i.e. whether homes are owner-occupied, Council-rented or in another category) has been shown to reflect differences within social classes. Blaxter (1990) comments that whilst we should not assume that health and well-being are necessarily superior for every owner-occupier, housing tenure can be a useful tool for, for example, comparing mortality rates. In the Health and Lifestyle Survey (Blaxter 1990), owner-occupiers as a whole were shown to have a lower mortality rate than Council or other tenants and to be healthier than Council tenants.

Blaxter points out that there was a much greater difference in health between owner-occupiers and tenants among women than among men. Women in non-manual social classes who were tenants reported much poorer health than did non-manual respondents in owner-occupied houses. Among the men in Blaxter's survey, those over 60 years old living in Council accommodation were much more likely to be in the category of 'poor or very poor' health than were the owner-occupiers in this age group, regardless of social class.

Research has shown that people who live in districts where housing is generally poor are less healthy than those who live in areas where there is good housing. Acheson & Hagard (1984) discuss research that demonstrates that those in poor housing areas have children who, at corresponding ages, are more likely than those in areas characterised by good housing:

- to be shorter
- to suffer from skin infections
- to die from pneumonia, enteritis and common infections of childhood
- to have defective hearing and vision.

However, the authors point out that evidence of this kind does not necessarily prove links between housing and illness or mortality. In inner-city areas, the worst homes are close together and possibly overcrowded, and are occupied by families who may have diets deficient in both quantity and quality. The links between poverty, deprivation and poor health need to be considered together with housing needs.

Housing plays a very important part in the health and well-being of elderly people. As Robertson (1991) comments, 'it is the key to the highly treasured independence and, like all needs for old people, is best planned for prior to retirement'. Warmth and safety to minimise the comparatively high rate of accidents to elderly people at home are of particular concern.

Homeless families

In recent years, there has been an increasing number of families living in bed-and-breakfast temporary accommodation. Such families often have high levels of health needs, yet tend to have difficulty in getting access to health care. Research cited by Robertson (1991) shows that children in homeless families commonly are delayed in development and are smaller than average. High levels of stress, poverty and the lack of laundry facilities, storage, cooking and play facilities are also major factors in the plight of homeless families. As with elderly people at home, the accident rate among children in temporary, unsuitable accommodation is unacceptably high. Robertson (1991) highlights the need for families in temporary accommodation to have access to information about:

- play facilities
- local GP services
- health clinics and other health services
- access to welfare rights
- social work arrangements
- relevant voluntary agencies.

SOCIAL CLASS AND HEALTH

Social class is the most commonly used indicator of social circumstances, and a great deal is known about the relationship between mortality and class (Blaxter 1990). In particular, as discussed in Chapter 8, research-based links have been demonstrated between infant and perinatal mortality rates and social class. Babies born to the manual classes are much more likely to die in the perinatal period than are those born to the professional classes. This disparity remains a challenge, as it has been unchanged for the last decade.

TRANSCULTURAL ASPECTS OF HEALTH

During the shortage of labour in the UK after World War II, many people migrated to the UK from the Indian sub-continent, Africa and the Caribbean to find employment. Health approaches in the early days concentrated on 'imported' diseases, which were sometimes seen as a threat to the indigenous white population. Special health care provision in the form of vaccination against tuberculosis, for example, is in some health authorities still offered only to Asian babies. Differences are also made in screening programmes for genetic disorders.

However, many minority groups object to specialist campaigns, such as the Asian Mother and Baby Campaign set up in 1984. The objection stems from the singling out of ethnic minorities in a racist approach, while little or nothing is done to help the minority communities who experience disadvantages in housing and work and prejudice from other people in the community, which may have negative effects upon health. Concentrating upon diseases such as sickle cell anaemia, despite their importance, diverts attention away from the major sources of ill-health within minority communities and will have little overall effect upon the health of the population.

Discovering the gaps

Questions that need to be asked by health professionals include (Hayes 1995):

- What attempts am I making to understand the needs of the ethnic population in my area?
- Do I have preconceived ideas and prejudices that detract from my effort to cater for ethnic minorities?
- Am I communicating effectively?
- Is it a two-way process?

Respect for religious beliefs, understanding of language difficulties and general knowledge of other cultures are important aspects of nursing today. Members of different ethnic, racial, religious and social groups need to be supported in maintaining independent lifestyles and adhering to their values within a common civilisation.

Nurses can help to promote health in diverse ethnocultural groups, for instance by learning about significant religious practices and the everyday patterns of hygiene, eating, types of food, sleeping, elimination and use of space. The stress of illness is increased if normal living patterns and practices are disrupted too much, so special nursing skills are required to adapt care within a varied cultural community.

WORK, UNEMPLOYMENT AND HEALTH

Many studies have shown that the environment in which people spend their working lives can have serious adverse effects on their health. It is not only in the traditional heavy industries, such as coal mining or asbestos manufacture in lethal dust-laden environments, that health is affected. The modern office block has brought with it many health and safety problems, including the so-called 'sick building' syndrome (Pike 1995).

The Health and Safety Commission (1992) places general duties on employers to ensure the health and safety of their employees by providing:

- safe plant and equipment, with maintainance, and safe systems of work
- safety in relation to the use, handling, storage and transport of articles and substances
- information, instruction, training and supervision
- maintainance of a safe working place – this does not apply to the homes of patients and clients of health workers as these are not under the employer's control, but it does not dilute the employer's duty to keep staff safe wherever they are
- facilities and arrangements for welfare at work. The employers of health-care staff need seriously to consider problems of violence, including racial and sexual harrassment, and demonstrate a commitment to ensure that staff are as safe as possible (Royal College of Nursing 1994b).

Mental health and work

Warr (1987) discusses nine features of the environment that help to determine mental health, and which are particularly applicable to the work setting. These are:

1. the opportunity for control
2. the opportunity for skill use
3. externally generated goals
4. variety
5. environmental clarity
6. availability of money
7. physical security
8. opportunity for interpersonal contact
9. valued social position.

Opportunity for control

Mental health is partly determined by the opportunities for a person to control events and activities. Warr (1987) points out that the opportunity for control consists of the freedom to decide and act in one's chosen way and the potential to predict what the consequences of such action might be. Not knowing what will happen can lead to feelings of helplessness, as discussed by Seligman (1975) in his theory of 'learned helplessness'.

Opportunity for skill use

Being able to use one's skills effectively is satisfying, and people who are unemployed or who are in restrictive job environments often cannot use the skills they have, or learn and develop new ones.

Externally generated goals

People who are in repetitive, boring jobs or not in work are not encouraged to set objectives or goals to strive for and have little upon which to structure their pattern of behaviour. They may as a consequence lack purpose and motivation.

Variety

Mental health may be adversely affected if work is monotonous and repetitive. For unemployed people, the lack of opportunities (possibly through poverty and a restricted role in life) to experience variety may have a negative impact on their mental health.

Environmental clarity

Warr (1987) identifies three main ways in which the environment may be unclear:

- in relation to difficulty in predicting a life course and the consequences of one's actions
- in a lack of feedback about one's own actions
- in a lack of clarity about the role one plays in society and what is expected of one.

Mental health can be impaired by these uncertainties, which may well be a feature in unemployment and in some job situations.

Availability of money

Low income is associated with high rates of illness and poor psychosocial health (Blaxter 1990). Blaxter's analysis suggests that this is true for all age groups; however, unemployment after the age of 30 was demonstrated in men to lead to a greater lack of fitness and to more long-standing chronic conditions than it was among those in low-paid work. Poor psychosocial health was also a feature of the unemployed in Blaxter's study. Warr (1987) points out that poverty is self-perpetuating in several ways. For instance, poor people cannot buy in bulk because they cannot afford the initial outlay, and they often cannot travel to cheaper retail outlets because they have no transport.

Physical security

In the framework we are considering, as was discussed in 'Housing and health', above, a physically secure living environment is an important determinant of health status. People need to have warmth, food, physical space and personal territory, as well as a sense of permanence in their surroundings (Seedhouse 1986).

Opportunity for interpersonal contact

An opportunity for interpersonal contact is important for four main reasons, as identified by Warr (1987):

1. It meets friendship needs and reduces feelings of loneliness.
2. It can provide help of many kinds, including social, practical and emotional support.
3. It provides the basis for comparison between the person's own situation and that of others.
4. It allows membership of formal and informal groups, so that achievements can be made that are not possible for one person alone.

Valued social position

Social structures are meaningful in relation to mental health, as they confer esteem from other people onto the individual. For example, a person may belong to a family, a work group, a local community and society as a whole. These positions may bring recognition, consideration and esteem from others in these groups. Membership of such groups involves responsibility and obligations and the necessity to play certain roles in each situation.

The nurse's working environment

It is as impossible for nurses as it is for other workers to maintain a healthy lifestyle in an unhealthy working environment. Rogers & Salvage (1988) criticise the NHS for its poor record in promoting a healthy working climate for nurses. Their recommendations for action are:

- the provision of a clean, attractive and safe working environment
- good staff facilities, including canteens, shops, recreational facilities, car parks and changing rooms
- childcare facilities on site for all staff who require them
- enough residential accommodation, well designed and maintained
- well-planned, flexible shifts so that family commitments can be met.

Rogers & Salvage (1988) also argue that district health authorities should establish and fund comprehensive occupational health services for all their employees. The main objectives would be to promote the health of all nursing staff by:

- monitoring, controlling or abolishing hazards in the workplace
- providing health screening facilities for nurses
- supervising employee nurses' health
- providing health education
- advising on occupational safety and environmental monitoring
- providing and maintaining a confidential counselling service
- advising on rehabilitation and resettlement where this is appropriate, for example for nurses who have experienced illness or disablement.

Nurses need to develop their own sense of self-empowerment so that they can feel responsible for their own health and well-being and enable others in their care similarly to make health-enhancing decisions for themselves.

Summary

Before one can tackle a person as a whole, including any 'ill-health', an understanding of what potentially comprises his 'health' is needed. Emphasis is placed on an holistic approach to care, taking into consideration physical, emotional, intellectual, spiritual and sociocultural aspects, and stressing the importance of the prevention of illness as much as its treatment.

Health means different things to different people. Health and ill-health are ranged on a continuum, with no clear demarcation line between values. What is considered 'normal' may vary with, for example, age or gender, and whether or not a person describes himself as healthy will also depend on his personal outlook. Thus, it may be problematic for the nurse to grasp the full impact of any changes in an individual's state. Her ability to do this may go a long way to speeding the patient's recovery.

However much a person works towards being 'healthy' in terms of diet, physical fitness, lack of stress and so on, inequalities will always exist as a result of, for example, social class, gender, race, age, employment and the presence, or otherwise, of disability. Nurses are in a prime position to identify these areas and work with clients to minimise the influence of as many as possible, empowering patients to be responsible for their own well-being.

REFERENCES

Acheson D 1995 Tackling health inequalities: an agenda for action. King's Fund, London

Acheson R M, Hagard S 1984 Health, society and medicine: an introduction to community medicine. Blackwell Scientific, Oxford

Aggleton P 1990 Health. Routledge, London

Antonovsky A 1987 Unraveling the mystery of health: how people manage stress and stay well. Jossey-Bass, San Francisco

Bernard M, Meade K 1993 Women come of age. Edward Arnold, London

Blaxter M 1990 Health and lifestyles. Tavistock/Routledge, London

Central Statistical Office 1995 Social Trends 25. HMSO, London

Clarke A C 1991 Nurses as role models and health educators. Journal of Advanced Nursing 16(10): 1178–1184

Cmich D 1984 Theoretical perspectives of holistic health. Journal of the Society of Health 54(1): 30–32

Department of Health 1994 Stroke. HMSO, London

Downie R S 1990 Ethics in health education: an introduction. In: Doxiadis S (ed.) Ethics in health education. Wiley, Chichester, pp 4–5

Doyal L, Gough I 1991 A theory of human need. Macmillan, London

Farrell E 1991 The mental health survival guide. MacDonald Optima, London

Graham H 1993 When life's a drag: women, smoking and disadvantage. Department of Health, HMSO, London

Hayes L 1995 Unequal access to midwifery care: a continuing problem? Journal of Advanced Nursing 21(4): 702–707

Health and Safety Commission 1992 Management of health and safety at work: management of health and safety at work regulations 1992: approved code of practice. HMSO, London

Hopson B, Scally M 1980 Lifeskills teaching: education for self-empowerment. McGraw-Hill, London

Horne E M 1990 Your healthy lifestyle. In: Professional nurse: patient education plus. Austen Cornish, London, pp 2–3

McBean S 1992 Promoting positive health. Primary Health Care 2(4): 10–14

Parsons T 1979 Definitions of health and illness in the light of American values and social structure. In: Jaco E, Gartly E (eds) Patients, physicians and illness: a sourcebook in behavioral science and health. Collier-Macmillan, London, pp 120–122

Pike D 1995 Health and the environment. In: Pike S, Forster D (eds) Health promotion for all. Churchill Livingstone, London, pp 176–177

Robertson C 1991 Health visiting in practice, 2nd edn. Churchill Livingstone, Edinburgh

Rogers R, Salvage J 1988 Nurses at risk: a guide to health and safety at work. Heinemann, London

Royal College of Nursing 1994a Public health: nursing rises to the challenge. RCN Public Health Special Interest Group Publication, RCN, London

Royal College of Nursing 1994b Violence and community nursing staff: advice for managers. RCN, London

Sarafino E P 1994 Health psychology: biopsychosocial interactions, 2nd edn. Wiley, New York

Seedhouse D 1986 Health: the foundations for achievement. Wiley, Chichester

Seedhouse D 1988 Ethics: the heart of health care. Wiley, Chichester

Seligman M E P 1975 Helplessness: on depression, development and death. Freeman, San Francisco

Warr P 1987 Work, unemployment and mental health. Oxford University Press, Oxford

Woods S, Edwards S 1989 Philosophy and health. Journal of Advanced Nursing 14(8): 661–664

World Health Organization 1946 Constitution of the World Health Organization. In: Caplan A L, Engelhardt H T, McCartney J J (eds) Concepts of health and disease: interdisciplinary perspectives. Addison-Wesley, Reading, MA

World Health Organization 1978 Report on the International Conference on Primary Health Care, Alma Ata, 6–12 September. WHO, Geneva

World Health Organization 1993 Health for all targets: the health policy for Europe, updated edn. WHO Regional Office for Europe, Copenhagen

FURTHER READING

Graham H 1993 When life's a drag: women, smoking and disadvantage. Department of Health, HMSO, London

Jacobson B, Smith A, Whitehead M (eds) 1991 The nation's health: a strategy for the 1990s, revised edn. King's Fund, London

Morris J 1993 Independent lives?: community care and disabled people. Macmillan, Basingstoke

Niven N 1994 Health psychology, 2nd edn. Churchill Livingstone, Edinburgh

Rankin-Box D 1995 The nurses' handbook of complementary therapies. Churchill Livingstone, Edinburgh

World Health Organization 1993 Health for all targets: the health policy for Europe, updated edn. WHO Regional Office for Europe, Copenhagen

7

Health promotion

Diana Forster

The overall aim of health promotion is summed up by Downie et al (1990) as 'the balanced enhancement of physical, mental and social facets of positive health, coupled with the prevention of physical, mental and social ill-health'. This chapter considers how nurses might contribute to reaching this wide-ranging and ambitious goal, by:

- **outlining the processes, principles and strategies of health promotion**
- **considering inequalities in health**
- **exploring an integrated approach to health promotion, encompassing environmental, social, organisational and individual levels of intervention**
- **investigating the relationship between health promotion and health education, and introducing three models of health education**
- **discussing communication, information technology and evaluation in health promotion.**

INTRODUCTION

This chapter considers the importance of health promotion, including health protection, health education and the prevention of ill-health, in relation to all branches of nursing. It focuses on the health-promoting goal of empowering people to influence and, if required, alter conditions that affect their health. Disabled people, for example, should have every opportunity to lead a socially and economically fulfilling and mentally creative life. For this to happen, more needs to be done nationally and locally to ensure that all disabled people receive the appropriate level and type of support they prefer.

Process and principles

Health promotion is the process of helping people to increase control over and improve their health – according to the Ottawa Charter for health promotion (Box. 7.1). This Charter was the result of the First International Conference on Health Promotion, held in Ottawa, and arising out of the theme of 'Health for all by the year 2000' (World Health Organization 1978).

Based on principles of equity and social justice in striving for health for all, the Charter encompassed five main elements guiding strategies for action:

1. building healthy public policy
2. creating supportive environments
3. enhancing community health action
4. developing personal health skills
5. reorienting health services towards new health-promoting functions.

Strategies

The strategies for action were meant to make health choices easier for individual people, organisations and groups. When hampered by factors such as poor health, low income, inadequate housing and lowered self-esteem,

---

> ### Box 7.1 Definition from the Ottawa Charter (World Health Organization 1986)
>
> Health promotion is the process of enabling people to increase control over, and to improve, their health. To reach a state of complete physical, mental and social well-being, an individual or group must be able to identify and to realise aspirations, to satisfy needs, and to change or cope with the environment. Health is therefore seen as a resource for everyday life, not the objective of living. Health is a positive concept emphasising social and personal resources, as well as physical capabilities. Therefore, health promotion is not just the responsibility of the health sector, but goes beyond healthy lifestyles to well-being.

---

people may not believe themselves able to take control or have any power to alter the conditions affecting their health and well-being. The whole approach is underpinned by the imperative to tackle inequalities in health and lifestyles. It is difficult for people to take responsibility for their health where healthy foods are too expensive, where housing is inadequate and telephones vandalised, where working conditions are unhealthy or unemployment is common. An elderly, frail person who is physically disabled and lives far from shops, or a young, unsupported mother with little money and poor housing, may require extra resources but not know how to gain access to them, or may not find them appropriate. Health promotion needs to be carefully targeted in such challenging situations, recognising that some people have a greater need for – and should therefore receive – more services than others.

Resources for health should be distributed according to need, and services should be accessible and acceptable to their users.

EUROPEAN TARGETS

The World Health Organization (WHO) European Region has set 38 targets covering a broad range of health promotion and disease prevention strategies that should be achieved by the year 2000 (World Health Organization 1993). The general aims, also discussed in the previous chapter, are to:

1. ensure the following prerequisites for health for everyone:

   - peace
   - social justice
   - wholesome food and safe water
   - decent housing and sanitation
   - education
   - secure employment

2. achieve equity in health
3. prevent premature death so that people live longer
4. reduce preventable disease and disability
5. add life to years so that older or disabled people enjoy a high standard of health for as long as possible

6. promote healthy behaviour
7. discourage unhealthy behaviour
8. encourage people to participate, enhancing family life, communities and other social groupings
9. create and preserve a healthy environment
10. develop appropriate health services
11. ensure that those responsible for research, management and training accept these goals and work towards them.

THE 'HEALTH OF THE NATION' STRATEGY

An ambitious plan of targets for the year 2000 was published in the 'Health of the Nation' strategy (Department of Health 1992). Although this was an English initiative, the development of strategies for health has also been underway in Wales, Scotland and Northern Ireland. Baggott (1994) argues that these other UK initiatives have attempted to follow more closely the WHO approach to health promotion, taking the context of people's lives more into account. However, the 'Health of the Nation' has the potential to broaden its scope, and many local and community initiatives have taken place, despite the initial failure of the document to address issues of poverty and health.

The key areas addressed should be ones for which effective intervention is possible, offering opportunities for improving health. It should be possible to set objectives and targets in the chosen areas to monitor progress and evaluate outcomes. Box 7.2 lists priority areas for health objectives for the year 2000.

Cardiovascular disease, cancers of all kinds, strokes and accidents are the leading causes of premature death in the European and North American regions of the world. In recognition of these facts, the 'Health of the Nation' declares its aims to reduce rates for diseases of the circulatory system (cardiovascular and cerebrovascular disease) by 40%, to reduce the death rate for breast cancer in the population invited for screening by at least 25%, and to reduce the incidence of invasive cervical cancer by at least 20%. By the year 2005, the death rate for

---

Box 7.2 Suggested key areas and targets for health promotion (Department of Health 1992)

Causes of substantial mortality:

- coronary heart disease
- stroke
- cancers
- accidents.

Causes of substantial ill-health:

- mental illness
- diabetes
- asthma.

Factors that contribute to mortality, ill-health and healthy living:

- smoking
- diet and alcohol
- physical exercise.

Areas where there is clear scope for improvement:

- health of pregnant women, infants and children
- rehabilitation services for people with a physical disability
- environmental quality

Areas where there is a great potential for harm:

- HIV/AIDS
- other communicable diseases
- food safety

---

accidents among children under 15 should be reduced by at least 33%.

PRIMARY HEALTH CARE

Arising from these national and international resolves has been an increasing move among health professionals towards primary care. Primary health care (also discussed in Ch. 6), public health and health promotion with individual people may be seen as parts of a continuum. Although the hospital and institutional setting is often characterised as being distinct from community care, people have many similar wants and needs, whatever the site of their care, and the challenge of health promotion is to adopt a more seamless, holistic approach.

In order to develop healthy public policy and achieve community and individual empowerment, there is a need to gain 'inter-sectoral collaboration', i.e. to form healthy alliances.

Healthy alliances

Healthy alliances stem from the WHO 'Health for All' strategy (World Health Organization 1993). A healthy alliance, such as Healthy City Project, should be a partnership of organisations or individuals that goes beyond health care and collectively attempts to change social and environmental circumstances affecting health. The NHS has a key role to play in mobilising action through healthy alliances with other organisations. These might include local authorities, schools, voluntary bodies, professional groups, institutes, community groups, local businesses or local media – newspapers, radio and television. Box 7.3 outlines a project in Avon.

Box 7.3 The Bournville Localities Project – Look After Your Heart – Avon (Chalmers 1993)

A 3-year health promotion project on the Bournville Estate, Weston-super-Mare, was developed to address the lack of health facilities and leisure activities for children. Local residents were helped to set up facilities such as a play park, child health clinic and a successful campaign for improved road safety. The project focused on the needs and wishes of local people, helping them to become more involved in the community and improving their environment. Only then did residents feel able to change their lifestyles and approach the issues of diet, exercise and smoking.

INEQUALITIES IN HEALTH

Chapter 6, about health, revealed that:

- making choices about being healthy or not is more complex than it seems
- many factors are outside an individual's control
- healthy choices are easier for some people to make than for others
- the health choices that people make are affected by their cultural background and by the social and physical environment in which they live
- nurses and other health promoters need to acknowledge their own difficulties in making healthy choices.

Health promotion is not simply about getting individuals to change but about changing many

of the social facts that we take for granted. There is much evidence to show that health among people who are socially and/or economically disadvantaged tends to be poorer. Those in social class V have worse health than do their contemporaries in non-manual occupations (Acheson 1995). Whitehead (1992) has also reviewed trends in both child and adult health. She reports that, although health status has improved over the past decades, those in non-manual occupations and their families have benefited most from these improvements.

Perinatal death rates (stillbirths and deaths in the first week of life) for social classes IV and V have been 50% above those for classes I and II. (For example, in 1990, the respective rates were 9.5 and 6.2 per 1000 births.) The national campaign against coronary heart disease, 'Look After Your Heart', will hopefully be effective in tackling the excess death rates among men in social classes IV and V. Its main aims include the development of programmes in various settings (Boxes 7.3 and 7.4), including places of work, where health promotion is concentrated upon:

- smoking and tobacco use
- diet and nutrition
- control of blood pressure
- the promotion of physical activity.

Box 7.4 'Look After Your Heart'

Over 500 organisations in the commercial sector have now signed up to the Health Education Authority's 'Look After Your Heart' (LAYH) Workplace Charter. The Automobile Association (AA) is one such example. The LAYH principles have been adopted, for instance, throughout the AA's staff restaurants. This involves providing staff with details about healthy living, as well as promoting and providing healthy choices of food (Proud 1994).

Health issues and ethnic origin

Although minority communities have patterns of mortality similar to those of the rest of the population, there are differences in the rates of some diseases (see Ch. 8). In order to promote the health of local populations, health authorities should obtain accurate information about the ethnic mix of the population, its cultural habits and health status, and take positive steps to eliminate any discrimination (Box 7.5).

Box 7.5

Free services developed to increase access to health services for the Chinese and South-East Asian residents of Greater Manchester include (Grant 1994):

- branch surgery sessions staffed by Chinese doctors who give advice and refer clients back to their own GPs as necessary
- a drop-in advice facility staffed by bilingual workers
- translating and interpreting services
- outreach interpreting (e.g. for clients in hospital) and translation of health education material
- facilities for self-help groups and seminars
- cultural information resource for mainstream health professionals.

The new impetus for improvement in health care for ethnic minorities has been emphasised in a guide for the NHS on ethnicity and health (Balarajan & Raleigh 1993).

Differences in access to health care may be due to lack of information about services, communication difficulties, provision of inappropriate or hard-to-reach services, and the different expectations of clients and health workers (Box 7.6).

Box 7.6 Quote from a member of an ethnic minority group (McGee 1994)

'There is a widespread belief that elderly members of ethnic minority groups will always be cared for within their families, that they do not need or want help from outsiders. As a member of an ethnic minority group I would argue that my sisters and I face the same problems in caring for our elderly parents as any indigenous family, yet the beliefs of professionals could mean that we are not offered the same help.'

AN INTEGRATED APPROACH TO HEALTH PROMOTION

Wilson-Barnett (1993) describes health promotion as a broad overarching concept that guides the way in which nurses and health carers should support and care for people. Nursing should be directed at general policy issues, as well as individual aspects of care and health enhancement. Goals for nursing and goals for health promotion should therefore be one and the same, so that health promotion is fully integrated into nursing care, as shown in the example in the next section.

The balance of good health

The new national food guide 'The Balance of Good Health' (Health Education Authority 1994) aims to help people to understand and enjoy healthy eating. It provides an example of the integration of goals for nursing and health promotion – healthy eating, nutrition and diet are vital for both. The guidelines apply to most people – vegetarians, people of all ethnic origins and people who are a healthy weight for their height, as well as those who are over- or underweight. However, it does not apply to children under 2 years of age as they need full-fat milk and dairy products, and for others there may, of course, be medical reasons for special dietary requirements.

The approach is based on the five commonly accepted food groups, which are:

- bread, other cereals and potatoes
- fruit and vegetables
- milk and dairy foods
- meat, fish and alternatives
- fatty and sugary foods.

The key message of the document is the balance of foods that should be consumed to achieve a healthy diet. For example, choosing a variety of foods from the first four groups every day helps to provide the wide range of nutrients that the body needs to remain healthy and function properly. Foods in the fifth group are not essential to a healthy diet but add extra choice and palatability. The guidelines discuss the difference in the amount of energy (or calories) people require according to gender, age, weight and level of physical activity. These guidelines are therefore a useful source of up-to-date, relevant information about healthy eating, diet and nutrition for nurses to share with their clients.

THEORIES AND PRACTICE

A range of models and approaches for nursing and for health promotion and health education has been developed over the years, and there is a need to integrate theoretical concepts with a practical application. One way of making health promotion interventions more effective is presented by Kelly et al (1993). These writers suggest the use of a checklist integrating four levels of health promotion, identified as:

* environmental
* social
* organisational
* individual.

They argue that the relationships between all four levels and the outcomes at all levels need to be considered, fitting in with the health alliance initiatives discussed earlier. Interventions need to be analysed to ensure that the health promotion has been effective.

Four levels of health promotion

Environmental

One of the greatest challenges facing nurses today is how to promote the health of people who live in conditions of social, economic and environmental deprivation. The health divide between rich and poor, the employed and the unemployed, is getting wider. The key to effective health promotion lies in looking beyond individual behaviours to the personal circumstances in which people find themselves.

Paradoxically, health promotion initiatives that fail to pay attention to low income and material disadvantage may increase health inequalities by improving the health of high-income groups, who are more likely to attend screening sessions or read health promotional literature, while failing to reach low-income groups and help them to improve their health.

Homes, transport systems and working conditions are examples of the environment that may be health promoting, health protecting or, instead, health damaging (Box 7.7).

> **Box 7.7 Some ways in which transport may affect health** (Hillman 1991)
>
> * Physically, owing to death and injury in road traffic accidents.
> * Psychologically, in distress from accidents and the fear of accidents.
> * Pathologically, as the pollution and noise from motor vehicles are sources of disease and mental impairment.
> * Ecologically, as exhaust emissions from traffic are a major contributor to global warming.

The environmental concern itself operates at several levels, including cellular, organ or bodily system (see Ch. 1) and the whole-person level, as well as at group and species levels. Thus the environment is a background influence to be considered in promoting health. The introduction of child resistant containers for medicine has been associated with a steep drop in childhood poisonings, and there are many other small- and large-scale possibilities in which preventive efforts reflecting environmental rather than behavioural changes alone could be effective.

 Activity 7.1

> Reflect upon your own setting – where you live, work or study. Can you identify one or more aspects that you would like to change to improve your own health and well-being? Which other people might join you in negotiating for change?

Many people have a part to play in promoting environmental health including:

* city planners
* social and health workers
* housing and traffic administrators
* teachers
* environmental health officers
* business employers
* community activists.

This is particularly important in a transcultural society, where a rich variety of lifestyles and values needs to be recognised (Box 7.8).

Box 7.8 **The Healthy Cities Project – an example**
(Ashton & Seymour 1988)

The rates for heart disease and strokes are 20–30% higher in Liverpool than those for England as a whole. As part of the Healthy Cities Project, a survey was carried out in the Liverpool Health District. It showed that, for many people, it is difficult to buy foods that would help to prevent heart disease and stroke because healthy food tends to be more expensive than unhealthy convenience food. The main priority for people on low incomes, the researchers found, was to prevent hunger and make their money last until the next Social Security cheque.

The researchers in Liverpool recommended that a victim-blaming approach be avoided, and that, as convenience foods were preferred, they should be improved in quality. It was also suggested that education and training in domestic science and cooking should ideally be provided for boys and girls of all intellectual abilities to enable them to maintain a healthy diet without constantly resorting to junk or convenience foods. The Liverpool study also showed that supportive policies for health promotion in reducing coronary heart disease need to be wide-ranging and should include:

- food labelling and education
- town planning, including supermarket sites
- agricultural and transport policies.

In the past, nursing was concerned mainly with the patient's immediate environment in the home or hospital. Today, nursing involves a concern for promoting a healthy environment for the person, family and community. One objective of the British government is to protect and promote the health and well-being of the nation by improving environmental quality. Information is available at a local level from the Health Promotion/ Education Department situated in each District Health Authority, and from the Environmental Health Officers in each local authority.

Social

An empowered community is one in which people are vigorously involved in creating the conditions necessary for healthy living. Medical services do not always meet the needs of the public and often take power away by treating people as passive recipients of care. In a holistic approach to care, health promotion focuses on cooperation rather than compliance with medical regimens, as shown in the example in Box 7.3, above.

The social structure includes patterns of group behaviour. Interventions at this level might include a number of methods for influencing people in groups, such as education, advertising, community development projects, pressure group techniques (e.g. demonstrations and media events), taxation and fiscal policy, and changes in legislation and law enforcement. The relationship between the person and society is an inter-dependent one – each influencing the other; for example, patterns of change may be seen most obviously in such factors as fashions in clothes and voting in elections. This dynamic and complex nature of social structures means that they are difficult to manipulate. Deliberate attempts to plan society may have unexpected and unplanned results. In relation to health, for instance, attempts to use advertising campaigns to reduce narcotic drug use may actually excite curiosity about the topic and instead increase drug usage. Merely providing information about the risks of smoking is often ineffective, as Graham (1993) illustrates in her research (Box 7.9).

While health professionals often identify pregnancy and early motherhood as times rich in opportunities for initiating behavioural change,

Box 7.9 **When life's a drag** (Graham 1993)

An open-ended question sought to identify why mothers who had tried to give up had started smoking again. The major reasons mothers gave for starting again clustered around the difficulty of managing their lives without cigarettes. One-third of the mothers (31%) said it was because they found it hard to cope with their everyday problems and stress. Other reasons focused on boredom and irritability and the related social pressures to smoke, either direct interpersonal pressure from partners or the indirect pressure of being in the company of smokers.

Graham (1993) found that 60% of the current smokers in those categories in her study had not attempted to stop smoking, although they understood the possible health effects on themselves and their children.

An integrated model of health promotion would include consideration of people's experience of social structures and the variety of influences upon them.

Organisational

A wide range of public and private services and institutions influence health for good or ill. The third level of potential intervention and analysis identified by Kelly et al (1993) is that of organisations. Organisations are not simply institutions, such as factories, hospitals, schools or health centres. They also consist of a set of interactions between people, patterned according to rules and procedures in relation to hierarchy and authority. Relationships are additionally based on informal interactions between people in organisations. People outside the organisation also form relationships with those within it, for example clients, consumers or users.

Some organisations, such as Health Promotion Departments and Public Health Departments, have an explicit health promotion function. Others, including schools, hospitals and health centres, have a commitment to the delivery of health promotion, including health education, although it is not their main function. However, all organisations should have a health-promoting role, aiming to create and sustain human dignity, creativeness and growth, and to provide a safe, stress-free working environment, as discussed in Chapter 6.

Individual

Individual behaviour is the last of the levels identified by Kelly et al (1993). The individual is considered in a holistic way as part of

- a family
- a community
- society
- the environment.

In recent years, nurses have come to acknowledge that the practice of nursing involves educating patients and promoting healthy lifestyles. Major health gains during the rest of this century, and no doubt in the next, will result far more from improvements in nutrition, physical fitness, personal habits, immunisation and environmental conditions than from traditional medical care. Nurses can teach people they have contact with about these issues (see Ch. 18).

Psychology and the individual

A number of psychological theories have found widespread acceptance in certain types of health promotion, including the health belief model and the theory of reasoned action.

The health belief model

Research suggests that four elements influence the likelihood of someone engaging in a healthy habit or changing a detrimental one (Bandura 1977, Becker 1984). The person must believe that:

- the disease or disorder is serious
- he is susceptible to the disorder
- the response will be effective in reducing the dangers and protect the person from the threat (i.e. he believes in the efficacy of the response)
- he will be able to carry out the recommended preventive health action (i.e he believes in the efficacy of the self in this respect).

Changing behaviour

Modifying health behaviours and beliefs is, however, not a simple matter; for example, the immediate costs of changing diet to avoid heart disease may not seem worth the effort. It may involve changing from preferred methods of cooking, eating less-favoured foods and perhaps increased shopping expenses.

Besides health teaching for individuals and groups, behavioural changes in relation to diet may be motivated by:

- advertising health aspects of foods

- labelling foods, as, for example, having a high or low fat content
- health warnings to raise awareness.

People often need to pass through stages of changing attitudes and assimilating information before they make actual changes in their behaviour. Those wishing to avoid the risk of HIV infection, for example, may need help in developing social skills enabling them to adopt safer sexual practices, such as effective condom use.

The motivation to change practices depends partly upon the social and cultural groups to which people belong, and how far HIV and AIDS, for example, are seen as threats to health. Successful helping requires that habitual practices are viewed from the client's own perspective. Actions that involve the risk of HIV infection, with its potential life-threatening, long-term consequences, may be regarded by outsiders as irrational and irresponsible, but to some clients unsafe sex may seem to offer security, love and the satisfaction of desire. The possible threats to health in an already uncertain and unpromising future then seem less important (Anderson & Wilkie 1992).

An understanding of health beliefs suggests that encouraging responsible attitudes towards sexuality involves empowering young people to resist social pressures – including sexual advances and advertising – and to act upon informed choices. Education in parenting skills and empowerment education in schools may be the best long-term solution.

The theory of reasoned action

Another model that has been found to be relevant to health promotion is the theory of reasoned action (Ajzen & Fishbein 1980). This separates beliefs from attitudes, for example in relation to making decisions about health, and emphasises the influence of significant others on a person's intention to act. The theory is based on the assumption that most health-related behaviour is under voluntary control. Behaviour is stated to be governed by two broad influences:

1. the person's attitude towards a certain behaviour – each attitude consists of a belief (e.g. that smoking can cause cancer) and a value attached to that belief, i.e. how important this is to oneself
2. people's ideas of what significant others will think of their behaviour.

These two influences combine to form an intention to act. People do not always behave in accordance with their expressed attitudes because of the influences upon them. Bennett & Hodgson (1992) provide the example of an ex-smoker who may have a number of negative attitudes towards smoking. However, when out for a drink with friends who smoke, he may himself smoke, because smoking is an acceptable norm for the group and drinking alcohol may also interfere with the previous intention of not smoking.

Similarly, a person may jump out of an aeroplane attached to a flimsy length of silk or nylon, despite having a negative attitude towards jumping – including fear at the point of leaving the aircraft – because she does not want to lose face with friends by going against the norms of the group.

Combining the four levels of health promotion

An integrated approach to health promotion is, therefore, involved in increasing access to health; the development of an environment, in its broadest social and physical sense, that is conducive to health; strengthening social networks and support; promoting positive health behaviour and coping strategies; and increasing knowledge and making information widely available.

For example, the initial government-sponsored HIV/AIDS television campaigns were directed entirely at individual behaviour, ignoring the environment in which people live, the social systems of which they are a part and the services available to them. It proved ineffectual to preach responsibility and safer sex without a service back-up to teach the necessary skills, including effective condom use, and without reference to relevant social systems. These included sub-cultures of drug abuse and various sexual opportunities. The ability successfully to change habitual practices is influenced by the social and cultural groups to which people belong, and the extent to which HIV and AIDS, for instance, are viewed as threats to health. Active participation and approaches that seek to raise self-esteem as well as provide factual information have been found to be the most effective ways of imparting health knowledge and promoting healthy lifestyles (Box 7.10).

Box 7.10 **Young people's family planning and counselling services** (Allen 1991)

These should be an integral part of mainstream family planning services.
  Two main types of service should be offered to young people:

- 'direct services', available at a defined base directly to people who attend there
- 'outreach services', which go out from the base to young people or those working with them.

Direct services with nursing input should include:

- a clinic service with a doctor available offering contraceptive advice and supplies, post-coital contraception, pregnancy testing, pregnancy counselling, referral for termination of pregnancy, AIDS counselling and health education of a more general nature in response to need.
- a 'drop-in' service offering a range of health-related options, with a counsellor present and geared to local cultural needs.

Outreach work should take place in collaboration with local Health Promotion Specialists, the Local Education Authority, AIDS coordinators, etc.

Characteristics of an integrated approach

Health promotion is characterised as:

- involving the population (or specific sub-groups) as a whole
- using many different but complementary methods and approaches
- being aimed at public participation, addressing problems that people themselves define as important
- being an activity in the health and social fields
- being often rooted in popular struggles and movements for social change
- valuing lay knowledge and not relying on expert-designed interventions in problem-

solving and decision-making (in self-help groups, for example)
- working best when in harmony with a healthy public policy.

Activity 7.2

Can you identify self-help groups that meet near to where you live or work? Find out from the local Community Health Council, Council for Voluntary Services or Social Services department what groups there are.

HEALTH PROMOTION AND HEALTH EDUCATION

The realisation that health and well-being are affected by a complex mixture of influences has developed over the past two decades. There has been a move away from traditional, simplistic health educational approaches, largely based on trying to persuade people to change their behaviour – perhaps stopping smoking or drinking, or taking more exercise – towards wider issues of health promotion. People in advanced industrial societies are faced with many choices that can affect their health, concerning such issues as food, sexual activity, exercise and the use of alcohol, tobacco and drugs. The emphasis on personal choice often implies that individuals are totally responsible for their health. However, this 'victim-blaming approach', as it is often called, takes no account of the social context, discussed earlier, in which decisions are made. For example, cocaine is used when it is socially available and other people are using it, so the individual choice is only one element in a complex social process.

Health education remains a vital tool concerned with the sharing and learning of knowledge, values and attitudes – with clients in partnership with their health educators. It is one component of the broader, umbrella concept of health promotion.

A definition of health education, in the context of empowering and supporting individual choice, is offered by Tones & Tilford (1994):

Health education is any intentional activity which is designed to achieve health or illness related learning, i.e. some relatively permanent change in an individual's capability or disposition. Effective health education may, thus, produce changes in knowledge and understanding or ways of thinking; it may influence or clarify values; it may bring about some shift in belief or attitude; it may facilitate the aquisition of skills; it may even effect changes in behaviour or lifestyle.

HEALTH EDUCATION AS A BASIS FOR HEALTH PROMOTION

Research has shown that health education often arises naturally from the routine interaction between nurse and patient. It has also been shown that health education is effective only if it is tailored to the needs of the individual. Swaffield (1990) comments, 'Unless you start from where your patient is you have no chance of taking him anywhere. And if you don't know where your patient is – ask.'

Health education is the process by which individuals and groups learn to promote, maintain or restore health and therefore be able to make choices and decisions for themselves. Its desired outcome is a change in behaviour or attitude, often in response to a new understanding of the impact upon health of such factors as:

- stress
- smoking
- exercise
- excess weight
- chronic disease
- air pollution
- recreation
- occupation.

Health education programmes may be devised in hospitals, clubs or schools to encourage children not to take up smoking, but for these programmes to be really effective, the whole community needs to be educated in the provision of more non-smoking environments. How long will it take, Macleod Clark & Latter (1990) wonder, before smoking in public places is banned entirely? Health promotion must go beyond the individual into society at large, influencing policies and health care plans. Nurses may be involved at all levels – in one-to-one teaching, counselling and advising, and in informing the whole community through pressure groups, campaigns and community programmes (Box 7.11).

> **Box 7.11 The nurse's role in preventing the spread of HIV and AIDS** (Stanford 1990)
>
> - Learn about HIV/AIDS.
> - Follow guidelines on the prevention of infection.
> - Inform the public about HIV/AIDS, and help dispel myths and prejudices.
> - Encourage people to accept responsibility for their sexual relationships and activities, and so protect themselves and their partners' health.
> - Encourage the use of condoms.
> - Encourage intravenous drug users not to share needles and syringes and to practise safer sex.
> - Inform the public about donating blood. There is no risk to the donor.
> - Allay anxieties about blood transfusions – the risk is negligible.
> - Encourage people with HIV to adopt a healthy lifestyle and tell them how to avoid infecting others.
> - Know where to refer patients for specialised help and counselling.
> - Promote a caring and responsible attitude towards people who have the virus.

Nurses need to be skilled facilitators; health education is a communication activity. It is not enough simply to relay information: the beliefs, attitudes and behaviour of individuals and communities must be changed if health education is to be effective.

HEALTH EDUCATION MODELS

Tones & Tilford (1994) describe three approaches to health education:

- the preventive model
- the radical model
- the empowerment model.

The preventive model

The preventive model may be considered under the headings of primary, secondary and tertiary health education.

Staying healthy – primary prevention

Primary health education encourages people to behave in ways that will help them to avoid disease or injury and maintain their quality of life. For example, parents who take their children to be immunised against such infectious diseases as diphtheria, polio, whoping cough, measles, mumps and rubella are seeking to prevent them contracting these potentially harmful illnesses. Health educators could teach parents that immunisation is designed to prevent the onset of certain diseases, and encourage them to undertake the appropriate immunisation schedules.

Primary health education also involves genetic counselling and ante natal care. Counselling may be offered, for example, to couples whose future baby might be at risk of developing a genetic disorder, such as sickle cell anaemia or Down's syndrome.

Road traffic accidents are the main cause of death in people under 30 years of age in the UK (Department of Health 1994), and nurses are greatly involved in caring for people who are injured on the roads. Primary health education can help to reduce the number of such accidents in many different ways. Accident prevention includes campaigning for safer roads and vehicles, as well as teaching people about safe practices. Nurses can encourage others to use seat belts and child safety seats in accordance with the law and never to drink and drive. Why should nurses not also become involved in changing laws where they think this is necessary, for instance, by making their views about penalties for driving offences, or about potentially dangerous situations for pedestrians, widely known?

Examples of educative efforts directed towards primary prevention also include:

- weight control to prevent the onset of diabetes
- nutrition education, to help maintain normal systolic and diastolic blood pressures
- education concerning the danger of over-exposure to sunlight as a risk factor for skin cancer
- 'stop smoking' programmes to help to prevent cancer of the lung and cardiovascular disorders.

Activity 7.3

1. Decide upon a target group. Visit your local Health Promotion Department and assemble:

   - leaflets
   - posters
   - facts about smoking and its possible effects
   - facts about helpful ways to stop smoking
   - details of audiovisual aids, including films, videos, audiotapes and slides.

2. Help your group to plan to stop smoking by:

   - discussing the benefits to their health
   - motivating them by discussing benefits to their appearance, for example having no nicotine staining of clothes, fingers or teeth.

3. Consider coping strategies, including:

   - avoiding places where others smoke
   - not having cigarettes and lighters at home
   - having a supply of non-fattening snacks on hand, such as fruit, celery or carrot sticks, or chewing gum, for when the smoking urge is strong
   - keeping busy and having relaxing hobbies, including exercising, sport, gardening or watching television
   - identifying people who can provide support and encouragement, for example local stop-smoking clinics and groups, and the GP, nurse, health visitor or district nurse (Kendall 1990).

4. Finally, evaluate your health-promotion role: did you help your group to stop smoking through your supportive discussion and sharing of knowledge?

The leading cause of death in the UK is coronary heart disease (CHD): of the total number dying each year in the UK, one in three men and one in four women die from CHD. It is also the main cause of death in men under 65 years old (premature death). Because smoking often starts in adolescence, health promoters have tried to tackle the problem by studying ways to keep teenagers from smoking. The most successful programmes seem to be those which provide anti-smoking information in formats that appeal to adolescents, portray a positive image of the non-smoker as independent and self-reliant, and use peer-group techniques (popular peers serve as non-smoking role models) and skills development to help teenagers to resist peer pressure.

Primary health education also has a major part to play in the area of mental health. Counselling individuals and families can help them to recognise or avoid problems such as anorexia nervosa in adolescents, to deal constructively with many situations that may cause stress and, more generally, to cope with life's crises as they arise. Health education and support may be available in local self-help groups or voluntary groups, advice centres or social or health services for people at risk of becoming depressed or suicidal, including those who are:

- unemployed – particularly young men
- bereaved
- physically disabled
- elderly
- socially isolated
- suffering from chronic, painful or life-threatening conditions.

School health. Much health education that takes place in schools is primary in nature, i.e. designed to promote a healthy lifestyle and to prevent, for example, the misuse of drugs, alcohol and tobacco, particularly during pregnancy. Stress, life events and family life are also topics for discussion.

Programmes and activities can be developed to teach children and young people how to take responsibility for their own health and lifestyle, not only to prevent illness, but also to enhance the quality of life itself. However, it is easy for those teaching health education merely to pass on knowledge and skills to their pupils, without evaluating the changes in pupils' outlook and behaviour. 'How can I motivate these young people to want to know what a healthy diet might be; and how do I encourage them to avoid such conditions as anorexia nervosa, bulimia and obesity?': these are questions that teachers, nurses and other health educators need to ask themselves when planning programme activities.

School nurses are introducing pupil-held records in many schools, reflecting the change towards viewing children as partners in health promotion (Box 7.12).

Secondary health education

Secondary health education is concerned with

Box 7.12 **The school health fax** (McAleer & Jackson 1994)

The health fax was piloted in 21 schools in inner London for pupils in year seven (11 plus). It was developed as a focus for interviews and as a tool to empower young people to share responsibility for their own health. In some pilot schools, many pupils used English as a second language, and travelled regularly between England and other countries. A readily accessible, up-to-date health record was found to be advantageous. Evaluation showed that most pupils liked the fax and appreciated having a comprehensive record of their own health status.

Activity 7.4

Select a health promotion topic currently in the news (e.g. substance/drug/alcohol abuse, healthy eating, AIDS). Build up an information/resource package on this subject for use within your work or college library, collecting as wide a range of information and promotional materials as possible, using all available sources. If other colleagues are interested in this project, take a group approach.

Consider supplying the package to other interested parties, for example youth clubs.

halting or reversing the development of an existing disease or condition.

Health screening. People may be encouraged to undergo health screening procedures so that a condition or disease can be identified at an early stage, often before any signs or symptoms have been noticed. The appropriate treatment or management of the condition can then begin. For screening to be effective for the condition or disease (Naidoo & Wills 1994):

- it should have a long pre-clinical phase so that a screening test will not miss its signs
- earlier treatment should improve the outcomes
- the test should be sensitive, i.e. it should detect all those with the disease
- the test should be specific, i.e. it should detect only those with the disease
- the test should be acceptable, easy to perform and safe

- it should be cost-effective, i.e. the number of tests performed should yield a number of positive cases.

Screening is now carried out to identify some of the possible errors in metabolism. All newborn babies in the UK are screened by a blood test for the disease phenylketonuria (PKU). This is characterised by an inability correctly to metabolise the amino acid phenylalanine. As a result, phenylketones are formed in large amounts, and the toxicity to brain cells causes mental retardation. However, detecting the disease aids the promotion of normal development, because a special diet limiting phenylalanine until the child is 7 or 8 years old prevents mental retardation. Having a child on a special diet imposes many strains on a family, and it is important that everyone involved in the child's care understands the diet and the reasons for the need for it.

Cancer. There is an increasing trend in testicular cancer in young men, and breast cancer accounts for 30% of all female cancers and will affect 1 in 12 English women at some time in their lives. Individuals can detect cancer of the breast or testicles in its early stages by self-examination, which can be taught by nurses either to groups or on an individual basis. People can also be taught to recognise early melanoma and to attend for treatment at a stage when prospects for cure are good – as is the case with several other types of malignancy. People can be encouraged to attend well-man and well-woman clinics, where health education and health promotion activities, including breast and cervical screening, are carried out.

Screening programmes for hypertension, diabetes, glaucoma and sexually transmitted diseases are examples of other vital aspects of secondary health education in which nurses can become involved. The community setting is the venue for essential preventive programmes, such as vision and hearing testing, screening for scoliosis and the assessment of children for disabilities or developmental delays.

Tertiary health education

The function of this aspect of health promotion is to prevent complications where disease already exists, thus preventing relapse and promoting rehabilitation of the patient, so that the best possible level of health might be achieved. Nurses taking part in tertiary health education may also be involved in helping patients to adjust to terminal illness, and in providing counselling for patients and their relatives and carers. In the treatment of incurable forms of cancer, the health education goal may be to help the patient remain as comfortable as possible.

In the public perception, AIDS is the territory of the young, its cause rooted in youthful behaviour, and its tragedy being the cutting short of young lives. However, in the UK, some 11% of people with AIDS are aged 50 and over (Kaufmann 1993). Those diagnosed as HIV-positive may have parents and grandparents who are, in their turn, deeply affected by the virus, and who need the kind of support usually only offered to younger people who need information, care and counselling.

Patients with chronic conditions such as diabetes need to adjust their dietary intake to ensure maximum health, and health education for them would include the stimulation of positive attitudes towards altering their diet. Nurses can help those whose illness is disabling to adopt a lifestyle that minimises limitations, for example through the introduction of mechanical and electronic aids. Simple adaptations, such as using easy-to-hold cutlery or modifying the living environment with ramps or rails, may be needed in addition to nursing and dietary advice. In the case of patients who have overcome an illness, nurses may need to provide support in the adjustment to a former state of health and in the abandonment of the 'sick role'.

Tertiary health education in mental health may involve helping individuals and their families to deal with the stress and management of established mental illness or handicap. Helping families to cope with current crises and to manage problems associated with long-standing illnesses can make a significant contribution to the rehabilitation of the whole family unit. The aim is to help the patient and his family to reach and maintain an optimum level of functioning. Support and education for the family is especially important in cases of handicapping conditions and long-term psychotic illnesses, such as schizophrenia (Simmons 1987).

The radical model

Tones & Tilford (1994) discuss criticisms of the preventive approach to health education. The radical approach rejects the so-called victim-blaming stance of the preventive model and attempts to 'refocus upstream'. This term refers to a parable that describes a doctor busily dragging drowning people from a flooding river who remarks, 'You know, I am so busy jumping in, pulling them to shore, applying artificial respiration, that I have no time to see who the hell is upstream pushing them all in'. The radical model seeks to focus not on the individual and his behaviour but on those social, economic and political factors that promote unhealthy practices and produce unhealthy food and hazardous products.

The large amount of information that was collected and analysed in the national survey discussed in Chapter 6 (Blaxter 1990) arrives at an inescapable conclusion: circumstances have greater weight than does behaviour in determining health status. This is not to suggest that a person's health would not be improved if he stopped smoking for instance, but that, in some circumstances, the improvement might only be a modest one. The avoidance of unhealthy behaviour, such as smoking and eating a poor diet, offers much more protection to health in parts of the country where the environment is already more conducive to good health, for example in non-industrial suburban or rural areas. Moreover, adopting a healthy lifestyle is much more difficult for those living in poverty.

The radical model applied to the prevention of CHD would focus not upon the individual, but upon the various social, economic and political factors that promote unhealthy products and practices. Public awareness of the ways in which commercial interests can be at odds with health interests such as dangers from factory emissions of smoke, might be heightened. A local campaign consistent with the radical approach might unite a parent–teacher association and a school's governing body to influence the school canteen to provide healthy food and discourage the consumption of foods high in saturated fat.

In some areas, many families, particularly those from ethnic minorities, live in high-rise flats or inner-city housing, where space for children to play is very scarce. Concern is often expressed about the high number of road traffic accidents among Asian children in large cities, and this sometimes prompts leaflets about road safety to be produced and circulated. However, many children have nowhere to play apart from narrow, traffic-filled streets. Health and safety could be promoted far more effectively through the provision of adequate housing and traffic-free play areas (Pearson 1986).

The empowerment model

This third health education approach reflects the idea that the individual's ability to choose for himself and determine his own lifestyle is an important aspect of both psychological and physical well-being. Health educators support change through the individual's own choices, rather than by coercion. True empowerment not only requires a basis of knowledge to support informed choices, but also demands the clarification of values and the chance to practise decision-making skills. People also need to be able to influence their own environment and to seek to change it, perhaps by working together in groups to influence policies at a local or national level.

In order to reach this level of empowerment, people will need support and guidance in acquiring the necessary skills. The ability to motivate patients to change their substance abuse behaviour, for example, is one of the most challenging skills that nurses need to develop. Through working with individuals, families and community organisations, nurses can help to influence change and promote health. On a one-to-one basis, nurses can motivate the patient by gradually building a therapeutic relationship in which they help the patient to set goals and to assume responsibility for his own recovery.

Nurses also need to be aware of the association of certain diseases, particularly AIDS, with drug abuse. The use of contaminated needles is now one of the major ways in which AIDS is contracted.

Nurses and other health workers concerned with the promotion of health should learn to detect signs of substance abuse, even when it is being concealed from them. Communication skills can enable nurses to recognise the barriers to communication put up by patients attempting to hide their behaviour.

COMMUNICATION IN HEALTH PROMOTION

The promotion of health through the practice of nursing involves communicating with individuals in hospital wards and units, health centres, homes for physically and mentally handicapped people, patients' homes and many other settings in the health care system. Nurses communicate with patients, clients, relatives and friends and professional colleagues, often without thinking about its effectiveness or quality.

Increased self-awareness can help nurses to recognise the skills they are using in their interactions, to develop those skills and to make their interactions more meaningful (see Ch. 17). Communication is basic to all stages of the nursing process (see Ch. 14). It is through communication that helping relationships are formed, problems identified and discussed and information on physical and mental health conveyed. Patient education cannot be successful without effective nurse–patient communication, as Macleod Clark & Latter (1990) point out.

Health professionals can be involved in promoting health at many levels, as discussed earlier. Baric (1990) considers community participation within primary health care as the most promising way of enabling people to take responsibility for their own health.

Helping people to recognise their own health needs, and to raise their competence in doing what they think is important for them and their community, depends on high levels of communication skills. People need constant access to information about health and about how they can individually and collectively assume control over health matters in everyday life.

Nurses face many possible dilemmas in communicating health knowledge to patients and other members of the community. In hospitals and other health care settings, therapeutic communication skills can help in the teaching and promotion of health only if the person feels safe with the health educator and is able to trust and respect her. One of the basic principles of health promotion is that it must start from where the patient is. Questioning and listening skills are vital in determining the patient's attitudes and priorities and in developing a therapeutic, health-promoting relationship.

Verbal communication problems

Because medical jargon is familiar to health professionals, it is easy for them to assume that other people understand it also. However, even an apparently straightforward term, such as 'abdomen', can be confusing for some lay people. An example of miscommunication through jargon is given by Friedman & DiMatteo (1989):

Doctor: Have you ever had a history of cardiac arrest in your family?
Patient: No, we have never had any trouble with the police.
Doctor: Do you have varicose veins?
Patient: Well, I have veins, but I don't know if they're close or not.

Surveys of patients in paediatric outpatient settings have shown that a large number of patients feel that doctors and nurses do not always understand their problems and use words that are too difficult for the patients to understand (Silverman 1987). Speech difficulties, such as stammers, can also cause problems in communication and should be taken into account.

Non-verbal communication problems

Touch is an important feature of communication and patient education. Porritt (1990) describes studies carried out in the 1940s that showed that children in hospital did not respond to treatment if they were not touched, patted and stroked. Children need consistent communication, including cuddling and touching, particularly during nursing procedures and while explanations are being given. Touch can, however, be intrusive in some intimate procedures of nursing care.

Non-verbal communication can be valuable in communicating with elderly patients (Macleod Clark 1991). When speech, hearing or sight are limited, the skilful use of touch can help to ensure that patients are aware that they are cared for and can enable them to learn to carry out some health care activities, such as washing or eating, for themselves. Macleod Clark (1991) suggests that most touch between nurses and elderly patients is related to practical procedures, fulfilling a practical rather than an emotional purpose. Touch has, however, been shown to raise patients' estimation of nurses as being helpful and ready to listen. Warmth, empathy and caring can be transmitted effectively through touch in people of all ages and contribute to the promotion of their health and well-being.

There are also cultural differences in normal eye contact patterns, which need to be remembered by nurses teaching people with backgrounds different from their own. Middle Eastern and Latin patients will tend to expect more eye contact than will Western European ones. Some Asian and American Indian cultures use less eye contact than do Europeans, and among these groups, it can be regarded as disrespectful to look into someone's eyes.

Nurses involved in developing relationships with physically and mentally handicapped people should not stare at deformities, but the strategy of maintaining constant eye contact in order to avoid doing so is also likely to be recognised by a patient. Interaction with a handicapped person, which includes eye contact, may be rigid, and this is often obvious to the patient (Friedman & DiMatteo 1989). Nurses should also guard against unwittingly placing increased distance, indicating distaste or disgust, between themselves and people who are handicapped or disfigured in some way, or whose appearance is otherwise abnormal. Fear of catching a contagious disease, and the fear of AIDS, may also lead to nurses maintaining a greater distance and avoiding opportunities to provide health education.

Smells and odours can become barriers to health promotion. Research suggests that a diseased person suffering from malodour is likely to be reacted to negatively (Friedman & DiMatteo 1989). Some nurses may increase the distance between themselves and a patient who produces unpleasant odours, perhaps as a result of the illness, drugs or treatment. Patients may notice this and feel embarrassed or unworthy, and do not listen to advice even if it is offered.

Macleod Clark & Latter (1990) emphasise the importance of recognising such possible problems in communication in health care and promotion, asserting that patient education cannot be successful without effective nurse–patient communication.

Activity 7.5

Watch a variety of television programmes. Observe some of the actors and speakers – sometimes with the sound turned down – and note aspects of their body language. Which non-verbal communication was helpful in conveying the message intended?

Health promotion and the media

The delivery of health education material through the mass media has several advantages, for example by being able to reach a large audience, as most of the population has access to radio and television programmes. However, mass media messages generally do not allow for interaction with the recipient, so the discussion or direct interchange that is vital in bringing about changes in attitude is lacking in this approach.

The following general principles should be observed to ensure adequate, effective message transmission about the prevention of drug abuse through the mass media (Gossop & Grant 1990):

• Target audiences must first be defined so that drug education programmes can be transmitted at the appropriate times for those audiences.

• Over-exposure should be avoided, and a stock of varied messages alternated, so that interest is maintained.

• The message should be transmitted by a well-known person if possible; for example, a well-known popstar denouncing drug abuse may have a strong influence on young people.

• Discussion between audiences and pro-gramme presenters, through studio audiences or telephone contact can enhance the health pro-motion message.

INFORMATION TECHNOLOGY IN HEALTH PROMOTION

The Public Health Common Data set is circulated annually to Family Health Service Authorities and District Health Authorities on magnetic media by the Institute of Public Health (Naish 1995).

The 1994 Data Set contained the following new indicators:

• the mean systolic blood pressure for 16 years of age and over
• the obesity prevalence in people 16–64 years of age
• underprivileged area scores
• an index of local conditions
• the Office of Population, Censuses and Surveys area classification
• age-standardised death rates from all causes.

Essential information, such as the above, can help in the attempt to identify risk reduction strategies and where they are needed. The appropriate use of computers and information technology can achieve major benefits, including:

• cost saving – by automating information-processing procedures
• quality of care – by providing fast and reliable access to information
• improved service delivery.

Optimum use of information management and technology could potentially produce a 40% saving on health care costs, but unfortunately the use of computers in the NHS has fallen far behind that in comparable businesses.

The NHS 'Information Management and Technology' (IM&T) strategy was launched in 1992. Its aim is to create a better health service,

and therefore promote health, through increased efficiency, accuracy and the provision of up-to-date information for all aspects of the NHS, including acute and non-acute hospital care, community care, primary care, commissioners and support services.

Staff should use information technology for quality audit and continuous improvement of the care provided (Benson & Neame 1994).

EVALUATING HEALTH PROMOTION INTERVENTIONS

Target 35 of the European WHO strategy (World Health Organization 1993) is headed: 'Health information support' and states:

By the year 2000, health information systems in all Member States should actively support the formulation, implementation, monitoring and evaluation of health for all policies.

Information in the health services is often geared only to the allocation of resources and the control of spending, rather than to the need to evaluate services and patient outcomes. Population-based data – on morbidity, disability, use of services, lifestyles and positive health promotion – have not received the attention their importance demands. More research is needed into developing indicators for well-being and perceived health status, morbidity, disability, the control and use of various resources, and the quality and accessibility of services.

The evaluation of group and one-to-one teaching programmes is considered in Chapter 18. Wider aspects of evaluation address aspects of quality. Quality assurance should build on current good practice and will lead to more effective work and greater job satisfaction. It can even be fun, as Evans et al (1994) assert. They have developed a pack that provides a theoretical framework for systematically assessing quality in health promotion work.

It is important to measure exactly what is being evaluated, as the example in Box 7.13 shows.

Box 7.13 Consumer audit (College of Health 1994)

The results of a questionnaire carried out by midwives at a London hospital showed that many women were happy with the hospital's policy of discharging them early (about 24 hours after delivery). When, however, the College of Health interviewed women who had had babies there, it became clear that women were indeed pleased to leave hospital quickly, but it was because they had experienced what they felt was very poor-quality care while in hospital, even when their stay was very short.

Summary

Health promotion is the process of helping people to increase control over and improve their health, with the goal of enjoying a fulfilling and creative life. The importance of health promotion is recognised by national and European targets to improve a range of diseases and conditions and tackle the widening inequalities in health that exist in Western society.

An integrated approach to health promotion encompasses environmental, social, organisational and individual levels of intervention, involving the cooperation of many different individuals and groups. If, for example, pollution or a lack of play facilities are not ameliorated on a local or national level, there is only a limited effect that can be gained by persuading an individual to change his behaviour. An understanding of the psychology behind personal health beliefs is also of great importance.

A major component of the process of health promotion is direct education, against a background of individual choice and empowerment; the preventive, radical and empowerment models of health education are described in the text. Education, in its turn demands effective communication, both verbal and non-verbal, and nurses thus need to be aware of the areas in which problems may arise.

A successful health promotion strategy demands evaluation of both personal and group outcomes; without this stage, refocusing of intervention cannot occur, and valuable opportunities for care of the population may be missed.

REFERENCES

Acheson D 1995 Tackling health inequalities: an agenda for action. King's Fund, London

Ajzen I, Fishbein M 1980 Understanding attitudes and predicting social behaviour. Prentice-Hall, New Jersey

Allen I 1991 Family planning and pregnancy counselling projects for young people. Policy Studies Institute, London

Anderson C, Wilkie P (eds) 1992 Reflective helping in HIV and AIDS. Open University Press, Milton Keynes

Ashton J, Seymour H 1988 The new public health. Open University Press, Milton Keynes

Baggott R 1994 Health and health care in Britain. Macmillan, London

Balarajan R, Raleigh V S 1993 Ethnicity and health. Department of Health, London

Bandura A 1977 Self-efficacy: toward a unifying theory of behavioural change. Psychological Review 64(2): 191–215

Baric L 1990 A new approach to community participation. Journal of Institute of Health Education 28(2): 41–52

Becker M H 1984 The health belief model and personal health behaviour. Slack, New Jersey

Bennett P, Hodgson R 1992 Psychology and health promotion. In: Bunton R, Macdonald G (eds) Health promotion: disciplines and diversity. Routledge, London, pp 23–41

Benson T, Neame R 1994 Healthcare computing: a guide to health information management and systems. Longman, Harlow, Essex

Blaxter M 1990 Lifestyle, health and health promotion: proceedings of a symposium on health and lifestyle. The Health Promotion Research Trust, Cambridge

Chalmers F 1993 Action in Avon. Healthlines 6: 18–19

College of Health 1994 Consumer audit guidelines. College of Health, London

Department of Health 1992 The health of the nation: a strategy for health in England. Cmnd 1986. HMSO, London

Department of Health 1994 On the state of the public health 1993. HMSO, London

Downie R S, Fyfe C, Tannahill A 1990 Health promotion: models and values. Oxford University Press, Oxford

Evans D, Head M J, Speller V (eds) 1994 Assuring quality in health promotion: how to develop standards of good practice. Health Education Authority, London

Friedman H S, DiMatteo M R 1989 Health psychology. Prentice-Hall, Englewood Cliffs, NJ

Gossop M, Grant M 1990 Preventing and controlling drug abuse. World Health Organization, Geneva

Graham H 1993 When life's a drag: women, smoking and disadvantage. Department of Health/HMSO, London

Grant L 1994 The Chinese health challenge. Healthlines 8: 22–23

Health Education Authority 1994 The balance of good health. Health Education Authority, London

Hillman M 1991 Healthy transport policy. In: Draper P (ed.) Health through public policy. Greenprint, London, pp 82–91

Kaufmann T 1993 A crisis of silence: HIV, AIDS and older people. Age Concern, London

Kelly M P, Charlton B G, Hanlon P 1993 The four levels of health promotion: an integrated approach. Public Health 107(5): 319–326

Kendall S 1990 Stop smoking: practical ideas for nurses and patients. In: Professional nurse: patient education plus. Austen Cornish, London, pp 9–10

McAleer M, Jackson P 1994 The school health fax. Nursing Times 90(31): 29–30

Macleod Clark J 1991 Communicating with elderly people. In: Redfern S J (ed.) Nursing elderly people, 2nd edn. Churchill Livingstone, Edinburgh, pp 67–78

Macleod Clark J, Latter S 1990 Working together. Nursing Times 86(48): 24–27

McGee P 1994 Developing a knowledge base for transcultural nursing. British Journal of Nursing 3(11): 544

Naidoo J, Wills J 1994 Health promotion: foundations for practice. Baillière Tindall, London

Naish J 1995 Public health common date set. In: Royal College of Nursing, Public Health Newsletter. Royal College of Nursing, London, p 3

Pearson M 1986 Racist notions of ethnicity and culture in health education. In: Rodmell S, Watt A (eds) The politics of health education: raising the issues. Routledge & Kegan Paul, London pp 38–56

Porritt L 1990 Interaction strategies: an introduction for health professionals. Churchill Livingstone, Melbourne

Proud T 1994 Catering for staff needs. Healthlines 9: 25

Silverman D 1987 Communication and medical practice. Sage, London

Simmons S 1987 Community psychiatric nursing. In: Littlewood J (ed.) Recent advances in psychiatric nursing. Churchill Livingstone, Edinburgh, pp 112–131

Stanford J 1990 Professional care for people with HIV/AIDS.

In: Professional nurse: patient education plus. Austen Cornish, London, pp 32–35

Swaffield L 1990 Patient power. Nursing Times 86(48): 26–28

Tones K, Tilford S 1994 Health education: effectiveness, efficiency and equity, 2nd edn. Chapman & Hall, London

Whitehead M 1992 The health divide. Penguin, Harmondsworth

Wilson-Barnett J 1993 Health promotion and nursing practice. In: Dines A, Cribb A (eds) Health promotion: concepts and practice. Blackwell Scientific, Oxford, pp 195–204

World Health Organization 1978 Report on the International Conference on Primary Health Care, Alma Ata, 6–12 September. World Health Organization, Geneva

World Health Organization 1986 Ottawa Charter for health promotion. WHO Regional Office for Europe, Copenhagen

World Health Organization 1993 Targets for health for all: the health policy for Europe, updated edn. WHO Regional Office for Europe, Copenhagen

FURTHER READING

Boud D, Cohen R, Walker D (eds) 1993 Using experience for learning. The Society for Research into Higher Education/Open University Press, Milton Keynes

Dines A, Cribb A (eds) 1993 Health promotion concepts and practice. Blackwell Scientific, Oxford

Ewles L, Simnett I 1995 Promoting health: a practical guide, 3rd edn. Scutari Press, London

Kiger A 1975 Teaching for health: the nurse as health educator, 2nd edn. Churchill Livingstone, Edinburgh

McBride A 1995 Health promotion in hospital: a practical handbook for nurses. Scutari Press, London

Pike S, Fôrster D (eds) 1995 Health promotion for all. Churchill Livingstone, Edinburgh

Webb P (ed.) 1994 Health promotion and patient education: a professional's guide. Chapman & Hall, London

8

Patterns of ill-health

Mary Walker

CHAPTER CONTENTS

Understanding patterns of ill-health is vital for the prevention and treatment of disease. This chapter aims to:

- outline the factors contributing to disease
- explain the epidemiological approaches to studying ill-health
- give an overview of the statistical parameters

- and methods of measurement used in epidemiology
- discuss the role of technology in data collection, storage and information retrieval
- consider the role of screening for disease
- examine the changing patterns of disease and the factors associated with a higher risk of some conditions.

For a concise profile of the epidemiology of some common diseases, the reader is referred to Peach & Heller (1984).

THE NATURE AND CAUSATION OF DISEASE

Ill-health and disease do not occur randomly in a population, but develop in subjects who are more susceptible than others, or who have had a longer or more intense period of exposure to adverse conditions. For this reason, it is possible to study the nature of disease and discover some of the patterns of its distribution. If it can be established that the occurrence of ill-health is associated with certain personal or environmental factors, it is then possible to go on to examine whether these factors are causal and, if they are, to seek methods of prevention.

It has been suggested that ill-health is what people suffer from and disease is what doctors treat. Consequently, while both doctor and patient usually agree that a problem exists, and can work towards a solution together, there are two situations in which this is not the case. First, there are those patients who feel unwell for whom the doctor is unable to provide a diagnosis. Second, there are those who consider themselves fit and well but in whom the doctor or nurse finds early evidence or signs of disease. In the case of an asymptomatic condition, such as high blood pressure, in which the patient generally feels well, early advice on weight loss, alcohol consumption and a change in lifestyle could help to prevent or postpone the need for drug therapy, and might even avoid the later more serious complications of a heart attack or stroke. But whatever the intention, whether it is preventive or curative, some understanding of the nature and causation of disease is needed in order that the disease process can be interrupted.

FACTORS CONTRIBUTING TO DISEASE

What makes a person ill? In the simplest possible terms, there are acute external factors, such as infective agents, poisons and trauma; chronic external factors, such as environmental carcinogens, for example radiation, asbestos and ultraviolet light; social and emotional factors, such as bereavement, unemployment and divorce, causing depression; and excessive consumption of products such as high fat foods, alcohol, tobacco and drugs. In other circumstances, there may be a deprivation of essential factors such as fresh food, vitamins, warmth, shelter and love, which can lead to malnutrition and physiological and mental ill-health. In circumstances in which a complexity of social, intellectual and psychological pressures exist, often associated with a dysfunction in the family, anorexia nervosa can occur. This condition is becoming increasingly common, particularly in young middle-class females (1% in 16–18-year-olds, and reaching 20% among dance students). Most conditions, whether they are acute or chronic, require a multifactorial model to explain fully their essential causative and exacerbating factors. These may be classified as biological, behavioural, environmental and medical dimensions of disease. The existence of iatrogenic disease (caused by the doctor) has been forcefully argued by Illich (1976). (Box 8.1)

THE DISEASE PROCESS

A simple infection provides a model of an acute disease process. A susceptible host, the human body, is invaded by a pathological agent (bacterium, virus or parasite), which, by multiplying and destroying the host tissue in a supportive environment, causes a set of symptoms associated with the invading agent. For example, a specific bacterium (Bordetella pertussis) is responsible for the paroxysmal coughing bouts so typical of whooping cough, whereas the varicella virus produces headache, malaise and a vesicular rash on the trunk, which is indicative of chickenpox.

Box 8.1 **The dimensions of disease**

Biological factors

- Genetic susceptibility to disease
- Congenital abnormalities
- Gender
- Age
- Nutritional state
- The immunity status of the host subject

Behavioural and lifestyle factors

- Exercise (physical fitness)
- Alcohol, drugs and smoking
- Dietary habits
- Sexual behaviour
- Religious and cultural beliefs

Environmental factors

- Air pollution
- Soil composition
- Water quality
- Allergens
- Climate
- Housing conditions
- Occupational hazards

Iatrogenic factors

- Side-effects from medication
- Complications from technical intervention
- Dependency on medical knowledge, in which people rely on doctors' skills for all problems, for example birth, ageing, pain and death, resulting in a loss of self-sufficiency

This virus may lie dormant in a host for several years and may at some later date, perhaps as a result of damage to a sensory nerve root, reappear as herpes zoster (shingles), a particularly painful skin eruption along a sensory nerve pathway.

Infectious agents enter the body through:

- the mouth, in contaminated food or water; for example salmonella or the cholera vibrio
- the nose, in air from droplet infections; for example influenza virus, tubercle bacillus
- insect bites; for example *Plasmodium falciparum* (causing malaria)
- wounds (broken skin), from soil and contaminated materials; for example *Clostridium tetani, Escherichia coli*.

These acute infectious conditions have challenged the health of mankind for centuries, and just as we come to understand their causes and learn

how to prevent them, new infections such as legionnaires' disease, listeriosis and AIDS emerge, and the search for causes and cures begins over again.

Tuberculosis (TB) is an acute infectious disease with a causative airborne environmental agent, the tubercle bacillus. This enters the host, usually through the respiratory pathway, and damages the lung tissue. Susceptibility to contracting the disease depends on the nutritional state, socioeconomic conditions and immunity status of the host. Many healthy people will come into contact with the infection but, because of their own biological immunity, will not develop symptoms of the disease.

Coronary heart disease (CHD) is an example of a common chronic disease in which more than one factor is usually necessary for the disease to be symptomatic. First, there has to be an underlying long-term exposure to high levels of cholesterol in the blood for the atherosclerosis to develop and cause narrowing of the coronary arteries. This may not be sufficient on its own to cause a heart attack, but the presence of additional risk factors, such as smoking, raised levels of blood pressure and emotional stress, are further aggravating factors, which act synergistically and considerably increase the risk of early coronary events (heart attacks). Without the essential underlying factor of atheroma, the additional risk factors would not produce a heart attack (Shaper 1988). In countries such as Japan, where heart disease is rare because the diet is low in fat, the blood cholesterol levels in the population are also low (less than 5.0 mmol/l), and atheroma is not advanced. However, smoking rates are high and hypertension is very common in Japan. Consequently, while it has one of the lowest rates of heart disease in the world, it has one of the highest rates of stroke.

When the cause of a condition is unknown, as in multiple sclerosis, the range of possible factors is a daunting one for exploration and research.

THE HEALTH–ILLNESS CONTINUUM

Health status is one of the most difficult concepts to measure because of the many different perspectives (personal, social and medical) and the multiplicity of factors involved in determining its level. Rather than thinking in terms of the presence or absence of disease at any one point in time, a 'health pathway' – a continuous line of changing levels of health status throughout life – may be described. The path begins with potentially perfect health at birth and descends to a state of zero health at death, with the possibility of any number of different routes between these two points throughout the lifespan. A less than perfect environment in the uterus, whether due to poor maternal nutrition, maternal infections that cross the placental barrier, smoking, drinking or other maternal behavioural factors, will affect the early growth and development of the fetus. Consequently, the health status of a newborn child could already be impaired at birth (as seen, for example, in human immunodeficiency virus (HIV) +ve babies; about one-quarter of babies born to HIV +ve mothers are infected). Congenital problems and genetic predispositions will also reduce health status at an early age and increase susceptibility to disease throughout life. Minor childhood infections temporarily depress health status, but rapid recovery is usual. Only after severe, recurrent infection in childhood might reduction in function be permanent, seen, for example, in deafness after repeated severe otitis media (middle-ear infections). As the individual moves along the health pathway, the duration and intensity of adverse factors, such as poor lifestyle habits, will accrue, contributing to the rate of development of disease. Personal behaviour, social support and medical intervention will all have an effect on health status and may raise or lower life expectancy.

Perfect health is a concept rather than a reality. At some point on the lifepath, health status will be at its optimum level, but at any point in time, some measure of disease or disability, be it recognised or unrecognised, may be present. There is a period in any disease process, before symptoms develop and a diagnosis is made, that is described as the subclinical, asymptomatic phase. In infectious diseases, this is often referred to as the incubation period. The period of symptom recognition, diagnosis and treatment is termed the clinical phase of the disease.

EPIDEMIOLOGY

There are two approaches to studying ill-health and disease: the clinical and the epidemiological:

1. The **clinical approach** deals with the individual patient and seeks to diagnose and cure disease. This approach requires a knowledge of the cause of the problem, and a proven and effective treatment.
2. The **epidemiological approach** is concerned with groups of people referred to as 'populations' and seeks to describe the distribution of disease, identify causes and help to prevent disease.

Epidemiology is an important subject for the nurse concerned with individual patient care for the following reasons:

• Epidemiology is a scientific discipline with its own terminology and methods, which are particularly important for understanding community aspects of disease.

• Epidemiology gives an overview of the major health problems in a community or population by measuring the occurrence (incidence) and distribution (prevalence) of disease.

• It seeks to explain the presence of disease by looking for possible causes; by understanding these, it can help in the development of preventive measures.

• It identifies high-risk groups in a community. Thus a nurse who knows the epidemiology of a disease will know who in a group is most likely to get the disease, when and where.

• Nurses have a key role to play in illness prevention and, as communicators, advisers and supporters of health promotion, they should have a knowledge of the theory behind their practice.

SOME IMPORTANT TERMS USED IN EPIDEMIOLOGY
Rates

These describe the frequency of a condition or event within a specified time period and allow comparison to be made between groups of different sizes. Knowing the number of people with a particular condition tells us nothing about the frequency of the problem; in order to find out whether it is a rare or a common condition, we must also know the size of the population it refers to and arises from.

A rate (Box 8.2) has:

- a **numerator** – the number of people with a particular condition
- a **denominator** – the number of people in the population at risk
- a **unit of reference** – per cent, per thousand, per ten thousand, for example
- a **time period** – for instance per annum.

A **mortality rate** (Box 8.2) is the number of deaths occurring in one year, divided by the number alive in the population at the mid-point of the same year in which the deaths occurred. This figure is multiplied by an appropriate factor – 100, 1000 or even 10 000 – chosen to ensure a convenient whole number in the answer. (The less common conditions would require larger samples.)

The total (crude) death rate for all ages and both sexes in Great Britain is approximately 1.1% per annum. In other words, in each year there are 11 deaths for every 1000 people alive in that year. Thus, in a population of 50 000 000, there will be approximately 550 000 deaths in any year. *At the 1991 census, the population of England and Wales was 51 100 000, and there were 570 100 deaths recorded in that year.*

Crude rates are calculated on whole populations, irrespective of age structure, and are used when making simple comparisons.

Age-specific rates provide an alternative means of comparing unlike groups, i.e. groups differing in their age composition, by selecting a limited age range (e.g. 50–54-year-olds) from each group and making comparisons between two similar subsets.

Age-standardised rates are used to make a more accurate comparison between two or more populations with varying age structures. In a town such as Bournemouth, with a very high proportion of retired and elderly people, there is a very high crude death rate. The population would need to be age-adjusted to match that of Great Britain as a whole in order for a fair comparison of death rates to be made. In other words, the crude death rate in Bournemouth is high, owing to its population structure. Age-adjusted rates would indicate whether death rates were still higher than average in this locality for reasons other than age.

Infant mortality rate (IMR) is the number of children under 1 year of age dying during a year, related to the number of live births in that population in the same year (Question 8.1).

Box 8.2 Epidemiological rates

Rate

numerator / denominator $\dfrac{X}{Y} \times 1000$ per year

Mortality rate

$$\frac{\text{No. of deaths}}{\text{No. in population}} = \frac{550\,000}{50\,000\,000} \times 1000$$

$$= 11 \text{ per } 1000 \text{ per year}$$

> In a general practice population of 10 000 patients, how many deaths would you expect to occur every year?

Incidence rate

$$\frac{\text{No. of new cases found in one year}}{\text{No. of persons in population that year}} = \frac{60}{300} \times 100$$

$$= 20\% \text{ per annum}$$

Prevalence rate

$$\frac{\text{No. of cases in population on one day}}{\text{No. of persons in population that day}} = \frac{30}{300} \times 100$$

$$= 10\%$$

> Each condition has both an incidence and a prevalence rate. These two terms are the most frequently confused. Explain in your own words the difference between an incidence rate and a prevalence rate.

Question 8.1

In 1991, the infant mortality rate (IMR) in Great Britain was lower than it had ever been before (7.3 per 1000 live births per annum; 20 years earlier, in 1971, it was 17.8 per thousand live births per annum). Can you think how this improvement has come about and how this figure compares with other countries? (OPCS 1994a.)

Within the national rate there are major variations in IMR between the social classes, such that the families of unskilled manual workers have more than double the rate of infant mortality compared with families in the professional classes.

Incidence rates (Box 8.2) refer to new cases of a disease or condition occurring within a given period of time. Thus the incidence of head lice in a school refers to all the first diagnoses made on children in 1 year, and the rate is calculated from the population at risk (i.e. on the school register) in that year.

The prevalence rate (Box 8.2) of a condition is the number of cases present in a population at a given period in time. For example, in a school of 300 infant children inspected on one day by the school nurse, 30 were found to have head lice. The prevalence in that school on that day was 10%.

Risk (Box 8.3)

Absolute risk describes the number of events occurring in a defined population in a given time period. It is another way of expressing the rate.

Relative risk compares two rates; in betting terms it describes the odds or probability of a member of one group getting a particular illness, compared with a member of another group.

DATA SOURCES

Demographic data

In order to measure ill-health or disease in a population, it is essential to have some basic

Box 8.3 Absolute and relative risk

Example 1
A review of neurosurgical patients with brain tumours carried out in over-65-year-olds in Wessex indicated that there were more cases in women (105) than in men (83). However, it was found that there were many more women than men over 65 years of age in the population at risk, so the rate in women was 5.9 tumours per 1000 women, compared with the rate of 7.3 per 1000 men. The relative risk in men was, therefore, 23% higher than in women, even though a higher absolute number of brain tumours was found in women.

Example 2
The absolute risk of a 40-year-old man having a heart attack is 0.2% per annum. In other words, two men in every 1000 aged 40 in Great Britain will have a first heart attack in a given year. The absolute risk of a 60-year-old man having a heart attack is 1.2%, or 12 in every 1000 aged 60 each year. Thus, the relative risk of a man of 60 having a heart attack is six times greater than that of a man 20 years younger (see below).

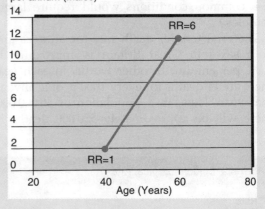

information about the population being studied. We must know:

- the size of the population
- its age and sex structure
- the time period of the data collection (usually one year)
- where the group is from (a region; a whole country)
- who is in the group (all persons; an occupational group).

Census

Great Britain has the best historical population data in the world. The National Census, begun in 1801, has been carried out every decade since then, apart from 1941 when World War II was in progress. The data are held at the Office of Population Census and Surveys (OPCS) in London. Publications such as 'Population Trends' and 'Social Trends' are produced at frequent intervals and may be obtained from many libraries.

The data collected are presented by sex, age, marital status, place of residence, occupation of the head of the household, educational attainment and many other characteristics, which can be used to describe the changing patterns of populations. In the 1991 Census, there was, for the first time, a question on ethnic origin and country of birth.

The population pyramid in Figure 8.1 compares the sex and age structure of the population of the UK in 1901 with that in 1989. In 1901, the average life expectancy was considerably lower (52 years), with very few people reaching the age of 60 and beyond. In 1901, the 0–20-year-old group was greater in number than the same age group in 1989, but at every other age the population was larger in 1989 than in 1901. Today, the average life expectancy at birth for men is 72 years, and for women, 78 years. The light blue shaded area indicates the growing number of people living to greater ages. By 1989, the adult population over the age of 15 had increased in all age bands, while the falling birth rate since 1973 had reduced the base of the pyramid by several thousands in the 0–15-year-old group.

Registration

Reliable vital statistics depend on compulsory registration. The Registration Act (1837) requires that all births and deaths be reported to a local registrar, usually by the next of kin. All birth notifications are sent to the Director of Public Health in each health district by a midwife or

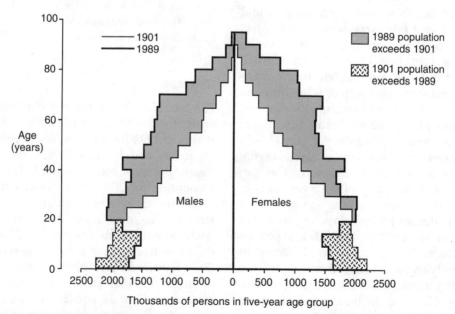

Figure 8.1   Sex and age structure of the population of the United Kingdom in 1901 and 1991. (Adapted and reproduced with kind permission of OPCS. 1974 Crown copyright.)

doctor within 36 hours of a birth. This information is then checked against the registrations in each district. Birth certificates are issued, which today entitle children to be registered with a doctor (GP) and receive free health treatment. In 1837, the primary purpose of registration was to prevent the practice of infanticide, which occurred particularly among the poor.

The death certificate, issued by the local registrar on production of the medical certificate of the death, records personal details as well as the cause of death, and is used by the relatives to obtain permission for cremation or burial, and for other legal procedures.

Emigration and immigration, marriage and divorce are also included in the registration acts, and these data provide useful measures of the changing social patterns in a community.

Using demographic data

National record-keeping maintains a check on the population growth between censuses. It can also be used to project population size and anticipate the needs of the nation in relation to education and housing. For example, in high birth rate 'bulge' years, extra demand will be put on child health services and nursery and school places, and this extra demand will affect all areas of social support and health provision as the group ages. Low birth rate periods will reduce need but will also deplete future manpower resources: the shortage of school leavers will affect levels of recruitment to essential services. More nurses are needed in our current population of increasing numbers of very elderly (over 75) people, yet fewer are available, owing to the changing population structure. This can be seen in the small group of 0–15-year-olds in 1991 (Fig. 8.1) who on reaching school-leaving age will be in demand from competing sectors of the job market. Plans have to be made and policies developed to meet these needs in all sectors of the community. A particularly important feature is the falling number of economically active people supporting a growing number of retired people.

Mortality data

The registration of deaths provides us with an accurate source of information on the personal details of the deceased, when and where he or she died, and from what cause. The OPCS codes the cause of death according to an International Classification of Diseases (World Health Organization 1994). A code number enables death rates to be compared by cause within and between countries. These national data on mortality by age, sex, place and cause have been available in Great Britain since 1837. However, comparing causes of death over time requires caution, because diagnostic habits have changed and our understanding of the causes of disease has developed. Consequently, coding categories are sometimes altered, which has a significant effect on the numerator (Clayton et al 1977).

The national data, which are published annually for Great Britain, are also available for smaller areas, and can be added together in units to form populations equivalent to health authorities, regions and other geographical areas. Comparisons can then be made between the death rates in different towns or districts across the country. This has been done by the Health Education Authority (1990) to demonstrate the very striking regional variations in coronary heart disease in England.

Causes of death

The bar chart in Figure 8.2 illustrates, in rank order, the top 10 causes of death in England and Wales in 1992 for all ages, displayed separately for males and females (OPCS 1994b). CHD is clearly the most common single cause of death, accounting for 30% of the total, with a further 11% due to cerebrovascular accident (CVA/ stroke). The next most common category of death is neoplasms (cancers) – 22%, of which digestive tract cancer is now the most common (7%), followed by respiratory tract cancer (6%). A further 5% of deaths are due to chronic obstructive lung disease (bronchitis, emphysema and asthma), more common in men than women,

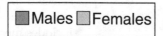

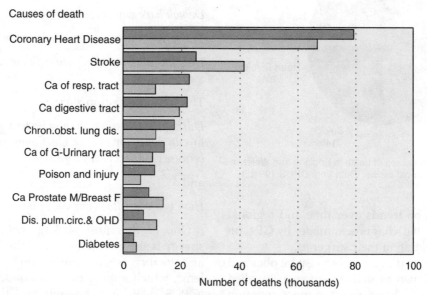

Figure 8.2 Top ten causes of death in England and Wales in 1992 for males and females of all ages. (Data from OPCS 1994b.)

as is lung cancer, a reflection of the lifetime smoking habits in men during and since the two World Wars. Poisons, accidents and violence contribute 3% to the total number of deaths, and one-third of this group is due to suicides (1%). Diabetes (1.4%), which affects between 1 and 2% of the British population occurs equally in men and women. It is less often a cause of death than its prevalence would indicate. This is because of the effective treatment available for this condition, but it is of some importance that people with diabetes have twice the risk of death from heart disease compared with non-diabetics of the same age. All the remaining causes of death combined make up 23% of the total.

It is essential to note the descriptive details of a table as the cases counted are derived from the population described. If a specific age group of young males aged 15–44 years had been used in the example above, a very different picture would have emerged. The most common cause

of death would be miscellaneous causes (30%) followed by accidents (29%), cancer (17%), suicides (14%) and heart disease (10%) (Fig. 8.3). However, the absolute number of deaths in this age group is small, contributing only 6% to the overall total in any one year (OPCS 1994b).

Morbidity data

The only morbidity information routinely collected on a national basis concerns certain communicable diseases, some congenital conditions, some occupational diseases and cancer diagnosis. Therefore, special surveys have to be mounted to collect data on most morbidity (non-fatal illness).

The General Practice Morbidity Survey (RCGP 1995) is carried out from time to time in a selected group of general practices. It provides information on consultation rates and the characteristics of those consulting. It also

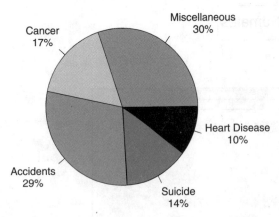

Figure 8.3 Major causes of death in England and Wales in 1992 for 15–44-year-old males. (Data from OPCS 1994b.)

provides data on trends over time and regional variations of the diagnoses made by GPs on patients presenting in their surgeries.

Information on diagnoses can also be obtained from hospital inpatient statistics (previously called HIPE). Table 8.1 shows the five most common diagnoses in rank order for the use of health services in three different situations. It shows clearly that a GP's perception of the health needs of the population will be very different from that of a doctor trying to find a bed for a new admission to hospital, or an epidemiologist concerned with the major causes of death.

The General Household Survey (OPCG 1989) has been carried out annually since 1971 on about 10 000 households in Great Britain, randomly

selected each year from the electoral register. It collects information on many social factors and includes measures of health status. The first health question asks:

Do you have any long-standing illness or disability?

Those who answer 'Yes' are then asked:

Does this illness or disability limit your activity in any way?

The second question asks:

During the two weeks ending yesterday, did you have to cut down on any of the things you usually do because of illness or injury?

and

Have you consulted your GP in this two-week period?

One of the most striking results from this survey is the increasing use of the health service and the increase in reported long-standing problems, which appear to have doubled since 1972 (OPCS 1989). It is possible that this increasing trend in health problems reflects an increased expectation of health status rather than a real deterioration in the nation's health.

Comparative data such as these must include information on the time, place and population from which they are derived. Without this, the information is of little value and can even be misleading, as there are many reasons why results might change over time or between places and surveys.

Table 8.1   Five leading diagnoses in rank order by place of presentation (Reproduced with kind permission from Barker & Rose 1979)

Mortality – males	Mortality – females	Hospital admissions	Hospital bed occupancy	GP appointments, all ages
Coronary heart disease	Coronary heart disease	Accidents	Mental illness	Upper respiratory tract infection
Stroke	Stroke	Mental illness	Geriatrics	Accidents
Lung cancer	Breast cancer	Coronary heart disease	Stroke	Psychiatric disorders
Bronchitis	Lung cancer	Bronchitis/ pneumonia	Accidents	Otitis media
Accidents	Accidents	Abortion	Coronary heart disease	Diarrhoea

Specific studies

Special studies are carried out to answer questions related to the frequency, distribution and causes of specific diseases. These are often funded by independent charities or trusts, such as the British Heart Foundation, the Cystic Fibrosis Society and Cancer Relief. Other funding may come from drug companies conducting clinical trials or from pressure groups concerned with environmental or social issues. Consequently, the sponsors may have a vested interest in the results, and it is therefore preferable for independent research groups to carry out the work, in order for the results to be more readily accepted as unbiased.

MEASURING DISEASE

The measurement of disease and health needs is not an easy task. Epidemiologists have developed and validated tools and methods in order to provide some standardised procedures by which the occurrence of ill-health might be quantified. Comparisons with measurements made in other countries, other centres and even between two observers should, at least, attempt to use a recognised and documented procedure. As well as using the same criteria to define what is being measured, an established baseline measurement is a critical starting point from which evaluation of change and development can take place.

Measurement scales

Measurement implies counting, and counting requires reliable scales. Different scales contain different qualities, some being much more informative or restrictive than others, for example:

• A **nominal** scale is a simple, mutually exclusive named category: 'Male' or 'Female'; 'Yes' or 'No'.

• An **ordinal** scale provides a name and a ranking; it is ordered, as, for example, for social class:

– non-manual
  I   Professionals
  II   Managers
  III   Clerical and technical
– manual
  III   Skilled   V   Unskilled.
  IV   Semi-skilled

• A **linear** scale contains a series of numbers with equal intervals, for example temperature on a thermometer in degrees fahrenheit, from −20 to +380°F.

• A **ratio** scale contains an absolute zero point, facilitating immediate comparison between two measurements if the same units have been used, for example height in metres or weight in kilograms.

Mortality can be measured simply using the nominal scale with two categories – 'Alive' and 'Dead' – for a given point in time.

Survival can be measured more informatively in terms of 'years survived since diagnosis', but this is a less reliable measure as it introduces the possibility of error owing to lack of precision and reliability in the date of diagnosis and in the different methods used for diagnosis.

Questionnaires

Questionnaires are a widely used tool for obtaining information on health status. There are two different approaches to collecting the data. The questionnaire may either be administered by an interviewer or self-completed by the subject. Whichever method is used, there is always the possibility of bias due to recall, misunderstanding or misinterpretation.

An administered questionnaire has the advantage of trained interviewers ensuring that questions are adequately understood and that all relevant questions are answered in full. However, untrained interviewers may introduce more problems than they solve by administering the questions in a manner that affects the respondents' replies. This can occur from unintentional emphasis on a multiple-choice answer or from the reordering or rephrasing of a question.

The presence of an interviewer may, in itself, provoke responses different from those that might be given anonymously.

Self-completed questionnaires need to be very clearly worded and unambiguous. It is absolutely essential that all questions are piloted before being employed, as they will invariably need modification and clarification before they are ready for survey use.

Open and closed questions

An open question leaves the subject free to choose the words of the answer and describe his views, attitudes, feelings and behaviours. This approach is more suitable for case studies and smaller ethnographic investigations aiming to establish a range of possible answers. In large studies wishing to establish levels of frequency (prevalence and incidence), the most practical approach is to use a set of questions with pre-coded answers. This type of closed question limits the range of answers that can be given. However, the choice of answers offered must be comprehensive (i.e. include all possibilities), and in most cases should be mutually exclusive (i.e. only one answer can be given).

A common error in question design is to ask more than one question in one sentence, which allows only one answer. An example of this is:

Have you been admitted or attended hospital out-patients in the last 12 months? Yes _____ No _____

Subjective assessment

Subjective measurement involves decision-making by the subject concerned; consequently, it is viewed with caution as having less scientific validity. The question 'How would you rate your current health status?' is one way of obtaining a standard measure of self-perceived health status in a group of people. It is standardised because it is a structured question that can be repeated accurately in different settings. It also requires that each person responding chooses one of a given range of answers, for example 'Excellent', 'Good', 'Fair' or 'Poor'.

The question above was asked in a mailed questionnaire to 7500 middle-aged British men as part of the British Regional Heart Study (BRHS), a national study of cardiovascular disease in 24 British towns. Ninety-eight per cent of the men replied, and of these, 21% considered that they were in excellent health, 56% good health, 20% fair health, and 3% poor health. Clearly, their opinion was subjective and depended on many factors, which must include how they were feeling on the day they replied. Nevertheless, 4 years later, the mortality rates in the four groups showed a remarkable trend. Those who considered they were in poor health were eight times more likely to die in the following 4 years (45 per 1000 per annum), compared with those in excellent health (5.5 per 1000 per annum) (Wannamethee & Shaper 1991). Self-perceived (subjective) health status is shown here to have a predictive value and should be taken into consideration when health assessments are made.

Objective assessment

An objective assessment assumes that an observer is involved in the measurement, but even an objective assessment made by a doctor or nurse on a patient has a subjective element to it. The interpretation of evidence or observation can vary quite markedly when no firm criteria are given as guidelines. The same wound might be described by one nurse as 'healing well' and by another as 'not healing'. A man with chest pain may be told he has angina by one doctor but not by another. There are always difficult, grey areas of uncertainty in which opinions do not coincide. These can be reduced to a minimum by the use of standardised protocols, clear criteria and automated methods of assessment.

Clinical measurement

A physical measurement made by a trained observer on a given subject should be the most repeatable and reliable type of assessment procedure. However, even here there are many areas open to variation and error. Taking a blood pressure is a good example of how many factors need to be considered even in a commonplace clinical measurement. These factors may be described as follows:

• The machine (sphygmomanometer) requires regular maintenance and calibration. Perished rubber and dirty mercury are common faults.
• The patient should be comfortable, preferably with an empty bladder and in the same position on each occasion when the blood pressure is taken, either sitting or lying and with the arm comfortably supported on a level with the heart.
• The cuff bladder should be the correct size for the arm – its length 80% and width 40% of the arm's circumference. For an average adult subject, the recommended bladder size is 35 cm × 12 cm, yet the most common bladder length available is 23 cm.
• The observer should be given some training on listening to and recording the Korotkoff sounds. A double-headed stethoscope is a useful teaching aid and a simple method of simultaneous observation for two people.
• The procedure should be controlled so that the air is released steadily from the cuff. The mercury column should fall at a rate of 2 mmHg per second. The systolic pressure should be recorded at the commencement of sound (phase I) and diastolic pressure at its disappearance (phase V).
• The environment should be quiet and warm.

Variation in method will affect the blood pressure reading. Even if perfect circumstances cannot be found, knowing what is desirable and being aware of any problems will allow the trained observer to interpret the results with appropriate caution. A standard procedure ensures

Question 8.2

Do you know the size of the bladder in the cuff you use to take blood pressures? Find out whether or not it is the recommended length and width.

that the method is repeatable and that approximately the same result is obtained, whoever carries it out. However, quite marked differences have been found even between trained observers using an automated machine (Bruce et al 1990), suggesting that the subject's response to the process is also a critical factor. A patient will very often have a raised blood pressure on the first visit to the doctor or nurse. This is called 'white coat hypertension', and it is always recommended that two readings should be taken, at least a minute apart, on each visit, and at least a second visit and repeat reading made before treatment for hypertension is commenced. Studies assessing the knowledge and technique of nurses and doctors of blood pressure measurement indicate a need for more training (Kemp et al 1994, Kennedy & Curzio 1995).

Having made the required measurement to the best of our ability, we then need to interpret it. Is it a normal or an abnormal result? What criteria should we use?

Normality

The measurement of blood pressure on a large sample of a population will give a series of readings on individuals that can be plotted on a bar chart or frequency distribution. Figure 8.4 is a distribution of systolic blood pressure readings made on 7735 middle-aged British men. The lowest level recorded was 95 mmHg and the highest 225 mmHg. The average or mean for this group, i.e. the sum of all the readings divided by the number of men in the group, is 145.2 mmHg. The average variation from this mean, i.e. the **standard deviation**, is +/− 21.0 mmHg. The distribution or pattern in Figure 8.4 could be described as 'normal'. The average (**mean**) value is in the middle of the range (**median** point) and is also the most common value found in the distribution (**mode**). The other values are distributed almost symmetrically around this mean, producing the bell-shaped curve called a **normal distribution** curve. This is a statistical term in common usage to describe what is 'usual' in a population.

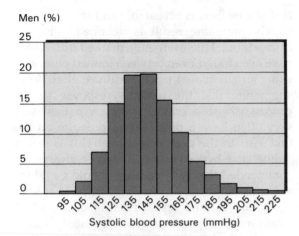

Men (%)

Systolic blood pressure (mmHg)

Figure 8.4 The percentage distribution of systolic blood pressure in 7735 middle-aged British men in the British Regional Heart Study (BRHS).

Where on the distribution shown in Figure 8.4 is the dividing line between normal and abnormal values? A statistician would work out the points that are two standard deviations from the mean. In this case, an 'abnormal' systolic blood pressure would be less than 103 and greater than 187 mmHg (i.e. 145 +/− 42 = 103 and 187 mmHg). An epidemiologist would choose to inspect the evidence in relation to the number of heart attacks or strokes occurring in people with varying levels of blood pressure. The epidemiologist would suggest that an abnormal level was one that carried with it an increased risk of developing the disease or condition being investigated. Thus, there are two very different meanings to the word 'normal': one describes what is usual, the other describes what is biologically normal, or a disease-free condition.

Figure 8.5 illustrates the association between the number of strokes that occurred in each of 5 groups of men with increasing levels of blood pressure. The 7735 men were ranked according to their systolic blood pressure (SBP) reading, from lowest to highest, and then divided into five equally sized groups with approximately 1500 men in each. The first four groups, with SBPs of less than 160 mmHg, each had few strokes occurring in 6 years, fewer than two per year. Men in the fifth group, with the highest readings, all had SBP levels of 160 mmHg or higher and

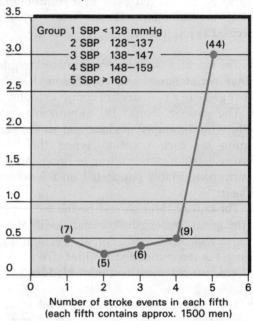

Stroke attack rate (%) over 6 years

Group 1 SBP < 128 mmHg
2 SBP 128−137
3 SBP 138−147
4 SBP 148−159
5 SBP ≥ 160

Number of stroke events in each fifth
(each fifth contains approx. 1500 men)

Figure 8.5 Stroke attack rates in five groups of men with increasing levels of blood pressure, derived from 6 years' BRHS data.

the largest number of strokes (44) occurring in 6 years. The relative risk of having a stroke was six times greater in the men whose blood pressure was 160 mmHg or more, compared with the groups whose blood pressure was less than 160 mmHg. A blood pressure level ≥160 mmHg is clearly associated with an increased risk of a stroke and is therefore biologically abnormal. If hypertension is defined as a systolic blood pressure of ≥160 mmHg, then in this sample, over 20% of middle-aged British men are hypertensive. Six per cent of men in this population had a systolic blood pressure of greater than 180 mmHg, and they had an even higher risk of having a stroke.

Changing perceptions

It is often stated that a normal blood pressure is 100 plus the age of the patient. This would allow older people to reach higher levels of blood pressure before treatment was considered necessary or appropriate. Today, evidence exists that strokes can be prevented in older people (60–80-year-olds) by moderate lowering of their blood pressure. Therefore, an SBP of 170 mmHg should not be regarded as normal and ignored in a 70-year-old person. Our perception of what is normal has had to change, so that a 'normal' blood pressure is one that does not carry an increased risk of disease.

SEEKING CAUSALITY

The epidemiologist attempting to identify the cause of a disease first makes observations and measures the distribution and occurrence (prevalence and incidence) of the disease, comparing the death or disease rates in different groups of people. If a variation in rates is observed between groups (Box 8.4), the personal and environmental characteristics that also differ between the groups must be examined.

An **association** found between a factor and a disease can be a positive starting point, but some

---

Box 8.4 An example of observed variation

Florence Nightingale was an obsessional record-keeper and avid gatherer of information, making astute observations and interpretations from her findings.

She noted from the figures she had collected that the rate of mortality in the army was always double, and in some cases more than double, that of the age-matched civilian population. For instance, in the parish of St Pancras, the civil mortality rate per year was 2.2 per 1000, while in the barracks of the Life Guards in St Pancras the rate was 10.4 per 1000. Furthermore, in the borough of Kensington, the civil mortality rate per year was 3.3 per 1000, while in the Knightsbridge barracks (in the same borough) the rate was 17.5 per 1000. Yet the men in the army were all strong young men who had been subjected to a medical examination to guarantee their physical fitness, while the civilian population included a group likely to have a higher risk of death. 'The living conditions in the Biritsh Army in time of peace are so bad that our soldiers enlist to death in the barracks' (cited in Woodham-Smith 1950).

Nightingale's report of 1857 was described as sensational by Sidney Herbert in his letter to government officials. The report was never published, but recommendations were rapidly introduced to remedy the abuses disclosed.

Question 8.3

It has been observed that more people die after eating grapes than after eating any other fruit. Does this mean that grapes are a causal factor in the disease process? Explain the possible associations for this finding.

---

associations between factors and disease may be misleading. For example, there is a pattern of high rates of car ownership in communities with high rates of heart disease. The car ownership factor is a marker for affluent lifestyle and is associated with many other factors that are related to heart disease, such as low levels of physical activity, high-fat diets, smoking and raised blood pressure. Car ownership itself has no direct causal relationship with heart disease (see Question 8.3).

Establishing a causal relationship

In order to establish a causal association between a factor and a disease there must be:

1. a clear *time sequence* of events, with the causal factor occurring before the onset of disease. e.g. the smoking habit preceding lung cancer
2. a *dose–response* relationship, with those at higher levels of exposure to the factor having higher rates of the disease; for example, heavier smokers have higher rates of lung cancer
3. *consistency* of results, i.e. replication of the findings in more than one situation or setting, such as lung cancer and smoking being related in all countries
4. a *plausible biological explanation* for the hypothesis, for instance, cigarette smoke contains identified carcinogens
5. verification of causation through *reversibility*, by means of test/intervention (Box 8.5): does removing the suspected agent from the disease pathway change the outcome? For example, does stopping smoking reduce the risk of developing lung cancer.

Considerable evidence is needed before new ideas can be adopted and new treatments used on

> ### Box 8.5 Historical example of testing a hypothesis
>
> John Snow, affectionately called the father of epidemiology, was a GP in Soho in the 1850s. He was a keen and inquisitive observer of events and was not satisfied with helplessly visiting his patients who were dying from cholera. He puzzled over why the cases occurred in some houses and not in others, because at that time cholera was thought to be an airborne disease.
>
> John Snow took a map and plotted all the points where his cholera patients lived. They clustered around part of Soho, except for one old lady who lived in Hampstead. He went to her home to find out whether she had visited Soho recently. He was told she never went out, but that her sons still lived in Soho and, at her request, always brought her water to drink from the well near her old home. John Snow returned to Soho and removed the handle from the Broad Street pump to prevent people from drawing the water. The cholera epidemic subsided in that area.

patients. Epidemiological data and statistical evaluation provide us with information to help us in our decision-making. Without this, our care and treatment of individuals would be based on guesswork. Fortunately, most problems are not unique, and the best we can do in any situation is to draw upon the wealth of experience and knowledge that is available.

In the over-simplified example in Box 8.4 are all the methodological steps of

- observation
- variation
- association
- experimentation by intervention
- identification of causation, leading to
- prevention.

Snow's work provided just one small piece in the puzzle, but it played an important role in adding to the evidence and understanding of one of the major causes of death and disease in Victorian Britain. With the introduction of the Public Health Acts of 1870, bringing clean water and sewage disposal to the population, cholera was eventually eradicated.

Probability

If we can demonstrate that a specific and more effective result will occur after an intervention has been made, more often than is likely to happen by chance alone, then we have evidence that helps to predict the probability of an outcome. The better we can predict the results of our actions, the more confidence we can have in proposing a new intervention or treatment.

A clinical trial is the best way of testing a new treatment, drug or intervention process. Only by demonstrating that one group of patients given the new treatment fares significantly better than another group (the controls), all else being equal, can we be sure that an action has been appropriate and worthwhile. Double-blind, randomised control trials are considered to be the most rigorous and convincing evidence that a particular intervention given to one group is truly more effective than a usual or placebo (dummy) treatment given to the control group.

The Cochrane Centre in Oxford is a specialised resource centre that reviews and indexes all the published and unpublished clinical trials. The availability of this resource is intended to encourage and enable health service personnel to use research-based evidence in their decision-making, as well as in their care of patients, through the implementation of new, effective and proven methods.

INFORMATION TECHNOLOGY AND THE SEARCH FOR EVIDENCE

Most nurses will have the opportunity, if not the obligation, to become familiar with some of the simpler computing facilities, such as word processing, data input and information retrieval.

The only satisfactory way of learning these skills is to switch on the computer terminal and begin, with advice and the manual not too far away. Once acquired, these new skills will offer a range of possibilities, giving confidence and the scope to undertake new roles never previously considered possible.

INFORMATION RETRIEVAL

Doing a literature search

In the library at the school, there is likely to be a special computer terminal (work-station) set up with a CD-ROM (compact disc with read-only memory). This allows access to the material in it for viewing, selecting, and then copying onto disc or printing out on paper any useful references that have been identified. It does not allow the user to write on or edit the material in any way. It is a condensed series of publications abstracted from more than 800 different journals in CINAHL (Cumulative Index for Nursing and Allied Health Literature), giving full references, which include the source journal, authors, title, abstract and keywords. The system may require the user to put a selected disc into the machine for accessing material from journals of nursing and allied health professions (CINAHL 1982–1994), the most recent publications from medical journals (MEDLINE 1990–1994) or any other resource.

Searching

Supposing you have been asked to write a research-based essay on a clinical problem of your choice. You decide to look at 'Rehabilitation after a stroke'. You have two critical keywords with which to select your papers – 'stroke' and 'rehabilitation'. (It is not always as easy as this to define the terms, but help is offered on the screen by the use of menus and inclusion or exclusion choices.)

Using the CINAHL disc, if you were to enter 'Stroke' as the first keyword, the programme would indicate an alternative term – 'Cerebrovascular disease'. If you accept this term, the search will then indicate that there are 883 papers with that word in the title, abstract or list of keywords given by the authors. Clearly the list is not sufficiently specific to meet your needs and has to be refined. The programme then offers a list of subheadings in order to help you narrow down your search. Rehabilitation is one of these subheadings and carries a list of 308

publications. CINAHL references include selected publications from medical journals. The range of references, in this case, is still too long. A further appropriate search term might be introduced to narrow down the field, such as 'Health promotion'. There are 1634 listed references under this heading, but when the two subject headings are combined with the term 'and', the search identifies seven papers containing both 'Cerebrovascular rehabilitation' and 'Health promotion' as keywords. After viewing the abstracts in turn and then reading the seven papers in full, there will be other references used by these authors that you may also wish to read and review.

If you finish your search with no suitable papers listed, you need to consider whether or not your technique was correct. Search steps are documented and can be repeated, but the smallest variation in chosen keywords will make a difference to the final trawl of papers. It is a rich hunting ground, and careful planning of the keywords is critical to the search. The success of this procedure is also dependent upon a simple, user-friendly programme, a very high-powered computer that can deliver the information quickly, and good accurate information being abstracted from published material, which is then entered into the computer in a systematic way for later retrieval by users.

NHS CENTRE FOR CODING AND CLASSIFICATION (NHS CCC)

The Terms Projects

Health care professionals from all disciplines need access to a common, agreed thesaurus of terms as the 'building blocks' for a computerised clinical record and reference system. The NHS CCC is the coordinating centre for developing an infrastructure and bringing together the needs of medicine (clinical terms), professions allied to medicine (PAMS) and nursing, midwifery and health visiting (nursing terms). The three projects have the support of all the Royal Colleges, professional societies and associations.

The Clinical Terms Project Working Group has put together a set of preferred terms, synonyms and abbreviations that are in current use in the manual record system. The terms will satisfy the clinical data requirements for care plans, protocols, decision support, research and audit. Each specialty will take the Read Codes as its starting point and build upon this from its own field. Since April 1995 some nursing terms and other terms required by professions allied to medicine (chiropody, dietetics, occupational therapy, physiotherapy and speech therapy) have also been included, and will be added to incrementally as the thesaurus develops.

Read Codes were developed in the 1980s in primary care to enable electronic patient records to hold clinical concepts in a concise, compact and unambiguous manner. They provide terms covering the breadth of health care and form a natural foundation on which to build. They are also being put forward as a standard for Europe.

The backbone of the system, which is hierarchical in structure, will be used by all the teams, but many additional codes will be needed to meet the requirements of a Language for Health in the National Thesaurus. New developments introducing qualifier terms will make the system more manageable; in addition, the possibility of a term having multiple parentage will reduce the need for duplicate coding.

An example of the Read Code, five-level alphanumeric system is given in Table 8.2.

A nursing statement 'Able to walk with the assistance of two nurses' would be coded for care plan purposes as:

Core term: *Ability to walk*
Qualifier: *Assistance required: one nurse/two nurses*

Aids required: Zimmer frame/one crutch/two

etc.

Work is in progress, but there is still a long way to go before a comprehensive system is ready to go into service in 1995 (Information Management Group 1993).

DATA COLLECTION

Hospitals and District Health Authorities collect data to provide administration statistics on admissions, discharges, length of stay, etc. These statistics are used as performance indicators to compare, for example, the activities of orthopaedic surgeons in the same hospital or the performance of similar departments between hospitals.

On a more individual level, patient details are kept on computer to facilitate appointment systems and retrieval of notes. Thus a patient who cannot remember his hospital number can be readily identified by his name and date of birth. The hospital number is a unique identifier but is only relevant to that hospital.

Record linkage

In some areas, systems have been introduced to provide a numbering system that goes beyond the hospital into the community and general practice. One pioneer example of this is the Oxford Record Linkage System. This level of sophistication depends on planning on a grand scale, in which all users must have compatible computing systems, use the same software and be fully committed to making it work. Freedom of choice is lost but is usually compensated for by financial incentives to purchase the equipment. When a patient moves outside the designated area he or she will have to be re-registered, and the note-taking begins again.

Funding is a major consideration in developing and implementing new technology. Many millions of pounds have been wasted within the NHS because of poor planning and serious misjudgement, at both high and low levels of man-

Table 8.2	An example of a Read Code	
Level	Read terms	Read code
1	Circulatory system diseases	G ....
2	Ischaemic heart disease	G3 ...
3	Acute myocardial infarction	G30 ..
4	Acute anterior myocardial infarction	G301.
5	Acute anteroseptal myocardial infarction	G3011

agement. At an individual level, GPs have been encouraged to invest in computer systems but have not always been well advised, and have purchased hardware and software packages without being fully aware of future need.

Age–sex registers

Computers in general practice are mainly used, at present, for patient registration details and other allied administrative chores, which include generating repeat prescriptions. The registration data also provide the fundamental population tool – the age–sex register – upon which so many important surveillance systems depend. Before computer technology was introduced into general practice, few GPs (less than 30%) kept a manual card index age–sex register. It created a large workload, owing to the need for continual up-dating of patients leaving and entering the list, but offered few obvious benefits. Today, with target-setting for cervical screening, child immunisation and visits to the elderly, the age–sex register provides the denominator of the target population. If it is not up to date, i.e. if it contains patients who no longer live in the area but are still registered with the doctor, reaching high response rates to screening programmes will be an impossible task. It is therefore in the interest of every practice to identify and remove all its 'ghost patients'.

Call and recall systems

An important new development is the prompt and recall system, which relies on good clinical and administrative data being systematically recorded on computer. The programme will identify the names of patients in a pre-selected group who are due for annual check-ups through-out the year. For example, patients with diabetes or requiring repeat cervical smears within 1 year can be offered an appointment as the date comes round. In the past, such procedures were difficult, if not impossible, to run efficiently, and were often not undertaken on a routine basis but left to the patient to initiate an appointment. This new proactive approach should provide a better

service, identifying problems at earlier stages of onset, before complications arise and irreversible damage occurs.

A considerable investment of time and thought is required to use computers wisely. There is still much time and effort being wasted in collecting information inappropriately and inaccurately, but expertise is increasing, and as more members of the team become proficient and a standard infra-structure is introduced, the database will improve.

Clinical data

Clinical data are much more difficult to deal with than is demographic and administrative information. A coding system – Read Codes – originally designed for use in general practice, is now universally recognised and recommended, and is being developed by the NHS Centre for Coding and Classification (see above). It will, as in all record-keeping, be totally dependent upon the accurate and complete entry of all relevant patient information. Missing and misclassified cases are always a threat to the validity of any database.

Expert systems

Computer software is being developed to aid in diagnosis, through examining symptom clusters and abnormal clinical test results. The general application of these packages is still some way off, but one diagnostic tool for high-risk identi-fication has been incorporated into commercially available software such as the EMIS package (Electronic Medical Information Systems).

A scoring system for the identification of men at high risk of a heart attack can provide a simple, quick calculation of a patient's risk factor profile. The computed score indicates the level of severity of risk of having a heart attack within the next 5 years. If the patient scores over 1000, he should be referred for further investigation and treat-ment. His risk of having a heart attack is 1 in 10, a 25-fold increase compared with a man in the lowest group scoring under 700 whose risk is 1 in 250. (It should be noted that the score can be calculated on a hand-held calculator and does

---

Box 8.6 **The GP score** (Derived from Shaper et al 1987)

For identification of a high-risk group of men who score more than 1000 points, in whom 54% of all heart attacks will occur in the 5 years following assessment.

7.5 × number of years of smoking history	_____
+ 4.5 × systolic blood pressure (mean of two readings)	_____
+ 265 points if a man has a doctor diagnosis of CHD	_____
+ 150 points if he has chest pain on exertion (angina)	_____
+ 80 points if either parent died of heart trouble	_____
+ 150 points if he is diabetic	_____
Total	_____

---

not depend on computers for its application in practice.) However, a template on the screen (Box 8.6) can provide a simple prompt format for data entry, and one key stroke will then deliver the calculated score.

SCREENING FOR DISEASE

Once the cause and natural history of a disease has been established, there is the potential for early detection and treatment through screening. However, certain criteria have to be met before a screening programme can be widely introduced. These criteria have been documented for the World Health Organization (WHO) by Wilson & Jungner (1968).

WHO CRITERIA

1. The condition being sought should pose an important health problem. It should have a high prevalence rate to be worth the effort.

It would be inappropriate (except in very particular circumstances) to subject thousands of subjects to a test that was unlikely to identify one case of the condition.

Can you give an example of a screening programme for a disease with a very low prevalence rate?

2. The natural history of the disease should be well understood and have a recognisable early stage with a known effective treatment.

It would be unethical to identify subjects with a condition before they were symptomatic if there were no benefits to offer.

3. There should be a suitable and reliable test.

A good screening test should have a high sensitivity, i.e. miss few positive cases, and a high specificity, i.e. pick up few negative cases.

It is very unsatisfactory to tell patients that they have a problem when, on further testing, they are found to be free from the condition. It is also very unsatisfactory if patients are inappropriately reassured.

4. The test should be acceptable to the population.

If a test is unpleasant or harmful it will reduce the acceptability and response rate to a programme.

5. Adequate treatment should be available to all those screened positive.

An invitation to a health-screening programme has an implicit promise that those who volunteer will benefit, either from appropriate reassurance or effective early treatment.

In cases in which there are high pick-up rates and large numbers of referrals, increased waiting times have sometimes reached unacceptable levels.

6. The cost of a screening programme should be balanced against the benefit it offers.

The costs include the individual psychological harm from induced anxiety, as well as the economic costs to society as a whole.

SENSITIVITY AND SPECIFICITY

Screening has become an important part of primary health care, largely because we have the knowledge and skills to identify and treat many of today's prevalent conditions at an early stage.

Table 8.3 An example of results from a screening test using >6 mg/dl of phenylalanine as the cut-off point for a test result being positive

	Diagnosis: PKU present	Diagnosis: PKU absent
Test +ve	14 true positives	67 false positives
Test −ve	0 false negatives	134 919 true negatives

Sensitivity is high when no true cases are missed 14/ 14+0 × 100 = 100%; +ve cases found/ total +ve cases

Specificity is high when few negative cases test positive 134 919/134 986 × 100 = 99.95%; test −ve/ total −ve cases

Question 8.4

Work out the sensitivity and specificity of mammography as a screening test for breast cancer if, in 10 000 women, there are 60 true positive cases, 735 false positive cases, 5 false negative cases and 9200 true negative cases. Think about the implications of your findings.

We are much less able to help people change their behaviours and lifetime habits in order to prevent the very early onset of chronic problems.

The mobile X-ray vans of the 1950s, used for identifying tuberculosis of the lungs, were one of the classic programmes of the past that played a key role in the early diagnosis and treatment of TB.

The Guthrie test, carried out by midwives on 7-day-old babies, using four drops of blood from a heel prick, is a very sensitive (100%) and very specific (99%) screening test for phenylalanine in the blood (Table 8.3). The identification of the 1 in 10 000 babies with high levels (over 6 mg/dl) of this metabolite confirms the rare but treatable genetic condition of phenylketonuria (PKU). If found early and treated, brain damage can be prevented.

This is an example of a rare condition that is worth screening for as the test is quick, cheap,

reliable both sensitive and specific and only slightly invasive.

CHANGING PATTERNS OF DISEASE

Patterns of disease may be described in relation to time, place and person.

TIME

Secular trends

These are changes in death and disease rates over time. Figure 8.6 illustrates the time trend by decade for mortality from tuberculosis from 1840 to 1990. Over this 150-year period, we observe a steady and remarkable fall in the death rate. This period saw the industrial revolution, which, despite its occupational hazards and air pollution, brought work and improved economic circumstances, better nutrition, a cleaner environment in relation to water and sewage, and a healthier lifestyle overall to the population. A further reduction in death from tuberculosis occurred when the appropriate drugs were developed in the 1950s and the BCG vaccine was introduced. The relative size of this improvement was small compared with what had already taken place

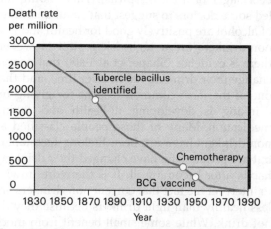

Figure 8.6 Mean annual death rates by decade from respiratory tuberculosis in England and Wales over 150 years. (Reproduced from McKeown (1986) with kind permission from Blackwell Scientific. Extended to 1990.)

from improved nutritional health status and natural immunity. However, tuberculosis is not yet eradicated. Its prevalence is now increasing in Great Britain, owing to immigration, particularly from the Indian subcontinent where it is still a major problem. Five hundred deaths from tuberculosis occurred in England and Wales in 1988, equivalent to 10 deaths per million persons, an imperceptible rise in level compared with the size of the historical epidemic. Although the death rate is not noticeably increasing, because we have a method of curing tuberculosis, there is nevertheless an increase in morbidity (ill-health) in the population, as approximately 5000 new cases are notified each year to the national Communicable Disease Surveillance Centre (CDSC) in London.

Cohort studies

Observing a cohort (an identified group of people) over time is one way of developing an understanding of how habits and disease patterns change as a group ages.

A debate has arisen over the finding that people who say they drink 1 or 2 units of alcohol daily have the lowest death rate, while those who say they are non-drinkers or heavy drinkers have higher death rates (1 unit of alcohol being equal to 1 glass of wine, sherry, etc. or $\frac{1}{2}$ pint beer/lager or a tot of spirits). This finding has led some doctors to suggest that small quantities of alcohol are positively good for health and that non-drinkers are a high-risk group! However, there is evidence (Shaper et al 1988) that people change their drinking habits over time, and that one of the most common reasons for giving up drinking is developing ill-health and taking medication. Many of those people classified as non-drinkers have not been lifelong teetotallers but are people who have changed their drinking habits after becoming ill. It is therefore unwise to interpret the fact that current non-drinkers are less healthy than light drinkers because they do not drink. While some small benefit from moderate alcohol consumption may exist for coronary heart disease, the overall increase in total mortality, accidents, injury and social distress is widely considered to outweigh the advantages. Alcohol in small quantities may not be harmful to health, but there is no adequate evidence at present to suggest that it is positively beneficial and should be recommended.

PLACE

International patterns

Disease and death rates are good indicators of socioeconomic conditions and levels of development in a country. We associate high infant mortality rates, high rates of infectious diseases and low life expectancy with Third World, poorer countries. Their health experience is similar to that of early 19th-century Britain. In contrast, low infant mortality rates, high rates of chronic disease (cancer and CHD) and life expectancy of 70 years or more are associated with the Western world and an affluent lifestyle.

When variations in disease patterns exist between countries with some similarity in lifestyle, those factors that differ can sometimes point to the causes of the disease. The Seven Countries Study (Keys 1980), begun in the 1950s, compared the rates of CHD in America, Japan, Italy, Crete, Holland, Finland and Yugoslavia. The most striking finding was the association of high CHD rates in those countries in which the men had a high intake of animal fat in their diet and concomitant high levels of blood cholesterol. This important work has led to a considerable amount of research on diet and heart disease, and provides the basic evidence from which the understanding of CHD and its risk factors has developed.

National patterns

Even within a country, there are geographical patterns of disease that require an explanation. The BRHS set out in 1978 to explain the marked regional variations in heart disease among middle-aged men in Great Britain. The rates in Scotland, North-west England and Wales are over twice as high as those found in East Anglia and South-east England.

A range of risk factors was measured in 7735 men from 24 towns in Great Britain (Shaper et al 1981), and the number of heart attacks occurring over 5 years in these men was compared with different levels of the various risk factors and between the different towns. The findings suggested that heart disease is common in Great Britain because the majority of middle-aged men have an unacceptably high level of blood cholesterol. This is largely due to a high fat intake in the diet, an average of 40% of calories being from fat (OPCS 1990). This is true in all towns, all social classes and all age groups and in every other subgroup that was considered. Therefore, blood cholesterol did *not* explain the regional variations, although it was the essential underlying causal factor in the disease process. Smoking was much more common in those areas with higher rates of CHD, as was hypertension. Blood pressures were on average higher in Scotland and the North compared with levels found in men in the South (Shaper et al 1987). Thus smoking and blood pressure, by their additional contribution to risk, in conjunction with other factors, in particular ubiquitous high serum cholesterol levels, helped to explain the regional variations in CHD in Great Britain.

Local factors

Environmental factors specific to local areas may also affect disease rates. Rural and urban communities may demonstrate differences due to conditions associated with the occupations carried out and with the hazards related to local industry. Examples of local environmental factors that have caused concern are given below.

Water pollution

Twenty tons of aluminium sulphate were accidentally tipped into the water supply in Camelford, Cornwall in July 1988, and, as a result, contaminated water was drunk by about 20 000 people. Around 10 000 people suffered from symptoms of diarrhoea, mouth blisters, skin rashes and aching limbs. The long-term effects are not considered likely to be severe, but

there is considerable anxiety and sensitivity to health problems in the area, which will continue to be monitored (Clayton 1989).

A contrasting example is the naturally occurring high levels of fluoride in water in some areas, which has been shown to prevent tooth decay; consequently, some authorities are now artificially raising fluoride levels in the water supply to improve the dental health of the community. This type of health policy has caused considerable public concern and debate, owing to the possibility of unrecognised side-effects and the lack of choice for the individual. It remains a policy issue to be decided on by each local water company.

Lead in air

Air pollution by lead from petrol fumes became a major national issue in 1983, partly as a result of American studies suggesting that raised blood lead levels were associated with reduced intelligence in children. Subsequent British studies did not confirm these findings (Pocock et al 1987), but the issue was taken up by pressure groups in this country, and lead-free petrol became available, subsidised by the government, despite the lack of positive evidence.

Cadmium in soil

In Somerset in 1980, soil used to grow vegetables was found to have high cadmium levels, owing to the dumping of waste sludge from local industry. This report caused considerable anxiety, but no adverse effects have so far been reported.

Occupational hazards

Radiation levels have caused considerable concern in communities living near nuclear plants such as that at Sellafield in Cumbria. Evidence of raised rates of childhood leukaemia in these areas have been found, and it has been suggested that radiation at the fathers' place of work, with subsequent transmission of a genetic defect passed by the fathers to their children at conception, is a possible causal factor. Causality has not yet been established, but research continues in this area (Gardner et al 1990).

PERSONAL CHARACTERISTICS

The following personal characteristics are known to be associated with changing patterns of health status.

Age

Perhaps the most obvious characteristic associated with increased risk of disease and death is age. This is probably due to age being a substitute measure for duration of exposure to an unhealthy environment or lifestyle, rather than having an effect *per se*. For example, high cholesterol levels in the blood do not damage the blood vessels and heart immediately. The problem develops slowly, but the longer and more severe the levels of exposure, the more the damage that is done with time.

Causes of death vary with age. In children under 14 years of age, congenital problems, infections and ill-defined conditions are the most common. In the 15–44 age group, miscellaneous causes, followed by cancer, accidents and suicide, predominate, while in those over 45, both men and women, heart disease is the most common single cause of death.

Gender

Some diseases, for example ovarian cancer in women and haemophilia in men, are sex-specific. Lifestyle is also associated with gender. In the past, men have tended to drink and smoke more than women and to undertake more dangerous work and leisure activities; consequently, they have experienced more chronic diseases, more accidents and a shorter life expectancy. At present, women can expect to live on average 5 years longer than men, but patterns are changing. Women and girls are smoking and drinking more than ever before, and we have yet to see the effects of these changing habits. In the past, childbirth was a major hazard for women. The dangers of this process have been greatly reduced by aseptic techniques, surgical intervention, good antenatal care and smaller families. However, the incidences of breast and cervical cancer are increasing, and we have yet to determine the reasons for this.

Occupation

Occupation is related to the aetiology of some diseases. Relatively high rates of nasopharyngeal cancer were found in carpenters and shown to be caused by the excessive inhalation of sawdust from certain types of hardwood. Today, butchers are also found to have a high rate of this condition, because of their use of sawdust on the floor. A high rate of lung disease (in particular pneumoconiosis) is found among miners as a result of inhaled coal dust. Occupational hazards in industrial situations cause high levels of back injury, limb trauma and skin diseases. Stress is one of the most common complaints occurring across a range of occupations, yet its measurement and identification as a causal factor are poorly substantiated. Confounding factors such as heavy drinking and smoking are very often present (OPCS 1981) (Question 8.5).

Question 8.5

Publicans and journalist are two small occupational groups with the shortest life expectancy. Can you suggest why this is?

A recent addition to the occupational diseases is the condition of repetitive strain injury (RSI). It occurs, for example, in data-entry clerks and typists and is thought to be caused from prolonged use of a visual display unit and keyboard, particularly where there is poor posture, unsuitable office furniture and lack of variation in activities. Patients complain of neck, arm and wrist pain, tingling in the fingers and other symptoms associated with neuromuscular damage, which can, in severe cases, be permanent. The condition received wide publicity in the press as the result of a court case in which the judge ruled that there could not be compensation for a condition that did not exist in the medical text books.

Social class

Social class was first defined by the Registrar General's Office (RGO) in 1911 (Leete & Fox 1977). Occupation is used to divide the population into the six RGO social classes described above (OPCS 1981). It is not used in Europe and America, where education and income tend to be better indicators of lifestyle by which to discriminate health status. However, in Great Britain manual workers (social classes IIIm, IV, V: skilled, semi-skilled and unskilled) have consistently been shown to have poorer health and shorter life expectancy than non-manual workers (social classes I, II, IIInm: professional, managerial, technical and clerical). Men and women in social class V are 2.5 times more likely to die before they reach retirement age than are men and women in professional occupations. Higher rates of illness and death consistently occur at earlier ages in those with poorer economic circumstances. This is particularly apparent for respiratory diseases but less marked for heart disease since standards of living have risen.

Ethnic origin

Certain conditions are found to be more common in some ethnic groups than others, even when they are sharing the same environment and have similar lifestyles. For example, Asians living in Great Britain have a higher prevalence of non-insulin dependent diabetes mellitus (NIDDM) than their Caucasian counterparts. This leads to higher rates of heart disease in Asians, even though they do not have higher levels of other CHD risk factors. Another example is the unexplained higher rate of schizophrenia found in Afro-Caribbeans, compared with Caucasians of a similar age and sex. Various suggestions have been made as to why this might be, but no firm evidence has yet been found.

Lifestyle

Today, the many factors that are consistently being identified as being responsible for ill-health are associated with manufactured products and individual lifestyle, in particular, smoking, drinking and dietary habits. The evidence is now incontrovertible that smoking alone is responsible for more disease than is any other single factor. It is the main cause of lung cancer, bronchitis and emphysema, and a contributing cause of heart disease, stroke, peripheral vascular disease and peptic ulcers (Health Education Council 1985). We can no longer make excuses about lack of knowledge of the evidence, but we have very litle knowledge about how to help people change long-standing habits.

Inequalities in health

Variations in all these personal characteristics lead, not unexpectedly, to varying levels of health status in different sections of society. For over 100 years, these findings have been recognized and reported on by the Registrar General in the decennial supplement, produced after each census. In the 1970s, inequalities in health became a political issue, as the differentials between the social classes for many conditions were found to be diverging (Townsend & Davidson 1982), despite an NHS that was largely considered to be equitable. Critics of the government were less certain about the equality of resource distribution and accessibility. They described the 'inverse care law', in which communities with better health status were better provided for, and poorer areas of the country, with higher unemployment levels and greater health needs, had fewer doctors per head of the population and fewer resources in terms of hospital specialties and capital spending. A working party was set up to examine the reasons for the increasing differentials in health status between social groups and the following explanations were offered.

Artefact. The differences are the result of changes in classification of social groups and the changing socioeconomic structures of the population. In other words, the differences seen are not real.

Natural and social selection. The increasing differentials are the result of the less fit and unhealthy moving down the social scale as they fail to find work. The differentials in health status are the cause rather than the effect of low income.

Materialist and structural reasons. Those with lower incomes are deprived of some of the basic necessities and are less likely to thrive when additional health problems occur and their needs increase.

Cultural/behavioural explanations. An irresponsible or incautious lifestyle can lead to poor health status. This victim-blaming approach is based on individuals being responsible for their own health. The failure to respond to information and education by changing behaviour is seen as socially irresponsible, and therefore the consequences as self-inflicted.

Each of these explanations may contribute in some way to the findings of health inequalities, but each argument has flaws that have led to public debate about the causes. The recommendations proposed by the Black Report (1980) carried many financial and resource implications that have largely been ignored. The working party that had been convened by a Labour government, reported to a new Conservative government who were not committed to carrying out reforms that they had not initiated.

CONCLUSION

The major causes of death and disease in Great Britain reflect our ability to prevent or cure most of the common infectious diseases. That leaves us with the many social and chronic age-related problems of hypertension, atherosclerosis, alcoholism, stroke, arthritis, depression and dementia, among others. It is the size of the problem that makes our high technology cures of hip replacements, heroic heart transplants and coronary artery bypass grafts unsuitable solutions. Given the cost for each single patient, such treatments constitute an impressive but inadequate use of limited resources. When Bevan and Beveridge conceived the idea of a National Health Service in the 1940s, they firmly believed

that, after a period of time, the health of the nation would improve and the demand for services (such as false teeth and other novel benefits) would gradually decline. They could not have been more wrong, and the same lessons are having to be re-learnt today.

Health problems that occur in epidemic proportions, such as cholera in the last century and heart disease today, cannot be treated only at the clinical level. Ways have to be found to identify their causes and prevent their widespread occurrence through appropriate health and social policies. This requires commitment and funding from government, the commitment of professionals to seek out causes, raise awareness of health problems and give advice on how they can be avoided or resolved, and the commitment of individuals to heed this advice. However, it must be understood that prevention is not a cheap option, for as the quality and quantity of life continues to improve, so also do our expectations.

Summary

Patterns of ill-health can be observed in groups of people, such as local communities or national populations, and provide an important insight into associations with the various biological, behavioural, environmental and medical factors related to the occurrence of disease. It is only with this information that a logical approach to seeking the causes of disease and its prevention can be achieved. This chapter explains some of the terminology encountered in epidemiology (the study of ill-health in populations) and the statistical measures used in the interpretation of the data.

Computers have now become more accessible, both technically and economically, and their role in the collection, analysis and retrieval of data has expanded. However, the results obtained are determined by the quality of information entered into the database and the reliability of the operator. This chapter offers an introduction to some common terms and databases and some of the uses of computers in health care today.

With the growing recognition and financial support for health service research and the increased accessibility of information, nurses will be expected to keep up to date with new findings, to be able to seek out and critically read the literature and then implement appropriate and effective evidence-based health care into their clinical practice.

This chapter attempts to provide the foundations for reading and understanding research methodology of a quantitative nature.

REFERENCES

Barker D J P, Rose G 1979 Epidemiology in medical practice, 2nd edn. Longman, London

Bruce N G, Cook D G, Shaper A G 1990 Differences between observers in blood pressure measurement with an automatic oscillometric recorder. Journal of Hypertension 8: 511–513

Clayton B 1989 Report of a select committee. HMSO, London

Clayton D G, Taylor D, Shaper A G 1977 Trends in heart disease in England and Wales. Health Trends 9: 1–6

Gardner M J, Snee M P, Hall H J et al 1990 Results of a case control study of leukaemia and lymphoma among young people near Sellafield nuclear plant West Cumbria. British Medical Journal 300: 423–429

Health Education Council 1985 The big kill: the smoking epidemic in England and Wales. HEC, London

Health Education Authority 1990 Mapping the epidemic. Coronary heart disease. HEA, London

Illich I 1976 Limits to medicine: medical nemesis, the expropriation of health. Marion Boyers, London

Information Management Group 1993 A national thesaurus of clinical terms in Read Codes DoH 3/93. DoH, London

Kemp F, Foster C, McKinlay S 1994 How effective is training for blood pressure measurement? Professional Nurse 9 (8): 521–524

Kennedy S S, Curzio J L 1995 A survey of Scottish Practice Nurses to assess their knowledge of blood pressure measurement technique. Practice Nurse (in press)

Keys A 1980 Seven countries study: a multivariate analysis of death and coronary heart disease. Harvard University Press, Cambridge MA

Leete R, Fox J 1977 Registrar General's social classes: origins and uses. Population Trends 8: 1–7

McKeown T 1986 The role of medicine. Blackwell Scientific, Oxford

OPCS 1974 Social trends No. 5. HMSO, London

OPCS 1981 Registrar General's occupational classification. HMSO, London

OPCS 1989 General household survey. HMSO, London

OPCS 1990 MAFF and DOH dietary and nutritional survey of British adults. HMSO, London

OPCS 1994a Population Trends No. 7. HMSO, London

OPCS 1994b Mortality statistics 1992. DH5 No. 19. HMSO, London

Peach H, Heller R G 1984 Epidemiology of common diseases. Heinemann, London

Pocock S J, Ashby D, Smith M A 1987 Lead exposure and children's intellectual performance. International Journal of Epidemiology 16: 57–67

RCGP, OPCS, DoH 1995 Morbidity statistics from general practice, 4th national study 1991–1992. HMSO, London

Shaper A G 1988 Coronary heart disease: risks and reasons. Current Medical Literature, London

Shaper A G, Pocock S J, Walker M et al 1981 The British Regional Heart Study: cardiovascular risk factors in middle-aged men in 24 towns. British Medical Journal 283: 179–186

Shaper A G, Pocock S J, Phillips A N, Walker M 1987 A scoring system to identify men at high risk of a heart attack. Health Trends 19: 37–39

Shaper A G, Ashby D, Pocock S J 1988 Blood pressure and hypertension in middle-aged British men. Journal of Hypertension 6: 367–374

Shaper A G, Wannamethee G, Walker M 1988 Alcohol and mortality: explaining the U-shaped curve. Lancet ii: 1267–1273

Department of Health 1980 Inequalities in health: report of a research working group, chaired by Sir Douglas Black, DHS. HMSO, London

Wannamethee G, Shaper A G 1991 Self assessment of health status and mortality in middle-aged British men. International Journal of Epidemiology 20: 239–245

World Health Organization 1994 International classification of disease, 10th rev. HMSO, London

Wilson J M G, Jungner G 1968 WHO Health paper No. 34. WHO, Geneva

Woodham-Smith C 1950 Florence Nightingale. Constable, London

FURTHER READING

Bowling A 1991 Measuring health: a review of quality of life measurement scales. Open University Press, Buckingham

Cochrane A L 1972 Effectiveness and efficiency: random reflections on health services. Nuffield Provincial Hospitals Trust, Oxford

Huff D 1980 How to lie with statistics. Pelican, London

OPCS 1986 Occupational mortality 1979–80, 1982–3. Decennial Supplement DS No. 6. HMSO, London

Petrie J C, O'Brien E T, Littler W A, De Swiet M 1986 Recommendations on blood pressure measurement. British Medical Journal 293: 611–615

Rose G, Barker D 1986 Epidemiology for the uninitiated, 2nd edn. British Medical Journal, London

Steiner D L, Norman G R 1991 Health measurement scales: a practical guide to their development and use. Oxford University Press, Oxford

Sudman S, Bradburn N M 1982 Asking questions: a practical guide to questionnaire design. Jossey Bass, London

Townsend P, Davidson N 1982 Inequalities in health. Penguin, Harmondsworth

9

Health care provision

Jon Evans   Neil Kenworthy

This chapter describes health care provision as it is now developing following the implementation of the reforms contained within the National Health Service and Community Care Act 1990. In doing this, it considers:

- the current management structure of the NHS, with special reference to the purchaser/provider split
- the roles of the NHS Executive, the Health Authorities and NHS Trusts

- the developing themes of rationing, targeting, research-based practice and new technology
- the Patient's Charter, the 'Health of the Nation' strategy, and the NHS and Community Care and Children Acts
- the changes in patterns of care, and the pathways by which this care is provided.

INTRODUCTION

Since 1948, the provision of the nation's health care has largely been the responsibility of the National Health Service (NHS); it is obtainable free of charge at the point of delivery, financed by the taxpayer.

Whilst concentrating on the 'here and now', it is also important to appreciate the enormous changes that have occurred over the years in the ways in which health care has been financed, managed and delivered.

Most countries have formal arrangements for health care provision, the extent and quality of which is usually directly related to the country's wealth, although the political and cultural values of the people and government are often significant. Numerous models for funding health care have existed across the world, ranging from total state provision to individual private purchase, with insurance schemes and general taxation being intermediary modes. In the UK, the NHS is funded almost entirely from general taxation, although there is increasing direct charging for some specific services, for example dental, ophthalmic and pharmaceutical.

In recent years, there has been a noticeable emphasis on preventive medicine, health promotion and health education. As a result, the general public has developed an increased awareness of, and an increased demand for, quality health care provision. Despite frequent media publicity claiming a scarcity of health care resources, such as shortages of beds, specialist nurses and medical staff, in actual fact, improvements in technology and treatments have brought about reduced patient stays in hospital and, in many cases, removed the need for hospitalisation.

Because the demand for health care will always outstrip the available resources, there will always be waiting lists and long hours spent in outpatient departments, and hence a need for the constant quest to improve efficiency and cost-effectiveness.

MANAGING THE NEW NHS

CHANGING THE STRUCTURE

The NHS, now some 50 years old, has been subject to reorganisation throughout its life. From the beginning, national health policy has been determined by the government, first by the Ministry of Health and now by the Department of Health. The organisation of hospital-based health care provision was overseen by Regional Hospital Boards and, at local level, Hospital Management Committees. General practice came under Executive Committees, and community health and ambulance services were the responsibility of local government (local authorities).

In the 1974 reorganisation, all the above services were brought under the control of the Department of Health and Social Services (national level), Regional Health Authorities (14 regions in England) and Area and District Health Authorities, with their associated Family Practitioner Committees, at local level. This created four tiers of controls.

A further reorganisation in 1982 abolished one of these four tiers, the Area Health Authorities, and redrew the geographical boundaries under newly constituted District Health Authorities. There was also the recognition of the need to develop the role of general medical and dental services, together with pharmaceutical and ophthalmic services. At the same time, the Family Practitioner Committees became constitutional bodies in their own right, separated from Health Authorities.

The last review of the NHS in 1991 determined the present strategies, leading to the current reforms. A prime intention of these strategies is to separate overall control and policy determination (the political function) from the planning and running of the health service (the executive function). The Regional Health Authorities acted as the bridge between the Department of Health, its newly created NHS Management Executive and the operational parts of the health service, i.e. the District Health Authorities. The latter managed all hospital and community health services, whilst Family Health Service Authorities replacing the Family Practitioner Committees, were created to oversee the GP services (Fig. 9.1).

These new structures were to form the framework within which a radical change in the way that health care was to be funded and delivered could take place. This radical step is the separation of the purchasing of health care

services from their provision – the concept of the internal market. District Health Authorities (DHAs), followed by some of the larger general practices (GP fundholders) became the purchasing authorities, with hospitals and community health services as the health care providers (now NHS Trusts). Each purchasing authority is allocated a sum of money per head of its population with which to buy health care. If this care is provided outside the patient's own health district, the money goes with the patient to provide the necessary care.

The key structural elements of the 1991 reforms were:

- the establishment of NHS Trusts (providers of health care services)

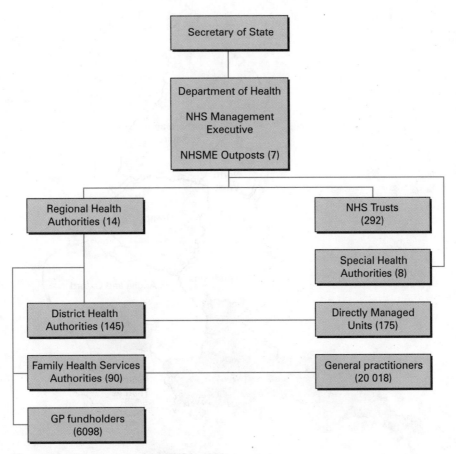

Figure 9.1 The structure of the NHS in 1991.

- the introduction of general practice fundholding
- the development of the purchasing function
- the encouragement of closer working between the DHAs and the Family Health Service Authorities (FHSAs), ensuring a better balance between hospital and community health services and primary care services.

Since 1991, the new structures have continued to be reviewed and refined, to the extent that the 14 Regional Health Authorities have been replaced by 8 Regional Offices of the NHS Executive, to which all NHS Trusts report (Fig. 9.2).

A further significant development has been the amalgamation in England and Wales of the DHAs and the FHSAs to become District Health Commissions, which are purchasers of health care (Fig. 9.3). The number of Health Authorities in each region varies, depending on the size and geography of the region. Structures in Scotland and Northern Ireland are somewhat different.

NATIONAL DIFFERENCES

Figures 9.1 and 9.3, above, describe the position in England, and whilst the key principle of purchasers and providers of health care applies also in Wales, Scotland and Northern Ireland, there are some structural differences in each country. Each Secretary of State for the countries is head of a national Office, i.e. the Welsh Office, the Scottish Office and the Northern Ireland

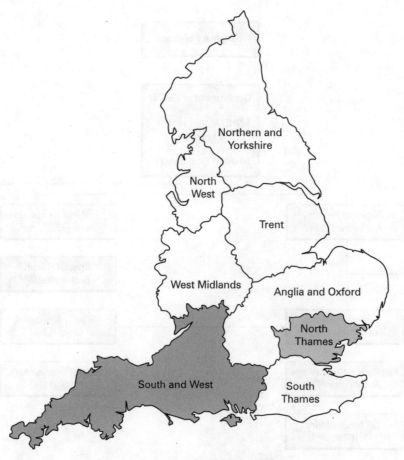

Figure 9.2 The eight regional offices of the NHS Executive in England.

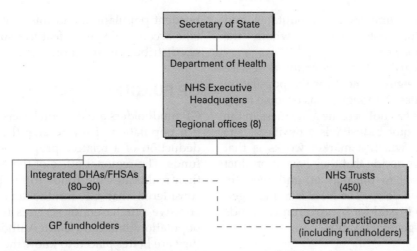

Figure 9.3 The structure of the NHS in England from 1996.

Office, and it is to departments within these Offices that the purchasers and providers of health care are accountable.

A significant feature of the Northern Ireland structure, in operation before the reforms and maintained afterwards, is the integration of health and personal social services under the Department of Health and Social Services (DHSS). This is reflected right down to provider level, the Health and Social Service Trusts (HSS Trusts). Between the DHSS and the Trusts are the purchasers of care, the four Health and Social Service Boards – Northern, Southern, Eastern and Western.

In Scotland, the purchasers are the Health Boards, and, as in Northern Ireland, they purchase hospital, community and GP care, except where there are fundholding practices. There are 15 Health Boards in Scotland – Argyll and Clyde, Ayrshire and Arran, Borders, Dumfries and Galloway, Fife, Forth Valley, Grampian, Greater Glasgow, Highland, Lanarkshire, Lothian, Orkney, Shetland, Tayside and Western Isles.

Prior to 1996, England and Wales had FHSAs that managed GP services. After April 1996, the merger of the DHAs and FHSAs in England and Wales to create single commissioning/purchasing authorities made all four countries alike in the area of health care purchasing. The five health authorities in Wales are Dyfed, Powys, Gwent, West Glamorgan and South Glamorgan.

THE PURCHASER/PROVIDER SPLIT AS A FUNDAMENTAL CONCEPT

The Secretary of State for Health is personally responsible to Parliament for ensuring that a health service is provided and, with the consent of Parliament, determines the structure and organisation of the NHS.

Since 1980, there have been major changes in the way in which the structure has changed in order to make the NHS become more effective, more up to date and more efficient in delivering high-quality care to meet the needs of patients.

The idea of the internal market, with separation between purchasers and providers of health care, comes from an American Professor of Management, Alain Enthoven, who was invited by the Nuffield Provincial Hospitals Trust in 1985 to comment on incentives to improve efficiency in health services management in the UK. He suggested that the separation of purchasing from providing health services, together with a greater influence of doctors on the policies of the NHS, would be the best way to improve its efficiency. Services would be bought for GPs by Health Authorities. NHS Trusts would be the providers, and competition would occur, with hospital and community health service providers having to look seriously at costs that, under previous systems, had received scant consideration. This inevitably lead to an increase in the numbers of accountants and information specialists, without whom the system could not work.

The NHS remains fundamentally a service provided by the government for the population of the British Isles. Although it has become more business-like, it has not become a business in the way that the motor industry is a business. The normal way in which a market works is that new competitors decide that they have a product they wish to sell to the market, and they set themselves up to do so. The NHS is a 'managed market', which is paid for by government funds raised through general taxation.

PURCHASERS OF HEALTH CARE

Members of the general public who pay taxes are contributors to the provision of the NHS and are therefore, in an indirect way, themselves purchasers of health care. In practice, however, the purchaser is that person or organisation paying directly for the service. DHAs, GP fund-holders, health insurance companies and the patient himself can all be purchasers of health care, either within the NHS or from independent health service providers. Individuals who buy health care, directly or indirectly through private insurance schemes, still have to contribute to the NHS through the payment of taxes; only the elderly are eligible for tax relief if they opt for private health care.

The largest purchasers of health care within the NHS are the DHAs. Each year, the NHS Executive allocates funds to the Regional Offices. The level of funding is based on the population of each region, taking into account age, morbidity and the relative costs of service provision and inflation. If the population of the region is increasing, the amount of money will increase. If the population is falling, the amount will decrease, although it may still look like an increase because of the inflation allowance. With the exception of some funds that are retained at the regional level to pay for services such as supporting teaching and the research and development institutes, the funding received from the Department of Health is passed on to the Health Authorities. Again, the basis of funding is the resident population, and this is also adjusted to take account of special features such as age and sex distribution, and morbidity.

GP FUNDHOLDERS

GP fundholders are the purchasers for their practice population. They receive their funding by deduction of a relative proportion of the DHA funds. The regional office of the NHS Executive then reallocates the funds to the practices. It is considered that GP fundholders can be more effective purchasers of services for the practice population than can Health Authorities, because they are better placed to know the needs of their patients.

There are limits to the sizes of practice that can become a fundholder. This limit was initially any practice or group of practices with a population of 9500, but this figure has been reduced from time to time and now (1996) stands at 5000.

There are also limits to the range of services that can be bought by GP fundholders. Initially, this was most of the general surgical services, all outpatient consultations except psychiatry, and some diagnostic services, such as X-ray and pathology. This range has been expanded and now covers general outpatient psychiatric referrals and community nursing and health visiting. There are still many services bought by DHAs for fundholding GPs, such as accident and emergency work, general medical services and long-stay services for the mentally ill and those with a learning disability.

Fundholding has now been extended to cover the small practices (3000 population), who can purchase community-based health services only. Also, national pilot schemes were set up in 1995 for groups of practices in a locality with a 30 000 population, whereby the GPs can band together and act as a small purchasing authority for all health services in the locality.

PARTNERSHIPS AND LOCALITY PLANNING

In 1991, the emphasis was on the introduction of the market and on competition. This has subsequently been shown to be not as effective as it might have been, because it negates all the previous years of planning and rationalisation of services, and can lead to duplication of services at an uneconomical level. Also, many GPs either have practices too small to enable them to become fundholders or they are unwilling to take the responsibility.

There is now a new emphasis, supported by all the political parties, the British Medical Association and leading health service academics, for a greater involvement of GPs in purchasing decisions, and for the Health Authority to work with many people, including GPs and patient representatives, in purchasing services for the health needs of the different localities within their geographical area.

NHS EXECUTIVE ROLES

ORGANISATION

The Secretary of State for Health considered that it was not desirable to set up a national health authority because this would mean a reduction in Parliamentary and public accountability; it was decided that the central management of the NHS should remain within the Department of Health. The NHS Executive has developed a clear identity as the Headquarters of the NHS, and there are, in England, eight regional offices, each headed by a Regional Director.

The Secretary of State is advised by an NHS Policy Board of eight non-executive members to ensure that there is a continuing link between Ministers and the Chairmen of Health Authorities and NHS Trusts.

The Regional Offices also have a chairman and non-executive members to act as a link with their constituent Authorities and Trusts and to oversee the work of the Regional Director and his staff in their regional strategic role.

STRATEGIC FRAMEWORK

The Central management of the NHS sets the strategic direction for the service according to the policies and priorities of the Secretary of

State. This will include:

- a statement of the results to be achieved by the NHS
- a strategic view of how services might be shaped and resources used to deliver the intended outcomes
- individual strategies for the main professional and functional areas
- a management strategy that integrates the individual professional and functional strategies so that they complement rather than compete with one another.

HEALTH CARE PRACTICE MONITORING

The NHS Executive will ensure, through the regional offices, that the services are monitored and controlled in line with the strategies that have been set.

HEALTH AUTHORITIES

ORGANISATION

From April 1996, the functions of the DHAs and the FHSAs were merged into a single authority called a 'Health Authority'. The membership consists of a chairman and non-executive and executive members. Their role is to work closely with NHS Trusts and integrate national policy with local needs. There are also local representative committees that reflect the professional concerns of the doctors, dentists, opticians and pharmacists on whose services the family health services depend. The non-executive members of the Authorities are drawn from, and expected to live in, the community they serve. In this way, local accountability is encouraged by publishing clear information on important issues, including purchasing plans, quality standards and local priorities.

The executive members are drawn from the Chief Executive, Director of Finance and three other directors, who may include the Director of Public Health, the Director of Primary Care and the Director of Planning and Purchasing. The

Chief Executive, with the other executive directors, is responsible for carrying out the policies and plans of the health authority.

RESPONSIBILITIES

Setting purchasing strategy – targeted to meet local needs

The purchasing strategy of the Health Authority has to be based on knowledge of what the local health needs are. The demand for health care is not the same as the need for it, and the demand always seems to exceed the supply. The Health Authority assesses the needs of the health district, using information that is contained in census data, hospital and community health service activity information, GP registers, such as those for diabetes or asthma, and many other sources. The Director of Public Health advises the Health Authority about health needs and the ways in which these needs can be dealt with. The Authority then produces the health strategy, which includes difficult issues, such as the balance between health promotion and treatment, the amount of resources to be allocated to child and maternal health compared with those for the elderly, and, most importantly, the ways in which the work can be shifted to the primary care services, where the onset of major diseases may be prevented, rather than waiting until the disease becomes apparent to the GP, thus requiring much more expensive treatment in a hospital.

The strategy is published annually, and comments are invited from the public, the Community Health Council, local authorities, voluntary bodies, GPs, NHS Trusts, and any other interested parties. It is most important that this consultation process is managed well because it is becoming clearer that the best way of ensuring a proper service to the community is when the health and local authorities work together with the community to construct an integrated set of local strategies that link health, welfare, housing, employment, recreation and other social policies.

The strategy must also contain standards for the provision of services, such as the waiting times in the Patient's Charter (Department of Health 1991, 1995), and a financial framework that shows how the money will be used to purchase services.

Purchasing services in accordance with local strategy

In the autumn of each year, the Health Authority learns how much money it is likely to receive for the following year's work. It will, within the overall strategy and in the light of pressing health needs, decide how it will buy services, and then produce a purchasing plan. This plan forms the basis of discussions with the health providers about contracts for services to be provided, so that, by the end of March in the following year, the GPs and other interested professionals will know what services they can use within their local community and with which hospitals the Health Authority has negotiated contracts.

In theory, Health Authorities can choose from a wide range of providers: NHS hospital and community Trusts, or the private sector in this or any other country. In practice, GPs have preferred local Trusts because this is more convenient for their patients, and there are a number of emergency services, such as accident and emergency and emergency admissions, that must be provided locally. Also, local Trusts are increasingly working towards partnership arrangements with their purchasers for longer-term contracts, which are more clearly in the patients' interests. The purchaser always has the right to 'shop around' if there are better services to be found elsewhere. The length of waiting lists and the quality of services for the patients play a more significant part in most purchasing plans than does the cost of services.

In the early days of the health service reforms, most of the contracts were negotiated on a block basis, i.e. a service would be bought for an unspecified number of patients for a fixed price. Now, however, the block contract is a rarity, and contracts are becoming much more specific. The most common contracts are negotiated on a cost and volume basis, with financial incentives for delivering the contract at a higher volume or a lower cost, and penalties for not achieving the cost and volume measures. Quality standards are also contained in the contracts, and these may also be subject to incentives and penalties. Another common form of contract, very much preferred by GP fundholders, is the cost per case contract, whereby a number of cases, perhaps for a single type of procedure such as a hip replacement, are bought at a specified price. There are many different variations across the country, and each Health Authority or fundholder makes the best arrangements it can.

Not all Health Authorities have a full range of services within their locality, in which case the patient or the GP will have to select a more distant hospital. For example, in many rural districts, services such as radiotherapy or neuro-surgery have to be provided from a university hospital or other major city hospital where there is a sufficient number of patients to make the capital investment worthwhile. These hospitals can employ the specialist staff who are able to produce a higher quality of service because of their specialist expertise. This is likely to become more common for some of the minor surgical specialties, such as ear, nose and throat and dental services, and for the more specialised surgical conditions that require particular skills and training, such as minimally invasive surgery.

Within a purchasing plan, the Health Authority will retain a sum of money for extra contractual referrals. These are cases where the GP chooses for particular reasons to refer the patient to an NHS Trust with which the Health Authority does not have a contract. The Health Authority may wish to confirm with the GP that there are good reasons for the extra contractual referral before agreeing to accept the financial responsibility.

Meeting quality and cost targets in contracts

Once the contracts have been placed, the purchaser has to ensure that they are delivered to the quality, quantity and cost criteria contained in the contract terms. Monitoring and evaluating the services depends on the purchaser getting information from the provider about how many patients have been treated and the

attainment of the quality standards in the contract. This is achieved by obtaining information routinely from the Trust, checking it either from the purchasing records or by visiting the Trust's premises, and checking in person. There will also be meetings throughout the year between the purchaser and the provider, at which the performance is evaluated, any problems resolved and possible variations to the contract negotiated. Where relationships between purchasers and providers are good and the initial tensions have been removed, the outcome is a better service for patients.

The Health Authority has to ensure that the patients' views are recognised in this process, and both purchasers and providers make arrangements to consult patients about contracts and services. Good health care, from the patient's point of view, may be judged by the availability and accessibility of a particular service, the range of hospital amenities, staff attitudes and the responsiveness of the hospital to personal needs. To the professional, good health care may mean fewer readmissions, the use of clinical audit and effective clinical budgeting. Both views are important and need to be recognised by the purchaser.

Patient registration

The Authority is responsible for maintaining an up-to-date list of all the patients registered with GPs within the geographical area covered. Patients regularly move house or change their GP for other reasons, and keeping the lists up to date can be difficult. The information is used not only for payment of GPs and their staff, but also as a current count of the number of people resident in the health district. In some holiday areas and university towns, there is a large number of temporary residents, and records have to be kept of all of those who require the services of the NHS.

Regulation of nursing homes

Most nursing homes are private organisations within which care is provided for the elderly, the mentally ill and those with learning disabilities. The general public and relatives of the patients are not able to judge the quality of the professional services provided within the homes, and Health Authorities have to license the nursing homes. This means ensuring that there are sufficient numbers of trained and untrained staff on duty, that the homes are safe and comply with fire regulations and that the patients are well cared for. There is an initial process of registration and two regular checks each year. Where there is reason to doubt the quality of the provision of the services to patients, there will be more monitoring visits, which will include spot checks carried out without notice, often at night or weekends.

Residential homes are licensed by the local authority Social Services department. They are not allowed to employ staff as nurses unless they are also registered with the Health Authority.

There are homes that have dual registration, and the Health Authority and Social Services department work closely together to ensure that there are common standards.

NHS TRUSTS

ORGANISATION

NHS Trusts were established as part of the health service reforms that began in 1991. The separation from the Health Authorities had to be recognised in the legislation, and the Trusts are set up as separate constitutional bodies, with their own management.

The membership of the NHS Trust board consists of a chairman and non-executive and executive directors. Their role is to work closely with purchasers, and they are expected to be responsive to the needs of their patients in delivering high-quality and cost-effective care, and to involve all staff, especially clinicians. NHS Trusts are also responsible for ensuring effective cooperation across service, education and research fields, which means working closely with their local university.

As with Health Authorities, the non-executive members are drawn from within the community they serve. In this way, the Authorities encourage local accountability.

The executive members are drawn from the Chief Executive, Director of Finance and three other directors, which must include the Medical and Nursing Directors. The Chief Executive, with the other executive directors, is responsible for carrying out the policies and plans of the NHS Trust and for fulfilling the demands of the service contracts.

RESPONSIBILITIES

Providing specified services

The NHS Trust derives its income from the contracts it has with purchasers, together with any other funding or income generation that is permitted under the Health and Medicines Act 1988. Trusts are also allowed to borrow money within certain limits from within government funds and increasingly to enter into joint ventures with the private sector under the Private Finance Initiative.

Within this total sum, the NHS Trust has to organise its services. The fact that there is a far greater emphasis on providing services to meet the needs of the GPs and primary care teams has meant a major review within most hospital Trusts of the quantity, quality and type of service they have previously provided.

Most Trusts are organised into clinical directorates, thus recognising the stated need to involve clinicians more closely in the affairs of the Trust. Each clinical directorate will have a business manager, who will ensure that the contracts the Trust has negotiated and which the directorate has to meet are managed effectively within the overall control of the clinical director. Some departments, such as Works and Estates, do not fit into the clinical directorate structure. These will often be managed by one of the executive directors.

The budget of the clinical directorate will include all the staff, for example the nursing and junior medical staff, and the cost of the ward and other accommodation they use to carry out the clinical work. The budget also has to contain enough money to 'buy in' the services of other directorates, such as diagnostic services and estate and management overheads.

Meeting 'value for money' targets

Each year, the NHS Executive, at the level required by the Chancellor of the Exchequer and the Treasury, sets value for money and efficiency savings targets. This is usually between 2% and 3% of the NHS allocation.

Purchasers reflect the efficiency saving in the price they are prepared to pay for the services they want to buy. The Trust then has to ensure that it becomes even more efficient through new ways of providing services or by elimination of waste.

Examples of new ways of providing services can be seen in the introduction of technological advances or changes in clinical practice. In the diagnostic services, the scientific instrument industry has introduced cheaper ways of obtaining the same results through the use of computers or lasers. In the surgical services, many operations that previously required the patient to remain in hospital for a number of days are now carried out on a day basis or even on outpatients.

Examples of the elimination of waste can be found in, among others, nursing services. Studies have shown that some patient care has been carried out by staff who are qualified and highly trained, but that it does not require the special skills of highly trained staff. Rearranging the skill mix of the staff on a ward or in a department can have significant cost advantages without any loss of quality in patient care.

Contributing views and information to local strategy

NHS Trusts are in a very strong position to make helpful comments on the Health Authority's local strategies. Trusts provide many of the services and they have much information about how disease patterns are changing, what patients think they should be getting, and how the professional staff feel about the future shape of services for the community.

The future of the NHS depends very much on the nature of the partnership between the purchasers and providers of the services, and the NHS Trust can only make really useful comments on the purchasing and other strategies if there is a similar partnership between the spokespeople and staff of the Trust. Both the Trust and the Authority also have to listen and hear the local voices within the community and understand what it is that the patients need and want, and then make arrangements to satisfy those needs and wants.

DEVELOPING THEMES IN THE NHS

Since the NHS reforms have been introduced, a number of themes have emerged.

RATIONING AND THE APPARENT SHORTAGE OF MONEY

The money that funds the NHS is raised from taxpayers, and if the general economy is in recession, there will be less money raised from taxation. The demand for health care seems to be inexhaustible, but the money is not inexhaustible. This means that when the demand for services exceeds the supply of money, there has to be some form of rationing. This is not a new phenomenon – there have always been financial and service shortages in the NHS – but, because the NHS has been getting more efficient, this has put off the apparent need for rationing. Since the reforms in the 1990s, the significant improvements in efficiency and the money saved have been redirected into increased levels of service and more patients being seen and treated.

Much of the improvement in efficiency had been taking place before the reforms, but one of the keys to the effective operation of the NHS since the reforms has been the considerably increased level of information that is now available. This information now makes visible that which was previously hidden, and it is now possible to demonstrate, in quantifiable terms, the size and nature of the gap between need and actual provision.

In the USA, there have been similar problems, but these had to be faced earlier. The US Federal Government is responsible for Medicare, the provision of services for the elderly, and the State Governments are responsible for Medicaid, services for those who are uninsured. The Federal and State Governments had to recognise the escalating costs and deal with them. The Medicare programme was managed, fairly successfully, by fixing the price that the Federal Government was prepared to pay for various operations, and the hospitals then worked within the price list. This, although it dealt with the problem of containing the cost, did not deal with the problem of rationing. The State of Oregon tried to seek the opinions of the Oregon residents to see what things they felt were of a high priority for the Medicaid budget and which were of lower priority. The idea was that certain high-priority procedures would be provided and others would not. This was the first time that words such as 'rationing' were used on a wide scale. It has now become apparent, from the much better availability of information, that the same process is possible in the UK.

There has always been rationing in the NHS. Doctors have rationed services in many ways, of which the most evident has been the waiting list, where cases are prioritised into urgent and those who can be delayed. However, the increasing voice of public concern about long waiting times has changed the nature of the NHS. Doctors are now saying that if a patient has been diagnosed as needing a particular treatment, putting the patient on the waiting list only puts off what is necessary, and the patient who can wait today tends to need much more urgent and expensive treatment tomorrow. Waiting lists are being reduced, although the backlog is still very great. In some areas, where large injections of additional funds are being made available, waiting lists are becoming quite short, and, in all regions, over 50% of cases put on the waiting list are treated within 3 months. However, the demand for

services and the increased capacity of the NHS to deal with them means that people who would not even have been put on the waiting list are now being put on the list, so the lists are growing.

Another area in which doctors have been quietly rationing treatment, perhaps covertly, has been the treatment of chronic renal failure by dialysis and transplantation. Doctors made choices about who would be treated and who would not – in effect, who would live and who would die. This has become unacceptable to doctors, as well as to the patients and their relatives, and they are voicing concerns that treatable terminal conditions, such as chronic renal failure, have suffered because of the expenditure of money on less important things, for example the cosmetic services of the removal of tattoos and liposuction.

This has been accompanied by the publication of Department of Health sponsored standards for the provision of renal services and has recently been extended to the treatment of coronary artery disease and new standards in the Patient's Charter for waiting times for coronary artery bypass grafting.

Thus rationing is now becoming explicit rather than being hidden away.

Almost all Health Authority purchasers are now having to think about and publish lists of services for which they will not pay because they wish to reserve funds for services they regard as a higher priority. One of the most controversial areas is that of infertility and in vitro fertilisation. This is regarded by couples who are infertile as a necessary service of the NHS. The issues brought about by rationing as a result of demand exceeding supply raise fundamental moral and ethical concerns, leaving very difficult choices to be made by NHS purchasing organisations.

TARGETING

Rationing has to be faced, and it is most important that public and professional voices are heard in the debate. The public pays for the NHS, and the professionals are much better informed about the issues, albeit from a professional point of view. The professionals must not be seen to be making up the public's mind.

Between the two sets of opinions, targeting of resources to achieve the highest standards of care must take place. This should meet as much of the health need as possible, with the greatest efficiency and to high standards of quality.

EVIDENCE-BASED PRACTICE

A responsibility placed on all who work in the NHS is that of ensuring that the services provided can be shown to be both the right ones for the patients and based on good diagnostic and other information. There are many treatments in the NHS that are based on little more than custom and practice.

One of the main themes of the NHS research strategy is to derive, from properly researched work, the evidence to support the highest quality of care, and ensure that this evidence is made available to practising clinicians working in NHS hospital and community Trusts.

NEW TECHNOLOGY

Much of the growth in the NHS occurs because, as technology advances, physicians and surgeons are able to perform more treatments than previously and in different ways. Most of the developing technology seems to lead to increased cost, partly because more can be done, and partly because the total number of cases increases, even though the individual treatment costs may reduce.

High-tech (hospital-based)

A number of new imaging techniques have been developing since the 1970s. This started with the advent of computerised automated tomography (CAT) scanning, and the recent introduction of nuclear magnetic resonance (NMR) scanning has meant that more imaging, and different ways of investigating soft tissue abnormalities, give doctors much more information, enabling them be more precise in their diagnosis and provide better services as a result.

Genetic screening for abnormalities has been introduced on a wider scale owing to continuing research; many previously untreatable conditions have been shown to have a genetic cause and are now becoming treatable.

The development of new drugs, such as those for peptic ulcer control, means that patients can be treated by the GP rather than by hospital admission and general surgery. In this case, the individual treatment cost is much lower, although more patients can. be treated. The hospital surgical resources can be used for other patients placed on a waiting list.

Low-tech (near-to-patient)

There have also been developments in the low-tech field that have profoundly changed the way in which patients can be treated, mainly by the primary care team. Screening for glue ear in general practice means that only those children who really have glue ear need to be referred to the ear, nose and throat department. Simple forms of external screening can also be seen. A cheap Doppler device can be used by GPs to detect whether there are circulatory problems, so only those showing symptoms need be referred to the hospital for a more precise diagnosis using the hospital's high-tech facilities. Another technique, bone densitometry, uses a low-tech device for the early diagnosis of osteoporosis, which is a matter of serious concern in general practice.

In the pathology field, there are developments in 'near-patient testing' and the use in general practice of much simpler tests than those used in hospital. This, providing there is effective calibration of the equipment, means that GPs can get good clinical diagnostic information far more quickly and with greater ease for the patient, who does not have to attend the hospital pathology department.

THE PATIENT'S CHARTER

The Patient's Charter was one of the first charters to be produced by an individual government department, following the introduction of the

Citizen's Charter, in November 1991. The first charter was mainly aimed at hospital services. Most Health Authorities have produced their own, which show how the Patient's Charter will be made effective in the locality. There have been a number of changes in the second edition of the Patient's Charter (DOH 1995), and a subsequent Charter has covered the field of primary care.

In the Charter, it is stated that patients of the NHS have Charter rights and that the NHS will work towards certain standards of service and care.

Rights

Every citizen of the UK has the following rights:

- to get health care whenever it is needed, regardless of the ability to pay
- to be registered with a family doctor
- to get emergency care at any time, through the GP or the local ambulance service and the hospital accident and emergency service
- to be referred to a suitable consultant when the GP thinks it necessary, and to be referred for a second opinion if the patient and the GP agree that this is wanted
- to have any proposed treatment (including any risks and alternatives) explained clearly before deciding to go ahead with the treatment
- to see the medical record and know that those working in the NHS have a duty to keep the record confidential
- to choose whether or not to take part in any research or student training
- to get detailed information on local health services, including quality standards and waiting times
- to receive treatment by a specific date that is no later than 18 months from the day the consultant places the patient on the waiting list
- to have any complaint about NHS services, whoever provides them, investigated, and to get a quick reply.

Further reference to the Patient's Charter occurs in Chapter 10.

Standards

The standards in the National Charter change and increase each year. They affect both the quality of the care provided, such as waiting times for specific conditions, and the quality of service offered, such as the maximum length of time that patients may have to wait in outpatient departments or GP surgeries. Most Health Authorities have also introduced standards of comfort in places such as waiting areas and for accessibility of services, such as beverages.

The standards are monitored regularly, are reported to Health Authorities and are published annually in local newspapers and public places. An up-to-date set of standards and the hospital's achievement rate should also be published where it can be seen by patients in hospitals and other service areas.

'HEALTH OF THE NATION – A NATIONAL STRATEGY FOR HEALTH'

In 1992, the Secretary of State for Health published the 'Health of the Nation – a National Strategy for Health'. This had initially been a consultative document inviting comments from a wide range of organisations and individuals. There were three intentions:

- to encourage a major change towards the prevention of ill-health and the promotion of good health
- to encourage people to change their behaviour with regard to smoking, diet, alcohol consumption, exercise, avoidance of accidents and, with the advent of AIDS, sexual behaviour
- to set objectives and targets for improvements in health.

This was the first time that any government, in this country or elsewhere, had taken such a step. It involves everyone: all government departments (not just the Department of Health), individual citizens and the NHS. It is recognised that health is an issue that affects everyone, and it requires everyone to play their part.

The targets are in:

- causes of substantial mortality: coronary heart disease, stroke, cancer and accidents

- causes of substantial ill-health: mental health, diabetes and asthma
- factors that contribute to mortality, ill-health and healthy living: smoking, diet and alcohol, and physical exercise
- areas where there is clear scope for improvement: the health of pregnant women, infants and children, rehabilitation services for people with a physical disability, and environmental quality
- areas where there is great potential for harm: HIV/AIDS, other communicable diseases and food safety.

Further discussion of 'Health of the Nation' occurs in Chapter 7.

THE NHS AND COMMUNITY CARE ACT 1990

In 1990, the government enacted the NHS and Community Care Act, community care being defined as the provision of services and support that people who are affected by problems of ageing, mental illness, learning disability or physical or sensory disability need to be able to live as independently as possible in their own homes or in 'homely' settings in the community. The Act lays the responsibility for implementing the Act on local Social Services departments, in close association with the NHS and other local and national government agencies and voluntary organisations.

There are six key objectives:

- to promote the development of domiciliary care, day and respite services to enable people to live in their own homes wherever feasible and sensible
- to ensure that service providers make practical support for carers a high priority
- to make proper assessment of need and good case management the cornerstone of high-quality care
- to promote the development of a flourishing independent sector alongside good-quality public services
- to clarify the responsibility of agencies and thus make it easier to hold them to account for their performance

- to secure better value for taxpayers' money by introducing a new funding structure for social care.

This Act, having been introduced, has always been subject to comment that it was not adequately funded. It has had an effect on the NHS, particularly within those health districts that had developed their services early and had reduced the number of hospital beds for the long-stay elderly and mentally ill. They now have insufficient resources for those patients whose care plans cannot be accommodated within the independent sector. The Act has also had an effect on the community nursing services, which are now becoming responsible for the home care of people who would previously have been accommodated in long-stay hospitals or nursing homes.

THE CHILDREN ACT

The Children Act came into force in October 1989. It brought together the public and private law relating to children, and deals with those areas where society intervenes in the actions of individuals (such as care proceedings) and where private law addresses the behaviour of individuals towards each other (such as with whom the children should live following divorce).

The Act makes it clear that it is the safety and rights of the child that are the first consideration. It:

- introduces the concept of 'parental responsibility'
- creates new duties and powers for Social Services departments to support families with children 'in need'
- contains a new framework for the care and protection of children.

RESEARCH AND DEVELOPMENT STRATEGY

In 1989, the Department of Health announced that it was intending substantially to increase the amount of money that would be dedicated to research and development. This amount had always been very low in relation to that encountered in industry, and it was felt that the level of funding had a direct relationship to the ways in which the NHS should both stay at the forefront of scientific medicine and develop better means of treating patients and of running the NHS for the benefit of patients.

A national Director of Research and Development was appointed, who, in 1991, published a national strategy. The result is that there is a national framework that directs research into areas of need, this research being carried out both on national programmes and on research programmes that have primarily a local need but whose results may be applicable elsewhere.

The new investment has been made, and the programmes are well developed, both nationally and locally. Attention is now moving to the development of the research work and the introduction of the research results into the everyday clinical work in hospitals and general practice. This is the foundation of the 'evidence-based practice' now being promoted to ensure good quality professional service and care. Close linkages between research and purchasing contracts, and the development of clinical protocols, means that the research results can be introduced more quickly than if this were left to individual practitioners who happened to read a specific article in a professional journal.

CLINICAL AND SERVICE AUDIT

Associated with the research and development strategy has been the development of clinical and service audit. The initial concerns of the Royal College of Physicians, very quickly picked up by the other Royal Colleges, meant that this was at first only a matter of professional interest related both to the safe practice of medicine and the education of doctors.

The importance of audit was soon picked up by the NHS Executive and managers in hospitals. Specific funding was made available and, in general practice, formalised through medical audit advisory groups in each Authority. The audits initially consisted of looking at a series of similar cases and comparing the treatments that were given with the outcomes for patients, and

using the audit process to help to improve the practice of those who were participating. This process is continuing, but attention is also being given to critical incident audit, whereby a 'near miss' is analysed and the procedures surrounding the case studied, and new and safer procedures, such as standardising on drug regimens, are introduced by the clinical team for all similar cases.

Audit is being widened to include not only the medical staff and their education, but also the other professional and managerial disciplines, so that whole services can be audited. The results of all these audits are now being reported to the management, and the results being used as an essential part of the quality control of an institution or service. This is also being extended into the field of purchasing and contracts. The results of specific audits can be very valuable to purchasers who wish to ensure that safe clinical practice for specific conditions is applied more widely.

JUNIOR DOCTORS' HOURS

During the early 1990s, the long-recognised issue of the hours worked by junior hospital doctors finally came to a head. The Secretary of State for Health, recognising that this was something that materially affected the quality of care provided in hospitals, and to a lesser extent in general practice, became personally involved in solving the problem once and for all.

Funds were specifically earmarked, a new deal for junior doctors was negotiated, and progressive reductions were made to the hours worked. This had a profound effect on the ways in which consultants and their junior staff were organised and also had an effect on nursing staff, who, in many cases, found themselves undertaking duties that had previously been the preserve of medical staff. (See Ch. 16.)

CONTRACTING WITH INDEPENDENT PROVIDER SERVICE COMPANIES, AND PARTNERSHIP SOURCING

A prominent element of the Secretary of State's White Paper reforms in 1991, and a major scepticism of those who opposed the reforms, was that the NHS would never be privatised. It was stated that there would always be a National Health Service funded through general taxation.

Although this remains the case, and the money that Health Authorities and GP fundholders use to purchase and provide health services comes from taxation, there have been changes in the level of involvement of private companies in the NHS, apparent in a number of ways.

Expenditure

The practice of competitive tendering for catering, cleaning, laundry and estate maintenance services is well established. It is now being extended to cover 'facilities management' of finance and information services.

Pharmaceutical and some diagnostic services are being provided by private companies in hospitals. This is likely to increase, providing the quality and cost measures can be guaranteed.

Waiting list funds are sometimes used to purchase from the independent sector some of the specialty treatments for which there is a long waiting time within the NHS. Often the independent hospital in the locality may be able to provide specialty treatment cheaper than the NHS.

Major capital projects have always been undertaken by the private building industry, but this is now being extended to include the operation of some of these new projects once they have been built.

Income generation

The NHS was first encouraged in 1988 to generate income from sources other than its own private pay beds and amenity beds. The early schemes were limited in scope and consisted mainly of renting space in hospitals for newspapers and flower shops, together with the use of hospital facilities for the purpose of advertising certain products. Subsequent schemes have become much larger and may consist of the management of car parking concessions on hospital sites, and similar ventures.

Partnership sourcing

Some major capital projects have become so large that the investment that an individual NHS Trust, or even a whole region, needs to make is beyond the means of the Trust. Private companies are being invited to join the NHS in joint ventures, contracts being arranged in such a way as to ensure that there is a benefit to both parties to the contract. Such schemes may be wholly driven by the need for capital funds, there may be a profit-sharing arrangement in a revenue generation scheme, or there may be genuine joint ventures in which both parties share the risk and the benefit evenly.

CHANGES IN CARE PATTERNS

The patterns of health care provision have changed significantly during the 1980s and 1990s as a result of the themes described above.

PRIMACY OF PRIMARY CARE

Historically, the hospital services have had the greatest demand upon, and the largest share of, resources. The hospital consultants have had a great influence on how resources have been used. The cost of these services and the fact that they are the result of poor health promotion and sickness prevention have changed this. There is now a wide recognition that the GPs provide the main gateway by which the patients receive care. The GP can influence and mediate the patients' health, rather than the consultant expert having to deal with a sickness that might otherwise have been prevented. The new contract for GPs, introduced in 1992, made incentive payments available to start health promotion clinics, introduce surveillance programmes for children and the elderly, and ensure that targets for vaccination and immunisation are met.

Purchasing agencies are under great pressure from the NHS Executive to develop the primary care services and give GPs and primary care teams greater influence than hitherto. Strenuous efforts are now made to seek the opinions of

GPs while putting together purchasing plans, and to use the information to draw up the specifications for the contracts in accordance with the stated and proven needs of general practice and primary care.

Some purchasing agencies are going much further still and are developing locality plans for small communities based around the general practice catchment population. Most purchasing agencies are very large and may have up to one million residents, whilst the individual communities may be urban or rural, industrial or service, rich or poor, white or non-white. In each case, the health needs can be markedly different, and a single service specification that averages the whole population covered by the Health Authority is unlikely to satisfy any of the real local needs and major concerns. Non-specific contracts for services are thus likely to be rather wasteful because they are not targeted on specific needs identified for small local communities.

DEVELOPMENT OF DAY CARE

Medical practitioners have developed newer and better ways of treating common conditions, which means that patients stay in hospital for shorter periods of time.

Day care, and particularly day surgery, is a natural next step, the length of stay reducing to simply overnight. Patients prefer not to stay in hospital any longer than they need to, and providing there is adequate follow up, either at hospital or preferably from community nursing and other specialist staff, the quality of care can be maintained at the highest possible level.

Economists and accountants have pointed out the cost advantages of day surgery, and the Audit Commission, with the advice of the Royal College of Surgeons, has suggested that the NHS should, for the most common cases in which it is safe to do so, move positively towards day-case surgery as the treatment of choice.

This advice has been taken, and purchasing authorities are setting day-case targets to be achieved by NHS Trusts. Where Trusts may be carrying out day-case surgery at a lower rate than the target, there may be financial incentives

to move from an inpatient regime to a day-case regime for a higher proportion of cases within the total number in the surgical services contract.

REDUCTION OF BEDS AND INCREASE OF CASES

Impact on provision in cities, especially London

The impact of shorter stays in hospital and the development of day care has lead to the recognition that fewer beds are needed to treat patients, and hospitals have been reducing their bed numbers. This has meant that, in the big cities, particularly London, the future of whole hospitals has had to be reviewed. The Tomlinson Report, which suggests the rationalisation of many of the London teaching hospitals, was adopted by the Secretary of State for Health, but there has been enormous resistance to the potential closure or amalgamation of much-loved teaching hospitals and their medical schools, particularly when their clinical performance remains among the highest in the land.

A number of strategies have been adopted by the big hospitals to retain their presence and the skills of their staff. For example, some of the teaching hospitals have been offering the provincial and rural purchasing agencies special rates for treating those patients whose condition does not really merit the attention of such highly specialised staff as work in teaching hospitals. This represents the operation of a market in a real commercial sense, but has the effect of keeping some over-provision of buildings and staff so that the NHS has the space to deal with more patients, but does not have the revenue resources, within the rationing and budget criteria previously mentioned, to pay for using this excess capacity.

There have been similar conclusions drawn in places such as Edinburgh, Glasgow, Cardiff and other provincial cities in England.

RURAL PROVISION

In the rural areas and the smaller towns, there have been similar reductions in the number of beds, and there have been closures of smaller hospitals where there is insufficient work to maintain a very local service with any degree of safety for the quality of professional care. However, the emphasis on locality planning and provision has to some extent reversed this, and local community hospitals are being provided which have a smaller range of services than the larger hospitals in nearby towns and cities. There is a need for purchasers to make sure that the balance between local provision and patient safety is right.

In addition, there are now incentives for GPs to provide a wider range of services; such as minor surgery, in their surgeries or cottage hospitals, so that people do not have to go to district hospitals. In an increasing number of cases, hospital consultants carry out their out-patient clinics in the cottage hospitals and GP surgeries. Many district hospitals are developing outreach services, which are locally provided and much more sensitive to local needs.

CARE PROVISION PATHWAYS

GENERAL PRACTICE AND PRIMARY CARE

In most cases, the first point at which an individual comes into contact with the NHS is through visiting the GP's surgery. All but 1% of the population are registered with a general practice, and, on average, each person sees his or her GP four times a year. Some 90% of medical problems are treated successfully by the primary care team or the extended primary care team, either at the surgery or the patient's home (Fig. 9.4). The remainder will require hospital care or some other form of secondary health treatment.

Practice nurses are employed by the practice and are increasingly developing their role to participate in patient consultation and the pre-scribing of medication, thus relieving some of the pressure on GPs. A significant proportion of general practices are now large in terms of registered patients, and, whether or not they have fundholding status, they can provide a wide range of additional health promotion and pre-ventive care services. Screening facilities, well-women and well-men clinics, drop-in fitness checks, dietary classes and anti-smoking clinics are examples of preventive services that are increasingly popular with the public.

Consumer choice and demand are important influences upon the development of GP services, with general practices now allowed to 'advertise' and promote the services they are able to offer.

When a patient goes to the GP's surgery, the result should be the preparation of a care plan that is proposed by the GP and in which the patient is an informed and willing partner.

Often all the services the patient will need can be provided by the primary care team, or the extended primary care team, within the patient's home or at the surgery.

Figure 9.4 shows the GP, the members of the primary care team at the centre and those specialists and other services who might make up the extended primary care team. This will, of course, be different for each team and be very much dependent on local circumstances, health needs and the community and hospital Trusts.

FUNDHOLDING

In fundholding practices, the options available to the GP in arriving at the care plan are determined by the GP and his practice because they fix the contracts with the NHS Trusts. The GPs in the practice are thus in a strong position to make sure that the patient gets the right service at the right time and in the right place.

NON-FUNDHOLDING

In non-fundholding practices, the Health Authority arranges the contracts, and although it is possible to make extracontractual referrals, the Authority has to give its approval before the provider Trust can be assured that it will receive the necessary funding for the patient's treatment. However, the developments in locality planning mean that, more and more, the benefits and strengths of fundholding will become

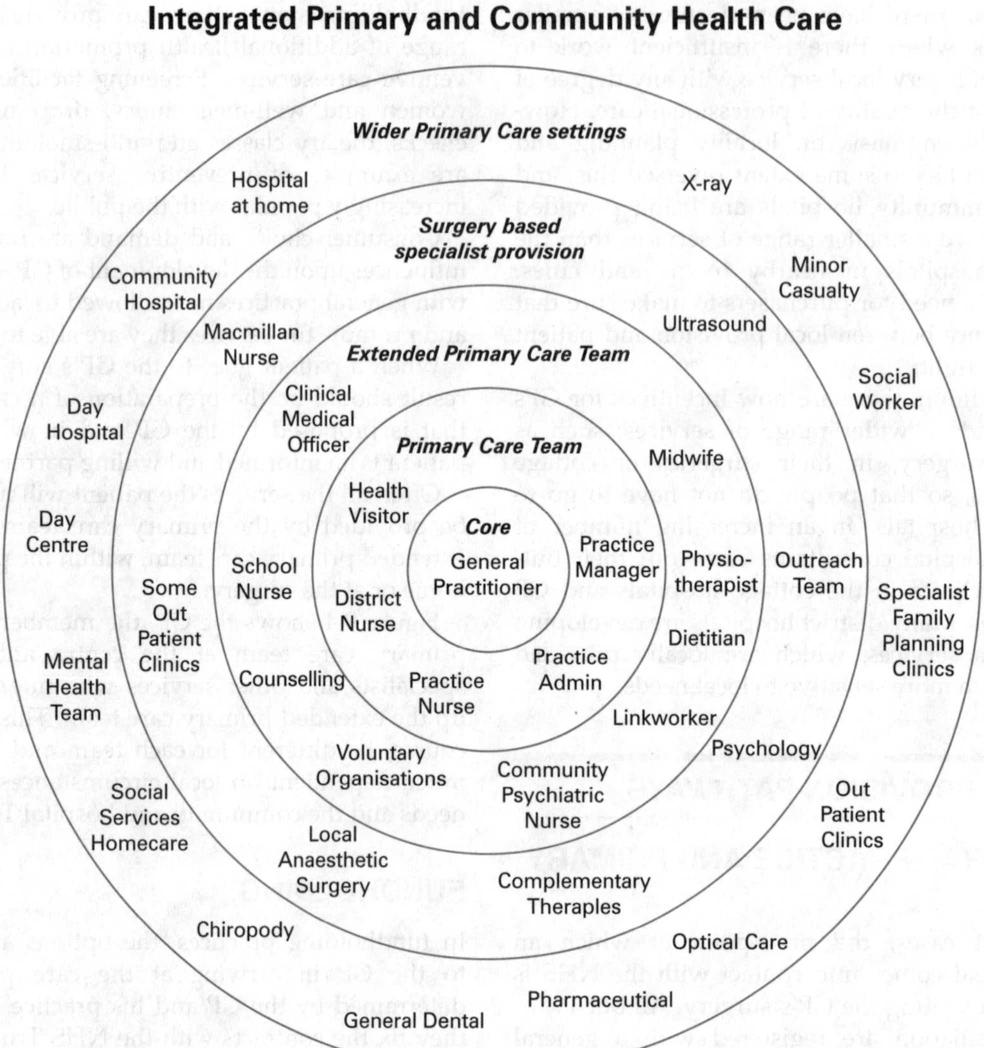

Integrated Primary and Community Health Care

Figure 9.4 The extended primary care team.

available to non-fundholders and their patients and primary care teams.

COMMUNITY HEALTH SERVICES

Community health services are normally provided by community Trusts, and the district nursing and health visiting staff are employed and managed by the Trust, although they are usually full members of the primary health care team. In a number of cases, the fundholding GPs are contracting with the NHS Trusts for the management of the Trust's district nurses and health visitors, and other professional staff alongside the practice nurses, as an integrated team within the practice. Professional training and supervision, and employment contracts, usually still rest with the community Trust. This means that there can be a more flexible use of all the nursing resources in the practice, more continuity of care and a better skill and grade mix than can be arranged if the management of the community nurses remains with the community Trust.

The extended team may have whole- or part-time members detached from the Trust's staff to work within the practice. For example, community psychiatric nurses, counsellors or physiotherapists may form parts of the extended primary care team, and similar arrangements can be organised with Social Services departments for attached social workers.

HOSPITAL-BASED HEALTH SERVICES

Referral

Within the care plan, it may be agreed that a specialist opinion or treatment is needed that cannot be provided within the practice. This will therefore need, with the patient's agreement, a referral to a hospital-based specialist or, if this is from a fundholding practice, an independent, non-NHS provider. The costs of this are borne by the Health Authority, whether this is within a contract or is an extracontractual referral. If this is a fundholding practice, the practice pays, although if the treatment is likely to be expensive, such as a coronary artery bypass graft, the Health Authority is required to pay for it.

Direct access

There are a limited number of services, usually for emergency treatment, the accident and emergency service being the most obvious, in which the decision to go to hospital is taken by the patient rather than the GP. In these cases, the Authority pays the provider through a block contract.

Ambulance and health transport

All ambulance services are NHS Trusts, and the responsibility for making sure that the emergency services are adequately funded rests with NHS purchasers. This may be done on a regional basis, as in London or the West Midlands, or it may be a county-wide service, such as in Lincolnshire, in which case the Health Authority will be responsible. Ambulance services have their own quality standards, based on the Patient's Charter, covering the length of time to activate an emergency crew or reach a patient requiring emergency transport to hospital. The development of very highly-trained paramedic staff has improved the survival rates of accident victims.

The ambulance service may, in addition, provide non-emergency service to other providers. For example, ambulances may provide routine transport to other NHS Trusts for bringing patients to day hospitals.

Ambulance services may also have contracts with other organisations, such as football clubs, for attendance at events.

Private sector

Recent years have seen a significant increase in the provision of health care outside the NHS. Over 6 million of the population have private medical cover, and there are over 100 000 private beds to meet their needs.

The cost of private health cover depends on a number of factors, the two main ones being age and the type of service required. Increased age attracts increased charges, although this can be offset by tax benefits for people over the age of 65. The services fall into three main categories:

- *Category A* services are those provided by some elite hospitals and clinics with national or international reputations, for example some independent hospitals, London teaching hospitals or provincial hospitals having designated high-quality accommodation and services and being recognised as leaders in a particular specialty or treatment.
- *Category B* services are those provided by the majority of hospitals in the independent sector.
- *Category C* services are those provided in some independent hospitals and most of the NHS hospitals that have private beds.

The premiums for category C services will be almost half those of category A services, category B coming somewhere in between.

Most types of insurance have some special discounts or conditions, such as no-claims bonuses. Health insurance is no different. It is possible to arrange reductions in premiums by making special payment arrangements or not calling on cover for low-cost treatment or care; equally, most insurance companies and provident societies will cap the payments they make to service providers for specific services such as physiotherapy, or they may not cover ambulance transport.

There are numerous attractions for private care, ranging from the immediacy of treatment to increased privacy and better facilities. Some patients opt for private care because they can arrange it around work commitments or holiday bookings. Others may seek the services of a particular consultant who has an excellent reputation.

One of the main reasons for there being a reasonably sized insurance market is that there were, and in some cases continue to be, many delays in getting treatment from the NHS. To some extent, this has been reduced by recent waiting list initiatives, and the NHS is now much more responsive to patient preference and personal choice. A number of employers have used private health insurance as part of re-muneration packages for their employees, and some companies have given private insurance on the grounds that they can then get their staff treated more quickly or at a time to suit the company. Medical insurance cover provided by employers for their staff normally ceases when the employee retires. In this case, the person has to decide whether to buy individual cover. Income tax relief on premiums for the elderly gives them some encouragement to remain within private sector provision.

Summary

The general principles of the 1946 National Health Service Act are still intact, but the processes by which care is provided have changed significantly. The health service has become more business-like since the 1991 reforms, which aimed at separating the political (Department of Health) from the executive (NHS Executive) function of the NHS, with District Health Authorities (DHAs) overseeing hospital and community health services, Family Health Service Associations (FHSAs) overseeing GP services and Regional Health Authorities (RHAs) acting as the bridge between these two tiers of control. From 1996, the RHAs have been replaced by Regional Offices of the NHS Executive.

A further important division, reflecting the concept of the internal market, is into purchasers (DHAs, FHSAs and GP fundholders) and providers (NHS Trusts and GPs, including fundholders), the aim being to improve efficiency and decrease costs in the NHS.

Government initiatives, such as the Patient's Charter and 'Health of the Nation' strategy, aim to ensure that all have access to appropriate health care of a designated standard when it is needed and that citizens also take some responsibility for improving their own level of health. Research-based care and its constant auditing will enable the maintenance of these standards and the targeting of resources where they are needed.

It has been said that the only constant thing in the NHS is change. Unless this is managed well and responds sensitively to the needs of patients and staff alike, only uncertainty will result. However, the in-creased efficiency from such changes will ensure that, whichever political party is in power, the NHS will continue to be regarded as a jewel in the nation's crown.

REFERENCES

Children Act 1989 HMSO, London
Department of Health 1991 The Patients Charter. HMSO, London
Department of Health 1992a The Health of the Nation. HMSO, London
Department of Health 1992b Report of the Inquiry into London's Health Service, Medical Education and Research (The Tomlinson Report). HMSO, London
Department of Health 1995 The Patients Charter, 2nd edn. HMSO, London
NHS and Community Care Act. 1990 HMSO, London

Providing a quality service

10

Peter J Nicklin

CHAPTER CONTENTS

All those associated with health care delivery, in particular nurses, would reasonably argue that, for them, quality has always been an issue of importance; in short, everyone agrees that quality is a good thing. What is more difficult is defining, describing and measuring quality.

This chapter will aim to:
* outline some of the imperatives that have made quality a watchword for health care providers
* discuss the principles of quality
* describe some of the tools and techniques used to measure and promote quality and how these can be applied to the delivery of nursing care.

THE QUALITY IMPERATIVES

In 1986 Charles Shaw observed that the NHS had previously been 'relatively unregulated either voluntarily or by statute about how it would perform its task' but concluded, 'attitudes are now changing. The question is no longer whether we should make an issue about the quality and effectiveness of the service, but about who, if anyone, will take the lead in assuring it'. A range of dynamically related pressures had conspired to change attitudes towards health care provision and of health care professionals. These include political and socioeconomic factors.

POLITICAL FACTORS

Restraining public expenditure, improving efficiency and obtaining value for money are fundamental to the government's economic policies. Previously, the professions, including nursing, delivered their services to an innocent public who accepted 'quality as given'. However, during the 1970s, there was a progressive loss of public confidence in a variety of professional groups, including those providing health care. Pollitt (1986) explains that 'perceived failures in public service programmes had shaken public confidence in professional competence, and left professional groups poorly placed to resist externally imposed tests of economy, competence and achievement'. During 1983, the DHSS published its Performance Indicator package for the NHS, and in the same year Roy Griffiths conducted his enquiry into NHS management (Griffiths 1983). The Griffiths Report, a milestone in NHS quality, claimed that the differences between the private sector and the NHS were greatly overstated and concluded that the 'similarities between NHS management and business are more important ... they are concerned with level of service [and] quality of product'. The drive for increased efficiency and improved quality was affirmed with the publication of 'Working for Patients' (Department of Health 1989), the creation of an internal market and its contracting procedures being intended to provide incentives for purchasers and providers of health care, not only to contain costs, but also to make explicit the quality of service to be delivered. The NHS reforms, among other measures, contributed to the UK's obligation to the World Health Organization that by 1990 it would 'have built effective mechanisms for ensuring the quality of patient care' (World Health Organization 1985) within its health care system.

SOCIO-ECONOMIC FACTORS

Improvements in social and economic conditions for the majority of the population have increased consumer choice and their expectations of the service they receive. No longer are the public inclined to be the passive recipients of an indifferent service. Corrigan et al (1988) explain that 'wealth allows choice and thus comparisons ... it is the enemy of blanket collective provision', and conclude, 'when there was not such wealth among the very large majority, collective provision for all its uniformity, brusqueness and remoteness, was not only tolerated but welcomed'. As a consequence, those responsible for the delivery of public services previously assumed that they 'knew what was best for the customer' – a tendency to see themselves as providing services *to* the public, rather than *for* the public. The emergence of consumerism has posed a significant challenge to the health service and health care professionals. The rights of consumers feature prominently in the policies of all the main political parties. In 1991, the government published the 'Citizen's Charter', which requires public service providers to publish explicit standards, and demands that 'services should be run to suit the convenience of customers, not staff'.

ADMIRATION OF THE PRIVATE SECTOR

Economic growth during the 1980s was accompanied by increased confidence in the private sector. The achievements of former public sector services, such as British Telecom and British Airways, since privatisation are cited as evidence for the government's concern that the NHS should become more 'businesslike'. The introduction of compulsory competitive tendering brought the health service into direct contact with the private sector and encouraged 'in house' providers to scrutinise the quality and costs of their services in a manner that was unnecessary in a non-competitive environment. Since the 'reforms' of the NHS, there has been a substantial increase in 'cross-sector flows', not only of services, but also of personnel. The boundaries between the public and private sectors have become increasingly permeable and have significantly influenced the character and style of health care provision.

'Quality as given'	------► Contracted standards
Organisational focus	------► Patient centred
Revenue allocation	------► Income generation
Non-competitive culture	------► Market orientation
Professional cultures	------► Corporate responsibility
Inputs	------► Measurable outcomes

Figure 10.1   The changing focus of health care.

These 'quality imperatives' have resulted in a discernible shift in the focus of public sector services. When applied to the NHS, they can be summarised as illustrated in Figure 10.1.

Political and socioeconomic forces have conspired to create a market in health care provision. As competition between NHS providers intensifies, there will be increasing pressure from purchasers for not only cost containment, but also demonstrable improvement in the quality of services delivered. In the past, quality might have been perceived as fashionable but not essential; in the future, it is likely to be the arbiter of survival.

The preceding paragraphs have summarised some of the pressures and incentives for quality improvement; as such, they have been concerned with '*Why* quality?'. But *what* is quality? In the subsequent sections of this chapter, an attempt will be made to define and describe the principles of quality in the context of health care. In preparation, Activity 10.1 should first be completed.

Activity 10.1

Identify any one item that you have purchased recently, for example your wrist watch, an item of clothing or your hi-fi system. Now, on a scale of 1 (low) to 5 (high), rate its quality. Then list the criteria used in making your judgement.

THE PRINCIPLES OF QUALITY

Quality is a notoriously difficult concept to come to grips with. When attempting Activity 10.1, you might have found that your quality criteria,

whilst appropriate in some circumstances, may not be applicable in others. Descriptions of quality include:

- getting it right first time
- fitness for purpose
- zero defects
- grade of goodness
- degree of excellence.

The growing literature on quality is replete with definitions and descriptions, but a recurring theme is a concern for the customer. In 1986, a somewhat exasperated Charles Shaw claimed that 'watertight definitions of quality and related words are too elusive to merit the time of practical people'. A useful working definition of quality is:

meeting or exceeding the comprehensively understood needs of customers.

CUSTOMERS AND CONSUMERS

In the public sector, it has been the convention to describe users of services as consumers, the term customer being reserved for those who pay directly (rather than indirectly through taxation) for a service or commodity. Whilst this distinction may be regarded as merely semantic, it has significant implications for quality. The NHS maxim 'free at the point of delivery' can be construed simply as 'free' and fuel the notion that the consumer is not paying, and is indeed receiving the service at no cost at all. Where there is no cash transaction between recipient and provider, both participants may be inclined to accept indifferent quality. There is no such inclination when a customer confronts a provider with his cheque book. It is salutary to note that, at the time of writing, NHS consumers (or customers) are paying £31 billion for their health care.

In the previous edition of this text (1992), Birch reminded us of who the consumer is – the patient (Box 10.1).

Whilst this usefully amplifies the pre-eminence of the patient, what are patients' needs if quality is about meeting these needs? Smith

---

Box 10.1   Who is the patient?

- The patient is the most important person on the hospital premises.
- The patient is not an interruption of work, but the purpose of it.
- The patient does not receive a favour at our hands – we receive one from him as the opportunity to care.
- The patient is not so much dependent upon us as we are upon him. None of us would be employed if it were not to meet his needs.
- The patient is not an outsider to our professional work/activities, but at the centre of them.
- The patient is not someone to ignore, talk over, put down, argue with or match our wits against.
- The patient may be anxious, frightened or agitated and ignorant of the simplest procedures. He requires empathy, reassurance and explanations.
- The patient is not a statistic but flesh and blood with feelings and emotions like our own, together with biases and prejudices.
- The patient would ask us to remember these truths today – it may be too late tomorrow!

(1986) proposes five tenets of consumerism, principles that can be readily applied to nursing practice:

- *Access*: Services should be accessible to all. The issue of access relates to many issues but is essentially about eliminating discriminatory practices that deny patients equitable access to services. This may relate to geographical location, opening hours, the provision of facilities for the disabled or the availability of certain specialist services.
- *Choice*: Patients should influence the range and style of services available. Satisfaction surveys or the view of patient interest groups can and should influence the services provided. These can range from clinical care to the domestic arrangements in a hospital ward.
- *Information*: Informed choice is subordinate to the availability of timely and accurate information. New technology permits any NHS Trust to produce its bespoke pre-admission video or discharge pamphlet, and such initiatives should be applauded. Such techniques, however, can only augment the skills and sensitivity of appropriately trained and knowledgeable staff.
- *Redress*: The Citizen's Charter requires that 'when things go wrong there must be a simple way of putting them right'. Health care providers must provide an explicit complaints procedure, known and clearly understood by all concerned. Complaints are feedback that not only require the organisation to apologise promptly and courteously, but also enable it to improve future performance.
- *Representation*: The interests of patients should be represented at all levels throughout the health service. Some would argue that the NHS reforms have reduced formal public representation; there remains, however, considerable scope for patient representation in the provision of health care. Community Health Councils have a statutory responsibility to represent the public interest, and pressure groups such as MIND, Age Concern, the British Diabetic Association and many others exert considerable influence. Professional organisations such as the Royal College of Nursing, Royal College of Midwives and Unison, in addition to representing their members, have a responsibility to inform and represent an 'innocent public'.

STAFF AS CUSTOMERS

Whilst it is self-evident that the public (or patients) are the prime customer of health care services, the notion that NHS staff are also customers is, for some, a novel if not surprising concept. However, regarding staff as internal customers and applying the principles of internal marketing is fundamental to service quality. Lewis (1988) asserts that 'personnel are seen as the first market of a service company and the objective of internal marketing is to get motivated and customer conscious staff'. Internal marketing has two related components:

- The values and attitudes of an organisation are conveyed by managers, either overtly or covertly, to their staff. If employees are treated with dignity, respect and courtesy, and their concerns and ideas are listened to, these values and behaviours will in turn be transmitted to patients and clients. It is salutary to note that the converse is also true. Of this phenomenon, Clemmer (1990) observes, 'it defies logic to expect exceptional behaviour from people who are not treated exceptionally'.

- The staff within an organisation, such as a hospital, health centre or general practice, provide and receive services from colleagues. This is described as an internal service chain. Consider, for example, a patient being admitted to hospital. A receptionist makes an appointment with the GP, the patient is examined by the GP, a practice nurse takes a specimen of blood and the specimen is despatched and tested at the hospital laboratory. On receipt of the result the doctor makes a referral to a consultant ... and so on, until the patient is perhaps admitted for elective surgery. This is a complex sequence of activities employing a range of individuals and their specialist skills. This sequence can be described as a quality chain (Fig. 10.2).

Each participant in the chain is simultaneously a customer and a supplier, receiving work from the previous stage as customer, and then applying personal skills and passing the work on, as a supplier. If this process is flawed at any stage, the work will have to be returned to the supplier and reworked. In our example, this might mean making another appointment, retyping a letter, taking another specimen of blood or cancelling the admission to hospital. Earlier, 'zero defects' was one description of quality, which spawned Crosby's (1978) claim that 'quality is free'. Mistakes cost money, and someone is paid for making them! It is estimated that 40% of the operating costs of service industries are associated with rectifying mistakes; to this has to be added the frustration, anger, blame, loss of esteem and, possibly, loss of a customer (or patient).

Pause for a few minutes and consider the questions in Activity 10.2.

This exercise reveals the length and complexity of a quality chain and demonstrates the requirement for suppliers to understand

Activity 10.2 Customers and suppliers

- Who are your customers?
- Who relies on you to provide information, specimens, staff, etc.?
- How satisfied are they with the service you provide?
- Who are your suppliers?
- Who supplies you with
  - equipment
  - information
  - staff
  - services?
- Are they meeting your needs?
- Do they know and understand your difficulties?

customers' needs and receive feedback on their performance.

QUALITY SYSTEMS

Not only is quality difficult to define, but the word itself is also embedded in a variety of concepts – quality control, quality assessment, quality improvement, quality assurance, quality management, total quality management. These terms are not synonymous but represent a quality systems hierarchy (Fig. 10.3). Applying this hierarchy to nursing, Wessex RHA (1991) defines these six levels of quality intervention, as given below.

Quality control

'Quality control' is a method for ensuring that specific standards of care can be attained. For example, in calculating a paediatric drug dose, a second nurse may check the calculation before the drug is administered.

Quality assessment

'Quality assessment' refers to measuring the

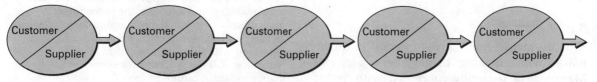

Figure 10.2 The quality chain.

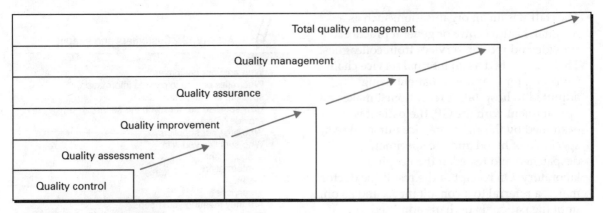

Figure 10.3   A quality heirarchy.

existing quality of a service. For example, a survey may be conducted by a general practice to assess patient satisfaction with appointment arrangements, the suitability of waiting room facilities and the punctuality of appointments.

Quality improvement

'Quality improvement' examines the current situation (quality assessment) and proposes solutions for improving the service. Such improvements can frequently be achieved without additional cost or resources. For example, simply improving signposting and the provision of wall-mounted site plans (with the helpful 'You are here' arrow) can substantially reduce the confusion and frustration of visitors to the complex world of the district general hospital.

Quality assurance

'Quality assurance' refers to a planned system of activities that, if carried out correctly, should result in a product or service satisfying agreed standards within prescribed resource limits and time scales. For example, BS5750 provides national standards that tell providers and manufacturers what is required of a quality system.

Quality management

'Quality management' gives priority to quality issues when making management decisions. Management is rightly concerned with 'reduc-

ing its costs', getting 'the biggest bang for its buck', 'sweating its assets' and so on, but it also aspires to reconcile cost containment with other issues. Shaw (1986) identifies six dimensions of quality management:

1. *efficiency*: resources are not wasted on one service or patient to the detriment of another
2. *effectiveness*: services achieve the intended benefit for the individual
3. *equity*: services are 'fairly' distributed to the population
4. *acceptability*: services are provided in such a manner as to satisfy the reasonable expectations of patients
5. *accessibility*: services are not limited by undue limits of time or distance
6. *appropriateness*: the service or procedure is what the population or individual actually needs.

For Shaw (1986), the key to quality management is 'appropriateness'. There is little, if any, point in providing patients with cost-effective, accessible, equitable care if there is no health gain. Shaw uses the following illustration:

Suppose that following a confusion of histology reports, a patient undergoes an unnecessary operation. The ward may be comfortable, the staff may be skilled and attentive, the procedure meticulously performed, no complications occur and an early and comfortable discharge is carefully organised with the community care team. Nonetheless, if the procedure or service is inappropriate, it cannot be 'good'.

Total quality management

'Total quality management' (TQM) embraces all the preceding sections. TQM is a culture that empowers individuals to provide the most appropriate care. Nicklin and Kenworthy (1995) assert that 'managers have subordinates, leaders have followers; managers tell people what to do, whilst leaders empower their people'. They proceed to describe the elements of empowerment that are fundamental to a TQM approach:

• *Capability*: Staff have the skills, knowledge and attitudes required for the job. This implies that employers link the strategic purposes of the organisation with the training of staff.

• *Confidence*: Employers work in a climate of trust, in a culture that is more interested in 'catching people doing something right' than in apportioning blame for errors. In such a climate, individuals will innovate, take risks and seek to achieve, rather than fear failure.

• *Congruence*, or alignment, is the essential component of empowerment. Empowerment is about 'doing the right thing' as well as about 'doing things right'. Crucially, empowered staff are clear about their organisation's objectives and values, and their personal contribution to their achievement.

QUALITY IN PRACTICE

Whilst the preceding sections have amplified or justified the quality imperative, clinicians and managers, although concerned with the why and what of quality, are practical people and require pragmatic options and solutions. This section will therefore concern itself with describing some tools and techniques that have proved (at least elsewhere) useful in measuring and promoting quality.

Reid (1988) observes that 'quality as a concept ... defies measurement', but proclaims that 'performance that dictates quality is capable of measurement if measured against some bench mark or predetermined set of criteria'.

STANDARDS

The NHS Executive (1993b) requires that standards of care should be specified, a useful definition of standards being:

qualitative and quantitative measures by which care can be measured or judged.

The literature of nursing has, in the past decade, been inundated with theories and models of standard-setting, the majority of which contain four critical elements. Standards should be:

1. *Meaningful*: This implies that standards are owned and acceptable. Some standards are derived from statute, contracts or regulations, whilst others may be determined locally. All those with a legitimate interest including patients should participate in standard-setting. Standards, if they are to be meaningful, must be acceptable, achievable and affordable.

2. *Measurable*: Standards, whilst being consistent and compatible with the organisation's objectives and values, should also be described in terms of observable phenomena and the conditions under which they should be achieved. As well as being meaningful and measurable, standards should be memorable, which probably means only five or six standards in any department, which everyone knows and would wish to be judged by.

3. *Monitored*: Standards need to be monitored. This may be achieved by a formal system of audit or random sampling. Technology may facilitate the collation, analysis and presentation of data. However, monitoring also requires 'aligned' staff who are constantly seeking and welcoming feedback on their performance against agreed standards.

4. *Managed*: The process of setting and achieving standards needs to be managed. Standards are too often developed on a wave of enthusiasm in the absence of a managerial infrastructure that will sustain them. Staff and their managers should be trained in the use of standards, and might require training to achieve them. Individual performance

review and personal development planning are prerequisites of the management of standards.

Quality is about meeting or exceeding customer needs. Standards are measures by which we can judge whether needs are being met, and are consequently the common feature of otherwise disparate approaches to quality management. The following are illustrations of techniques in common use.

Audit of nursing services

The NHS Management Executive (1991) has defined nursing audit as:

part of the cycle of quality assurance. It incorporates the systematic and critical analysis by nurses, midwives and health visitors, in conjunction with other staff, of the planning, delivery and evaluation of Nursing and Midwifery care, in terms of their use of resources and outcomes for patients and clients and introduces appropriate change in response to that analysis.

In its 'Framework of Audit for Nursing Services', the NHS Management Executive identifies two basic concepts:

- audit areas
- the audit cycle.

The six audit areas are:

1. *clinical care*: clinical nursing procedures and techniques
2. *workload management*: prioritising the clinical care that is required
3. *deployment*: identifying the skills required and the grade of staff who will most efficiently and effectively deliver the required care
4. *personnel management*: the selection, training, development and retention of staff to deliver care
5. *organisational arrangements*: the preparation of policies and procedures that facilitate the delivery of care
6. *environmental support*: the provision of supplies and services required to enable the prescribed care to be delivered.

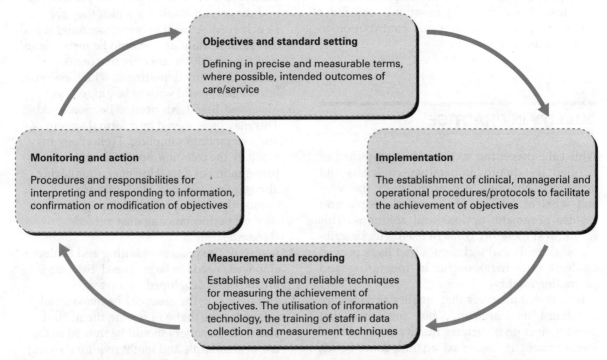

Objectives and standard setting

Defining in precise and measurable terms, where possible, intended outcomes of care/service

Implementation

The establishment of clinical, managerial and operational procedures/protocols to facilitate the achievement of objectives

Measurement and recording

Establishes valid and reliable techniques for measuring the achievement of objectives. The utilisation of information technology, the training of staff in data collection and measurement techniques

Monitoring and action

Procedures and responsibilities for interpreting and responding to information, confirmation or modification of objectives

Figure 10.4 The audit cycle. (Reproduced with kind permission from North Lincolnshire Health Authority 1992.)

Area	Clinical care		Sheet		
Category	Therapeutic care		A	1	2
Issue	Resting and sleeping for patients				
Version	1.0	Revision date		Revised by	

Objective
To minimise patients' distress, irritation and discomfort caused by lack of sleep.

Standard(s)
- All patients will enjoy a sleep pattern which is as close as possible to their normal routine.
- Disturbed and inadequate sleep patterns will be restored to normal for each individual whenever possible.

Implementation
- Staff are educated in general aspects of sleep and factors that disturb normal sleep, skills of assessment and planning for adequate sleep in hospital.
- Sleep standards are communicated to all staff, patients and relatives.
- Care routines are flexible to accommodate individual sleep programmes, including pre-sleep rituals.
- Pain-relieving measures and therapeutic interventions for comfort are provided whenever necessary.
- Physical standards in the environment and staff activities are altered, when necessary, to reduce noise and interference.
- Patients and relatives are made aware of opportunities for relatives to stay overnight.
- All primary nurses are responsible for reporting and supplying sleep audit data.

Measuring and recording
- Observation and interviews with patients, daily reporting and appropriate alteration of care plans will be employed.
- The views of random samples of patients and/or their relatives will be obtained by confidential questionnaire every 3 months.
- The views of a cross-section of care staff (all professions) will be sought every 3 months.

Monitoring and action
- Care routines are altered, if necessary, in accordance with patient satisfaction surveys.
- Primary nurses are responsible for making procedural alterations for their named patients.

Cross-refs				Data source(s)	

Figure 10.5 Specimen Clinical Audit: resting and sleeping. (Reproduced with kind permission from North Lincolnshire Health Authority 1992.)

These audit areas or 'layers' acknowledge the complex and dynamic relationship between direct care, other agencies (including management) and the environment in which care is delivered.

Each of these six areas can be audited using a four-stage cycle (Fig. 10.4).

Figures 10.5 and 10.6 are specimen audits of clinical care and personnel management employing the audit cycle.

Monitor

Monitor is possibly the best known of the UK nursing quality systems. It is the anglicised

Area	Clinical care			Sheet	
Category	Supportive care		A	1	2
Issue	Religion				
Version	1.0	Revision date		Revised by	

Objective
To allow complete freedom to every patient to practise their religion.

Standard(s)
- Facilities will always be available for patients to continue with worship or other religious activity.
- Patients and/or their families will be able to carry out specific religious rights and customs associated with feeding, hygiene, dress and prayer.
- Clergy and leaders of ethnic religious groups will have 24-hour access to patients, at the request of the patient.
- Whenever appropriate, specific rites and customs will be carried out following the death of a patient.

Implementation
- On admission to care all patients will be asked about their requirements for religious activity, if any.
- All care staff are educated in the specific aspects of religious practices of Christians, Jews, Moslems, Hindus (... and any other).
- All staff are aware of the procedure to be followed if a patient refuses medical treatment for religious reasons.
- Primary nurses are responsible for reporting and supplying audit data.

Measuring and recording
- Regular discussions with patients and relatives to ascertain level of satisfaction with ability to continue religious practices.
- Seek views of a random sample of patients by confidential questionnaire following discharge from care.
- Seek views and knowledge of staff by discussion.

Monitoring and action
- Results of patient satisfaction questionnaires will be recorded and used to inform planning for any change in arrangements.
- Ward manager to initiate discussions for change in overall arrangements for patients to pursue religious practices.

Cross-refs				Data source(s)	

Figure 10.6 Specimen Clinical Audit: religion. (Reproduced with kind permission from North Lincolnshire Health Authority 1992.)

version of the Rush Medicus Index, having been developed by the North West Staffing Project (Goldstone et al 1983) during the early 1980s. Although initially constructed for evaluating the quality of acute surgical and medical care, Monitor has subsequently been refined and developed for paediatrics, care of the elderly, midwifery, mental health and district nursing.

Monitor is a patient-orientated approach to quality assurance, consistent with contemporary systematic approaches to nursing care (i.e. the nursing process), although it has also been used successfully where the mode of operation is task allocation. Monitor assesses the quality of:

- care planning
- physical care
- non-physical care
- evaluation of care.

The Monitor methodology takes account of

differing levels of nursing care dependency, which are defined and subsequently categorised as:

I   Minimal care – requires minimal nursing supervision, but may require treatments or clinical observations

II Average care – requires moderate supervision, may require assistance with personal care needs in addition to treatments and observations

III Above-average care – greater than average supervision and assistance. Requires almost complete assistance to meet personal care needs. Requires medical support and sometimes the use of special equipment

IV Maximum care – requires very frequent to continuous care, combined with close supervision by medical personnel and the support of technical equipment.

Monitor contains in excess of 450 questions about care. Information is collected by trained observers who examine care records and interview patients, in addition to observing direct nursing care. According to its authors, typical areas of scrutiny include:

• assessment and planning: for example, is there a statement written within 24 hours of admission on the condition of the skin?
• physical care: for example, is adequate equipment for oral hygiene available?
• non-physical care: for example, do nursing staff call the patient by the name he prefers?
• evaluation of care: for example, do records document the patient's response to teaching?

Illustrative of the Monitor questionnaire is Figure 10.7.

The Monitor scoring system is the average of all patients in all categories (I–IV) and provides an index (%) of care provided in a particular ward or care environment. Additionally, there is a questionnaire that interrogates ward management and organisation and yields a 'ward index'. A typical data matrix is illustrated in Table 10.1.

The data in Table 10.1 reveal that Henderson Ward scores 76% and that patient care scores

Table 10.1 Typical Monitor data matrix

Results for Henderson Ward (male surgical)

| | Dependency category | | | | |
	I	II	III	IV	Weighted average
Planning care	50	41	30	56	47
Physical care	75	70	62	68	68
Non-physical care	75	77	25	65	70
Evaluation of care	70	70	54	64	66
Totals	66	67	47	60	63
				Ward score	76

63%; such scores are typical, but the value of Monitor is in not so much the data it provides, but the questions it raises for managers and clinicians. The anomalies of care in different categories in Figure 10.1 are self-evident and merit discussion and exploration.

Activity 10.3

If you were the manager of Henderson Ward, what questions and issues would the data in Table 10.1 raise?

Whilst well regarded, Monitor is undeniably time-consuming and costly to operate. Consequently, the costs and benefits of Monitor have to be carefully and systematically weighed.

Quality Pointers Tool (QPT)

The QPT (Baghurst 1993) was developed conjointly by the North Western Region and the University of York. It is designed to be less time-consuming and cumbersome than other techniques, whilst remaining a valid and reliable indicator of nursing quality. According to its authors, the 'objective nature of QPT' means that problems can easily be verified, resulting in speedy remedial action.

The QPT is based on a 44-item questionnaire that scrutinises:

Source of information		Patients code or initials	6									
			7									
Section B meeting the patient's physical needs			8									
			9									

1 Protecting the patient from accident and injury

Observe patient	a Is the patient's identification bracelet worn on his wrist or leg as appropriate?	No										
		Yes	✓									
		24										
		Score	1									

Ask nurse	b Are assigned nursing staff informed of the patient's present condition?	No										
		Yes	✓									
		25										
		Score	1									

Observer must know patient's present condition. Then asks nurse what patient's condition is. If nurse answers incorrectly record 'no'.

Observe bed	c Is the patient's name displayed on his bed?	No										
		Yes	✓									
		26										
		Score	1									

Inference	d Is all care of the patient accurately done and appropriately prescribed?	No										
		Yes	✓									
		Not applicable										
		Not available										
		27										
		Score	1									

Answer 'no' if any procedures are not both accurately done and specifically prescribed e.g. a catheter irrigation when it is not ordered or not needed. Applies to medical or nursing orders.

Observe environment	e Is the bed at a suitable height for the patient (except when treatments are being done)?	No										
		Yes	✓									
		Not applicable										
		28										
		Score	1									

Figure 10.7   'Monitor' – specimen questionnaire. (Reproduced with kind permission from Goldstone et al 1993.)

- ward shift details
- levels of care
- staff development
- nursing duties.

The questionnaire items were generated by asking nurses about the activities and issues that influenced the quality of nursing care. These items were subsequently refined and validated. The results of the questionnaire, which can be completed in 5 minutes (or less), can be produced either numerically or graphically, providing a Care Quality Score, defined in Box 10.2.

Figure 10.8 displays some questions randomly selected from the QPT.

Figure 10.9 is a specimen report generated by the QPT PC software c YHEC.

Subsequent QPT scores can be compared with previous ward ratings, the ratings of other wards in the hospital or a 'reference data set' derived from QPT users throughout the UK.

QPT questionnaires and software are available for general medical and surgical wards, and

Box 10.2 The Care Quality Score

1. Dangerous: The level of care was so low that patients were at risk of accident or deterioration in condition due to a lack of observation and/or insufficient staff for essential needs.

2. Barely safe: The level of care was such that, although serious risk of deterioration or accident was avoided, only essential needs could be met.

3. Less than adequate: The level of care was such that patients were not at risk from accident or deterioration, but it was unsatisfactory since generally some needs could not be met.

4. Adequate: The level of care was generally acceptable, although occasionally some patients' needs could not be met.

5. Good: The level of care was such that most needs of all patients could be met.

6. Excellent: The level of care was such that all needs of all patients could be met, and it would be difficult to have improved the standard of care.

are currently being expanded to embrace mental health and community nursing.

The QPT is a simple-to-use instrument, but its methodology is based exclusively on the perceptions and judgements of nurses. A powerful adjunct to the QPT would clearly be similar data derived from patients. The QPT team are currently developing a Patient Perception Tool (of quality) to be used in conjunction with the QPT.

Activity 10.4

If you were developing a Patient Perception Tool (of quality), identify the 10 key questions that might be crucial indicators of quality from the patient's perspective. THEN ask some of your current patients to comment on your questions.

Patient satisfaction surveys

In Activity 10.4, you were invited to identify 'crucial quality indicators' from the patient's perspective. Inviting patients to comment on their care and the services they receive is not an unusual or novel undertaking but an obligation.

Section 3: Ward Management

Staff deployment
1. Were there any nursing staff present during the shift who had never worked on the ward before?

3. Did you have to delay collecting any patients from theatre owing to lack of ward staff?

Paperwork
6. Did you delay dealing with all paperwork (this includes legal requirements)?

Communications
10. Were you able to answer all incoming phone calls?

General oversight of ward
12. Were you able to check/re-order non urgent stocks?

Supervision and teaching
19. Were you able to check the charts of all patients?

21. Did learner nurses undertake any tasks or procedures unsupervised for which they had insufficient training or experience?

Section 4: Nursing Duties

Care planning and assessment
24. Was the preparation of a care plan for any new patient deferred to the next shift owing to pressure of work?

Procedures/technical
27. Was the administration of PRN drugs delayed for any patient owing to pressure of work?

28. Was the drugs round delayed long enough to affect the timing of the next drugs round?

Ward routine
39. Were any stores/clean laundry not sorted and shelved owing to pressure of work?

Communication/support
42. Were any patients wishing to discuss their care/condition refused immediate nurse attention owing to pressure of work?

Figure 10.8 Questions randomly selected from the QPT.

The Citizen's Charter (HM Government 1991) demands that 'the people affected by services should be consulted. Their views about services they use should be sought regularly and systematically to inform decisions about the services to be provided'. You may even have participated in developing a survey instrument or been involved in the collection of responses. The majority of hospitals and NHS Trusts have developed their own patient satisfaction surveys. Typical items in these include:

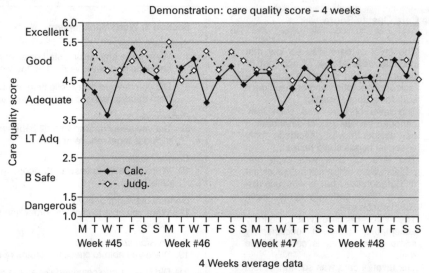

Figure 10.9   Specimen Care Quality Score report. (Reproduced by kind permission of York Health Economic Consortium, University of York)

- staff attitudes
- the provision of information
- access to services
- the quality of the environment
- the perceived outcome for the patient
- the quality of food
- visiting regulations and restrictions
- waiting times.

The strength of locally devised satisfaction surveys is that they are 'local' and consequently reflect local circumstances, culture, difficulties and aspirations. Additionally, those responsible for developing the survey instrument, for example patient interest groups, clinicians, professional organisations and managers, will be committed not only to its design, but also to responding promptly and effectively to its results. However, Wedderburn Tate (1995) reports that, while managers may be interested in such feedback, satisfaction surveys rarely affect the care process. She argues that 'in house' surveys may lack scientific rigour and can be biased by 'what staff already know', resulting in positive results that are of little value. She commends the use of externally validated methods conducted by experienced researchers, the results of which can be compared with other hospitals. Such comparisons using common

instrumentation can enable an organisation to participate in 'benchmarking'.

Benchmarking

Benchmarking has, according to Bendell et al (1993) 'become a vogue phrase of the 1990s', and, like other terms imported from the USA and subsequently applied to the British public sector, it has lost something in the translation, and consequently is used with varying degrees of ambiguity. However, the Xerox Corporation's definition of benchmarking seems clear enough:

the continuous process of measuring products, services and practices against the toughest competitors or those recognised as industry leaders.

If this definition were applied to patient satisfaction, what would it mean?

- Identify the benchmarking issue, in this case 'patient satisfaction'.
- Identify hospitals or health care providers who are competitors or are regarded as being exceptional in satisfying their patients.
- Determine the data to be collected; these may be from nationally published sources or could be derived from a site visit to the 'market leader'.

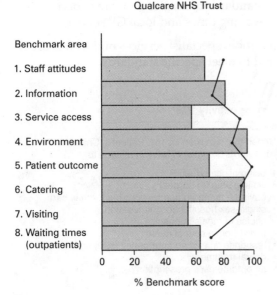

Qualcare NHS Trust

Key

☐ Qualcare Trust score
•—• Benchmark partner score

Figure 10.10 Benchmark data – patient satisfaction survey.

• Measure the 'performance gap', i.e. the discrepancy between your performance and that of the exemplar or competitor.

• Set targets for future performance.

• Agree an action plan for improving performance.

• Implement the plan and monitor its performance.

• Evaluate performance and recalibrate the benchmark.

In Figure 10.10 the results of the fictitious Qualcare NHS Trust's, patient satisfaction survey are compared with those of their benchmark partner(s). Such information can then be used to target improvements or consolidate and sustain areas of above average performance.

Complaints

Actively eliciting the patient's perceptions of the service they receive or want is an important adjunct to providing a quality service. However, what of a patient's wish to provide unsolicited feedback? Whilst many, indeed the majority of,

patients appear satisfied with the service offered and received, things occasionally go wrong, and in these circumstances 'at the very least, the citizen is entitled to a good explanation or an apology' (HM Government 1991). According to the NHS Executive (1993a), complaints should be regarded as 'positive feedback to organisations', provide valuable information about perceived weaknesses and help organisations to raise the standards of service. Consequently, all health care providers should have systems for managing complaints.

A complaints system should:

• be easily accessible and well publicised
• be simple to understand and use
• allow speedy handling, with established time limits for action, and keep people informed of progress
• ensure a full and fair investigation
• respect people's desire for confidentiality
• address all the points at issue, and provide an effective response and appropriate redress
• provide information to management so that services can be improved.

Activity 10.5

Think of an occasion when a patient has made what *he* considers to be a serious complaint. Using the seven characteristics of a complaints procedure (above) as a checklist, how would you rate:

• your own performance
• your unit or ward performance
• your organisation's policy for managing complaints?

The Patient's Charter

In the preceding sections, there have been several references to the Citizen's Charter, published as a White Paper in 1991. It aims to raise quality, increase choice, secure better value and extend the accountability of public services. Subsequently, charters for a comprehensive range of public sector services have been published, including those for education, transport, the Post Office, the police, the Inland Revenue, social services and the NHS. The Patient's

Charter, first published in 1991 and revised in 1995, sets out the rights and standards that patients can expect from GPs, hospital services, community services, ambulance services, maternity services, dentists, and optical and pharmaceutical services.

Under the provision of the Patient's Charter (1991), users of the NHS have a *right* to:

1. Access to services:

   - receive health care on the basis of their clinical need, rather than on their ability to pay, their lifestyle or any other factor
   - be registered with a GP and be able to change their GP easily and quickly if they want to
   - get emergency medical treatment at any time through their GP, the emergency ambulance service and hospital accident and emergency departments
   - be referred to a consultant acceptable to them when their GP thinks it is necessary, and be referred for a second opinion.

2. Personal consideration and respect:

   - choose whether or not they want to take part in medical research or medical student training
   - expect all the staff they meet face to face to wear name badges
   - expect the NHS to respect their privacy, dignity and religious and cultural beliefs at all times and in all places.

3. Providing information:

   - have any proposed treatment, including any risks involved in that treatment and any alternatives, clearly explained to them before they decide whether to agree to it
   - have access to their health records, and to know that everyone working for the NHS is under a legal duty to keep records confidential
   - have any complaint about NHS services (whoever provides them) investigated, and to get a quick, full written reply from the relevant chief executive or general manager.
   - receive detailed information on local health services. This includes information on the

standards of service they can expect, waiting times and local GP services.

In addition, specialist services of the NHS are required to meet specific standards.

Activity 10.6

Under the provision of the Patient's Charter (1995), what *rights* do patients have in relation to:

- being allocated a GP
- waiting time for surgery
- having a named nurse responsible for their care
- single-sex hospital accommodation
- choice of meals in hospital
- a visit from a district nurse
- response time of an emergency (999) ambulance
- dental treatment
- an optometrist's prescription?

Activity 10.6 can be a salutary exercise. Earlier it was claimed that standards should be owned, known and understood. How many NHS staff and users could correctly answer the questions posed in Activity 10.6? The Patient's Charter is available in 10 languages other than English and, for people who are blind, partially sighted or deaf, in a variety of forms, including Braille, large print, audiocassette and videotape. Details of the Patient's Charter are available free on 0800 665544.

In a previous section, the concept of *internal marketing* was discussed; therefore, in concluding this section on quality in practice, it is appropriate to consider techniques and methods that assume that staff (and students) are also customers and should be the recipients of a quality service.

Ward Learning Climate Indicators

The Ward Learning Climate audit tool was developed by Sheffield Hallam University in collaboration with the Sheffield and North Trent College of Midwifery and Nursing (Orton 1993). The audit instrument aims to assess the quality of the learning climate for student nurses and midwives. Rigorous and comprehensive research revealed six key issues that characterise a good learning environment for students (Box 10.3).

Box 10.3 Ward Learning Climate – key characteristics

1. *Placement orientation*: Students are welcomed to the placement and have a named mentor. Their orientation programme provides explicit information on the placement's policies and procedures.
2. *Supernumerary status*: Students and staff have a common understanding of their respective roles. Students are not used merely as a 'pair of hands', and are encouraged to negotiate aspects of their experience.
3. *Theory and practice*: The relationship between the college and clinical placements is effective; students are well supported in clinical areas and have opportunities to participate in care that is based on appropriate research. What is taught by the college is relevant to clinical practice.
4. *Attitudes of staff*: Placement staff are approachable, supportive, well informed and positive about the student's course of training. Students are encouraged to work with the ward team, ask questions and be given appropriate feedback on their performance.
5. *Mentors*: The student has sustained access to a named mentor. The mentor is supportive, agrees and identifies learning opportunities for the student, and is able to respond effectively to the range of learning styles of individual students.
6. *Assessment*: The requirements of clinically based assessments are agreed and understood by the student and mentor, and progress is regularly reviewed.

Activity 10.6

As a student nurse or midwife, you have made judgements about the quality of your clinical placements. Identify and list the characteristics of a 'good' clinical placement.

How do these compare with the views of your peers, mentors, clinical supervisors and teachers?

The Ward Learning Climate Indicators are identified by the administration of a 55-item questionnaire to staff and students. Results are scored and presented graphically. A software package has been developed that requires minimal computer expertise and substantially reduces the time-consuming process of scoring questionnaires. Figure 10.11 is a summary of a specimen ward learning climate, and Figure

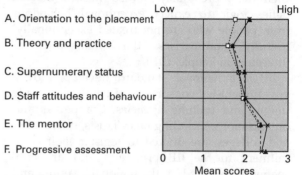

Ward Learning Climate Indicators for:
Summary

A. Orientation to the placement

B. Theory and practice

C. Supernumerary status

D. Staff attitudes and behaviour

E. The mentor

F. Progressive assessment

Figure 10.11   Ward Learning Climate Indicators summary chart. (Reproduced with kind permission from Orton 1993.)

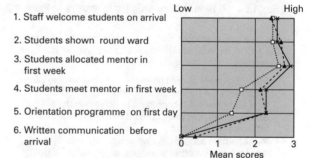

Ward Learning Climate Indicators for:
A. Orientation to the placement

1. Staff welcome students on arrival

2. Students shown round ward

3. Students allocated mentor in first week

4. Students meet mentor in first week

5. Orientation programme on first day

6. Written communication before arrival

Figure 10.12   Ward Learning Climate Indicators – scores for 'placement orientation'. (Reproduced with kind permission from Orton 1993.)

10.12 displays the scores for the 'placement orientation' characteristic.

Investors in People

Clemmer's previously quoted maxim that 'it defies logic to expect exceptional behaviour from people who are not treated exceptionally' usefully summarises the philosophy of 'Investors in People' (IIP).

IIP is a national standard developed by a government-led consortium of employers, trade unions and training agencies. Companies and organisations, including NHS Trusts, universities and colleges, are invited to register their commitment to the IIP principles and are subsequently assessed by the regional Training and Enterprise Councils (TECs) (and Local Enterprise Councils (LECs) in Scotland), who decide whether or not they meet the standards and are eligible for the IIP award.

There are four principles to the national standard, each having between five and seven assessment indicators (24 in total). The National Standards for Investors in People are identified in Box 10.4.

Your college of nursing, or the hospital in which you are receiving clinical tuition, may be an 'Investor in People' or have registered its commitment to the award. Activity 10.7 is a checklist of some IIP characteristics.

CONCLUSION

Quality is a notoriously difficult issue to come to grips with, particularly when the concept is applied to an issue so emotive, value laden and controversial as health care delivery. The issue of quality, however, must be addressed and a common understanding and language developed, so that all those involved in health care, including patients, can gauge the performance of their NHS against reasonable, rational and affordable criteria.

A note of caution, however. Many nurses, possibly as a result of nursing's heritage, believe there is only one standard, only one type of quality – the best. This the author challenges. Quality is not about providing the best possible service or the best possible care; it is about providing services and care that achieve appropriate outcomes and meet expectations at the lowest possible cost. The problem with the

---

Box 10.4   National standards for Investors in People

An Investor in People makes a public commitment from the top to develop all employees to achieve its business objectives.

- Every business should have a written but flexible plan which sets out business goals and targets, considers how employees will contribute to achieving the plan and specifies how development needs in particular will be assessed and met.
- Management should develop and communicate to all employees a vision of where the organisation is going and the contribution employees will make to its success, involving employee representatives as appropriate.

An Investor in People regularly reviews the training and development needs of all employees.

- The resources for training and developing employees should be clearly identified in the business plan.
- Managers should be responsible for regularly agreeing training and development needs with each employee in the context of business objectives, setting targets and standards linked, where appropriate, to the achievement of National Vocational Qualifications (or

relevant units) and, in Scotland, Scottish Vocational Qualifications.

An Investor in People takes action to train and develop individuals on recruitment and throughout their employment.

- Action should focus on the training needs of all new recruits and continually developing and improving the skills of existing employees.
- All employees should be encouraged to contribute to identifying and meeting their own job-related development needs.

An Investor in People evaluates the investment in training and development to assess achievement and improve future effectiveness.

- The investment, the competence and commitment of employees, and the use made of skills learned, should be reviewed at all levels against business aims and targets.
- The effectiveness of training and development should be reviewed at the top level and lead to renewed commitment and target setting.

Activity 10.7

These are some of the characteristics of an 'Investor in People'. How does your organisation rate?

Yes   No

- Have you received a summary or abstract of your organisation's business goals?
- Do you regularly receive a report or briefing on your organisation's progress?
- Is there a student/staff committee that is consulted on the organisation's goals and plans?
- Are you able to relate the objectives of your job directly to the goals of your organisation?
- Is your performance regularly and systematically reviewed by your boss?
- Have you formally agreed a personal development plan with your boss?
- Is your organisation committed to your training and development, so that you are able to meet organisational goals?
- Are the outcomes of your training (and development) evaluated?

. . . standard raising has little to do with static protocols and rigid systems, rather it has more to do with stout hearts and gut reactions, with fostering a sense of the individual within the system.

Summary

Nurses and patients alike are concerned with the quality of nursing care. What is difficult, however, is to define, describe and measure that quality.

The forces behind the current focus of quality have been both political and socioeconomic, the general public no longer accepting a role as the passive recipients of an indifferent service, be it related to consumer goods or health care. These forces have conspired to create competition between NHS providers, with the result that quality has now become an indispensible part of any health care service.

Many authors have attempted to define the principles of quality, but a recurrent theme has been concern for the customer, whether a patient or a member of staff. This chapter considers some aspects of this customer focus and describes a taxonomy for the management, measurement and monitoring of quality.

However, discussions of the theoretical aspects of quality are of no use if they are not translated into practice, and a selection of tools and techniques for doing this is outlined in the text.

Only if quality is an active component of health care can patient's reasonable expectations be met and appropriate care outcomes be achieved.

best is that it is inclined to be the most expensive. Health expenditure in the UK is touching 32 billion, and with little effort could cost twice as much. Costs have to be contained, and excessive, exceptional, elaborate or even luxurious care for one patient may deny another any treatment at all.

In the preceding paragraphs, much has been said about quality, and, as an academic discipline, its gurus have generated a disproportionate number of memorable sound bites. However, it should be remembered that the route to quality is through the familiar landscape of daily nursing life. Quality can only be achieved if everyone in the care team believes in it, if everyone contributes to it and above all if every practitioner is committed to improving their own standards of practice; in the words of Alison Kitson (1987):

REFERENCES

Baghurst A 1993 Quality Pointers Tool. NWRHA & YHEC, University of York, York
Bendell T, Boulter L et al 1993 Benchmarking for competitive advantage. Pitman, London
Clemmer J 1990 Firing on all cylinders. Piatkus, London
Corrigan J 1988 Socialism, merit and efficiency. Fabian Society, London
Crosby P B 1978 Quality is free. McGraw Hill, Maidenhead
Department of Health 1989 Working for patients. HMSO, London
Department of Health 1991, revised 1995 The Patient's Charter. DoH, London
Goldstone L A, Ball J A et al 1983 Monitor – an index of the quality of nursing care for acute medical and surgical wards. Newcastle upon Tyne Polytechnic, Newcastle
Griffiths R 1983 NHS management enquiry. HMSO, London
HM Government 1991 The Citizen's Charter. HMSO, London
Kenworthy N, Snowley G et al 1992 Common foundation studies in nursing. Churchill Livingstone, Edinburgh
Kitson A 1987 Raising standards of clinical practice – the fundamental issue of effective nursing practice. Journal of Advanced Nursing 12(3): 321–329

Lewis B 1988 Customer care in service organisation. International Journal of Health Care Quality Assurance 2: 1

NHS Executive 1993a Citizen's Charter Unit – complaints task force. DoH, Leeds

NHS Executive 1993b Achieving an organisation wide approach to quality. DoH Leeds

NHS Management Executive 1991 Framework of Audit for Nursing Services. DoH, London

Nicklin P, Kenworthy N 1995 Teaching and assessing in nursing practice. Scutari Press, London

Orton H 1993 Charting the way to excellence. Pavic, Sheffield

Pollitt C 1986 Beyond the management model. Financial Accountability and Management 2: 3

Reid E 1988 Recent advances in nursing. Longman, London

Shaw C D 1986 Introducing quality assurance. King's Fund, London, p 11

Smith M 1986 The consumer case for socialism. Fabian Society, London

Snowley G, Nicklin P, Birch J 1992 Objectives for care, 2nd edn. Wolfe, London

Tate C Wedderburn 1995 What do patients really think? Health Service Journal 105: 18–20

Wessex RHA 1991 Quality – using information in managing the nursing resource. Greenhalgh, Macclesfield

World Health Organization 1985 Target for health for all. WHO Europe, Copenhagen

FURTHER READING

Collard R 1990 Total quality success through people. IPM, Wimbledon

Koch H 1992 Implementing and sustaining total quality management in health care. Longman, Harlow

Marr H, Giebing H 1994 Quality assurance in nursing. Campion, Edinburgh

Nicklin P, Lankshear A L 1989 Quality matters. Nursing Times 86: 31

Snowley G, Nicklin P 1992 Objectives for care. Wolfe, London

3

Nursing: fundamental principles and skills

Nursing provides a multi-functional service for patients in addition to the traditional delivery of 'tender loving care'. In this section of the book the student is introduced to the concepts of professionalism and nursing ethics, together with accounts of the increasing range of skills now demanded of the qualified nurse.

11 The development of the nursing profession

Stephanie Kirby

The image of the nurse and the history of nursing are inextricably intertwined. Celia Davies (1980) asserts that nursing cannot be seen in a vacuum, but in its social context. To understand issues that influence nursing today and that have implications for the future direction of nursing, it is necessary to understand the historical background to those issues.

To do this, Chapter 11 discusses:

- women's traditional role in healing
- the influence of religious beliefs, social changes and war
- the part played by Florence Nightingale and other reformers in the development of nursing
- the developmental care of the mentally ill and mentally handicapped, and children
- the setting up of the professional Register, the inception of the NHS and the changes leading up to a new preparation for nurses.

Activity 11.1

Ask your friends and family to give the name of one famous nurse. Do you have a spread of varied names, or does one name consistently appear?

Activity 11.2

Browse through the get well cards at your local newsagents. What pictorial images of nurses do they convey?

Activity 11.3

Compare and contrast how the nurse characters are portrayed in current soaps and dramas, for example 'Neighbours', 'Casualty', 'Coronation Street' and 'Cardiac Arrest'.
    Do discernible images and stereotypes emerge?

These images of nursing are shaped by the history of nursing:

1. Images of nursing are often synonymous with images of women, who were historically the largest proportion of the nursing workforce, and the history of nursing is linked to women's history. Traditional gender roles have influenced the classification of nursing in the past as women's work, with its consequent low status and low remuneration.

2. Changing religious and social attitudes have influenced the pattern and organisation of care throughout the centuries. Social change is, in turn, influenced by demographic trends.

3. The prevalent knowledge base also governs the extent of care and treatment that can be offered to clients. For example, oral histories give testimony to the changes in nursing activity brought about by the introduction of penicillin in the 1940s.

4. War accelerates the acquisition of knowledge; it poses new problems that require new solutions; it demands new approaches to logistics and manpower planning. It was the experience of war and the threat of an influx of unqualified volunteer staff that added weight to the pro-registration party. The appalling conditions of the wounded in the Crimea, brought home to the public by the new developments of the telegraph and the war correspondent, led to Florence Nightingale's call to Scutari. Similarly, the equitable distribution of goods owing to rationing in World War II and the provisions of the Emergency Medical Service, paved the way for the Welfare State and the National Health Service.

5. The legislative framework of health care policy affects the work of all nurses in a variety of health care settings. The variety of professional and trade union representation among nurses is linked to the past experiences of the different branches of nursing. Nurses in the voluntary hospitals, the Poor Law infirmaries and the asylums faced very different conditions of service, which necessitated different responses and varied routes to professional identity. The demands of the political framework within which all nurses are obliged to deliver care continue to shape and develop the nature of nursing.

WOMEN AND HEALING

Versluysen (1980) argues that, statistically, it is women who have always been the main healers in English society. Until the last 15 years, there has been little historical work on the role of the woman healer. Such women traditionally delivered babies, tended the sick and infirm, and passed the secrets of the traditional herbal remedies on to the next generation by word of mouth. Most people are familiar with the image of the traditional herbal healer or 'wise woman'. Brooke (1993) identifies another image of the innovative woman healer, who worked alongside her male colleagues, often having the credit for her work purloined by them.

Many ancient traditions saw woman as the powerful creator figure. In Ancient Egypt, a highly organised and respected female healing tradition centered around the worship of Isis, the restorer of life and source of healing herbs. It may have been male practitioners who developed the skills of preserving the dead, but it was the female healers who became skilled in the treatment of obstetric and gynaecological conditions, as the Kahun papyrus dated circa 1900BC testifies (Brooke 1993). Female political hegemony and the position of women healers were closely linked. The schools of these women healers were instrumental in the training of the physicans of Classical Greece. The Greeks developed a questioning approach to the study of disease and health, based on the philosophical approach of the philosopher Aristotle (382–322BC) and the empirical work of Hippocrates (circa 460BC). Many people are familiar with Hippocrates' contribution to medical ethics. He also compiled detailed descriptions of many diseases and, for the first time, attributed a natural, rather than supernatural, cause to epilepsy. Unfortunately, one of Aristotle's legacies was the expounding of the theory of humours in the body, namely blood, water, yellow bile and black bile. Excesses of these were said to correspond to different individual temperaments. Treatments were aimed at correcting inbalances of these humours. They included purging, blood-letting and the application of leeches, which formed the basis of the physician's treatments until the 19th century.

The male ascendency continued, women in Classical Greece being forbidden the study of medicine. To gain access to this knowledge, the young Athenian girl Agnodice studied at the school in Alexandria disguised as a man, and subsequentially treated women patients. She was discovered, denounced by her male colleagues, tried, found guilty of the illegal practice of medicine and sentenced to death. It was the threatened mass suicide of her female clients that saved her, allowed her to continue to practise and indeed then allowed all Greek gentlewomen the right to study medicine. This gave many women a degree of economic freedom (Brooke 1993). Aspasia, another Greek female physician, practised in Rome. Texts survive, written many hundreds of years later, which are based on her knowledge of gynaecological conditions.

The Romans, whose Empire stretched from North Africa to Britain, built on many of the traditions of the Greeks. They venerated Aesculapius and his family as the promoters of health and health care. The female members of his family, his wife Epione and daughters Panacea and Hygeia, were seen very much as his helpmates, in subservient roles.

Galen of Pergamon (AD129–199), who was physician and friend to the Emperor Marcus Aurelius, was an influential figure in the study of health. He drew attention to the relationship between health, lifestyle and occupation. He misunderstood the nature of the circulatory system, but, like Aristotle, his influence was so great that his misconceptions were not challenged until the 17th century, much of mediaeval medicine being based on his teachings.

In Rome, many women from aristocratic families practised healing. Octavia, the wife of Mark Antony (circa 83–30BC), wrote a book of prescriptions. It was the advent of Christianity, which was eventually adopted as the state religion of Rome, that provided an outlet for the energies of many women in nursing activities.

Question 11.1

- Why is it only so comparatively recently that the achievements of these women healers have been discussed?
- Why should the study of medicine be forbidden to women in Classical Greece?

THE INFLUENCE OF RELIGIOUS BELIEFS

With its emphasis on good works and charity, Christianity promoted the help of the sick. In the 1st century, the Church organised groups of married women or deaconesses to visit the sick and needy in their own homes. Nursing became a chic activity for upper-class Roman women. Fabiola (died AD399) was praised by St Jerome for her compassion to the sick, for washing 'their putrid matter that others could not bear to look upon'(cited in Baly 1995). She founded an infirmary for the sick poor of the city. This activity came within accepted thought of Christian duty. The espousal of Christianity meant that after the fall of the Roman Empire in the 5th century, elements of Greek and Roman thought were preserved in Western Europe. However, there was at times a return to demonology. St Augustine of Hippo (AD345–430) held the belief that disease and demons were linked, and this influenced the treatment of the mentally ill for many hundreds of years.

Monasticism contributed to the care of the sick and poor in guest houses and infirmaries, particularly those outcasts of mediaeval society – lepers. Both men and women in religious orders developed skills and knowledge in healing and herbal remedies. Friars, too, were important as 'they provided most of the organised care for the sick in England in the fourteenth century, and their hospitals became the basis of later foundations' (Baly 1995).

Women had to be circumspect in relation to the authority of the church. Midwives had to be licensed to practice by a bishop; there was a constant fear that midwives would carry out demonic practices, and there was much speculation on the fate of the placenta. Suspicions culminated in the notorious witch hunt craze that swept Europe and the New World between the 15th and 17th centuries. Even a woman held in high esteem, such as Hildegard of Bingen, had to resort to the female stance of humility when making her works public (Flannagan 1988). During the Crusades, hospitals such as St Bartholomew's, St Thomas' and the Hotel Dieu in Paris were built along the pilgrim routes.

Plagues and venereal disease were brought back from the East. Together with famine, these were the main cause of death in mediaeval Europe. The poor were generally cared for in their own homes, with friends and neighbours rallying round in a crisis. In addition, wise women and herbalists were available for a small fee or a service in kind to the poor. In times of great outbreaks of famine or plague, local women were also employed as searchers to report cases of plague, who then needed to be isolated: Marye Jerome and Anne Lovejoy were employed by the town of Reading (Clark 1982).

From the 14th to the 16th centuries, there was a revival of classical learning in Europe known as the Renaissance. Together with religious, economic and social changes, this can be seen as the watershed between the old and modern worlds. Educated men and women of that time 'truly believed that they were living in a period of great change and they felt themselves to be different from the Middle Ages, which they regarded as barbarous' (Baly 1995).

New knowledge gained from the work of scientists such as Copernicus (1473–1543) led to a questioning approach by many of the educated classes. The authority and teachings of the Roman Catholic Church were brought into question. Martin Luther, a German monk, led a movement that eventually caused the division of the universal Christian Church in Europe. By the 1530s, Europe was divided into two aggressive faiths – Protestant and Catholic – each sure of the God-given righteousness of their cause. This ideological divide had profound effects on the attitudes to the provision of care to the poor and sick for 300 years and beyond. In England, King Henry VIII took the opportunity that the Reformation afforded him to break with Rome and divorce his childless wife. One consequence of the Reformation in England was the dissolution of the monasteries, which took place during the late 1530s and early 1540s. Valuables were transfered to the royal treasury, and land was sold off. The cathedral churches survived, but about 10 000 monks and nuns were displaced. Attempts were made to replace monastic learning with secular institutions, such as grammar schools, but no widespread hospital system replaced the hiatus left by the dissolution of the monasteries.

The Protestant attitude to illness, like that of the Catholic Church before it, saw suffering very much as the will of God but did not emphasis the value of good works on the road to salvation. In its harshest form, it followed the doctrine of the work ethic, which emphasised the value of hard work and its worth to the individual. It also gave less importance to the place of saints and the Virgin Mary.

Two factors assisting the spread of the new religion were:

1. the new invention of printing, which provided a cheap and readily distributable vehicle for the dissemination of new ideas
2. the growth of urban society, where the new faith had great following, many of the town dwellers being attracted by the notions of self-advancement in the work ethic.

Activity 11.4

Visit a Roman Catholic and a Protestant church locally.
Compare and contrast the decorative features.

SOCIAL CHANGE FROM TUDORS TO VICTORIANS

MERRIE ENGLAND

Following this ideological change, there was also a period of economic upheaval. Inflation appeared, fuelled by the import of cheap silver from the Americas. The rising population made labour an excess commodity and forced wages down. Fears of social unrest and disturbance from packs of sturdy beggars grew. Contemporary descriptions of these rogues, cutpurses and Bawdy Baskets, who plied 'their lyues in lewed lothsome lechery' (cited in Pound 1971), give evidence that some amassed more from this trade than a labourer could earn honestly.

During the course of the 16th century, legislation was passed that sought to tackle the issues of poverty and vagrancy, culminating in the Poor Law Act of 1601. This became the anchor of social policy for the next 300 years. The 43rd Elizabethan was designed to operate within a rural economy based on the parish. Justices of the Peace (JPs) were given the power to appoint Overseers of the Poor and collect a compulsory poor rate from the parishioners. Almshouses and hospitals for the poor were built. Fathers of the parish illegitimate children were encouraged to marry their mothers; if they would not, the overseers were to foster the children or put them out as apprentices. For those vulnerable to the fluctuations of the market and poor harvests, the parish kept a stock of materials such as wool and thread on which they could work and receive a grant of money or outdoor relief. Those who refused to mend their ways were sent to the Bridewell House of Correction. As each parish was responsible for its own poor, it was essential that no responsibility was taken for vagabonds and vagrants from other parishes. Much time and energy was spent in getting vagrants back to their parish of origin, with a subsequent reduction on the poor levy for the parish ratepayers.

The overseers' budget ran to the provision of nursing services of a kind. Sometimes nurses were provided for the poor by religious and charitable ladies, who, like Vicountess Falkland, hired nurses to serve them. Sick nurses were also engaged by the well-to-do to attend upon themselves or their servants.

> **Box 11.1 Women nursing for wages in Elizabethan England.** (Cited in Clark 1982, from the Sussex Archive Collection)
>
> To Goody Halliday for nursing him and his family 5 weeks £15
> To Goody Nye for assisting in nursing 2 shillings and 6d
> To Goody Peckham for nursing a beggar 5 shillings.
> For nursing Wickham's boy with the smallpox 12 shillings

URBAN GROWTH AND INDUSTRIALISATION

During the 17th century, the population of cities such as London and Bristol experienced a period of sustained growth. England developed trade and industry, and by 1760, when George III ascended the throne, corn had to be imported to supplement home-grown crops. There was growth in transport, canals, roads and manufacturing industries, known as the Industrial Revolution. Scientific advances were made that enabled production to become mechanised. Medical science also developed, with the work of pioneers such as John Hunter (1728–1793), who investigated the mechanics of wound healing, and Edward Jenner (1749–1823), who developed a vaccine for smallpox from the cowpox virus.

In the growing cities, disease and squalor made life expectancy low. High infant mortality meant that one child in three died before the age of 6. The parish still operated in the cities as the unit of social administration. Some needs of the population were met by the foundation of charity hospitals. The old royal hospitals of St Bartholomew's and St Thomas' had been refounded after the dissolution of the monasteries. Five new charity, later called voluntary, hospitals were founded in the 18th century by philanthropic individuals; these were Guy's, the Westminster, St George's, the London and the Middlesex.

Baly (1995) calculates that by 1789, there were about 30 similar charity hospitals in the provinces, which gave a ratio of about 1 hospital bed per 5000 of the population. Teaching of medical students took place in these institutions, and the medical students also performed many tasks that later came to be nursing duties. Matrons were appointed by the governors and were responsible for household affairs, including linen rooms and the control of female staff. Nurses were of lower status and mainly lived outside the hospital, those who lived in usually sleeping in small rooms off the wards. This author remembers being shown the site of these rooms at the voluntary hospital where she trained. They were similar to the rooms that domestic servants of the time would have occupied. Nurses received some money and an allowance of beer.

The admission of the sick to the charity hospitals was strictly regulated. Letters had to be provided vouching for the ability of the patient to pay for his own funeral. Not all the patients were bed cases; in the Gloucester Infirmary, patients were expected to help with the farm animals (Storr 1983). Fever cases and the destitute had to rely on the free dispensaries that were often set up in private houses. As the medical profession developed, new hospitals were opened, with the aim of providing patients for teaching purposes. The physicians and surgeons who gave their services freely, their income coming from their private patients, insisted on seeing interesting acute cases.

The voluntary hospitals were part of a reciprocal system in their local communities. Tradesmen had contracts to supply them with goods, whilst employers paid contributions to the upkeep of the hospitals with facilities for their workforce. One such scheme operated to provide Liverpool dockers with emergency care in the event of accidents at work. Local dignitaries endowed beds, which were named in recognition of this financial support. With the growth of the cities and industrial development, the old systems of social provision were stretched to breaking point. Migrants left the country to seek work in new factories, and although many lived in better built-houses than the country cottages they had left, basic facilities were lacking. People were subject to a grinding routine, often working 12–16 hours a day and being exposed to unguarded machinery, overcrowding and poor sanitation. The old system by which the poor had been given outdoor relief was considered to be burdensome to the ratepayers and regarded as encouraging idleness.

Prevalent philosophies of the time were dominated by the thinking of the Utilitarian movement of Jeremy Bentham (1784–1832) and the market-driven economics of Adam Smith (1723–1790). A rise in population that could not be sustained by available resources was predicted by Thomas Malthus (1766–1834). The memory of the French Revolution (1789) and its consequences also filled the ruling classes with a fear of popular unrest.

THE NEW POOR LAW 1834

It was against this background that a commission was set up in 1832 to investigate the working of the Poor Law. The man most associated with this work was Edwin Chadwick (1800–1890), a follower of Bentham. Chadwick was an austere person who gained many enemies in the course of his work, both in poverty and public health legislation. For him, poverty, poor health and crime were all forces that stopped the full potential of national production. The report of the commissioners was dominated by the notion that most paupers were able-bodied.

By the Poor Law Amendment Act, which came into force on 21 April 1834, parishes were grouped together to form Unions, to build workhouses in which to subdue these able-bodied poor. The principle of less eligibility was established. This made conditions inside the workhouse worse than the most intolerable outside it, which would, it was believed, deter idleness.

Every penny bestowed that tends to render the condition of a pauper more eligible than that of the independent labourer is a bounty on indolence and vice. (Edwin Chadwick, (1834), in the Report of the Royal Commission)

Boards of Guardians were elected by the ratepayers to supervise the details of poor relief with the aid of Relieving Officers. The administration was patchy and varied in different unions. Guardians also found that they still gave outdoor relief to many. Only a small proportion of those for whom the system had been designed were catered for within its institutions.

Box 11.2 The pauper population, 1846. (Midwinter 1968)

1846:
  1 331 000 paupers
    199 000 inpaupers
  1 132 000 outpaupers
of these 375 000 able-bodied

From the outset, the Commissioners recommended that the categories of children, the sick, the insane and the able-bodied be separated, with strict segregation of the sexes in the able-bodied group. Many failed to do this, resulting in a jumble of the sick and insane with the able-bodied. The workhouses, or bastilles as local people called them, were objects of fear and loathing, only to be resorted to as a last desperate measure. As such, they have become enshrined in the popular memory. There were some well-organised Unions under the control of the workhouse Master and Matron, where possible a married couple, with a full complement of seamstresses and porters. As the 19th century progressed, many workhouses were enlarged and renovated, some becoming objects of civic pride, such as new libraries and Town Halls. Leading architects of the Victorian era, such as Gilbert Scott, started their careers by winning contracts to design new workhouses.

There was an ideological conflict involved in the care of the sick poor and their children. If the sick were given care and children were educated in the workhouse, what would that do to the test of less eligibility? The standard of nursing in the workhouse infirmaries was brought to public attention by the work of a Victorian woman activist, Louisa Twinning. She had visited an elderly acquaintance in the Strand Workhouse in 1853 and was appalled by the conditions she found. The sick poor were nursed by other pauper women, many of whom were over 60 years of age. Few could read the labels on the medicine bottles. They were both physically and intellectually limited in their ability to care for the sick.

Miss Twinning organised groups of ladies to visit the workhouses. She used her talents, energies and considerable resources to campaign for workhouse reform. Some schemes had been started in the 1860s to train nurses for the workhouses. Florence Nightingale herself had sent Agnes Jones to a Liverpool workhouse infirmary at the request of William Rathbone in 1865. Miss Jones had done stirling work there, reforming the nursing provision, but had died during a typhus epidemic at the infirmary. By the 1870s, both metropolitian and rural districts had been pressed into providing purpose-built infirmaries for the sick poor. In 1873, The Metropolitian Poor Law Act allowed these newly built infirmaries to admit and train probationer nurses. However recruitment to the Poor Law hospitals remained a problem, as many of the patients in them were the old and chronically sick. As we have already noted, those cases perceived as acute and interesting were admitted to the voluntary hospitals. Many of the Poor Law hospitals built in the wave of construction after the 1873 Act, although refurbished, remain in use today. Often they are the very buildings that still house specialties such as care of the elderly. Many older patients remember these buildings as workhouses. Although these hospitals were incorporated into local authority administration in 1929 and into the National Health Service in 1948, the stigma of the Poor Law remained with them for many years.

Activity 11.5

Investigate the history of the institutions where you have clinical placements.

- Were they originally voluntary hospitals or Poor Law infirmaries?
- Speak with older patients. Ask them to share their memories of the hospital with you.

The sick and poor were seen as a threat to the health of the nation, which was especially felt at the time of epidemics of cholera. Cholera was no respecter of class. Because it was waterborne, it also affected those well-off enough to have access to piped water supplies. Fuelled by the epidemics of the 1830s and 1840s, the 1848 Public Health Act, which owed its inception again to the work of Edwin Chadwick, was the first in a series of items of legislation that laid the foundations of a public health structure, being consolidated by further Acts of 1872 and 1875. The Local Government Act of 1871 brought together public health and the Poor Law. However, it was not until the last half of the 19th century that the countrywide provision of safe water supplies was properly organised.

During the course of the 19th century, attitudes towards the poor changed. Gradually, thinking developed that saw poverty not as the result of idleness in all cases, but as a result of sickness and other circumstances. The belief grew that there should be protection for less fortunate members of society.

DEVELOPMENTS IN THE CARE OF SICK CHILDREN

'Children constituted a quarter of the workhouse population' (Baly 1995). Digby (1978), writing on the Norfolk workhouses, finds little recorded concern for the health of pauper children. Many suffered from scabies and eye infections. Their poor diets reflected contemporary ignorance of the nutritional need of babies and children. Infant mortality in the workhouses is difficult to access accurately as little significance was attached to babies dying

in the workhouses. Indeed, as already mentioned, high infant mortality was familiar in Victorian society. There were philanthropic institutions, such as the Foundling Hospital in London, founded by Captain Thomas Coram in 1756. The 19th century saw the foundation of other voluntary bodies, including Barnado's, with the aim of protecting children from the results of rapid industrialisation and *laissez-faire* labour legislation.

Sick children were nursed at home by members of their family, or, in more wealthy households, by domestic servants or hired nurses. In the mid-19th century, the belief developed, led by the physician Charles West, that children could be helped to recover in special hospitals where they would be separated from adults. His foundation at Great Ormond Street in London is world famous. Other children's hospitals were established in provincial towns, and separate children's wards opened in the general hospitals. As an indication of changing attitudes to the needs of sick children, these wards were decorated with specially commissioned tile murals of nursery rhymes and fairy tales 'to amuse and cheer the young patients' (Mitchell 1984).

Technical advances and social welfare legislation of the late 19th and 20th century fostered the conditions that helped to eradicate many of the killer diseases of childhood. The sick child of the 1990s is confined to hospital only when acutely ill and nursed with families as partners in care in the home environment as much as possible.

Further information on the development of children's nursing can be found in Chapter 21.

THE LEGACY OF FLORENCE NIGHTINGALE

If the 19th century saw the gradual development of a collectivist approach to social welfare provision, there was still scope for the work of philanthropically disposed individuals. A notable individual, without whom no account of the development of nursing would be complete, was Florence Nightingale (1820–1910). Miss Nightingale achieved celebrity status in her own lifetime. The experience of the Crimean War, which led to her fame, took place in just 2 years of her long, busy life.

Born in Florence in 1820, she was the daughter of wealthy middle-class parents. Both were from the non-conformist Protestant Unitarian religious tradition, with reforming philanthropic beliefs. Florence was a lively, intelligent young girl. Both she and her sister Parthe had the benefit of a thorough education, unusual for genteel young ladies of the time. As a result, she was able to converse with many of the leading social and political figures of the day. For all this, Florence found the restraints and enforced idleness of her life irksome.

At the age of 17, she received the first of her calls from God. Although as yet unsure of God's purpose for her, this experience had a profound influence on the future direction of her life. She developed an interest in the social issues of the day and studied the reports of the public health commissions, in which field she was to become an expert (Baly 1995). In 1845, her parents refused to allow her to train as a nurse at the Salisbury Infirmary. She later recalled that 'it was as if I had wanted to be a kitchen maid'. During a tour abroad, she visited the hospital run by Pastor Fliednor at Kaiserworth in Germany, staffed by lay deaconesses. The following year, she returned there to undertake 3 months' nurse training. Although she denied that she had learnt anything at Kaiserworth, Florence was impressed by the atmosphere and by the fact that many of the deaconesses were peasant women. This was to influence her views on the nature of the most suitable women for nursing.

In 1853, Florence was appointed superintendent of the Establishment for Gentlewomen during Illness in Harley Street, London. During her employment at the Institute, she revolutionised its management, installing piped hot water, lifts and many labour-saving devices. She was emphatic on the need for nurses to concentrate on nursing tasks and not be diverted by domestic chores. Using the results of a questionnaire she

had circulated to hospitals in Germany and France, she was already lobbying her friend Sidney Herbert on the need for nursing reform.

In 1854 came the start of the Crimean War, which was to make Florence Nightingale a household name. Britain, France and Turkey were fighting Russia, and the allies defeated the Russians in October at the battle of Alma. Reports by The Times war correspondent, William Russell, criticised the British medical facilities for the wounded. Summers (1988) has discussed at length the problems facing the army in the Crimean War. She argues that many of these were caused by logistics and related to the fact that this was the first major European war for over 50 years. Florence's abilities were ideally suited to tackling these problems. For the first time, the British public, thanks to Russell, knew about conditions in a war zone.

In response, Sidney Herbert, Minister at War, appointed Florence to superintend the introduction of female nurses into the military hospitals in Turkey. The expedition left England within 2 weeks of Herbert writing to Miss Nightingale. Thirty-eight nurses had been interviewed and recruited in this short time. This was a remarkable achievement and another sign of Florence's organisational abilities. In November 1854, the Nightingale party arrived at the Scutari barracks, where the wounded arrived from the last stage of their long, painful journey across the Bosporus from the battlefields.

Initially, the military doctors would not allow the nurses into the hospital. Ten days later, however, as casualties poured in from the battle of Inkerman, the nurses were fully stretched at their work. Miss Nightingale's persistence, her powerful connections at home and her control of £30 000 all contributed to this turn-round. She transformed the filthy, dilapidated barracks, which at one stage had 4 miles of patients on mattresses on the floor and 1000 diarrhoea cases, into something resembling a therapeutic institution, applying the principles of sanitary science to the situation. Although she was mistaken in her understanding of the spread of infection, improved ventilation and less overcrowding undoubtedly contributed towards reducing the mortality rate of the wounded. Her grasp of the importance of adequate nutrition is evident in her cooperation with the famous chef Alexis Soyer.

Miss Nightingale's personal dynamism was reflected in the hours she worked. She contracted Crimean Fever, and the common soldiers feared she would die. She recovered and returned to her work, determined to improve the lot of the soldiers. Baly (1995) records the high esteem in which the men held her. She, for her part, recognised their human dignity. It is not the first impression that springs to mind when discussing Miss Nightingale, yet the soldiers described her as 'full of fun'.

Back in England, Florence set about campaigning to improve the health of the army. The 1860 Royal Commission resulted in the establishment of an Army Medical School and improvements in barracks and army hospitals. Florence provided the commission with a formidable collection of statistics. For this achievement she became, in 1860, the first woman to be elected a Fellow of the Statistical Society. She enjoyed an excellent working relationship with Dr William Farr, compiler of statistics for the Registrar General. She developed a revolutionary new way of collecting statistics, known as Model Forms. These were later adopted by several London hospitals and government departments. 'Throughout her long life Florence Nightingale used figures ... She knew that without hard facts she could achieve nothing' (Nuttall 1983).

THE NIGHTINGALE SCHOOL

In 1855, while Miss Nightingale was still in the Crimea, Sidney Herbert set up a committee to collect money from a grateful nation; £45 000 was collected in the form of a fund to enable Miss Nightingale to train nurses. She was not enthusiastic about this, her energies being with the need of the army, and few hospitals relished the patronage of Miss Nightingale.

Her attention was drawn to the proposed move of St Thomas' Hospital from its Southwark site in London. Mr Whitfield, the Medical Officer,

was in favour of a relocation to the suburbs, as was Miss Nightingale. As the support of the Nightingale Fund would strengthen his case, Mr Whitfield joined forces with Miss Nightingale. St Thomas' became the compromise site for the Nightingale Nursing School.

From the outset, the agreement was subject to adaptation. Florence had envisaged a nursing school similar to a medical school. Mr Whitfield insisted that the 15 probationers, as assistant nurses, would be under the supervision of the Matron, Mrs Wardroper. The fund paid for the board and lodging of the probationers, who worked under the instruction of the Sisters. No-one questioned whether the Sisters could actually teach. The probationers (Box 11.3) had to sign a contract that bound them to St Thomas' for at least 4 years after their training. Miss Nightingale felt this to be rather like a servant's contract.

Box 11.3

Probationers were expected to be (Howlett 1993):

- sober
- honest
- truthful
- trustworthy
- punctual
- quiet and orderly
- clean and neat.

The first 10 years of the school were hardly spectacular. Baly's (1995) analysis of the register shows that comparatively few of the probationers were nursing at the end of 4 years. Many were dismissed for insobriety and other defects. This may have been a reflection on the candidates themselves or on Mrs Wardroper's judgement. Despite these facts, publicity for the school was good.

By the 1870s, most of the London teaching hospitals had a training school along Nightingale lines.

From 1867, Miss Nightingale decided to devote more time to the school. Pressure from ladies and the demand for trained nurses led to the introduction of the grade of Special Probationer in 1867, intended for ladies. They paid £30 per annum for their board and lodging but received the same training as the ordinary probationers. At the end of the year, they expected to be appointed to superior positions as ward sisters, matrons or lady superintendents. Florence's ideal probationer nurse was a woman of the upper servant class, a tradesman's daughter or a farmer's daughter, who had some education but was used to earning her own living. However, the 'specials' provided more money for the now-depleted fund. Miss Nightingale felt that the scheme was rather like educating the lady with her cook!

Another part of Miss Nightingale's plan for the school was the appointment of a Home Sister to be responsible for helping the nurses with their studies and for their general well-being and life in the nurses' home. Mr Whitfield was replaced by Mr Croft, who introduced a much more systematic form of lectures and examinations for the probationers. In 1873, he had his own lectures printed for nurses' use, and from 1874, he instituted regular monthly examinations to test the progress of the probationers.

The most famous Nightingale export of the first 10 years of the school was Agnes Jones, who, as mentioned above, was sent to the Liverpool Workhouse Infirmary. The fund started to diversify and influence training elsewhere. In 1872, the fund sent a team of nurses to Edinburgh and later to St Mary's Hospital, Paddington. Miss Nightingale also extended the school's influence to the Poor Law hospitals. In 1881, she sent Miss Vincent to the St Marylebone Workhouse Infirmary.

The fund also undertook to train nurses for home nursing. Florence worked with William Rathbone in establishing a movement to nurse the poor in their own homes. Rathbone, a wealthy shipping magnate, was so impressed by the work of Mrs Robinson, a nurse who had cared for his wife in her final illness, that he hired her to nurse the sick poor of Liverpool. It soon became apparent that this was more work than Mrs Robinson could manage alone. Rathbone contacted Miss Nightingale in 1861 with the request to supply nurses for home nursing. Florence suggested that the Liverpool Royal Infirmary train its own nurses for this purpose. Mr Rathbone donated a new building as a school of nursing. The resulting school began in 1862 to train nurses for care both at home and in hospital. Liverpool was divided into 18 districts, each with a committee of lady volunteers and a trained nurse. In 1882, Queen Victoria donated the greater part of the Womens' Jubilee Fund of £70 000 to an extension of the district nurse scheme. William Rathbone and Miss Nightingale continued their work together until his death in 1902.

Florence sought to inspire and encourage the probationers. She sent them gifts of flowers and fresh fruit from the country. Every summer, they spent a day at her brother-in-law's country house. It must be remembered that 'It is important to see Florence Nightingale in the context of the social change of her day' (Baly 1995).

Although there had been institutions that trained nurses in England (notably St John's House, founded in 1848, which in 1856 provided the nursing staff for King's College Hospital, London), the Nightingale School was the first secular nurses' training school with no religious affiliation. For years to come, the Nightingale School based nurse training on the acute general hospital. Other systems, such as the Liverpool scheme, covered the wider sphere of home and hospital. The old personnel on the wards at St Thomas' Hospital taught the student nurses.

The Nightingale School maintained the myth of its success by its publicity while the reputation of Miss Nightingale was extended beyond her own lifetime by biographers who wrote of her in almost saint-like terms. The reformers allowed the myth to develop that there were no responsible nurses before 1860. They frequently compared the new product with Dicken's Sarah Gamp. It must be born in mind that the fictional Mrs Gamp was a caricature. 'Indeed it is worth considering whether, had Mrs Gamp not existed, would reformers not have felt it necessary to invent her?' (Rafferty 1995).

Other women contributed to the welfare of allied soldiers in the Crimean War. One of them was Mary Seacole, a nurse and healer of mixed

Scottish and Jamaican descent. Although she had considerable experience in the treatment of fevers and wound care in the Caribbean and Central America, Mary's services were rejected by the authorities in England. She set up her own establishment, the British Hotel, near Sebastopol – a mixture of a hotel and hospital. She visited the battlefields, dispensing comfort and provisions to the wounded. In 1856, she returned bankrupt to England. She published her book 'Wonderful Adventures of Mrs. Seacole in Many Lands', one of the few published writings of any black woman before the 20th century. She was helped by fundraising attempts on the part of the soldiers she had nursed and finally by a pension from Queen Victoria. Mary died in 1881 and was forgotten. Since her centenary in 1981, there has been renewed interest in her, and her achievements have been acknowledged.

Nursing and hygiene certainly improved under the Nightingale system, and a career structure for nurses was established, opening up nursing as a respectable occupation for middle-class women. Yet even in her own lifetime, Florence was expressing doubts about the direction nurse training had taken and had reservations about the growth of the influence and power of the hospital matron.

REGISTRATION AND THE DRIVE FOR PROFESSIONALISM

The success of the Nightingale reforms led to a rapid expansion in the number of nurse training schools. These were set up first in the London voluntary hospitals, followed by the provincal voluntary hospitals and the workhouse infirmaries. Hospitals, both voluntary and public, were poor, and probationer labour was cheap. Lady probationers added prestige, and as more middle-class people became hospital patients, there was a demand for more and better nurses. It was in the interest of the hospital budget for their training to be as long as possible. Advances in medical science, such as antiseptic surgery

and anaesthesia pioneered by Lister, Pasteur and Simpson, also demanded a more conscientious type of nurse. These new requirements found an ideal person as a result of demographic changes. Late marriage, a fall in birth rate and the emigration of young men overseas in the growing empire meant that, by the 1870s, there was a large pool of young, middle-class women who saw nursing as a worthy career for themselves. Only teaching and the newly developing Civil Service rivalled nursing as an occupation for this group until after World War II. However, it was the reformed schools that were the hospitals of choice for these women, rather than the Poor Law infirmaries.

By the 1880s, the new nurse leaders were beginning to ask whether nursing should be tested by public examination and only those passing this examination be entered on a register and entitled to call themselves nurse. Indeed, medical practitioners had been required to do this by the provisions of the 1858 Medical Act, and there had been a significant improvement in standards. Miss Nightingale was opposed to state registration, as she felt it would impose a lower uniform standard. Miss Luckes, matron of the London Hospital, was also anti-registration, believing that it was a waste to train every nurse applicant with a uniform training for each different type of nursing.

The main protagonist for state registration was Ethel Gordon Manson (1857–1947). In many ways, she was a product of the reformed training schools. From a professional family, Miss Manson trained as a lady probationer at Nottingham and Manchester. She was appointed as a sister at the London Hospital, and in 1881 at the age of 24, she was appointed Matron of St Bartholomew's Hospital. This experience convinced her of the need for a uniform training to raise standards and guarantee a professional status for nursing. Her marriage to Dr Bedford Fenwick in 1887 allowed her to continue in the struggle for state registration, supported by her husband, who was himself a political activist.

The registration debate has been described as 'a battle for status conducted against a background of rampant snobbery and militant feminism' (Abel Smith 1960). Mrs Bedford Fenwick was a keen supporter of the movement to enfranchise middle-class and professional women. The issue was debated with ferocity in the pages of the nursing press, including Sir Henry Burdett's publication, the *Nursing Mirror*. The Bedford Fenwicks acquired a vehicle in 1893, when they took over the *Nursing Record*, changing its name in 1903 to the *British Journal of Nursing*. Mrs Bedford Fenwick was editor, a post that she occupied for nearly 50 years.

Some nurses saw registration as a means of boosting their professional status, whilst others felt that their livelihoods would be at risk if they had not trained in a reformed school. Mrs Bedford Fenwick, with her support of women's rights, did nothing to endear herself to the bulk of the medical profession. She certainly saw herself as part of the managerial section of nursing, founding the Matron's Council of England and Wales in 1894. In 1902, the Midwives Act required all practising midwives to undergo training and register with the Central Midwives' Board. This gave fresh impetus to the movement for state registration.

From the turn of the century until 1914, Registration Bills were introduced into Parliament and were blocked. It was the impact of the changes during World War I (1914–1918) that eventually hastened the state registration of nurses. Young women volunteered to nurse for the war effort. With a hasty basic training, these Voluntary Aid Detachment (VAD) nurses were sent to assist trained nurses. Many became highly skilled, as they had to learn quickly in the devastating conditions. In their uniforms with a red cross on their aprons, these women were called 'nurses'. It was the threat of the dilution of nursing with these women in peace time that united nurses in favour of registration.

As a prelude to state registration, a College of Nursing was set up in 1916. Its aim included the promotion of:

• the education and training of nurses.
• the professional status of nursing.

This was the embryonic Royal College of Nursing, which today continues to strive for the maintenance of standards in patient care (see Ch. 16). Even with peace in 1919, there was still not complete agreement in the pro-registration lobby, and the head of the newly created Ministry of Health, Dr Addison, was forced to step in and draft his own Registration Bill. The inability of nurses to be clear about their objectives meant that an outside body decided their professional future.

The 1919 Nurses Registration Act was passed for England and Wales, Scotland and Northern Ireland. Each country was to set up a Register of qualified nurses and compile a syllabus for instruction and subjects for examination. Mrs Bedford Fenwick became State Registered Nurse (SRN) no. 1 on the Register for England and Wales. There was a time lapse to allow nurses who had undergone a period of training before the Act to register. The first examinations for the Register were conducted in March 1925, after which no applicants, other than those who had taken the examination, were accepted. In 1921, the General Nursing Council (GNC) set up a Disciplinary and Penal Committee, which had the power to remove those not felt to be fit and proper persons to remain on the Register. The Council also had the power to prosecute those fraudulently posing as registered nurses.

The Register comprised several parts, the main part containing the names of all nurses satisfying the conditions of admission to the Register. There were supplementary parts for:

• male nurses
• mental nurses
• children's nurses
• fever nurses
• nurses trained in the care of mental defectives.

Internal discipline and the protection of the public, two important tenets of professional identity, were in the hands of the GNC. However, nurses had given the right of control of standards of entry and the requirements of basic training to the government, and this regulation is one of the most crucial characteristics of professional status. It was to be another 60 years before this control was regained.

Question 11.2

1. What type of preparation is best for a nurse?
   - A bedside, hands-on approach.
   - A university degree course.

2. Who should be referred to as a nurse?
   - A staff nurse.
   - A student nurse.
   - A nursing assistant.

   Which one of the above do patients call 'nurse'?

DEVELOPMENTS IN THE CARE OF THE MENTALLY ILL

PENNY FOR THE KEEPER

During the registration debate, the main players assumed that registration, when it came, would be based on general nursing. Indeed, mental nurses were on one of the supplementary registers. What had been the developments in the training of mental nurses up until the 1919 Registration Act, and why had mental nurses not been considered in the same light as general nurses?

Before the 1830s, only a small number of the mentally disordered were confined to institutions. In a well-to-do household, the mentally ill person might be coped with by hiring an extra servant to deal with them, as for the first Mrs Rochester in 'Jane Eyre'. Paupers might receive outdoor relief, or another villager might be paid to attend them. St Mary's Bethlem, had been in existence in London since the Middle Ages. In Georgian London, it was still a popular Sunday afternoon pastime to view the lunatics, on the production of a bribe for the keeper. King George III's mental state had brought mental disturbance into high public profile.

Ideas about the nature of mental illness began to change around the mid-18th century. The belief in demonology changed, influenced by the new philosophical trend of the Enlightenment. Guy's Hospital, London, started to provide accom-modation for lunatics in 1728, and St Luke's, Muswell Hill, was founded in 1751 to provide treatment for mild cases of mental disorder. There were also private madhouses, which were run very much on a profit-making basis. William Tuke's pioneering work at The Retreat in York, treated inmates on a regime of 'moral treatment'. This stressed self-discipline and provided work and a structured routine, which Tuke believed would help inmates' minds to become reordered.

THE BUILDING OF THE COUNTY ASYLUMS

The institutionalisation of the mentally ill gathered momentum alongside developments of the Poor Law. It was soon discovered that among the indiscriminate entrants to the work-houses, there were the mentally ill, who could not be treated according to the new regimes. The Lunacy Act of 1845 set up a Board of Com-missioners in Lunacy as a permanent body with power of inspection. It became compulsory for boroughs and counties to make provision for the insane, and within the next two decades, many did. These new buildings were in the same style as the newly built workhouses and prisons – solid and stark – many still surviving today. Many of these buildings were in remote locations with estates that might extend to 600 acres. They had their own farms and workshops. As Dingwall (1988) explains, this made them self-sufficient but also more socially isolated. For some, these institutions did provide asylum, protection from a changing world, but they also isolated and protected the public from aware-ness of the mentally ill. It may have been intended to implement the therapeutic regime advocated by Tuke in these county asylums. However, the asylums very soon became insti-tutions where the maximum number of inmates could be housed in the most cost-effective manner. There would be a medical superin-tendent in charge of the institution. In the case of John Conolly, at Hanwell Asylum, he was a pioneer of new methods. The conditions of the inmates often depended on the individual idio-syncracies of the medical superintendent.

Between the superintendent and the inmates were the attendants, or, as they had been called earlier, the keepers. Their names give clues to the nature of their duties. The preferred name for the male staff eventually became 'attendant', while the female staff were always referred to as 'nurses'. Recruitment for attendants was dominated by working-class men. Four main groups predominated:

- agricultural labourers, their skills being needed for the farms, and because they were in surplus owing to the declining agricultural sector
- Ex-servicemen, because the work was physically demanding and they were used to giving and receiving orders
- servants, for the same reasons as the military men
- families of attendants, because they were used to the conditions.

Wages and conditions were modelled on those of domestic and farm servants. Attendants worked long hours, slept in on rota and received little time off. Night staff were introduced gradually from about 1860. In fact, the attendants shared the conditions of the inmates, remote from the medical superintendent.

Doctors of the mentally ill gradually began to adopt more vigorous approaches to their treatment. These included treatments such as baths, showers, wet-packing and the administration of drugs. With these developments, the need for a more educated attendant, who could be a better aid to medical superintendents, became evident. In 1885, a group of Scottish medical superintendents produced the famous Red Book. This was a 64-paged text entitled 'A Handbook for the Instruction of Attendants on the Insane' and was, with some modification, the standard text used in the training of mental nurses until 1954. By then, the word 'attendant' had been changed to 'nurse' to reflect the fact that both male and female staff were referred to as 'nurse'.

As Nolan (in Baly 1995) explains, the publication of this book moved the attendants' knowledge base from the oral to the written domain. In 1885, a national training scheme leading to a Certificate in Psychological Medicine was started for doctors. The Medico-Psychological Asssociation (MPA) started a training for attendants in 1891. It was hoped that training the attendants would add to their sense of loyalty to their particular asylum and maximise productivity. The attendants, however, hoped that training would help them to better themselves.

These expectations on the part of the attendants were not met. They found that despite acquisition of the MPA certificate, their pay and conditions of service remained unchanged. An added insult was the trend to try to recruit general trained women nurses to senior positions on the female side of the asylums. Having discovered that training and self-improvement could not better their lot, the asylum nurses turned to the trades union movement. Relations between workers and superintendents deteriorated at the turn of the 20th century. In an attempt to mollify the attendants, the superintendents had sponsored the Association of Workers in Asylums (AWA), founded in 1897. Whilst most of the female asylum staff remained in the AWA, the male workers joined the National Asylum Workers Union (NAWA). This was far more militant and politically orientated, becoming affiliated to the Labour Party in 1914 and to the Trades Union Congress in 1923. This was, as Carpenter (in Davis 1980) asserts, the only option open to them.

The 1919 Nurses Registration Act, with its Supplementary Register for mental nurses, confirmed the idea that mental and general nursing were separate branches of a common occupation. Its personnel and the path they took to representation were vastly different. This pattern is still reflected in present-day trade union membership within nursing disciplines.

THE CARE OF THE MENTALLY HANDICAPPED

The care of people with learning disabilities, called at varying times the 'feeble minded' or 'mentally deficient', was not finally separated from asylum work until the Mental Deficiency Act of 1913. This provided legislation for the separation of mental handicap from mental illness. Colonies were to be developed where the mentally handicapped could be trained in some way to reduce the financial burdens of their care. This development was slow to start, and by the beginning of World War II in 1939, only half of the projected places for the mentally handicapped had been created.

It was after the creation of the NHS (see below) that the provision of specialised services for clients with learning disabilities grew. In 1946, the 'colonies' were, for a brief period, under NHS control and renamed Mental Deficiency Hospitals. The concept of community integration developed earlier and more steadily in this field than in other specialties. During the 1970s and 1980s, Education Acts transferred the education of these clients back to local education authority control. The philosophy of normalisation espoused the integration of children with learning disabilities and special education needs into mainstream schools. 'By the end of the 1980s there had been a 50% reduction in inpatient beds and a vast increase in residential and day care provided by statutory, voluntary and private sector agencies' (Nolan, in Baly 1995). (For more information on the development of nursing people with learning disabilities, see Ch. 22.)

NURSING WITHIN THE LEGISLATIVE FRAMEWORK – THE 20TH-CENTURY EXPERIENCE

THE SEARCH FOR SUITABLE RECRUITS

It has been demonstrated that the development of professional nursing has been connected with prevailing social philosophy and the legislation resulting from it, much of that legislation having itself been accelerated by war. One of the effects of World War I was the stimulus to the registration movement, and the formation of the GNC. During the 1930s, there was widespread

Question 11.3

Do you have any clinical placements in institutions for the mentally ill?

If your answer is yes, how long does it take you to walk around the grounds?

If your answer is no, why not, and what has happened to the mental hospital in your locality? Where have the clients gone?

dissatisfaction within nursing over pay and conditions, and problems with recruitment. A series of reports sought to remedy this by improving conditions of service. Regimes with their petty disciplines, which at times verged on the infringement of personal liberties for nurses, were blamed by the Lancet Commission, which reported in 1932. The Athlone Committee, set up in 1937, recommended in 1939 measures to restore nursing's competitive position in the labour market. These included a 96-hour fortnight, universal and transferable superannuation provisions and a national negotiating machinery on pay and conditions. The outbreak of World War II proved a reliable excuse for the shelving of the Athlone proposals.

WAR-TIME NURSING – A GOVERNMENT SERVICE

With the advent of war, nursing became part of the complex machinery of the Home Front. A degree of state control hitherto unthinkable was exercised. In 1938, an Emergency Hospital Service was set up. The country was divided up into sectors. A Sector Matron and administrative staff had charge of each sector, which was built around a teaching hospital. Urban hospitals were cleared. Patients well enough were discharged or evacuated with nurses. During all these removals and upheavals, nurse training went on, and the State Final Examinations continued to be set and marked for candidates. During the war vacancies remained static. Recruitment efforts were made for the civilian hospitals, which had suffered as many nurses preferred to join the military services.

A committee set up in 1943 under the chairmanship of Lord Rushcliffe examined the conditions of service and payment of nurses and extended government control over them. This became the starting point for the Nurses and Midwives' Whitley Council, which negotiated nurses' pay settlements for the next 40 years. The committee recommendations improved the status and pay of trained nurses to a level commensurate with teaching. The 1943 Nurses Act made provisions for the control of nurses as a labour force. It also brought into being, as a temporary expedient, the enrolment of a group of assistant nurses and brought them under the jurisdiction of the GNC.

The creation of the grade of State Enrolled Assistant Nurse (SEAN), later changed to State Enrolled Nurse (SEN), was originally a temporary expedient to cover the nursing shortage caused by the demands of war. Candidates were still being prepared for this temporary grade over 40 years later.

The SEN had been envisaged as a bedside nurse, working under the supervision of an SRN. This distinction gradually became eroded. Many SENs found themselves with no clear definition of their role and were exploited – in charge of the ward one shift and tidying the linen cupboard the next. They saw student nurses whom they had advised qualify and gain senior positions, whilst their own careers could progress no further. The proposals for Project 2000 (see below) provided an opportunity for existing SENs to convert to Registered Nurse and abolished the second-level preparation.

THE EFFECTS OF WORLD WAR II

During World War II, technology changed the nature of nursing practice. Nurses who worked in war conditions testify to the way in which observations on the progress of wounds led to the wholesale adoption of new techniques. Plastic surgery and the treatment of burns changed radically, owing to the experiences of health workers caring for the victims of air warfare. New drugs, such as penicillin, ousted practices such as the application of poultices. Early ambulation became an accepted feature of nursing owing to the pressure on beds. After World War II, nurses found themselves affected by legislation with an immense scope: the foundation of the Welfare State and, in particular, the implementation of the NHS, by the Labour government of Clement Attlee.

NURSING AND THE NHS

During the war the whole nation had suffered, fought and shared hardships. There had been an equitable distribution of food and equipment by rationing, and greater state intervention than ever before. Evacuating young children and their mothers from the large cities to safer areas had shown the middle classes just what the social conditions were for many of the population. There was a determination not to return to the conditions of the 1930s but to move towards a fairer and more equitable society. The harsh philosophy of the Poor Law had softened towards the end of the 19th century, and there had been attempts to introduce a more organised state system of poor relief. In 1911, Lloyd George had introduced the Old Age Pension and the National Insurance Act. These schemes were not comprehensive, and progress towards welfare provision between the wars was slow, one of the reasons being the economic constraints of the slump of the 1930s. In some areas, enlightened local authorities were able to make some progress, but provision was patchy.

In 1942, Sir William Beveridge (who had been associated with the Lloyd George reforms as a young man) published his report on the future shape of welfare provision after the war. The Beveridge Report on Social Insurance and Allied Services was a best-seller. Beveridge's plan was targeted to eradicate the five giants of:

- want
- disease
- ignorance
- squalor
- idleness.

To defeat them he designed a comprehensive welfare system based on three assumptions:

1. a free national health service
2. child allowances
3. full employment.

The pledge to adopt and implement the Beveridge recommendations was one of the keys to the Labour victory in the 1945 election.

The NHS came into existence on July 5th 1948. The NHS was full of compromise engineered by the talent of the famous Minister of Health, Aneurin Bevan. There were to be two subsequent reorganisations of the Health Service in 1974 and 1982 to try to remedy some of the shortcomings of its administration. The inauguration of the NHS was a tremendous achievement, and it has been universally admired world wide. For many, its existence took away the desperation of not being able to care for their loved ones through lack of money. A health service free at the point of delivery to all was felt to be the mark of a civilised society. If the clients were pleased, however, many of the staff were apprehensive. In the transition to the start of the service, many nurses had been worried about their jobs and uncertain whom they would be employed by. Nurses, as today, had a great deal of loyalty to their training hospitals, and many saw the advent of the NHS as the loss of supremacy of the voluntary hospitals.

However, it soon became obvious that Beveridge's hope that, once the bulk of cases were treated, prevention would be the order of the day would never be accomplished. Changes in population distribution, especially the growth in number of the aged and infirm, and increased expectations in health care meant that the original cost estimates for the NHS were far exceeded.

NURSING FOR NEW NEEDS

Nursing had to adapt to new needs. The 1949 Nurses Act completed the integration of nursing into the legal framework of the NHS. Many of its stipulations were dilutions of the 1947 Wood Report, which had tried to update nursing education for the second half of the 20th century. Wood called for a changed training with less

repetition and not just geared to provide hospital workforces. The Register itself was still divided into parts, but at least male nurses were integrated on it with their female colleagues. By 1959, there were experimental courses in existence combining training for different parts of the Register. These showed that there was much overlapping and repetition in nurse training.

Resolving the conflict between demands and resources was to occupy the nursing profession for many years to come. How was that conflict tackled? During the 1960s, there were attempts to integrate a management structure into nursing, when senior nurses realised that they often had no say in local policy decisions. The report of the Committee on Senior Nursing Staff (Salmon Report) based nursing management on three tiers, sisters being the lower tier or first-line managers. Many nurses did not take with confidence to their new roles, and there was no provision for a clinical career pathway.

THE BRIGGS REPORT – TOWARDS PROJECT 2000

Amidst the background of industrial unrest in 1970, a new Committee on Nursing was set up under the chairmanship of Professor (later Lord) Asa Briggs. This committee had the brief to review the manpower needs in the light of demographic changes and in the context of a move towards more care in the community. The committee reported in 1972 and recommended that there should be a common portal of entry into nursing at the age of 17. Entrants would follow an 18-month foundation course, specalising for a further 18 months in a particular branch of nursing.

To oversee this, there should be one statutory body for pre- and post-registration education, to replace the multiplicity of bodies then in existence in the UK. The recommendations of the report were accepted by the Labour government elected in 1974.

In April 1979, The Nurses, Midwives and Health Visitors Act was passed, with the United Kingdom Central Council for Nursing, Midwifery and Health Visiting (UKCC) and four National Boards functioning from July 1983.

It was in 1986 that the UKCC put forward its proposals for the new preparation of nurses – Project 2000. This report also contained information in its papers on the changing health care needs of society. Using this material, it attempted to provide a rationale for the proposed changes in nurse education. Project 2000, with its common foundation and branch programmes, its espousal of the one level of professional nurse and higher-education status for student nurses, was the culmination of the recommendations of both the Wood and the Briggs Reports. Thirteen demonstration districts commenced Project 2000 in September 1989. By 1993, all Colleges of Nursing had fully established their links to higher education and had changed to Project 2000 courses.

NURSING AND THE BUSINESS CULTURE

If nursing was having to meet the new demands imposed by the NHS from 1948, it also adapted within a context of changing social and political thought. Nursing's knowledge base grew during the post-war era. New tools and approaches were developed for delivering care. The nursing process and primary nursing, backed up by research-based theory, both contributed to a more individualised, patient-orientated approach to care. The routine so treasured by the Nightingale nurses had been replaced by the Care Plan agreed between client and nurse.

Nursing has also had to adapt its care delivery to meet the demand caused by the reorganisations of the NHS in the 1980s and 1990s. The first Thatcher government in 1979 introduced the ideas of the business world to the NHS. The NHS Management Enquiry (Griffiths Report) published in 1983 confirmed this with the introduction of general managers, some of whom had no nursing or health care background, to hospitals and units. (For more discussion on management issues within the Health Service see Ch. 9.)

The NHS, which Mrs Thatcher in 1987 proclaimed was safe in Conservative hands, was the target for major media coverage of its deficiencies. In 1989, Mrs Thatcher announced a fundamental review of the NHS. The review team, unlike those involved in earlier reports on nursing and health, consisted of a small team of senior ministers, civil servants and political advisors, chaired by the Prime Minister herself, and was conducted in private. 'Working for Patients', published in 1989, reaffirmed the key principles of the NHS but introduced the new concept of an internal market. With the purchaser/provider split, Health Authorities would use money to purchase services for their population, and there would be independent provider units, otherwise known as NHS Trusts. This internal competition, it was claimed, would improve quality and force costs down. These proposals, embodied in law as the 1990 NHS and Community Care Acts, represent the most radical reorganisation of the NHS since 1948.

We may reflect on the impetus to change brought about by this legislation in the future, we cannot yet step back to consider them objectively. Would innovations such as the named nurse concept have been the natural development of primary nursing or a reactive response to the Patient's Charter? Only time will tell. How will the skill mix of nursing evolve in the 21st century? Will academically prepared nurses be a few supervisors, 'hands on' care being provided by those prepared by the National Council for Vocational Qualifications (NCVQ) awards? Will informal carers be relied upon ever increasingly in the community? The power and influence of nursing was greatly reduced by the reforms of the 1980s. Will there be new opportunities for nurses to lead in health care away from the old management structures? To go forward, nurses need to know where they have come from. Nurses have always adapted to new clinical demands. In taking on new responsibilities, they must not lose the essentials, the core skills of nursing care. These are the key activities that have given the nursing profession its unique role in the health care provision of our society.

Summary

Today's media image of the nurse is heavily influenced by the history of nursing over the centuries. In ancient tradition, women held the roles of healer and carer of the sick, young and infirm, the doors to training as physicians, however, being barred to them by their male counterparts. With the rise in the independence of women and the growth of the feminist movement, these supposedly low-status positions have gained new recognition.

Other carers of the sick, especially the mentally ill, were those in religious orders. As the supremacy of the Church was challenged by science, lay carers became more important, although religious beliefs coloured the treatment of the mentally ill and handicapped for more than 200 years. Subsequent changes in social pattern, brought about by legislation, industrialisation and war, also affected the delivery of health care.

During the 19th century, a more philanthropic approach to social health and welfare developed, aided by various social activists and encapsulated in the work of Victorian women reformers in sowing the seeds of professionalism in nursing.

Consequent on this was the impetus for state registration and the setting up of the NHS. In the latter half of the 20th century, there have been organisational changes in the running of the nursing profession, and a restructuring of nurse education, which will give the profession its next step forward. This will tackle the new climate of the 21st century whilst retaining a clear idea of nursing development and always recognising the core skills of nursing that have been cherished over the centuries.

REFERENCES

Abel-Smith B 1960 A history of the nursing profession. Heinemann, London

Baly M 1995 Nursing and social change, 3rd edn Routledge, London

Brooke E 1993 Women healers through history. Womens' Press, London

Carpenter M 1980 Asylum nursing before 1914: a chapter in the history of labour, Ch. 6. In: Davies (ed) Rewriting nursing history. Croom Helm, London

Chadwick 1834. Cited in Hennessy P 1992 Never again. Jonathan Cape, London

Clark A 1982 Working life of women in the seventeenth century. Routledge and Kegan Paul, London

Davies C (ed) 1980 Rewriting nursing history. Croom Helm, London

Digby A 1978 Pauper palaces. Routledge and Kegan Paul, London

Dingwall R, Rafferty A M, Webster C 1988 An introduction to the social history of nursing. Routledge, London

Flannagan S 1988 Hildegarde of Bingen, 1098–1179: a visionary life. Routledge, London

Howlett B 1993 The origins of the Nightingale school. The Florence Nightingale Musuem, London

Midwinter E 1968 Victorian social reform. Longman, London

Mitchell S 1984 The country life book of nursery rhymes. Hamlyn, Feltham

Nolan P 1995 Mental health nursing – origins and developments, Ch. 20. In: Baly (ed) Nursing and social change, 3rd edn. Routledge, London

Nuttall P 1983 The passionate statistician. Nursing Times 28 August 25–27

Pound J 1971 Poverty and vagrancy in Tudor England. Longman, London

Rafferty A M 1995 The anomaly of autonomy: space and status in early nursing reform. International History of Nursing Journal (1): 43–54

Storr F 1983 The first hundred years of nursing in the Gloucester Infirmary 1755–1855. History of Nursing Society Journal 1(3) 3

Summers A 1988 Angels and citizens. Routledge & Kegan Paul, London

Versluyen M C 1980 Old wives' tales? Women healers in English history, Ch. 8. In: Davies (ed) Rewriting nursing history. Croom Helm, London

FURTHER READING

Baly M 1986 Florence Nightingale and the nursing legacy. Croom Helm, London

Dick D 1987 Yesterday's babies. Bodley Head, London

Fraser D 1984 The evolution of the British welfare state, 2nd edn. MacMillan, London

Hector W 1973 Mrs Bedford Fenwick. RCN, London

McGann S 1992 The battle of the nurses. Scutari, London

Nolan P 1993 A history of mental health nursing. Chapman & Hall, London

Webster C 1993 Caring for health: history and diversity. Open University, Milton Keynes

12

Nursing ethics

Isabelle Whaite

In their everyday practice, nurses constantly encounter situations that demand an ethical response. To help nurses to clarify their thinking in this area, this chapter aims to:

- **arrive at an understanding of the term 'nursing ethics'**
- **investigate the moral values underpinning nurses' actions, and their relationship to the facts**
- **consider ethics with respect to various aspects of nursing practice**
- **explore ethical theory and its underlying philosophical approaches**
- **examine how moral decisions may be made in practice.**

UNDERSTANDING WHAT IS MEANT BY NURSING ETHICS

As yet little is known about the quality of nurses' experiences in the practice of nursing ethics, as there is a paucity of research. Nurses have yet to tell their own stories about their experience in order to enable the true essence of nursing ethics to be fully understood. This chapter will explore the meaning of nursing ethics as we understand it so far, question its utility as a basis for nurses' decision-making and behaviour in practice and consider the relevance of the study of ethics for the nurse and for practice.

ETHICS IS THINKING AND DOING

You will already have your own ideas about what is meant by nursing ethics (Activity 12.1).

Activity 12.1

Just imagine you are asked by someone from another planet what is meant by nursing ethics. What would you tell them? You can write down the words, phrases and/or sentences you would use and that are representative of what the term 'nursing ethics' currently means to you.

You might have come up with several ideas that reflect your understanding of the term 'nursing ethics'. Your response may well include Codes of Conduct, values and beliefs, the law, confidentiality, personal viewpoints, respect for persons, doing good, not doing harm, being honest and many other aspects.

Nurses often find it easy to produce such lists of words, phrases and sentences, but what is not so easy is to explain what is meant by them. Does everyone share the same meaning of a word or phrase? Surely, the same words can have different meanings for different people. Too often, it is assumed that all parties in a debate or discussion are thinking and talking about the same phenomenon, when in reality they are not. Clarification of the meaning of the words and terms we use and an explanation of how these are linked to each other are needed if we are to give a meaningful explanation of nursing ethics to someone else.

A starting point in this clarification process is that nursing ethics is about what nurses do in practice. The emphasis and focus for the study of ethics is on action as well as knowledge: how actions are good or bad, or right or wrong, and their consequences. In giving health care, nurses and other health carers increasingly find themselves in situations where they are asking themselves what is the morally right thing to do.

Rowson (1990) writes that when we evaluate behaviour as right, wrong, good and bad, we can do so from a number of points of view, of which morality is only one. These viewpoints include those of law, social convention, professional codes, religious codes and politics, and a practical approach.

An example of judging behaviour from a socially constructed viewpoint is a college lecturer taking all his clothes off when addressing the assembled students. This behaviour would be considered as wrong, insofar as it does not conform to the customary way of behaving in such an organisation or in society itself; it defies social convention. But would it necessarily be morally wrong?

Moral values underpinning thoughts and knowledge in nursing practice

Is the moral point of view different from the one in this example, which is based on social convention? What is moral goodness or badness in relation to conduct? The answer to this may well be found in the evidence provided to support any judgement made. A judgement of what is right or wrong in a legal sense can be supported with evidence from the statute book. A judgement of right or wrong in a social convention sense can be supported with cultural codes, rules and etiquette. The evidence to support a judgement about whether or not action is right or wrong in a moral sense is not so accessible.

Although all of these points of view may provide some evidence for making a moral judgement, they are not sufficient in themselves, and different evidence for the moral truth needs to be found, based on a set of external or internal rules and principles from several sources. What are the standards that underpin such moral action or conduct? What is the source of our moral knowledge, and what influences the choices we make about action to take in a particular situation? Action is underpinned by attitudes, values and beliefs. A major focus of study in nursing ethics is to identify, clarify and critically analyse and evaluate these moral values and beliefs, which have the moral sense of goodness, badness, right and wrong attached to them. For instance, justice is associated with the moral sense of goodness, whereas injustice equates with badness and vice in the moral sense.

Thus nursing ethics is the study of not only how our actions are good or right in the moral sense, but also moral thinking, the moral values that we ascribe to our knowledge or thoughts. It is the study of how we decide what we ought to do – making moral choices – as well as what we actually do in practice.

Moral values held by the individual are unique and personal to that individual. When a decision is to be made between competing and conflicting values about what is the morally right thing to do, evidence has to be provided to support the action chosen.

Identifying, clarifying and choosing the values we prize and ascribe to our knowledge and thoughts is an important process in the study of nursing ethics. Morality includes reasoning about the whole area of value judgements we make in our whole lives, including those of nursing

practice. This involves the nurse in abstract thinking and reflection, where knowledge is arrived at through such processes as logical reasoning or problem-solving.

Facts and values as evidence for moral decisions

As well as moral knowledge, knowledge gained by direct observation of the external world, known as the empirical or scientific way of knowing, also underpins thoughts and knowledge in nursing practice. This knowledge is arrived at through observations we make about phenomena in the environment. From what we observe in a particular situation, we arrive at knowledge, through the process of induction, i.e. generalising from the specific to the general. This involves the nurse in concrete thinking and empirical testing, systematically measuring directly observed phenomena to arrive at knowledge of the facts believed to be true.

Hume (1978) argues that beliefs and values are something separate from the body of empirically derived knowledge. Unlike statements of fact, beliefs and values cannot be proven or disproven using scientific methodology: the moral worth of any action can never be observed. We cannot discover empirically whether or not action is right or wrong in a moral sense, which makes statements about morality qualitatively different from statements of fact. Using the 'is ought' distinction described by Hume (1978) can prevent us falling into the trap of confusing evidence of what is (fact) with evidence of what ought to be (evaluative evidence, based on value judgement). Hume explains that it is possible for two people to agree about all the facts observed in a situation yet to differ in the values that they assign to these facts, as it is man who adds moral content. Nowhere in the facts is it possible to discover rightness or badness in the moral sense. These evaluative judgements are based on one's own values of what ought to be. It is false logic to base moral truth on fact.

The 'is ought' distinction is well recognised in the study of ethics. All statements can be divided into factual or partly factual, and evaluative or partly evaluative elements. A skill is to distinguish what is factual and what is evaluative. Value statements are often smuggled into factual statements and are stated as fact. This is very important to notice and to challenge when reasoning about what ought to be in a moral sense.

Hume's proposition is that one cannot reach a decision about what ought to be done in a moral sense based on the facts. It does not follow the rules of logic to look at a fact and then to say in a factual way that it is morally wrong (Box 12.1).

Box 12.1 Facts and values – the 'is ought' distinction

Consider the following statement:

- Jean took £10 from her grandmother's handbag.

This is factual because it can be tested out empirically: we can observe the act.
Now consider this statement:

- Stealing from another person is morally wrong.

This is evaluative. If, however, one were to think that this evaluative statement smuggled in here is fact, one could wrongly conclude as fact the following:

- Jean was wrong to take £10 from her grandmother's handbag.

Here we have a value statement that has been smuggled in without being examined. To the description of the facts has been added one's own values of what ought to be, which is now passed off as fact, i.e. what is. Unbeknown to the observer, Jean's grandmother may well have instructed her to take the money!

To further illustrate the gap between fact and value, which cannot be bridged by logical argument, consider Activity 12.2.

Activity 12.2

Consider the following two statements:

- Ann told a lie to her daughter Fiona to prevent her being upset.
- The man took the gun and shot the intruder.

Take each statement in turn. Divide the statements into factual or partly factual, and evaluative or partly evaluative elements. What conclusions might you come to if the value statements you smuggle in are not examined and are wrongly claimed as fact?

When we evaluate action as right, good or bad from a moral point of view, different evidence is needed. The facts are insufficient in themselves as evidence for whether or not action is right or wrong in a moral sense.

In addition to the 'is ought' distinction, there are some other common errors in reasoning that do not follow the rules of logic. It is useful to be aware of these, both in one's own thinking and reasoning and in that of others (Box 12.2).

Box 12.2 Some fallacies or errors in reasoning in ethics

- *The 'is ought' distinction:* a skill is to identify what is factual and what is evaluative. Value statements are often smuggled into factual statements and stated as fact. This is important to notice and challenge.
- *Using force:* making another person accept the conclusion of an argument on the basis of force alone, without supporting evidence for your conclusion.
- *Using personal blame:* blaming another in a personal way for a decision he has taken rather than trying to understand the reasons for the decision.
- *Appeal to the majority:* the false claim that since everybody does something or thinks in some particular way, it must be right.
- *Authority versus expertise:* people within the hierarchy being invested with moral expertise they do not have, based simply on their position of power in the organisation.
- *Preaching dogma:* the refusal to allow any evidence that contradicts one's own conclusions or arguments about moral rightness or badness; protecting one's choices and actions against criticism; the nurse or doctor refusing to question any ethical argument or conclusion or to allow questioning of her own conclusions.

Being aware of some of the common errors in reasoning in nursing ethics can help in developing moral thinking and the ability to reason in the search for the truth about moral knowledge.

ETHICS AND THE PRACTICE OF NURSING

Among the more general reasons for the growing interest in nursing ethics is an awareness that questions of values and moral choice are central to many developments in health care. Biomedical and technical advances have created higher expectations of the effectiveness of health care.

Resources in the NHS are not unlimited, and with increasing demands, rationing of health care resources is inevitable. This means that, increasingly, decisions about the allocation of health care resources at all levels of the organisation are not always seen to be in the interest of particular groups or individuals. In addition to these general developments in health care, interest in nursing ethics reflects development in the philosophy and practice of nursing.

The new nursing and evidence-based practice

Nurses face many challenges. Health care is being delivered in an environment in which the pace of change is relentless. Social, educational, legislative and epidemiological changes, together with manpower and employment developments, all impinge on the delivery of nursing care. Improving health care and making care services better is heavily dependent upon nurses, midwives and health visitors (Department of Health 1993). Knowles (1984) writes that 'the half life of the knowledge, skills, attitudes and values required by nurses ... is shrinking fast'.

Against this backcloth, the nursing profession is presented with opportunities for new and enlightened developments in care. The profession of nursing needs to acquire and demonstrate an understanding both of the social need that gives rise to a call for nursing, and of a body of knowledge that can be drawn upon in order to create the nursing response. Nursing as a discipline must be informed by different kinds of knowledge, nursing knowledge first, according to Schon (1987). Ideas and methods of knowledge development come from disciplines outside that of nursing, including biology, social sciences and the humanities. These, together with study of the social and political context of contemporary society, are brought into ways of thinking and doing nursing. Taking into practice knowledge from other disciplines has enabled nurses to discover the knowledge of nursing within the practice situation, which is the site and context for knowing nursing. The discipline of nursing is concerned with discovering, creating, structuring, testing and refining knowledge needed for the practice of nursing; this must occur within the discipline.

Carper (1978) writes that knowing nursing means knowing in several areas all at once, including:

- personal knowing, using knowledge about oneself and one's own and others' experiences of the self
- empirical knowing, which is factual, research-based knowledge needed by the nurse in order to be competent in a given situation
- ethical knowing, which includes values and beliefs underpinning choices and decision-making in practice, and identifying conflicting values and one's obligations in a given situation
- aesthetic knowing, which is how the nurse uses all of the knowledge brought to the practice situation and created within the practice situation to form possibilities and ultimately the nursing response.

A view of nursing as a unique discipline with knowledge to be found in its practice including personal, ethical, empirical and aesthetic knowing all at once is presented here. Studying knowledge from disciplines outside the discipline of nursing, together with the study of nursing and the knowledge created within the nursing situation, will enable nurses, through this increased knowledge, to develop critical thinking in relation to contemporary views from nursing. This will make them effective, innovative practitioners able to respond to changing needs for health care and calls for nursing, to recognise the value of nursing knowledge and its impact on patient care, and to provide evidence of their impact on patient care.

Professional responsibility and accountability

Salvage (1990) writes that the key to new nursing is to be held in its clinical base. As the traditional hierarchical occupational model for nursing must be replaced by a professional one, the professional nurse must be prepared to fulfil such a skilled, responsible and demanding role through an improved educational programme.

The new nurse should have greater autonomy and work in partnership with patients. Nursing is viewed as a kind of therapy in its own right, within the therapeutic potential of the relationship.

The new nursing draws heavily on psychological theories of psychoanalysis and humanistic psychology. As yet, insufficient is known about the professional–patient relationship based on partnership, and there is a lack of clear evidence that this is what patients want. Nevertheless, according to Salvage, nursing is involved in some kind of 'occupational evolution'. Nursing knowledge and nursing as a discipline is firmly on the agenda in health care, although not all developments are universally accepted within nursing or by other health care professions. There is a great deal of debate about directions in which it is considered the profession of nursing should or should not be developing.

Ethical dimensions of care

By the very nature of their work, nurses are involved with and intervene in other people's lives, often at times when they are at their most vulnerable. This provides the opportunity for nurses to do a great deal of good or harm in a moral sense. The possibility of nurses doing good or harm depends partly on factual knowledge and partly on the values underpinning their knowledge and thoughts. Factual knowledge and personal, professional and universal values must be consciously and critically evaluated for their potential to do harm or good. Consider Case example 12.1.

Case example 12.1 Intervening in other peoples' lives

Grace has severe learning disability and has lived in a hospital for most of her life. She is now living in sheltered community accommodation and likes to get out into the garden, where she can walk independently. She is finding this increasingly difficult owing to worsening of osteoarthritis of both hips.

The health care professionals have decided that Grace is not a suitable candidate for a hip replacement operation, so have decided not to refer her to an orthopaedic surgeon.

Reflect on Case example 12.1 and imagine yourself as Grace's keyworker. What do you feel about the decision that has been made for Grace by the health professionals? What would you like to say and how would you intervene? What is the possibility of your intervention doing good or doing harm in a moral sense? Perhaps you could identify the facts of the case. Do we know them? What are the possible value judgements that may be smuggled in and claimed as factual evidence to justify not giving Grace the operation?

Professional values in nursing practice and ethics

A code of ethics states the primary goals and values of the professional nurse. When individuals become nurses, they make a moral commitment to uphold the values and special moral obligations in such a code. The Nurses, Midwives and Health Visitors Act (1979) gave power to the United Kingdom Central Council for Nurses, Midwifery and Health Visiting (UKCC) to give guidance on Standards of Professional Conduct. As a result, the UKCC formulated a Code of Professional Conduct in 1983, which was revised in 1984 and 1992 (see Ch. 16).

The professional nurse is expected to work within the guidelines and to embrace the values and beliefs expressed within the Code of Conduct. Within the limits on decision-making offered by the Code of Conduct, the professional nurse has to decide for herself what she ought to do. The study of ethics provides some frameworks for professional nurses to use in practice to help in clarifying thinking, logical reasoning and problem-solving when determining what should be done. It also aids nurses in reflecting in and on their practice, and in studying what they actually do when they make moral decisions in practice.

VALUES AS THE BASIS FOR MORAL THOUGHT AND ACTION

As stated above, a major focus of study in nursing ethics is to identify, clarify, critically analyse and evaluate one's own and others' values and beliefs underpinning moral decisions and choice of action in practice.

Values are those assertions or statements that individuals make, through either behaviour, words or actions, that define what they think is important and for which they are willing to suffer or even die. Uustal (1980, quoted in Tschudin 1992) states that 'A value is a personal belief or attitude about the truth, beauty or worth of any thought, object or behaviour.'

Value choices constitute almost the whole of human freedom. We often choose to do something because of the values we hold.

FORMATION OF VALUES

Values that we ascribe to our knowledge and thoughts can be shaped by political ideology, societal and cultural values, peer group, family and community values, organisational, institutional and professional values. Whether or not we are aware of them or have consciously chosen or assimilated them, our lives are lived by certain standards and values. These values influence what we choose to do in our own life domain with our body, life, property and privacy, and are also a basis for judging the actions of others. Activity 12.3 considers consciously chosen values.

Activity 12.3

Try to bring to mind a particular value you learned from your parents and which has influenced your thinking and choices of action in the way you have lived your life.

- Is this value one that you still apply in your life to guide your actions?
- What are your own grounds for continuing to hold or not hold this value that your parents instilled into you?

It is possible to discover that not all values instilled in us by any of the external agencies, including parents, are necessarily our own. Rogers (1951), in his theory of personality and behaviour, considers that the child learns to respond to the environment in a way that pleases his parents and avoids their displeasure. The child learns to deny his own valuing system and is conditioned into accepting the values framework of parents and other influential persons and institutions. Rather than offend influential others, we may leave unquestioned some of these values imposed upon us and which we have assimilated into our own value frameworks as our own. Through the experience of living, personal values can change. They are not static (Activity 12.4).

Activity 12.4

Think of the choice you made to become a nurse.

- What other alternatives did you consider?
- Why did you choose nursing?
- What did you value about nursing?
- Did anyone influence your choice?
- What did they value about nursing?
- Has anything changed for you since you started to study nursing?
- What do you value about nursing now?
- What do you not value about nursing now?

Personal value systems

It is not always easy to identify the particular values and standards by which we live our lives. With the increasing complexity of moral issues and dilemmas confronting health care professionals has come a greater openness in discussion and debate about values. Carper (1978) identified ethical knowledge as a major element of nursing's knowledge base. To be effective in practice, the nurse will be required to know the value basis for that knowledge base in order to justify, defend or challenge decisions made by herself and others and the subsequent action taken in practice.

Getting in touch with this personal value base is a crucial first step in the study of nursing ethics. Tschudin (1992) advises that values can be brought into consciousness through discovering meaning. This means not being content with superficial levels of meaning and merely responding to prevailing circumstances, but striving and searching to discover a richer level of meaning about life, its purpose, the worth of one's self, who and what we are and ourselves with others. The source of our values is to be found through the discovery of meaning in our lives, which comes out of learning about ourselves: finding out the kind of person we are, our likes and dislikes, personality, temperament and whether we are thinking or feeling people. Through the study of the psychological and social theory of the formation of values, we will be helped to further our understanding of what has influenced our own personal value systems.

Through reflecting on what we do in work, recreation and hobbies, we can discover meaning about ourselves, our purpose, our aims and what we seek to accomplish. Our values and meaning in life come out of what we do in our lives.

Frankl (1978) believes that we discover meaning in our lives through experiencing nature and culture, being open and receptive to our experiencing, and hearing nature's stories and the experience of people from different cultures within our society. From this develop our values and meaning in life.

Frankl (1978) also believes that we discover meaning and values through the experience of our own and others' suffering. Suffering as a result of pain, disease, poverty, injustice, bereavement and disablement affects us. It shapes us, challenges us and is a source of our values (Activity 12.5).

It should be increasingly obvious that today's nurses cannot remain indifferent to the fact that nursing ethics is applied to the public and political domain as much as to the personal and clinical practice of nurse and patient. By virtue of the nurse's unique knowledge of health, illness, nursing and health care, she has a professional responsibility to influence and inform decisions about ecological and environmental issues, social and health policy, housing, health education, health promotion, research, resource allocation and the politics of health, both nationally and internationally. Thus today's professional nurse is not solely confined to nursing ethics individualised within a caring relationship with patients.

Activity 12.5

1. As a nurse, even if it meant a great personal cost to you, would you give up driving your car when air pollution was reported as not meeting an acceptable safe standard?
2. Is it better to keep an area of land to preserve various species of animals, plants and birds, or to build a new motorway so that more people can enjoy better access by car?

What values emerge for you in reflecting on these two questions? Discuss them with your colleagues. Do you all share the same opinions?

3. Pain, disease, poverty, bereavement, disability and injustice are all associated with suffering.

- Have you suffered any of these? Did your experience result in you changing your views and values?
- Has the experience of observing others' suffering caused by any of these resulted in you changing your views and values?

Values are not static: in searching for and discovering meaning, they can change. Discuss your answers to the above question with a colleague.

Learning values through observation, reasoning and experience

Knowing nursing includes the area of ethical knowing. Factual knowledge, personal, professional and universal values all must be consciously and critically evaluated for their potential to do good or harm.

Values that are based on prejudice or bias, and values that are assimilated without question, can result in behaviour and a choice of action that has the potential to do harm. This may occur when giving individualised care at a local level or developing and implementing community policy at a national level. The tendency is for the personal value system of individuals involved to override all else. Getting in touch with meaning can lead to uncovering of such values, which are sometimes not easy to defend if they have been unconsciously assimilated or are based on prejudice. Consider Case example 12.2 with this in mind.

Tschudin (1986) states that when nurses give no thought to the choices they make, but just

Case example 12.2

Helen Brown, aged 60, is the major care provider for her daughter, aged 18. Her daughter has been diagnosed as suffering from schizophrenia. She is 6 months pregnant and her behaviour is currently very difficult to cope with.

Helen's son has learning disability and has lived in an institution for many years. He is aged 28 and is now living with Helen. On the whole, he is coping well, but he becomes very moody when his sister's behaviour becomes difficult for his mother to cope with.

Helen's husband is unemployed and lives with his family in a two-bedroomed flat in a deprived inner-city area.

The community psychiatric nurse is visiting Helen's daughter. Helen looks tired and very distressed. She explains to the nurse that she is unable to cope with her daughter's behaviour and its effect on the whole family. Her daughter is uncommunicative, stays out at night and is not attending to her personal hygiene.

In response, the nurse congratulates Helen on how well she is doing in such difficult circumstances. He reminds her of both the government and Health Authority policy, which is 'to keep patients in the community and out of hospital'; his consultant would not support admission of Helen's daughter to hospital. The nurse bids Helen farewell and promises to call again within the next week to see Helen's daughter, who was not present during his visit.

During a post-visit review, the nurse is challenged by the student nurse who had accompanied him on the visit. He confirmed his grounds for not taking action. Adherence to the rules of the Health Authority and consultant psychiatrist would avoid the displeasure and gain the approval of his seniors, despite the distress and threat to the well-being of his client and her family. The nurse confessed that he had not given the situation further thought beyond this. He valued highly the approval of the consultant psychiatrist who expected his directive to be obeyed.

Being challenged to reflect on the experience, he found difficulty in sustaining the grounds for his choice of action. Blindly following the rules was not a good enough reason. In touch with his professional values, he realised that a policy and system that treats some people so unfairly is not meeting basic fundamental needs and must be questioned and challenged. This, he admitted, was not something he felt confident to do.

The nurse was eventually able to negotiate for Helen's son to spend 2 weeks at a community residential home; he was happy with this. This relieved the pressure on Helen, who was able to give more time to coping with her daughter's erratic behaviour, which she was well used to and with which she usually coped well. Helen also felt much happier and supported as a major carer.

respond to the prevailing circumstances, 'they have no claim to be considered dependable, honest or trustworthy. Persons who are flighty, apathetic, moody, rebellious, conforming and submissive may be people who have not come to grips with their own values'. In Case example 12.2 thoughtless action, when political values that are in conflict with professional values have been assimilated without question, has a greater potential to do more harm than good to the whole family if it goes unchallenged. Our values and meaning in life come out of what we do. Thus reflecting on what we do in practice enables us to learn about ourselves as people and as nurses.

Model for value clarification

Value clarification is an attempt to bring into conscious awareness the values and underlying motivations that guide one's actions. A strength of value clarification is that one expresses value preferences and priorities in an open and honest way. Questioning our value choices will help us to see how and why we make our decisions. Sometimes it is not easy to defend our choices when challenged.

Raths et al (1966) provide a seven-step model for value clarification (Box 12.3).

Box 12.3 Value clarification

When you value something, you:

choose	• freely
	• from alternatives
	• after considering the consequences of each alternative
prize	• are proud and happy with choice
	• affirm this and tell others
act	• to act on one's value choice
	• to integrate the value in the way life is lived.

The nurse who knows her value basis has at some stage thought about it, compared it with alternatives and acted on this choice. In reality, the process may not always be so clear as the simple model outlined in Box 12.3.

A drawback of value clarification is that one's preference does not provide justification for one's choice. It does not mean that no matter how carefully we have arrived at our choice, it is the the one that is morally good and praiseworthy. A preference as a basis for action may well bring about morally bad and blameworthy action. A teacher may prefer students to keep quiet and just listen to him. Such a value about the nature of people as students that guides this teacher's choice of behaviour may well, however, be damaging for the students.

Ethical theory, a branch of moral philosophy, offers different ways of viewing how phenomena and actions possess ethical values. The study of philosophical medical ethics based on moral theory provides a further tool for nurses to develop a more comprehensive understanding of the specific meanings of moral value and moral worth when applied to thinking, values and beliefs, and underpinning knowledge, thoughts and choice of action in practice.

ETHICAL THEORY AS THE BASIS FOR MORAL THOUGHT AND ACTION

PHILOSOPHICAL MEDICAL ETHICS AS A BASIS FOR NURSING ETHICS

It would seem the bioethical model of teaching ethics currently predominates both medical and nursing curricula. Gallagher & Boyd (1991) report on a research survey they undertook to examine how ethics is taught to midwives, nurses and health visitors throughout the UK. The study was undertaken in conjunction with the Institute of Medical Ethics, in collaboration with the Royal College of Nursing. The emphasis and focus throughout the study was clearly within the parameters of medical ethics thinking. In their recommendations, the authors try to put nursing ethics within the mould of medical ethics and imply that teachers who should teach nursing ethics must be experts in ethical analysis and reasoning.

Gillon (1986), writing about philosophical medical ethics, describes it as 'the analytic activity in which the conceptions, assumptions, beliefs, attitudes, emotions, reasons, argument, underlying moral decision making are examined critically'. The ultimate aim of this activity is to construct and defend a comprehensive consistent moral theory for medical practice, based on universal principles applying to and capable of justifying conduct in practice.

Devising ethical theory

Seedhouse (1988) sees it as the work of moral philosophers to devise and refine technical ethical theory. The aim of the moral philosopher is to design a theory that is internally coherent, that contains principles that are consistent and complement each other, and that will enable a person to act morally, whatever the situation in life. A major concern with technical ethics is the process of clarification and criticism. Inconsistency, contradictions, illogical arguments, assumptions and generalisations are inappropriate. Following on from this initial stage is the formulation of hypotheses, which have to be clarified and criticised in order to be tested and justified.

Seedhouse (1986) refers to Wittgenstein, who concludes that philosophy is more concerned with retaining awareness that 'clarifications are incomplete' than it is with obtaining right answers. With tight analysis, it would seem that the aim of ethical inquiry is to clarify issues, distinguish between fact and value statements and uncover when rules of logic are broken. Trying to think out answers to moral questions for yourself is to practise philosophy. This is much more important than hitting the right answer by guesswork or passively taking in what the teacher says. The effort to get your answers is, in itself, of intrinsic value.

The bioethical model

Moral philosophers put forward two very different theories in technical ethics, deontology and utilitarianism, both of which offer ways of viewing how phenomena and actions possess ethical values. The study of these theories provides a further tool for nurses to develop a more comprehensive understanding of the specific meanings of moral value and moral worth when applied to thinking, values and beliefs and choice of action in practice. The bioethical model is based on these moral theories and principles.

DEONTOLOGY AS A FOUNDATION FOR MEDICAL AND NURSING ETHICS

This category of moral theories is about a view of morality that prescribes sticking to moral rules or duties because they are right in themselves, and that certain duties are right acts in themselves and fundamental to the idea of morality. Deontology is not concerned with the results of actions. Without exception, the deontologist acts on the basis of a perceived duty, whatever the consequences. The act itself is judged as a right and moral way to act.

Deontological theories are justified on several grounds. One is that people have a moral duty to obey 'God's' moral laws. A problem here is that different people understand 'God's law' to mean different things, depending on which God one recognises. Another ground for justifying such theory is the claim that natural law, the laws of nature, include moral laws that bind everyone. Again the question about what we mean by nature and natural laws arises. However, so long as the deontologist can state what the duty is, it does not matter where it comes from, and it does not need to be empirically defined. One could find in today's society evil deontologists who consider that harming people of particular race or ethnic group is a duty to purify the race. A moral deontologist follows duties as a priority, claiming that they are morally important and worth following despite the consequences. Examples of duties followed by deontologists include keeping promises, telling the truth, not killing, doing no harm and always doing good. Deontologists are concerned with the way in which people act and how they intervene in other people's lives.

A problem with this theory is that following duties without exception does not always produce the best consequences in the short term or, in some instances, the long term. A deontologist may select only one duty or, alternatively, a range of duties. Selecting only one duty is hardly a guide to acting morally; selecting a range of duties inevitably causes conflict at times between competing principles. For example, it might be that to tell the truth and to do no harm in a particular situation are in conflict: to do no harm, one might be compelled not to tell the truth. In this situation, the deontologist must either list a hierarchy of principles and decide which of these are of supreme importance and which are of less importance, or select a single primary duty. The deontologist will be challenged to give a good reason why he has acted in a particular way. For example, if you have promised a person confidentiality, and he tells you that he has stolen money from his mother, you will have to apply moral reasoning in order to decide which of your duties should take precedence. You may also believe that retributive justice should always be administered. Keeping your promise to the person means that it is possible that justice will not prevail in this case, whereas breaking your promise means that retributive justice may well be administered.

In this situation, you would apply moral reasoning in order to decide which of your duties should take precedence. Once you do this, you will have to consider factors that are not purely questions of duty: you will be confronted with considering the consequences. Whilst deontologists would consider it sensible to consider the consequences of actions, they would not overrule moral duty on the grounds of consequence in order to bring about the most favourable outcome in the short term. They would consider that there are certain duties that are of supreme and abiding importance. If, in the above scenario, a case is made to support the principle of justice as a supreme duty, the moral grounds for supporting the choice of action are that the act itself is judged as a right and moral way to act. It is purely a question of duty, rather than of consequences. Deontologists consider that it is wrong to override moral duties to bring about the most favourable consequences.

Act deontology

This is one of several types of deontology. 'It considers that each context, situation, persons involved and judgement made in a moral sense is unique. The overriding duty in act deontology in every situation is that the person who is to make a moral choice and decide what ought to be done does so based on honest personal judgement. This will depend on how he sees each unique situation. It is not being true to oneself as a moral agent blindly to follow rules or do what one is told to do. Everything rests on the person who is to judge and to decide in each situation.

Within the complex world of health care and nursing, Seedhouse (1988) argues that act deontology is impracticable, as it would be well nigh impossible to base health care practice on such a philosophy that advocates individuals making their own decisions. It could be extremely confusing and chaotic if there was no consistency in moral intervention.

Seedhouse argues that some aspects of people's lives and situations have common features. Thus it is possible to make some generalisations and to provide health care workers, including doctors and nurses, with some rules and principles of conduct to guide them in ethical practice.

Rule deontology

Instead of claiming that a person's moral choice depends on how he sees each unique situation, and on personal integrity in being honest and exercising true personal judgement as a moral agent, rule deontology asserts that a person's moral choosing should depend upon a set of rules that should be followed without exception. An advantage of this approach is that the rule deontologist's actions will be more predictable. Codes of professional practice could be described as a version of rule deontology.

Problems could again arise on occasions when it would be better to break the rule. For example, one might reason that it would be better to break a promise in view of new evidence coming to light since the time of making the promise.

If a set of rules are chosen, there may again be a situation in which conflicts between them are revealed. How then does the rule deontologist choose between the rules that are now in conflict? One solution offered is to rank the rules in order of worth or importance. Again, the problem with this is that a situation may arise in which it could be logically argued that it would be better to break the supreme, primary rule or duty. Deontology does not offer guidance about how and when to do this. Arguments based solely on competing duties or rules does not seem to provide good enough reason for preferring one rule and rejecting another.

Kantian ethics

The philosopher Immanuel Kant (1724–1804) proposed a rule deontology perspective. If a particular rule or duty is right in one situation, it is right in all situations; it is a general rule. The person deciding what ought to be done in those situations has a duty to obey the rules. Kant claimed that we do many things out of a sense of duty because of external influences such as the anticipation of reward or the fear of sanctions; in these situations, there is no sense of moral duty. Acting out of a sense of duty comes from the willingness to do so from within the person. There are no pressures, it is a natural inclination to act morally. Each rule or principle that is acted on out of 'a good will' is truly a morally good decision. It is a universal moral law, right in all circumstances. Such universal ethical principles are always followed, irrespective of the consequences.

UTILITARIANISM AS A FOUNDATION FOR MEDICAL AND NURSING ETHICS

There are two main approaches to the ethics of consequences – consequentialism and utilitarianism. A consequentialist will decide how he should act by considering alternative actions and assessing the likely outcomes of proposed actions, i.e. whether the act will produce more benefits than disadvantages. The choice of the course of action to take will be based upon which action will bring about the greatest amount of benefit and the least amount of harm.

Utilitarianism was the approach proposed by Jeremy Bentham (1748–1832) and John Stuart Mill (1806–1873). The consequence thought to be beneficial was the greatest balance of good over evil, good being defined as happiness or pleasure. Defining these in measurable terms is problematic, and other measures of utility are now considered. In health care, benefit is usually described in terms of health status, added life years, quality of life years, health gain, and freedom from pain and disability. Whatever the definition of benefit, it must be measurable.

Exploring the meaning of the examples given here, and the value basis of decisions based on a calculation of outcome, raises much controversy and disagreement among health care professionals, health service managers and health economists. Defining these in measurable terms is equally problematic. In the calculation of the balance of benefit over non-benefit, all those involved are considered to be of equal importance to all others in the assessment. All persons are taken account of in the calculation of the effect of the chosen action. This is seen as a strength of the theory, in that it is a position that challenges individual self-interest and bias.

The action taken is justified according to the outcomes achieved in terms of the best consequences. Acts are morally right only if they have utility (are useful) in bringing about the best consequences.

Act utilitarianism

The person taking this approach will look at each situation from the perspective that the context, situation, persons involved, benefits and judgement made is, in a moral sense, unique.

Seedhouse (1988) argues that, in the complex world of health care, it is unrealistic to expect people to go through new calculations each time. Much work is being done in the area of producing measurable outcomes where difficult decisions are to be made about rationing of health care resources. Much controversy surrounds this work, including the view that taking such an approach means that not all persons are

valued equally nor treated fairly. Major critics of utilitarian theory claim that this approach can lead to decisions that seem to be patently unjust.

General utilitarianism

The person taking this approach will ask what the consequences would be if everyone were to pursue a particular course of action. It is a useful question to ask in that it enhances our view of reality in terms of the far-reaching consequences of actions.

Rule utilitarianism

The person taking this approach will calculate the best consequences to result from obedience to predefined rules, to which no exception is acceptable. Always to keep a certain predefined rule will be to produce the greatest good. The rule has greater utility in terms of consequences and has been established based on a process of calculation of which rules, if always followed, produce the greatest balance of good over evil.

In health care, following the theory of rule utilitarianism provides a basis for ethical practice that has been arrived at through a thorough review of past experiences. One shortcoming is that, sooner or later, the rule utilitarian will be faced with a rule to which it would be better not to adhere, in that it will not result in producing the greatest balance of good over evil. Rules are rigid; they are also created by people who may well be biased and prejudiced in some way.

DEONTOLOGY AND UTILITARIANISM COMPARED

It would seem there are problems with the philosophical basis of the theories of utilitarianism and deontology as a basis for medical and nursing ethics. Neither are sufficient in themselves for providing adequate theory for moral decision-making and for justifying moral action taken in practice. Despite this, philosophical medical ethics as a basis for nursing ethics must be one area of study in any programme of nursing ethics.

Activity 12.6

You have promised your friend that you will come to her farewell party, as she is leaving the next day to live in New Zealand. You agree to go round before the party to help with preparing the food.

Just as you are leaving your home, a colleague studying on the same course as yourself telephones you to say that he is having difficulty finishing an assignment that is to be handed in the next day. He is very worried as it is a re-submission following failure to achieve a pass at the first attempt. He reminds you that he once helped you with some course work and asks you to go to his home that evening. He has no transport and lives 20 miles away.

Will you help him to finish the assignment, or will you be with your friend and help with the farewell party?

- How would a utilitarian decide what to do?
- How would a deontologist decide what to do?

Focus on the process of arriving at a decision.

Think about the two opposing theories and consider Activity 12.6.

PRINCIPLES OF BIOMEDICAL ETHICS

Traditionally, the moral principles of beneficence (to do good) and non-maleficence (to do no harm) have been the basis of the doctor–patient and nurse–patient relationship. The professional's duty, as an expert, was to act in the best interests of the patient, and the patient was seen as taking a relatively passive role within the relationship.

More recently, however, thinking in philosophy has moved towards the need to address the patients' wishes. Respect for autonomy is a principle that is becoming central to the doctor–patient or nurse–patient relationship in health care.

It could be said that resource allocation is the 'problem' facing health care today. The care services are facing new demands as a result of changing patterns of need and the expectations of clients, and rationing of resources is inevitable. Finding methods of rationing health care resources based on a moral principle of justice is a major challenge to all health care professionals working at all levels of the health service.

The principle of autonomy

The concept of autonomy has come from the philosophical work of freedom.

A basic distinction to make is between negative freedom and positive freedom. Negative freedom means the absence of constraint or coercion, a person being said to be free to the extent he can choose his own goals. Berlin (1969) questions the value of this notion of freedom from interference to 'men who are half naked, illiterate, underfed and diseased'. There are situations in which individual freedom is not everyone's primary need. Thus, it is argued, personal freedom is not enough; what is needed is positive freedom – the means or power to act. Seedhouse (1988) argues that the measure of freedom a person has is the extent to which he has knowledge; he considers knowledge as another necessary condition in order to be free.

Autonomy has different meaning for different people. Gillon (1986) writes about the control a person has over his own life and choices as 'the will'; the will of the person must be respected. Seedhouse (1988) expresses concern that if autonomy of will is all there is, we could, in health care, risk neglecting opportunities to help people enhance their lives. Seedhouse argues for the notion that autonomy is a quality, a part of being human. Autonomy as a quality can exist only so far as certain conditions are present; to be able to understand one's environment, to make rational choices and to be able to act on the choices made.

Autonomy is a matter of degree. It can be considered on a continuum with 'no control' and 'total control' at the extremes. The greater the degree of autonomy, the more a person is able to do in his life. Autonomy is a quality that can be possessed to a greater or lesser degree in different areas, situations and times in our lives. Admission to hospital can result in fear and distress and reduce a person's degree of autonomy, and thus his ability to function in that particular situation and at that particular time. Working with patients to produce the conditions necessary for autonomy is a large area of nurses' work.

A dilemma exists when it is felt that it is more important to act in the best interest for a patient rather than to respect his autonomy. Overriding a patient's autonomy is serious, and an action that must be justified.

The principle of justice

The basic point of view is that we should value people equally and treat everyone alike unless there is a difference between people that is relevant to treating them differently. In health care some differences are relevant to one's treatment of people. A person may be very ill or distressed and need more physical and emotional care than others who are more independent. Health care workers sometimes disagree over which variations between patients they think are relevant to treating them differently.

There are different ways of understanding the meaning of justice. An egalitarian view of justice in health care is concerned with the distribution of health care resources according to individual need. Individual needs must be met by equal access to services and an adequate level of health care to meet individual needs. Justice, here, is based on need.

A libertarian view of justice holds that the most important value is individual liberty and choice. Here, the best kind of State is one that protects individuals, leaves them alone and lets them enjoy the rewards of their labour. Justice relates to how hard one has worked or how well one has done – justice according to merit.

A rights view of justice implies that someone has a duty or obligation to the person exercising his right. There are different sorts of right talked about, including natural rights, legal rights and moral rights (deontology). Clearly, a patient has legal rights not to suffer harm as a result of negligence on the part of any health care professional.

There are differing points of view regarding the nature of rights, so justice may be apportioned on the basis of different rights.

If we want to be just, there is a need to resolve the conflict between the different principles of justice, which is illustrated in Case example 12.3.

Case example 12.3

Consider two girls. The owner of the snack bar promises each girl £5 for cleaning the kitchen. When the job is done each girl has a right to £5 – this is what was agreed. This puts justice according to right above all else.

What if one girl does an excellent job and the other girl does a poor job? The owner of the snack bar then judges that the girl who did an excellent job deserves more reward than does the other girl, so he pays the first girl £8 and the second girl £2, thus putting justice according to merit above all else.

Then the snack bar owner learns that the hard-working girl comes from a well-to-do family, whereas the second girl is from a large family and is known to go hungry at times so that her small sisters can eat. The owner of the snack bar now judges that the second girl, who did a poor job, obviously needs more money, as she is going hungry in order to feed her sisters. Thus, he pays both girls £5, with an extra £2 for the second girl to buy food. This puts justice according to need above all else.

How would you be just? Which of the principles of justice would you put first? Defend your position. Don't forget the rules of logic.

CARING AS THE BASIS FOR MORAL THOUGHT AND ACTION

The concept of caring has occupied a prominent position in the nursing literature and has been presented as the essence of nursing practice by many nurse theorists and writers, including Leininger (1981, 1984), Benner & Wrubel (1989), Noddings (1984), Tschudin (1992) and Gilligan (1982).

Benner & Wrubel (1989) claim that inherent in nursing practice is the moral sense of caring. Caring as a basis for nursing ethics is a central value that underpins a special way of being and doing within the nurse–patient relationship that can promote good and enhance patients' and nurses' lives. Many of the writers above refer to the implicit moral sense of caring, a universal value that guides practice.

The writers from the caring movement strongly oppose importing into nursing theories from other disciplines, including moral philosophy.

There is concern that the moral sense in nursing practice that relates to day-to-day choices and their potential to do good or harm is lost. Instead, there is detached, decontextualised reasoning about particular problems, usually of a dramatic nature, using rules and principles from moral theory. Noddings (1984) claims that ethical decisions cannot be made in this detached mechanical way.

Seedhouse (1988) refers to 'ethics in the general sense'. The person who deliberates in a general sense of ethics realises that all thought and action can and should produce moral reflection; all action has potential for good or harm. Two often, he claims, nurses confine themselves in ethics to dramatic ethical dilemmas, well deliberated in the public arena, which are only the tip of the iceberg. So much of ethics in everyday practice goes unnoticed without reflection; this is the bulk of the iceberg that remains out of sight.

The writers from the caring movement highlight particular features of the caring relationship, including ways of relating, the existence of particular conditions within the relationship, specific aims for interacting and the presence of particular qualities or characteristics of the care-giver.

Gilligan (1982) found in her studies that there was an emphasis on empathy and concern for the well-being of the other within the caring relationship. In one study, nurses and patients described a sense of fulfilment as a direct result of nursing care delivered out of a moral sense.

Noddings (1984) writes about being non-judgemental and accepting the patient, empathy and person-to-person relating as particular conditions existing in a caring relationship. In order to create these conditions, the care-giver needs to develop self-awareness and empathy as a quality and a skill. This means not only trying to step in and out of the patient's inner experiencing private world to glean meaning, but also developing the skill to convey to the patient the ascertained meaning of his inner private world.

Certain qualities and characteristics of the care-giver are described by several writers. Roach (1987) identifies compassion, competence, con-fidence, conscience and commitment. Leininger (1981) refers to 27 differing caring constructs, including compassion, concern, empathy, love, nurturance, presence, support and trust. Other writers have identified knowledge, patience, honesty, trust, humility, hope and courage. Total caring requires one to be free of self-centredness. Through self-actualisation and the development of these qualities and characteristics, the nurse will strive for the good of the self and others, and good in general.

All of the values expressed by those of the caring movement are open to serious challenge, and none enjoys the status of demonstrable truth. There is a danger of wholesale adoption of the humanistic existential ethic, which leads to subtle indoctrination of that ethic.

Foot (1978) questions adopting an ethic of caring that is so dependent upon putting others interest before one's own. She challenges this in the light of a society that would seem to refuse to value caring, placing instead greater value and emphasis on individualism and egoism, and having little regard for selflessness and concern for the well-being of others.

The caring model as a basis for nursing ethics would seem to be orientated by the values of the agapistic or altruistic models developed by ancient and mediaeval philosophers, such as Aristotle and St Thomas Aquinas. One source of appeal might well have been the emphasis on the development of natural virtues, including providence, wisdom, temperance, courage and justice. Ethics is about virtues of character that are acquired through man's rational thought, desire and action. To develop a virtue is to express one's essence as a rational responsible agent, so, to that extent, the cultivation of virtues must be part of a rational agent's good.

Virtue of character is a mean state between excess and deficiency of action and feeling, and ethical action is about responding appropriately. This is determined by the reason of the wise, i.e. rational, person. Being generous is part way between being extravagant and miserly, and courage is a mean between foolhardiness and cowardice.

VIRTUE ETHICS – A REVIVAL

Several philosophers who have become increasingly frustrated with the impersonal form of the dominant moral theories of utilitarianism and deontology have started to revive virtue theory. The question of what one ought to do in any given situation is not to do with calculations of consequences, balancing interests or resolving conflicts of rights. It is about what kind of person is making the decision. Virtue theory seeks to describe the types of character we might find admirable and praiseworthy, raising questions about what a good person would do in a particular situation.

The argument put forward in support of the revival of virtue ethics is that notions of moral duty and obligation are no longer compatible with today's world views. It is felt that modern societies have inherited fragments of conflicting ethical traditions and that people are feeling confused. Questions need to be asked on whether or not we can resurrect in modern life the virtues of Aristotle and the code of an 18th-century aristocrat, where societies were not democracies. Stressing the perfection of the individual and the future of man, how does this fit with the view that all men are equal? Does a man who does not measure up to this perfectionist ideal of character have less worth? Is this view compatible with moral equality and justice?

Many would argue that it is not possible for an ethical theory which is based entirely on a virtuous character to do all the work of ethics. The idea of a core of all virtues suggests there is only one good way to live and for society to develop, but there are many ways to live and possible different worlds in the future, each requiring different systems and practices, and people with different kinds of virtue, for its development.

However it is a deep fault of non-virtue theories that so little attention is paid to the major areas of life that form character. Much more needs to be learned about caring as a virtue guiding decisions and action in practice.

MAKING MORAL DECISIONS IN NURSING PRACTICE

Few studies of nurses' experiences of ethical decision-making and ethical behaviour in practice are to be found in the literature.

STUDIES IN MORAL DEVELOPMENT

Studies in moral development are based on the cognitive theory of moral development proposed by Kohlberg (1984). This work advanced and extended the work of Piaget on the moral development of children. The theory holds that the underlying cognitive structures or principles that an individual uses to resolve moral dilemmas develop through a series of six sequential stages, each embodying a qualitatively different kind of moral reasoning and representing a form of thinking about morality. In the initial stages, where rudimentary levels of decisions are made, anticipation and fear of punishment and obedience have a major impact on decisions. Moving up the scale, conventional acceptance of society's values and rules has a major impact on decisions made. At the top end of the scale, moral decisions are made on the basis of universally valid ethical principles. Stages five and six are the highest stages of cognitive development, which not everyone achieves.

A cross-section of society, including doctors and nurses, will reveal a sizeable number at many of the moral stages. At each succeeding stage, there is greater appreciation of the welfare of others and a greater desire to resolve moral dilemmas in a fair and equitable way.

An implicit assumption is that those who have reached a higher stage of moral reasoning are more likely to act morally than are those at the lower stages. There is, however, no empirical evidence to support this. The cognitive theory itself is criticised with respect to moral development and reasoning being a purely cognitive process. Hoffman (1979) demonstrated a tendency of children as young as 2 years old to empathise with others and express this in a rudimentary way.

Studies examining nurses' reasoning ability have been based on Kohlberg's work and assumptions that a relationship exists between hypothetical reasoning, practical reasoning and actual behaviour in the real, lived, experienced world of nursing practice. These studies in the literature asked nurses to say what they *ought* to do and what they *would* do in response to a hypothetical situation, but none of the studies investigated what nurses actually did in practice. Hofling et al (1966) found that what nurses said they ought to do and would do, if asked to give medication over the telephone by a doctor not known to them, did not match up with what they actually did in practice. With only one exception, all the nurses in this study were prepared to administer a drug ordered over the phone by a doctor unknown to them, despite confirming that this was not what they ought to do nor would do in practice. Crisham (1981) reported that nurses with the most education achieved higher scores of principled thinking than did those with less education. In another study, it was found some senior nurses did not score beyond the level of reasoning that displays obedience to authority and the need to maintain harmony with institutions and those in authority.

Although limited, these studies raised important issues. Factors other than the ability to reason were reported by the researchers as having the potential to determine moral action in practice. Influence could be from the environment, the work setting, the personal characteristics of the nurse, the perception of the role and role relationships, differing values and beliefs among professionals, conflicting loyalties, organisational values, supportive and unsupportive environments, power and power relationships and forms of power sharing.

INFLUENCES ON THE ETHICAL DECISION-MAKING PROCESS

Erlen & Frost (1992) describe a common experience of nurses in relationship with doctors –
'perceived powerlessness' – which led to nurses describing themselves as ineffective in influencing moral decisions. On the other hand, Uden et al (1992), when comparing doctors' and nurses' experiences, found that doctors reported feeling isolated, lacking support and feeling insecure in their work because they were criticised by nurses. Doctors described nurses as not being willing to explore problems deeply.

Swider et al (1985) took a large sample of 800 nurses and found that 60% of patient decisions made were based on organisational needs and rules, 19% were centred around the doctors' directives and only 7% were patient centred, i.e. what the patient would want.

As yet, the experience of nurses in practice is a little-known phenomenon. There are other factors, besides the ability to reason at a high-principled level and follow rules of logic, that may well have an influence on moral reasoning and the practice of nursing. This is a rich and challenging field for nursing research.

THE NATURE AND ISSUES OF POWER WITHIN RELATIONSHIPS

The study of power and politics goes hand-in-hand with ethics. To be a professional nurse means that one exercises a public role. The professional nurse is dealing with different power relationships and the use of that power, both within her work, in clinical practice, research, management education and politics, and outside the nurse–patient relationship, with colleagues, other disciplines, managers, the organisation, professional bodies, pressure groups, unions and politicians at local, national and sometimes international levels.

The practice of ethics in all of these relationships is intimately tied up with the power issues of control, compliance, conformity, manipulation, coercion, facilitation, enabling, negotiation, domination and the use of authority.

Whatever the philosophical basis for nursing ethics in practice, political knowledge and ability is essential for informing decisions and choice of action. Ethical decisions so often come into conflict with the realities of power between professionals, different influential groups, persons at different clinical and management levels, and individuals and communities.

The nurse with a public role has a responsibility to try to use her political influence actively to shape health policy and influence public opinion on health matters. Nurses have a responsibility to the wider community and to society. Working with people every day can give nurses first-hand experience and information about whole communities, their health status, inequalities and health care needs.

PRESCRIPTION FOR ETHICAL REASONING, DECISION-MAKING AND ACTION

The focus in this chapter has been on the individual making a judgement about what is morally right or wrong to do in a particular set of circumstances. To assist individuals in this process, several different prescriptions are offered as frameworks and guiding principles for nurses in their decision-making, when making moral choices and when taking action in nursing practice.

Ethics is not a subject with a shallow end in which you can paddle around the edges; you need to jump in at the deep end. Tschudin (1992) quotes Joseph Conrad: 'it is not the clear sighted who lead the world. Great achievements are accomplished in a blessed, warm mental fog.' The search for meaning is never easy, but there is a way through the fog, given commitment and determination.

Getting in touch with one's personal value base is a crucial first step in the study of nursing ethics. Keeping in touch thereafter is equally important. Questioning their value choices will help nurses to see how and why they make the choices they do.

All of the values expressed by the caring movement are open to serious challenge. There is still a need for nurses to examine the appropriateness of caring as a basis for nursing ethics in practice. Thus it must continue to be an area of study in any programme of nursing ethics.

Linked to caring as a basis for nursing ethics is the attempt at a revival of virtue ethics, which holds that certain characteristics and virtues are an alternative basis for guiding moral thought and action. Much is still to be learned through empirical research about the many areas of life in which character is formed.

The research basis for a prescriptive theory in nursing ethics is sparse. A review of the literature indicates there is an urgent need to explore the relationship between hypothetical reasoning, practical reasoning and actual behaviour in the real lived world of practice, and to explore, through empirical research, all the factors that would seem to be influencing moral choices made in practice.

Finally, the professional nurse, in her work in clinical practice, research, management, education and politics, is dealing with the issues of power and politics in all relationships at all levels. Ethical choice decision-making and choosing courses of action so often create tensions and come into conflict with the realities of power and politics in any of these relationships and in particular situations. There is a need for the study of power and politics to go hand-in-hand with the study of nursing ethics: one cannot practise nursing ethics without political knowledge and ability in today's complex health care system.

Through the use of narrative, nurses must tell their stories about their experiences in the practice of nursing ethics. A reflective diary or log can be used to reflect on and record significant events or situations where there are moral issues or problems (Box 12.4). This can help the nurse to tell her own story and to learn about her own and others' moral values and choices, emphasising the importance of the individual.

The description of ethics in practice is still awaited. It would seem that the prescriptions we already have are insufficient in themselves to provide an adequate theory upon which to decide moral decisions and to justify moral action.

Box 12.4 **Format for reflection**

Date:

Description of day:

Events of day	Reflection and comments
Events – give description	a) The significant moments for me were ....
	b) What I thought at the time ....
	c) What I felt at the time ....
	d) What I feel remembering it now ....
	e) What did I learn ....
	f) What will I change (do differently) ....
	g) When I tried the change (repeat cycle a–f)

End of day or end of week overview

My discovered needs are:

Summary

On entering the nursing profession, students will bring with them a personal idea of the ethical dimensions of care, which will be refined and challenged the more often and more deeply they enter relationships with their patients and colleagues. By seeking out and monitoring the development of their own value bases, nurses will become sensitive to the difficulty of ethical decision-making and will be able better to act as the patient's advocate in the ever-changing field of health care.

Identifying the source and personal importance of our values may be hard, but doing this helps us to challenge our reasons for holding them, and enables us to understand our and others' individual responses to different situations.

Aspects that need to be addressed are one's view of goodness and badness, the relationship between values and facts, professional accountability and knowledge, autonomy, justice and rights, and the philosophical principles that seem to direct our action.

Much has been written on ethics and its related subjects, but as yet there is little literature on the application of ethics to nursing practice. With today's emphasis on research-based care, this will be a fruitful and fascinating area for future study.

However, all are essential areas of study in nursing ethics. This body of knowledge and understanding can then be taken into practice, so that the student and the professional nurse can learn about and begin to articulate the moral sense of nursing practice, thus contributing to the development of nursing's ethical knowledge base. From a description of what occurs in practice, a new prescription sufficient for practice may well be written.

REFERENCES

Benner P, Wrubel J 1989 The primacy of caring: stress and coping in health and disease. Addison Wesley, California

Berlin I 1969 Four essays on liberty. Oxford University Press, Oxford

Carper B 1978 Fundamental patterns of knowing in nursing. Advances in Nursing Science 1: 13–24

Crisham P 1981 Measuring moral judgement in nursing dilemmas. Nursing Research 30 (2): 104–110

Department of Health 1993 Vision for the future. Department of Health, London

Erlen J, Frost B 1992 Nurses' perceptions of powerlessness in influencing ethical decisions. Western Journal of Nursing Research 13 (3): 397–407

Foot P 1978 Virtues and vices. Basil Blackwell, Oxford

Frankl V 1978 Man's search for meaning. Hodder & Stoughton, London

Gallagher V, Boyd K 1991 Teaching and learning nursing ethics. Scutari Press, London

Gilligan C 1982 In a different voice: psychological theory and womens' development. Harvard University Press, Cambridge, Mass.

Gillon R 1986 Philosophical medical ethics. John Wiley, Chichester

Hofling C, Brotzman E, Dalrymple S, Graves N, Chester M, Pierce M D 1966 An experimental study in nurse physician relationships. Journal of Nervous and Mental Diseases 143: 171–180

Hoffman M 1979 The development of moral thought, feeling and behaviour. American Psychologist 34: 958–966

Hume D 1978 A treatise of human nature, 2nd edn. Nidditch P (ed) Oxford University Press, Oxford

Knowles M S 1984 Andragogy in action. Jossey Bass, San Francisco

Kohlberg L 1984 Essays in moral development, vol. 11, The psychology of moral development. Harper & Row, New York

Leininger M (ed) 1981 Caring: an essential human need. Proceedings of Three National Conferences. Charles Slack, New Jersey

Leininger M 1984 Care: the essence of nursing and health. Charles Slack, New Jersey

Noddings N 1984 caring: a feminine approach to ethics and moral education. University of California Press, London

Raths L, Harmin M, Simon S 1966 Values and teaching. Merrill, Columbus, Ohio

Roach M 1987 The human act of caring. Canadian Hospital Association, Ottawa

Rogers C 1951 Client centred therapy. Constable, London

Rowson R H 1990 An introduction to ethics for nurses. Scutari Press, London

Salvage J 1990 The theory and practice of the new nursing. Nursing Times Occasional Paper 86 (4): 42–45

Schon D A 1987 Educating the reflective practitioner. Jossey Bass, San Francisco

Seedhouse D 1986 Health. Foundations for achievement. John Wiley, Chichester

Seedhouse D 1988 Ethics. The heart of health care. John Wiley, Chichester

Swider S, Mcelmurry B J, Yarlinga R R 1985 Ethical decision making in a bureaucratic context by senior nursing students. Nursing Research 34 (2): 100–112

Tschudin V 1986 Ethics in nursing: the caring relationship. Heinemann, London

Tschudin V 1992 Values. A primer for nurses Workbook. Baillière Tindall, London

Udén G, Norberg A, Lindseth A, Marhanga V 1992 Ethical reasoning in nurses' and physicians' stories about care episodes. Journal of Advanced Nursing 17: 1028–1034

United Kingdom Central Council for Nursing, Midwifery and Health Visiting 1992 Code of professional conduct for the nurse, midwife and health visitor. UKCC, London

FURTHER READING

Beauchamp T, Childress J 1979 Principles of biomedical ethics. Oxford University Press, Oxford

Boykin A, Schoenhofer S 1993 Nursing and caring: a model for transforming practice. National League for Nursing, New York

Davey B, Popay J 1993 Dilemmas in health care. Open University Press, Buckingham

Department of Health 1987 A strategy for nursing: report of the steering committee. Nursing Division, Department of Health, London

Harris J 1985 The value of life. Routledge, London

Hugman R 1991 Power in caring professions. Macmillan, London

MacIntyre A 1981 After virtue, 2nd edn. Notre Dame, Indiana

Singer P (ed.) 1993 A companion to ethics. Basil Blackwell, Oxford

Thompson I, Melia K, Boyd K 1994 Nursing ethics, 3rd edn. Churchill Livingstone, Edinburgh

Williams A 1992 Cost effective analysis: is it ethical? Journal of Medical Ethics 18: 7–11

13

Legal aspects of nursing

Helen Caulfield

A good foundation in legal principles for nursing will increase each nurse's confidence in practising nursing skills, and an enhanced ability to identify potential legal problems will enable the nurse to become the advocate of his or her patients and clients. This chapter on the legal aspects of nursing aims to:

- **consider the importance of the law to nursing**
- **describe sources of the law and the system by which the legal process works**
- **explore criminal and civil law with respect to various aspects of nursing practice and different client groups**
- **outline the legal requirements for particular types of health care documentation.**

IMPORTANCE OF THE LAW

Nurses face increasing dilemmas in their practice, which require an assessment of the professional, ethical and legal aspects of many situations. Some may be obvious: what is the nurse's role when the police arrive at an accident and emergency department and ask for details about a patient's condition? Some, however, are more subtle: what about the patient with AIDS who is in great pain and requests the nurse to increase pain-relieving medication to an extent that both know the patient will die? How do nurses in the community respond to a patient who assaults them – do they have to continue providing nursing care or does the law also allow a measure of self-defence? When a nurse wishes to provide care to a child who flatly refuses to receive any treatment, how does the nurse respond, and what is the legal position of the child's refusal?

Many nurses faced with these and other situations will look to their professional Code of Conduct for guidance, or they may ask managers for assistance. Knowledge of the legal principles involved will also be important to help nurses recognise the lawful boundaries applicable to these health care situations. Employers and other members of the health care team will also know that they are required to act within the law and that failure to do so could mean a potential action in civil or criminal law.

The role of nursing is becoming more independent in some areas, and it is increasingly important that nurses working in these fields are aware, on an individual basis, of the legal principles that apply to their work. Such knowledge leads to greater confidence on the part of the nurse.

Patients and their families have an increased awareness of their rights and appear to be more willing than in the past to challenge health care decisions. Publications such as the Patient's Charter increase patients' confidence to demand greater standards for the care and treatment proposed for them. There is a perception that litigation will play an increasing part in the provision of health care services, and more people are turning to the courts for assistance on the extent and degree of health care that should be provided.

Legislation is now playing a fundamental role in determining boundaries for the provision of health care. Along with legislation providing for NHS Trusts and extended community care, other Acts of Parliament deal with, for example, access to health records, transplantation, abortion, provision of mental health care and child care.

It is becoming more important for nurses to be aware of these developments in the law, and just as important for nurses to ensure that their own practice is reflected in future legislation. The nurse who acts as the patient's advocate will influence social policy-making by demanding high standards of health care provision, and a working knowledge of legal principles in this field will enrich the nurse's own approach to his or her work.

SOURCES OF LAW

LEGISLATION

A statute is an Act of Parliament that sets out the law in a formal document. Examples of statutes are the Children Act 1989, the Human Embryology and Fertilisation Act 1990, the Access to Medical Records Act 1990 and the Medicinal Products – Prescription by Nurses etc Act 1992. Each Act of Parliament follows a formal and detailed procedure of debate and voting in the House of Commons and the House of Lords. Statutes form a body of law that set out in detail how individuals must act. If someone fails to act in accordance with any part of a statute, a criminal penalty may be imposed. For example, a driver who is found with excess alcohol in his blood may be charged with a criminal offence under the Road Traffic Acts, which set out the relevant legal limits.

Delegated or secondary legislation allows for more detailed statutory rules to be drawn up without requiring debating time in the House of Commons. The Nursing, Midwives and Health Visitors Act 1979 creates a legal duty for the United Kingdom Central Council for Nursing, Midwifery and Health Visiting (UKCC) to hold professional conduct hearings into allegations of improper conduct on the part of a nurse. The rules that govern the conduct hearing itself are provided in a statutory instrument (The Nurse, Midwives and Health Visitors Rules 1993). The effect of this statutory instrument is to oblige the UKCC to follow a certain procedure in its investigation and hearings of these matters.

A further source of legislation comes from Europe, which requires member states to implement Community law through their own Acts of Parliament. European legislation, which is also known as European Directives, encompasses a variety of issues, including the 1990 European Directive (90/269/EEC) on the manual handling of loads and Directive 92/85/EEC on the protection of the rights of pregnant workers.

COMMON LAW

Where no legislation exists to determine the law on a particular subject, common law will be used.

Common law is made by judges who sit in court and determine how a legal dispute between two or more parties is to be resolved. The law relating to negligence, for example, is not defined in a statute but has evolved over time through various court decisions. These decisions form a body of law. Patients who allege that negligent treatment has led to injury will have their disputes heard in court, and the legal principles that apply will be those of the common law of negligence.

In many health care situations, an application can be made to the court for guidance on legal issues where no legislation exists. In 1993, the legal issues surrounding the withdrawal of treatment from a patient in a persistent vegetative state were discussed in court in the case of *Airedale NHS Trust* v. *Bland* (1993). Among the arguments raised were questions of whether it was lawful to withdraw artificial hydration and nutrition from the patient, knowing that it would lead to his death. This was the first time this situation had been raised, and no other legislation existed to clarify the issues involved. Such cases become legal precedent, so that future decisions can refer back to the judicial reasoning that took place in earlier cases. The principles laid down by the court in Bland's case have already been followed in at least one other situation (*Frenchay Healthcare NHS Trust* v. *S* 1994).

DIFFERENCES BETWEEN THE LAW AND THE NURSING PROFESSIONAL BODY

The UKCC is the regulatory body of the nursing, midwifery and health visiting professions, and was set up by an Act of Parliament – the Nurses, Midwives and Health Visitors Act 1979 – later amended by a further Act (The Nurses, Midwives

and Health Visitors Act 1992). The UKCC is charged with acting as Parliament's representative in regulating the profession. The UKCC has drawn up a Code of Conduct (revised in June 1992), which sets out the extent of the professional duty required of a nurse, midwife or health visitor. It is a requirement of the UKCC that the professions adhere to the Code of Conduct, and failure to do so will potentially lead to a nurse, midwife or health visitor being disciplined or even removed from the Register.

The UKCC determines professional duty, which may differ from the nurse's legal duty. A nurse's legal duty can be defined by looking at relevant statutes and common law. There is, for example, no legal duty for a nurse to promote the interests of a patient, but there is a professional duty to do so under the Code of Conduct, paragraph 1. If a nurse appears in court for any reason, he or she may be found liable in negligence, or guilty of a criminal offence, and whilst the courts have power to order a nurse to pay compensation or to impose a criminal sentence, they do not have power to order that a nurse be prohibited from working as a nurse. The UKCC alone holds the power to determine whether or not the nurse has behaved in a professional manner.

The UKCC will not require a nurse to behave in a manner that is unlawful, and the principles behind each section of the Code of Conduct are based on the common law.

The result of this is that a nurse has a professional duty to the UKCC that may be different from the legal duty owed to clients, colleagues and employers (Wright & Caulfield 1994).

LEGAL FORUMS

Disputes that need to be resolved within the legal system will be heard in public. It is rare for a legal case to be resolved by a judge in private, although in cases where a vulnerable person is involved, such as in child abuse or mental health cases, it is common for the person to be referred to by their initials so that their full identification is protected. It is always open to the parties involved in the dispute to reach an agreement before the public hearing. This avoids any resultant publicity and helps to keep legal costs down. There are several types of legal forum, each governed by its own procedures.

Courts

There are civil courts and criminal courts, ranging from magistrates courts to high courts. Each have their own system of resolving particular cases and are considered in more detail below.

Industrial tribunals

Industrial tribunals deal with disputes relating to employment, including discrimination and redundancy. Each party is required to pay its own costs at the end of a case. The tribunal has power to hear employment cases and make rulings, which include the power to order reinstatement or a payment of compensation if a finding of unfair dismissal or discrimination is made. The Arbitration and Conciliation Advisory Service (ACAS) will attempt to arbitrate between both sides to assist in reaching a settlement before the hearing.

Inquest

The purpose of an inquest is to investigate the circumstances of a death that may not have been natural or expected. A coroner directs the hearing and can put questions directly to a witness. A jury sit and listen to the evidence and return a verdict in relation to the circumstances of the death. Any nurse who is required to attend an inquest should notify his or her manager to ask for guidance. Most employers should provide legal assistance to any nurse in this situation. Where it seems that there may be a conflict, the nurse should contact his or her professional body or trade union.

Public enquiry

A matter of national concern can be handled by a public enquiry, set up and funded by the government, in which witnesses are asked to give evidence in a formal setting. A report is published after the enquiry has ended and recommendations will be made to remedy the problems leading to the crisis. Nurses who are requested to give evidence should seek assistance in handling both the hearing and any consequent publicity. The Clothier Report in 1994 looked into the background of the murders committed by the nurse Beverly Allitt and published recommendations dealing with, among other issues, proposals for the type of health screening for prospective employers to consider.

Lawyers

The people who work within the legal system are called lawyers and may be solicitors, barristers, judges or legal executives. Solicitors are able to advise clients directly about the legal position on a case and are based in offices accessible to the public. They can represent clients in some courts and generally advise on a wide range of issues from conveyancing to divorce. Barristers are self-employed lawyers instructed by solicitors who may require detailed research into the law or to use the specialised advocacy skills of a barrister in court. The general public cannot approach a barrister directly and must go through a solicitor. After 10 years, a barrister may wish to become a Queen's Counsel (QC) and then take on more complex cases. Murder trials must be presented by a QC.

Judges are generally barristers, although more solicitors are being encouraged to apply for such positions. The role of the judge is to direct the hearing in a civil or criminal trial and ensure that the correct rules of law and procedure are applied. In a criminal case, the judge will determine the sentence if the defendant has been found guilty. In civil cases, the judge will decide the level of compensation to be awarded to a successful plaintiff.

Legal executives work in solicitors' offices, and although they are not as highly qualified as solicitors, they can deal with their own cases and see clients. Lawyers or doctors can apply to become coroners and preside over inquests; they are subject to their own rules of procedure and conduct.

CRIMINAL LAW

The criminal law is found in statutes. Anyone breaking the rules in a particular Act of Parliament could be guilty of a crime. For example, if a nurse steals sheets from the linen cupboard of a hospital and is discovered, he or she could be guilty of theft under the provisions contained in the Theft Act 1969. The police have powers to investigate a suspected crime. If the police believe that there is a criminal case, papers are sent to the Crown Prosecution Service, where an independent assessment takes place to decide whether or not prosecution should take place. If it should, the case is initially heard in the magistrates court.

Every town has a magistrates court. Magistrates (who are not lawyers) are drawn from the community and have power to decide a person's guilt or innocence and to pass sentence. When a case comes before the magistrates court that is beyond the legal powers of the magistrates to deal with, for example a charge of murder or rape, the magistrates refer the case to the crown court. In the crown court, barristers represent both the defendant and the prosecution. A judge directs the hearing before a jury of 12 people, again non-lawyers chosen from the community. It is the task of the jury to decide *beyond reasonable doubt* whether or not the defendant is guilty, and they carry out their deliberations in secret. If a finding of guilt is made, the judge can hear evidence from the defendant (a plea in mitigation) before deciding on an appropriate sentence.

The function of criminal law is to determine the boundaries of behaviour acceptable to society and within which members of society are allowed to act freely. The criminal law system is designed to allow the defendant to dispute the allegations before a representative section of society.

CRIMINAL LAW AFFECTING NURSING

A crime occurs when the legal provisions in a statute are broken. It must be shown beyond reasonable doubt that a crime has been committed, to the satisfaction of a jury, before the person charged can be convicted. Whilst it is unlikely that nurses will face the prospect of prosecution for a criminal offence in their professional careers, the advances of clinical care are constantly being tested against provisions that make up the criminal law. For example, it is an offence under the Suicide Act 1961 to assist a person to commit suicide, and there are difficulties for health professionals in interpreting this, particularly where a patient may be requesting extra medication to cope with a painful illness, which may be sufficient to end his life.

Most of the problems in assessing whether clinical treatment may or may not be criminal occur at the beginning and the ending of life, and the law has gone some way in assessing the extent of the nurse's legal role in these areas.

Abortion

The criminal law relating to abortion is found in the Abortion Act 1967, with amendments subsequently made in s. 37 Human Fertilisation and Embryology Act 1990.

It is an offence under this Act to procure an abortion unless certain conditions have been fulfilled. Where two doctors have formed an opinion in good faith that the pregnancy would involve a risk of injury to the physical or mental health of the pregnant woman or to any of her other children, and as long as the pregnancy has not progressed beyond its 24th week, a termination of the pregnancy may be lawfully carried out by a doctor. It is possible to terminate a pregnancy after the 24th week if a risk exists of grave permanent injury to the pregnant woman, including a risk to her life, or where there is a substantial risk that the child might be born with severe physical or mental handicap.

Abortion is therefore unlawful unless the criteria set out in the statute are fulfilled. The moral and ethical debate surrounding the termination of pregnancy will continue to influence any future legislation, and much debate centres on the rights of the fetus and the point at which the fetus becomes a person. The law gives full legal status to an infant born alive. A stillborn delivery has no legal standing, as the law does not give any legal rights to an embryo or fetus until it is capable of being born alive.

The Abortion Act 1967 allows a person with a conscientious objection under s.4 of the Act to withdraw from participating in treatment connected with a termination, except where treatment is needed to save the life of the woman or prevent grave permanent injury to her health.

The role of nurses in abortion is problematic and possibly not fully recognised by the legislation or subsequent judicial cases. Whilst it is clear that a nurse may rely on s.4 conscientiously to object to participating in the treatment connected with an abortion, this would seem to apply only to the abortion itself. It is less clear whether or not a nurse could refuse to care for a woman who was transferred to a general medical ward following an operation. Case example 13.1 considers how far this legislation extends.

Case example 13.1

In the case of *R.* v. *Salford Health Authority ex p. Janaway* in 1988, a doctor's receptionist refused to type the letter referring a patient for a termination. She justified her refusal by claiming conscientious objection under section 4 of the Abortion Act 1967. The court found that the receptionist was so removed from the actual treatment that s.4 did not apply to her. This test of proximity is a difficult one to assess in relation to nurses, particularly where they may be expected to move around a hospital in a far more flexible manner than a doctor, who may be assigned to a particular ward.

Death and dying

Allowing the patient to die can be complex in law. There is a legal difference between letting something happen and active intervention to ensure that it occurs. The law accepts that each person has the legal right to determine what will happen to his or her body, and interference by a third party may be unlawful.

There is no legislation that allows euthanasia, and the intentional killing of another person is murder. Where a health care practitioner wishes to assist a patient to die through some form of intervention, a charge of manslaughter may be brought if the intervention was unlawful. This

will be the case even where the patient requests assistance, for example by an increased level of medication in order to cause death. In *R.* v. *Cox* (1992), a doctor was convicted of attempted murder after he gave an injection of potassium chloride to a patient with an incurable illness, knowing that she would die almost immediately.

It is lawful to provide treatment to relieve pain and suffering even where this may have the unintended effect of hastening death, and treatment for these purposes will not constitute manslaughter. In the Cox case, the injection of potassium chloride was intended to cause death rather than to relieve pain and suffering, and was as such a criminal offence.

Where the patient is unable to be involved in the decision-making process, the legal concept of 'best interests' has been used to decide the most effective care that should be provided. This has arisen in relation to the selective non-treatment of severely handicapped neonates. When a child is born with severe physical and mental handicaps, the choice is to provide intensive therapy, usually involving surgery, to alleviate symptoms and prolong life, or to make a decision to provide only pain-relieving medication when there is a possibility that the child will die. When such cases come to court, the argument of best interests is used to determine which treatment programme should be followed. In *Re C* (1989), the court directed that a hydrocephalic child should be treated in such a way that she would end her life peacefully. It was considered to be in the best interests of the child that she be given non-invasive treatment.

In the *Bland* case cited above, a different situation was presented to the court. The patient had been in a persistent vegetative state for over $3\frac{1}{2}$ years following injuries sustained at Hillsborough Football Stadium. He was on a ventilator, and was receiving artificial hydration and nutrition. The court was asked to consider whether the withdrawal of artificial hydration and nutrition would be lawful. Legal argument took place in the high court, the court of appeal and the House of Lords, where it was agreed that there was no prospect of recovery from this condition and that the withdrawal of the treatment would be in the patient's best interests. It was accepted that, by removing this treatment the patient would die, and that it was lawful for the doctors to proceed in this manner as continuation of the treatment would be futile. In the absence of any subsequent legislation, it will be for the court to decide the criteria to be used in assessing the legal definition of a patient's best interests when deciding whether treatment should be given or withdrawn.

Assault

It is a reflection of the changing nature of relationships that there is an increasing number of recorded assaults by patients on nurses. These occur most commonly in community, psychiatric and accident and emergency nursing. Most employers have a policy that means the assailant is not reported to the police, and no prosecution takes place. Very often, the attack may be the manifestation of the illness that is being treated.

Where a prosecution does take place, it will be heard in the magistrates court, and the nurse attacked will be required to give evidence. If the assailant is found guilty, the magistrates have powers to order that an amount of compensation be paid to the nurse by the assailant.

If the injuries sustained are serious and result in the nurse taking time off work to recover physically or psychologically, it is possible to make an application to the Criminal Injuries Compensation Board, which can make a separate award of compensation for injuries received as a result of a violent attack without the necessity for a criminal prosecution.

Nurses are legally entitled to use a measure of self-protection if they fear an attack from a patient. The measure of self-defence must be in proportion to the threat or attack itself: it would be reasonable for a nurse to push a patient who was threatening to strangle him or her, but it would not be reasonable for a nurse to do this if the patient were shouting abuse. Most hospitals have introduced control and restraint courses, from which nurses can learn non-violent means of deflecting perceived or actual attacks. When any attack takes place, even if there is no injury, it is imperative that it is reported immediately so

that appropriate steps for the safety of the nurse and the patient can be taken.

CIVIL LAW

Civil law is designed to resolve differences between individuals. As a consequence, civil law encompasses a wider range of issues than does criminal law, including negligence, employment, divorce, child care, libel, defamation and any other matter that is not criminal in nature.

Because civil law is concerned with disputes between parties, court hearings do not require the use of magistrates or a jury (with the historic exception of libel hearings, which need to be heard before a jury). Matters that involve claims of up to £3000 are heard in the small claims court without the active involvement of lawyers. Civil law cases that do require the use of lawyers will be heard in either the county court or, if the matter is more complex, the high court.

CIVIL LAW AFFECTING NURSING

The majority of health care situations that need legal involvement will be civil matters. It will be far more common for a nurse to be affected by civil law than criminal law decisions. Some of the most important areas of civil law are assessed here. The development of health law is constantly reshaping nursing practice, although the basic principles set out below should remain unchanged.

Consent

It is an established part of law that no treatment can be given to a person without consent – this is a fundamental foundation of the law. Any clinical professional who touches a patient or client without consent commits a battery that is both a civil and a criminal offence. It is extremely rare for a health care professional to be prosecuted under the criminal law for battery, but civil actions brought by patients for an unlawful touching are more common (*Devi* v. *West Midlands RHA* 1981, *Marshall* v. *Curry* 1993). If a nurse gives an injection to a patient who has not consented to being touched, the nurse will have acted unlawfully and will have committed a battery.

It is important that the consent itself must be obtained in a way that does not render it invalid. If a nurse tries to persuade a patient to agree to invasive treatment by, for example, threatening the patient, it will automatically mean that any agreement given by the patient becomes invalid, as the consent was not obtained voluntarily. In this situation, even where the patient says yes and signs a consent form, the consent will have been obtained in an unlawful manner and any subsequent treatment will also be unlawful.

In order for a consent to be valid it must consist of three elements:

- The person giving consent must have the capacity to do so.
- The consent given must be informed.
- The consent must be given in a voluntary manner.

1. The person giving consent must have the capacity to do so. It is vital that a person giving consent has the capacity to understand what is involved in the proposed treatment. It is accepted that adults over the age of 18 automatically have the relevant capacity to understand and make their own decisions about medical and nursing treatment.

2. The consent given must be informed. Informed consent has caused much discussion among health care professionals. Just how much information needs to be given to a person before he or she has enough on which to make a decision? The most famous case on this point is that of *Sidaway* v. *Board of Governors of Bethlem Royal Hospital* (1985) (Case example 13.2).

There is no duty imposed by law on a health care professional to inform the patient of all the likely risks or advantages in the proposed treatment, and the courts have held that the extent of what to tell the patient lies within the doctor's discretion. If the patient asks questions, these should be answered truthfully, but again the doctor can use discretion on the amount of information that should be volunteered, and he or she can withhold information for good reason (although this may require later justification if the case ever comes to court).

Case example 13.2

Amy Sidaway agreed to an operation. She was not told that there was a very small risk that her spinal cord might be damaged. In the operation the risk materialised, and she suffered partial paralysis. She argued that she would not have consented to the procedure had she been told of the risk, and her claim in court was that her whole consent was invalid as she had not received sufficient information to make an informed consent. This argument was rejected by the House of Lords, who found that the doctor had fulfilled his duties in relation to informed consent by telling the patient of the material risks, alternatives to the treatment and the nature and consequences of the proposed treatment. In addition, there is a duty on the doctor to assess whether the particular patient requires any further information.

How does an individual nurse decide what information should be given and what could be held back? The test for this was formulated in the case of *Bolam* v. *Friern Hospital Management Committee* (1957), in which the court decided that the standard of care required of a nurse is to act in accordance with a recognised body of nursing opinion and practice. The standard is therefore determined by the nursing profession itself and not by reference to an individual patient. This standard of care has been criticised for failing to give sufficient weight to the patient's own circumstances, and it has been suggested that a nurse or doctor should provide the patient with all the information in his or her possession in order to enable the patient to make an informed decision. This has been largely rejected by the courts as being impractical and overburdensome on the health care professional.

3. The consent must be given in a voluntary manner. Consent must be freely given and no threats or implied threats used. Threats such as the use of a compulsory section under the Mental Health Act 1984 if treatment is not accepted nullify the consent. Whether treatment is voluntary will depend on what information is given to the patient and how this is presented. Coercion or manipulation of the patient would tend to imply that the consent has not been obtained voluntarily.

Once these three criteria have been established, a valid consent can be given to treatment or care.

Most hospitals require patients to sign a consent form before agreeing to invasive treatment, and some health professionals have mistakenly placed too much emphasis on such a signature being obtained. A signed consent form does not prove that the consent is valid, but it is usually good evidence that a discussion on consent has taken place. In this context, a consent form is important evidence, but it should never be considered the sole factor needed to be taken into account in establishing proper consent with patients.

Particular aspects of consent in relation to different sections of society need separate consideration, and are dealt with below.

Young people

Those over the age of 18 years are allowed to make their own decisions about treatment and care. Between the ages of 16 and 18 years, adolescents can consent to treatment under the provisions of the Family Law Reform Act s.8 (1). The more problematic area concerns adolescents under the age of 16. The legal position is established in *Gillick* v. *West Norfolk and Norwich AHA* (1985), which allows adolescents under 16 years to consent to treatment provided they have sufficient understanding and intelligence to enable them to understand fully what is proposed. Adolescents of sufficient understanding to make an informed decision have the right to consent to examination and treatment. They also have the right to refuse the treatment or care. The question of deciding whether or not an adolescent is capable of understanding is determined by the doctor, although it is likely that nurses, for example, would be able to give treatment to children when they have made a professional assessment that the child has the understanding to know what is proposed and involved in the nursing treatment.

Where the child is not capable of giving consent, the guardian of a child under the age of 16 years may give valid consent on behalf of the child.

The court has, however, indicated that such a child does not have the final say in refusing treatment, and has held that any refusal of treatment by a child is not conclusive (*Re W* 1992). It is open to the parents or guardians to override

that refusal and to consent to the treatment proposed by the health professional. Where a nurse is confronted with a strong difference of opinion between a child and a parent or guardian over proposed treatment, the nurse should always seek advice to ensure the correct weight is given to the child's wishes. In some situations, it may be necessary to ask the court to decide between the conflicting wishes. For example, if a 14-year-old girl involved in a road accident refuses any blood transfusions because of her religious beliefs, her parents may want to override her refusal so that treatment can proceed. It may be difficult for the doctor or nurse to determine how far the child's wishes should be taken into account. In this type of situation, a court would be able to hear the evidence and make a decision to be followed by all parties.

Adults

In contrast to the rights of a child to refuse treatment, the Court of Appeal upheld a case in 1992 that affirmed in strong terms an adult patient's right to refuse medical treatment (*Re T* 1992). In this case, a woman aged 22 years old was involved in a car accident and, while in hospital, told medical staff both orally and in writing that she did not want a blood transfusion should one become necessary. Her condition deteriorated and she was placed on a ventilator. When it became apparent that a blood transfusion would be required, she was unable to give specific consent or refusal. The Court of Appeal upheld the view that a competent adult patient has a right to refuse medical treatment even if the outcome will be that the patient will die. Any health care professional who ignores a valid refusal and carries out treatment will commit a battery. The impact of this case means that a terminally ill patient can refuse to receive any further treatment, and the doctor or nurse who accords with these wishes will not be held responsible for committing the crime of aiding and abetting a suicide.

What about the patient who is admitted in a state of unconsciousness who is clearly unable to provide consent to any proposed emergency treatment? It would be difficult to support a view that any subsequent touching or treatment would constitute battery in the absence of consent, because it is simply not possible to obtain this from the patient. The law accepts that treatment should be given where it is in the best interests of the patient to save life or preserve health, and that, in these circumstances, there is no necessity to obtain consent. It is, however, not possible for non-urgent medical or nursing treatment to be given to such a patient and in these circumstances, it would be unlawful to proceed with that treatment. It is necessary in those situations to wait for the patient to regain consciousness and then obtain consent.

There may be an issue of conflict between a mother and her unborn child where the mother's refusal of treatment puts the life of the child at risk. The high court was asked to consider this issue in 1992 (*Re S* 1992). A woman in labour refused a caesarean operation because of her religious beliefs. The health authority asked the high court for a declaration that the operation would be lawful, despite its being against the mother's wishes. The health authority argued that the operation was necessary to save the life of the child. The court granted this declaration and ordered that the caesarean operation proceed, on the basis that it was in the interests of both mother and child to have the operation as, without this intervention, it was likely that both would die. This decision has caused concern that the interests of the unborn child may take precedence over those of an adult woman, and this case goes against the principles laid down in other cases that give legal respect to the wishes of an adult.

Elderly care

Nursing older people brings its own complications when assessing consent, particularly with the onset of dementia. Where this occurs it could well be that capacity based on understanding will vary. The older person suffering from dementia may have periods of complete lucidity in which he or she can determine exactly what is wished in terms of medical or nursing care. On other occasions, this may not be possible. In these situations, it will be necessary for the nurse to assess the patient's ability to understand the proposed treatment or care before each procedure takes place. Dementia may be a situation in which medical technology will allow a clearer assessment of these periods of fluctuating capacity, but, in the meantime, it remains one of the hardest areas to resolve in terms of capacity and consent.

This particular difficulty is highlighted in a situation in which a patient refuses to have a particular type of treatment or care. Some difficulty may exist for nurses who are motivated to act in the best interests of the patient. When the older person's choice accords with nursing practice, the level of competence of that person is rarely assessed. Since the older person agrees with the treatment that is being proposed, many nurses automatically assume that the patient has capacity to consent. Because the treatment being proposed will always be in the patient's own interests, it is assumed that a patient who consents to that treatment is showing the necessary capacity to understand what is involved. Difficulties arise when a patient refuses certain treatment. In such a situation, it seems that nurses demand a much higher level of understanding in order to satisfy themselves that the patient has capacity, even though he or she is now actively choosing a course not deemed to be in his or her best interests.

The importance of a refusal from an older person seems to be that it triggers a fresh evaluation of understanding, but it does not mean that because the person refuses to agree with the nurse's proposals that he or she has necessarily lost the understanding that is crucial to give consent. There have been no cases dealing with this problem yet that would provide legal guidance.

Mental health

Adults who are incapable of giving consent because of mental illness can receive treatment under the provisions of the Mental Health Act 1984 for that disorder. However, there may be some situations in which a person with a mental disorder may require medical treatment for some other condition. The dilemma here is that the person has no capacity to consent on their own behalf, and, because they have reached adult status, there can be no guardian to make the decision for them. In such circumstances, there will be a hearing before a judge to determine whether or not the proposed treatment is in that person's best interests. Cases have involved a proposal to sterilise an adult mentally ill woman who was unable to provide legal consent or refusal. The court assessed the operation would be in her best interests (*F* v. *West Berkshire HA* 1989).

The court has held that some patients with mental disorder can refuse treatment for a condition unrelated to that disorder (Case example 13.3).

Case example 13.3

In September 1993, doctors at Broadmoor Hospital discovered gangrene in a patient's foot and informed him that unless the foot and part of the leg were amputated, he faced imminent death. The patient, who suffered from chronic paranoid schizophrenia, was transferred to the local hospital. He refused to consent to the amputation. He applied to the court for an injunction restraining the hospital and the surgeons from amputating his leg, both then and in the future, unless he gave his express, written, valid consent. The judge was satisfied that the patient understood the proposed treatment and believed what he had been told about it, and that the patient was capable of balancing the risks. Although his general capacity was impaired, the judge found that it was not established that the patient did not understand the nature, purpose and effects of the treatment he refused (*Re C* 1994). The ruling in that case gives clear authority for the legal binding status of advance directives, which has importance particularly for mental health patients who may wish to give an advance directive about their future treatment. A patient who suffers from psychotic states of mind may have rational and lucid periods, in which he or she has sufficient capacity to make a decision to decide on future mental, medical and nursing treatment.

Negligence

The possibility of an action in negligence is one that is feared by more nurses than any other area of law. When a procedure goes wrong and involves injury to a person, the possibility of an action in negligence must always be considered. The same applies equally if a nurse is himself or herself injured in the course of employment, and it is open to the nurse to consider bringing a claim of negligence against the employer. The law on negligence has been determined through common law, and the following principles emerge that need to be established before a claim in negligence can be successful.

1. There must be a duty of care owed by one person to another. This principle was established in the case of *Donohoe* v. *Stevenson* (1932). In that case, a woman in a tea shop drank a bottle of ginger beer and discovered the remains of a decomposed snail at the bottom. She was ill as a result. The court held that the manufacturer of the ginger beer owed a duty of care to its ultimate consumers to provide them with a beverage free from impurity. The principle of the duty of care applies in a nurse–patient relationship as well as an employer–nurse relationship, and a duty of care exists between these parties that could give rise to an action in negligence.

The extent to which one person may owe a duty of care to another has been discussed in relation to nervous shock suffered by a person who witnesses an accident. Whilst anyone may suffer nervous shock by witnessing injuries occurring to another person, the courts have held that in order to justify a claim that the person causing the accident owed a duty of care to prevent nervous shock, it is necessary to show a family relationship with the injured person.

2. The duty of care is broken when one person fails to do what a 'reasonable' person would or would not do in the circumstances. The test to determine whether or not a person has acted as a reasonable person is judged by an objective test called the Bolam test (from *Bolam* v. *Friern Hospital Management Committee* 1957). The standard of care required of a nurse in establishing whether or not a duty of care has been broken is to assess what a reasonable nurse would or would not have done in the circumstances according to a recognised body of nursing opinion. If a patient on a 24-bedded ward falls out of bed and breaks a leg, it is open to the patient to claim that the staff owed a duty of care to ensure his safety and well-being. In order to prove that the duty of care has been broken, it will be necessary for the patient to demonstrate that reasonable steps could have been taken to prevent him falling out of bed.

3. The injury caused must arise directly from the duty of care that has been broken. This is best illustrated by the case of *Barnet* v. *Chelsea & Kensington HNC* (1969) (Case example 13.4).

Case example 13.4

Three night watchmen presented at a casualty department complaining of vomiting. The nurse on duty took their details and telephoned the casualty officer, who listened to the nurse's report and gave telephone advice that the men should go home and seek GP treatment. The nurse accurately relayed this information to the night watchmen. Shortly afterwards, one night watchman died, and the post mortem revealed that all three had been subject to arsenic poisoning after someone had laced their flasks of tea, which they had drunk earlier that night. The widow sued the hospital in negligence.

The court held that both the nurse and the casualty doctor owed a duty of care to the night watchmen. It was found that the nurse had behaved as a reasonable nurse, according to the Bolam test, in taking advice from the casualty officer and relaying this to the night watchmen. It was therefore ascertained that the nurse had not broken her duty of care, and therefore any claim in negligence against her failed at that point.

The casualty officer's decision not to come and investigate the night watchmen was held to be sufficient to break the duty of care, as it was demonstrated that a reasonable casualty officer would have examined the men. However, independent medical evidence showed that the night watchman would have died in any event because of the arsenic poisoning, and the lack of intervention on the part of the casualty officer was not a material cause of death. It could not be demonstrated therefore that the death was directly attributable to the negligent omission of the casualty officer. In these circumstances, the action in negligence failed.

It is worthwhile considering at this point the different standards that might be applied to nursing practice by the law and by the nursing professional body. In Case example 13.4, it is shown that the law requires all three elements of negligence to be proved before an action can succeed. In this case, therefore, even if the nurse had broken her duty of care, the law would not have made a finding of negligence against her, because the death was not connected with her action. It is interesting to note that the UKCC does not require that the third legal element of negligence be proved before they can investigate

whether a nurse has been guilty of misconduct, and the UKCC may indeed investigate the actions of a nurse without reference to any legal position in a finding of negligence.

In an action for negligence, there is a time limit of 3 years from the date the injury occurs or the person becomes aware of the injury to the date on which the court must be notified that a claim is being brought. No claim in negligence for personal injury can be made outside this 3-year period. Where children have been injured potentially as a result of negligence, they are allowed to reach adult status before the 3-year period runs. Therefore if a 6-year-old is involved in a road traffic accident in which somebody else was responsible, that child is allowed to reach the age of majority, i.e. 18, and then have a further 3 years, i.e. until the age of 21, before notifying the court of an intention to sue for negligence.

In most nursing practice, the principle of vicarious liability will mean that any omission or error made by a nurse that may result in an action for negligence will not be brought directly against that nurse but against the nurse's employer. The principle of vicarious liability means that the employer is responsible for all the actions of its employees that are carried out in the course of employment. However, the fact that a nurse may not be named on the court documents does not mean that he or she will not be very closely involved in any subsequent proceedings, and that nurse will generally be required to give evidence in court.

In an emergency situation, it may not be possible to assess how a reasonable nurse should act in the circumstances. Where a patient is involved in a road traffic accident and a nurse comes across the scene outside the course of his or her employment, there is no positive duty on the nurse to become involved in helping the injured victims. If the nurse chooses to become involved and apply what first aid knowledge he or she has that may help the situation, no action in negligence can be brought against that nurse if the steps taken make the condition of the patient worse. Although the general public may mistakenly assume that any nurse is also a qualified first aider to deal with accident situations, this is not always the case.

Confidentiality

Confidentiality is a fundamental part of the nurse–patient relationship. Information given to a nurse in the context of a nurse–patient relationship must be protected. The law on confidentiality also applies to other professionals who are in a professional relationship, and covers lawyers and their clients as well as, for example, banks and their customers. The law will uphold and protect confidentiality in situations where a relationship is established in which one person agrees to give information about themselves to another in the trust that it will be kept confidential.

Any information given to a nurse should not be passed on to a third party without consent. It is accepted that the nurse may be required to pass some patient information to other members of the health care team if it is necessary for the team to know of the patient's condition to provide effective health care. In this situation, it is implied that the patient gives consent for the nurse to pass on the relevant information.

If a nurse passes information about the patient to a third party outside the health care team, a breach of confidentiality will have occurred. It is possible for the patient to bring a civil action against the individual nurse and to sue the nurse for breach of confidentiality. Equally, it is open to a patient who is told that information is about to be passed to a third party to bring a civil action and seek an injunction, in which the court will be asked to make an order preventing the information being passed to a third party (Case example 13.5).

Where a breach of confidentiality has occurred that is successfully pursued in court, it will result in a payment of compensation to the aggrieved patient.

No breach of confidentiality will occur when a court order requires specific disclosure of patient information. A court order demanding disclosure overrides the duty of confidentiality, and nurses are under a legal duty to comply fully with the

Case example 13.5

In 1988, a journalist discovered details of two hospital doctors who had been diagnosed as having Aids. The journalist intended to publish details about the doctors. The hospital employing the doctors sought an injunction to prevent publication. In court, the journalist argued that such disclosure was justified on the grounds that it affected the public interest, but this argument was rejected by the court, which ordered an injunction to prevent publication of the article (*X* v. *Y* 1988).

terms of any court order. No breach of confidentiality occurs in these circumstances.

Equally, where a patient consents to information being passed to a third party, no breach of confidentiality occurs. Consent is the key issue, and the law requires that no disclosure to a third party is made without this consent.

The only defence allowed to a breach of confidentiality is that it is justified in the public interest. The burden falls on the person breaking the confidence to prove that his or her actions were so justified.

The UKCC Code of Conduct follows these legal principles, and the UKCC has published a separate document dealing with this subject (United Kingdom Central Council for Nursing, Midwifery and Health Visiting 1987).

The prime difficulty for nurses in the area of confidentiality is in determining whether or not information can indeed be passed to a third party if the patient specifically declines to give consent. Individual nurses will need to assess whether or not there is sufficient public interest arising in any case to determine whether a breach of confidentiality would be justified. Even where a nurse makes this assessment, a court may take a different view of the justification and rule that a breach of confidentiality had occurred that was not justified.

The justification for a breach of confidentiality in the public interest has evolved through civil cases in which confidentiality has been a key issue. The courts have, in the past, held that such breaches are justified where a person had been involved in criminal activity or behaved so disgracefully that it was judged in the public interest to expose that behaviour. In these cases, no breach of confidentiality has occurred. These cases have generally involved confidentiality connected with banking practice.

There are also circumstances in which there may be no wrongdoing on the part of an individual but where it is considered vital to make confidential information known on a public basis. An example of this would be a significant breakthrough in medical technology, such as the first successful heart and lung transplant.

There have been no legal cases that deal with a nurse's proposed or actual breach of confidentiality. In *W v.* Edgell (1990), the case concerned a doctor's breach of confidentiality. In this case, the patient sued Dr Edgell for disclosing a psychiatric report to the medical director of a special hospital. The report indicated that the patient was unfit to be considered for discharge. The patient had specifically refused to give consent for this report to be disclosed to the medical director, and when Dr Edgell took this step, the patient sued for breach of confidence. It was not disputed in the court that the report had been disclosed to the medical director against the specific wishes of the patient. The doctor argued that this breach of confidence was allowed on the grounds that disclosure was justified in the public interest. He maintained that there was a fear of real risk to public safety were the patient discharged. The court of appeal accepted this defence and made no order of compensation. They commented that only the most compelling circumstances would justify a doctor acting in this way, and that the defence of disclosure in the public interest should only be used in the strictest circumstances possible. The court felt that, in every case, the doctor should seek to obtain the patient's consent before breaching confidentiality.

The UKCC takes a similarly guarded approach to breaches of confidentiality in dealing with the public interest element. It considers that disclosure in the public interest could be justified if the nurse became aware of issues affecting society in which criminal activity of a serious nature, such as child abuse or drug trafficking, was involved.

Some contracts of employment include a clause requiring the nurse to keep confidential all information learned about the work environment, and in some cases, the nurse is required to respect this confidence even after the employment contract has terminated and the nurse is working elsewhere. In addition, many hospitals now have policies for staff to follow when police or journalists make enquires about a patient. The decision of whether or not to provide such people with information about a patient is not one that any member of staff should make without assessing the employer's policy on this issue. There is no requirement to pass information to police making enquiries, even when they are investigating criminal activity, unless the nurse in charge feels that such criminal activity falls within the boundaries provided by the UKCC in defining the public interest. In addition, that nurse should also be able to justify his or her own actions at any later stage should the patient make a claim that a breach of confidentiality has occurred.

DOCUMENTATION

Should patients be allowed to keep their own medical and nursing notes and read what is written on them? In the past, patient records have been kept secret even from patients, and disclosure was generally only allowed with a court order. Recent legislation allows the patient to have greater access to the information written in certain circumstances, which is viewed as increasing patient autonomy.

The Secretary of State for Health assigns by delegation to the Health Authority or NHS Trust the duty to keep records on patients. The paperwork on which these records are completed belongs to the Health Authority or NHS Trust; it does not belong to the patient, and the patient has no right of automatic access to the records that are kept.

Legislation allows the patient to have access to the information kept in certain circumstances, as outlined below.

Data Protection Act 1984

This Act and the subsequent Order allow the patient to have access to electronically stored data by giving sufficient notice in a required form. The Act does not apply to manually kept records.

Access to Medical Reports Act 1988

This Act only applies to reports made for insurance or employment purposes, and does not cover any notes made about a patient's condition. A patient has a right to see a medical report compiled by a doctor with responsibility for his clinical care if this is then to be sent to an insurance company or employer.

Access to Health Records Act 1990

This Act provides a right of access by patients to records kept about them that were created on or after 1 November 1991. A request can be made in writing, enclosing the set fee plus reasonable photocopying charges, and the patient can then receive copies of these notes. No fee can be charged for records that are less than 40 days old. This Act only applies to manual records. It means that there is no right to access manually kept information created before 1 November 1991.

It is open to the holder of the manually or electronically stored records to refuse disclosure if, in the opinion of the holder, it is decided that disclosure would cause serious harm to the physical or mental health of the patient. The Act does not require the holder of information to justify such a decision.

Wills

Adults of sound mind can sign their own Will, and it is open to anyone to write out the Will for themselves, although it is always better if a solicitor drafts the will to avoid any possible misinterpretation or confusion about the wishes of the person making the Will. Anyone can witness a Will being signed, although they lose their entitlement to benefit from the Will if this happens. If a patient wants to leave a gift to a nurse in a Will, the nurse should check his or her employer's policy and seek professional advice to avoid the possible implication of fraud. A nurse who is receiving a benefit from the Will should not witness it.

The rules for signing a Will need to be complied with exactly for the Will to be valid. The person making the Will is called the testator. He or she needs to sign the Will in the presence of two independent witnesses, who then need to sign their own names on the Will in the presence of the other witness and the testator. It is not sufficient for two people to attend as witnesses and sign the Will at separate times; if this happens, the whole Will becomes invalid.

Accident and incident reports

It is important that all incidents involving a nurse are recorded on the appropriate accident or incident report, even where no injury has been sustained by the nurse. Accident reports are necessary in assessing risk that may arise in the place of work, and the available statistics may need the employer to take some steps to reduce the occurrence of incidents that lead to injury.

Summary

In his or her everyday practice, the nurse increasingly faces a range of professional, ethical and legal dilemmas, of varying degrees of complexity. Having a good basic knowledge of legal principles will enable the nurse to be more aware of potential problems and be able to act as the patient's advocate. To this end, this chapter describes in some detail the sources of the law and how the legal process operates. This is then specifically applied to nursing, special mention being made of particular client groups and areas of practice.

The use of legal remedies will form an increasing part of practice for nurses in the future. As patients' rights continue to be developed, the nurse's role will be further shaped by legislation and legal precedent. It will be important for all nurses to have a good working knowledge of the basic legal principles that apply to their practice. As nurses move into fields of specialisation, the law applicable to each area will assume an even greater importance.

REFERENCES

Airedale NHS Trust *v.* Bland [1993] 1 All ER 821
Barnet *v.* Chelsea & Kensington HMC [1969] 1 QB 428
Bolam *v.* Friern Hospital Management Committee [1957] 2 All ER 118
Devi *v.* West Midlands RHA [1981] CA 491
Marshall *v.* Curry [1993] 3 DLR 260
Donohoe *v.* Stevenson [1932] AC 562
F *v.* West Berkshire HA [1989] 2 All ER 545
Frenchay Healthcare NHS Trust *v.* S (1994) The Times, 19 January 1994
Gillick *v.* West Norfolk and Norwich AHA [1985] 3 All ER 402
The Nurses, Midwives and Health Visitors (Professional Conduct) Rules 1993. SI 1993 No. 893. HMSO, London
R. *v.* Cox (1992) 12 BMLR 38
Re C (A minor) (wardship: medical treatment) [1989] 2 All ER 782
Re C (adult: refusal of medical treatment) [1994] 1 All ER 819
Re S (adult: refusal of medical treatment) [1992] 4 All ER 671
Re T (adult) (refusal of medical treatment) [1992] 4 All ER 649
Re W (a minor) (medical treatment) [1992] 4 All ER 627

Sidaway *v.* Board of Governors of Bethlem Royal Hospital [1985] 1 All ER 643
United Kingdom Central Council for Nursing, Midwifery and Health Visiting 1987 Confidentiality. UKCC Advisory Paper. UKCC, London
W *v.* Edgell [1990] 1 All ER 835
Wright S, Caulfield H 1994 Defining nurses' and doctors' duty of care. Nursing Standard
X *v.* Y [1988] 2 All ER 648

FURTHER READING

There are relatively few books and articles available on the application of the law to nursing practice. The majority still cover medical practice. The following suggestions deal with nursing issues.

Mason, McCall Smith 1994 Law and medical ethics, 4th edn. Butterworths, London
Brazier 1992 Medicine, patients and the law, 2nd edn. Penguin, London
Montgomery 1989 Nursing and the law. Macmillan, London
Dimond 1995 Legal aspects of nursing, 2nd edn. Prentice Hall, London

14 Concepts of individual care

Peter Draper

The main purpose of this chapter is to explore the nature of nursing. To achieve this, the chapter will:

- examine the historical development of models of nursing care
- discuss the meaning and application of various concepts, models and theories that nurses use to plan their work and explain it to others
- outline the way in which such models are applied through the nursing process
- explore nursing theory, the relationship between concepts, theories, models and nursing practice.

There are two reasons why we should consider the nature of nursing. The first is that nursing models, the nursing process and other theoretical ideas have a major impact on modern nursing practice, and their influence will be seen in many of the clinical areas visited during professional education. The second reason is that the boundaries of nursing practice are constantly changing in response to the pressure brought to bear by new legislation and changing work patterns among other members of the health care team. If we, as nurses, are to remain in charge of our professional destiny, it is important that we are able to discuss the nature of our work and defend it to others.

What, then, is nursing? This is a question that has fascinated practitioners since the days of

Florence Nightingale. One way of gaining an answer to the question is to observe a group of nurses at work and to write down the things that one sees them doing. A list produced in this way might include activities such as measuring blood pressure, talking to people, helping patients to take a bath, conducting assessments and reading nursing journals. Such a list would emphasise the *doing* aspects of nursing work. It would be useful because a good deal of nursing time is spent on activities of this type, but many practitioners would argue that this would only be a partial answer to the question 'What is nursing?'. For a full answer, we would need to know not only *what* nurses do, but *why* they do it. Why, for instance, do nurses appear to spend so much time assessing patients and completing records? Why do they encourage patients with diabetes to test their own urine? Why do nurses read books on research methods?

The most fruitful way of answering these questions is to review and discuss some of the answers given by nurse practitioners and academics in a body of literature known as 'nursing theory'. In doing this, we will begin by putting our discussion in its historical context.

MODELS OF CARE: A CRITICAL HISTORY

Although nursing has not always existed as a distinct occupation in the way that it does today, there have always been people (usually women) who have accepted the responsibility of caring for the sick, nourishing children, bringing infants into the world and attending to the dead. There is a sense, therefore, in which nursing is a universal human activity.

Nursing was probably first practised on what we might loosely call a 'professional' basis by the Knights of St John Hospitaler. The Knights of St John were warrior monks who offered nursing care to people sick and injured during the Crusades. From that time onwards, some have regarded nursing as a vocation to be practised

by the members of religious orders who regard the care of the sick as a duty towards God. It is likely that these ancient practitioners possessed considerable skill in the use of herbs and other pre-scientific remedies.

The roots of the modern nursing profession are closely intertwined with the development of medicine, the invention of the hospital as a specialist centre for the treatment of disease, and the social position of women in the Victorian and pre-Victorian eras. Hospitals were the response of an industrial age to the problem of disease. As repositories of sickness, they enabled patients to be brought together for treatment and scientific study in a way that was convenient for medical practitioners. The demands of private work undertaken to compensate for honorary appointments in the voluntary hospitals meant that doctors were only ever intermittently present on hospital wards. Nurses, on the other hand, were able to provide continuous patient supervision (Rafferty 1993).

As hospitals grew in size and complexity, the pattern of relationships that developed between various groups of employees mirrored the social structure of wider society. The male-dominated medical profession exercised unquestioned authority in hospitals, reflecting the position of the father in the Victorian home. The nursing profession was almost exclusive in its employment of women. Nurses in the hospital, like women in the middle-class Victorian home, were concerned with domestic matters, such as cleanliness, the administration of food and the moral health of their charges. The distribution of work between nurses and doctors that evolved in the Victorian era, and the medical approach to understanding disease, still influences the organisation of work in the modern health service (see Ch. 11).

Historically, the medical profession has not only had the power to determine the nature of nursing work, but has also defined the way in which disease is understood and treated. The medical approach (or the medical model, as it is sometimes called) views people with diseases in much the same way as an engineer views a faulty machine: symptoms are the result of physiological and anatomical defects, and can be eliminated if the underlying disorder is corrected. It should be recognised that the medical approach to disease is enormously powerful and has been very successful in certain respects. It has enabled medical scientists to understand what is going wrong in all sorts of disease states. For instance, medical scientists have discovered that all of the acute symptoms of diabetes mellitus can be explained by the failure of the pancreas to produce insulin and can be corrected if insulin from an external source is given. However, the medical model also has its limitations. Many diseases have complex causes that include social influences as well as anatomical and physiological defects. Case example 14.1 will help you to understand this point.

Case example 14.1 shows us that the causes of ill-health are complex, and that the medical approach, for all its power, has clear limitations.

The medical approach has been the dominant influence on the organisation of health care within hospitals. As such, it has had and continues to have an effect upon the way in which nursing is organised. Sometimes, this influence has been positive. At other times, however, it has had a harmful effect upon patients. Research has shown that the medical model is particularly inappropriate as a way of organising the care of people whose health problems have a pronounced social component, such as frail, older adults with chronic ill-health (Robb 1967, Baker 1978) or people who have a profound learning disability. The medical model also has little to offer to people who are suffering from the predictable consequences of acute illness, such as bereavement.

In the 1970s, nurses began to question the dominance of the medical model. At this time, considerable effort was invested in devising and developing approaches to organising care that emphasised the distinctive nursing contribution to illness and the promotion of wellness. The first major change to occur was the introduction of an approach to the management of patient care that focused on the problems patients faced, rather than the diseases from which they were

Case example 14.1 Tommy's broken leg

Tommy Jones is a boy of 10 admitted to the hospital with a broken leg, after being hit by a car whilst cycling to school. The fracture, which affects the tibia (shin bone), is a simple one, meaning that the skin is not broken.

A medical approach

Tommy is admitted to hospital. The leg is X-rayed, and a fracture is discovered. Tommy is given an anaesthetic, the broken bones are realigned, and the leg is encased in plaster to splint it. Analgesics are given for the pain, and Tommy is taught how to walk with crutches. After a few days in hospital, he is discharged home with an appointment at the orthopaedic outpatient department. Three months later, the cast is removed, and Tommy is discharged.

A social approach

The immediate cause of Tommy's broken leg is the car that hit him. Tommy is one of thousands of children injured in similar accidents every year. Behind the statistics lies an increase in the popularity of the motor car as a form of personal transport. A number of organisations, including the oil and motor vehicle industries, have a financial interest in promoting the popularity of motor cars. Another factor in Tommy's accident is the lack of cycle paths or traffic-calming devices in place on the route he takes to school.

Commentary

On the basis of this brief case study, we can draw a number of conclusions. The case study shows that the causes of health problems, including alterations in the correct functioning of the body and a number of social issues, are very complex. It also shows that the medical approach is a very effective way of dealing with health problems once they have arisen. However, the case study also illustrates the fact that health problems are affected by events that lie well beyond the influence of the medical approach to illness.

suffering. This approach, which was known as the nursing process, is discussed towards the end of this chapter. The nursing process was also accompanied by the introduction of holistic philosophies of care, under which attention was paid not only to the patient's disease, but also to the whole person.

However, the most important result of nurses' challenge of the dominance of the medical model has perhaps been the development of alternative, nursing models of care. The articles and books in which nursing models are described, discussed and debated have become known as 'nursing theory'. The next section of this chapter discusses the nature of nursing theory and considers the contribution that it has made to nursing practice. British nurses have debated this relationship for at least 15 years, and it is an issue about which many hold strong views. Some passionately believe that the use of nursing models brings clear benefits to patients and nurses alike. Other nurses are deeply sceptical, arguing that nursing theory is an elaborate waste of everybody's time. It is therefore important to approach the literature with a cool head and a clear eye. We must always weigh the evidence upon which claims are based, and, most importantly, we must understand that the theory–practice debate is part of a much bigger debate about the nature and future of the nursing profession itself. We must therefore adopt a critical attitude, which means looking constantly for the evidence upon which claims are based and testing the arguments that are put forward.

CONCEPTS, THEORIES AND MODELS OF NURSING

In this section, we will discuss some of the most important developments that have occurred in nursing in recent years, concentrating specifically upon models of nursing, and the nursing process. It is important to have a clear understanding of the nursing process and models of nursing because they have a profound effect upon the way in which nurses organise nursing work. We will begin by discussing the meaning of three important words – concept, theory and model – and will then take a detailed look at the work of two important nursing theorists: Sister Callista Roy and Nancy Roper (and her colleagues). There will then be a discussion of the nursing process. Finally, we will examine the work of three writers (Fawcett, Argyris and Bright), whose insights

enable us to understand how the abstract ideas developed by nursing theorists are related to nursing practice.

THE NATURE OF CONCEPTS, THEORIES AND MODELS

Fawcett (1984) suggests that concepts, theories and models are related to each other in a hierarchical way: concepts form the base of the hierarchy and are the building blocks from which theories are constructed: theories are, in turn, the building blocks of models. We will start at the bottom of the hierarchy as we look at the characteristics and purpose of concepts.

Concepts

Concepts are tools that help us to make sense of the world around us. Imagine that you were blindfolded and taken to a place that you had never visited before: perhaps a ward in a hospital in a strange town many miles away from your home. When the blindfold was removed, you would look around and notice familiar objects such as beds, lockers, and trolleys, and activities such as nurses walking about or chatting to patients, visitors arriving and leaving, and domestic staff cleaning the floor. These clues would enable you to reach the reasonable conclusion that you were in a hospital ward. The important thing to note about this exercise in imagination is that it reveals our ability to recognise that *particular* objects we have never seen before, such as this locker, this trolley or this bed, can be mentally grouped with other, similar objects because of certain features that they have in common. We refer to these mental groups as *concepts*. Another way of understanding concepts is to think of them as shelves in a library. In a well-organised library, each shelf will contain a number of individual books that are all on the same topic – research, for example. An alternative way of arranging the library would be to have all the books in a mixed up heap in the middle of the floor. In this case, however, it would take us hours to find the books that we wanted. In a similar way, if we did not use concepts to organise our experience, we would find the world to be a confusing muddle.

Not all concepts refer to physical objects such as beds and chairs; some relate to things that we cannot directly experience with our senses, but which are nonetheless important. An example of such a concept from nursing would be 'mental health', which, although it cannot be touched or seen, is an important goal of professional nursing practice. As nurses, we often use concepts such as comfort, pain, reassurance and the quality of life to help us communicate with colleagues and patients. These concepts help us to understand what is happening to patients and clients and to communicate with one other in an effective way. However, nursing scholars are interested in concepts not only because practitioners find them to be useful, but also because they are the essential building blocks of theory.

Theories

Nurses are interested in doing things that enhance the health and well-being of their patients and clients; they want to dress wounds in a way that makes them heal, devise behavioural programmes that enable people to overcome their phobias, and advise parents of children with learning disabilities how to cope with patterns of challenging behaviour. Unfortunately, it is not always obvious what is the helpful thing to do. Should we dress a wound with sugar, with gauze or with nothing at all? If a child's behaviour is challenging, should we beat the child with a cane, lock her in a cupboard or use a system of rewards? Theory can play an important role in helping us to make these decisions.

Let us take as an example two theories that relate to the development of pressure sores. Until quite recently, most nurses accepted the theory that the most effective way to prevent sacral pressure sores from developing in susceptible patients was to give the sacral area a vigorous rub several times a day in order to stimulate the circulation (we will call this Theory 1). However, the practice of vigorous rubbing has now been abandoned because a more recent theory proposes that it actually damages the fragile micro-circulation, thus making pressure sores more likely to develop (we will call this Theory 2). We can use these example to help us understand some of the general features of theories.

The first thing to note is that theories contain concepts. Our theories contain concepts such as 'pressure sore', 'vigorous rubbing', 'micro-circulation' and 'damage'. Second, these theories do not just contain concepts, but also have something to say about the way in which the concepts are related to one another. For example, Theory 1 claims that rubbing makes sores less likely to occur, whilst Theory 2 claims that it makes them more likely to occur. Third, there is often more than one theory competing for the same territory (in this case Theory 1 and Theory 2). Fourth and finally, particular attention should be paid to the fact that good theories are testable: that is to say, the theory is written in such a way that we can investigate its claims, either by doing an experiment or by assessing the evidence for and against it in some other way.

The final point to be made here is that there are different levels of theory. Microlevel theories are about specific issues and contain relatively few concepts. An example is Melia's (1987) theoretical category of 'learning and working', which she uses to help explain the process by which student nurses become socialised into their chosen occupation. At the other end of the scale, there are grand theories. Darwin's theory of evolution through natural selection provides us with an example of this. Grand theories enable us to explain the relationship between many different concepts and have successfully withstood many attempts to demonstrate that they are false. Grand theories often provide an organising framework for whole branches of science.

Models

Models of various kinds play a useful role in everyday life. Physical models may have two dimensions (think for instance of a map) or three dimensions (such as an anatomical model of the heart), but however many dimensions they have, all physical models represent the most important parts of an object and give us information about the way in which those parts are related to one another in space. Models also vary according to the function we want them to serve. Maps of the London Underground show the stations but they do not represent the distances between them in an accurate way. Ordnance Survey maps, on the other hand, show distances very accurately, but do not usually show the presence of underground tunnels.

The models that we are interested in are not physical but conceptual models. Where three-dimensional models contain physical parts, conceptual models are made up of abstract parts, such as concepts and theories, and where physical models give information about spatial relationships, conceptual models give information about the relationships between ideas.

NURSING MODELS

In recent years, a number of nurses have constructed conceptual *models of nursing*. These are systematic attempts to identify the important parts of nursing practice and to show how they relate to one another. Conceptual models resemble physical models in that they are developed for a purpose (or for several purposes). The reasons for which nurses have found it useful to construct nursing models fall into two groups. First, models have been found to be useful because, in various ways, they help nurses to do their work. Nursing models often contain patient assessment schemes, they offer useful frameworks for curriculum development, they may stimulate ideas for research and so on. Second, nursing models have made an important contribution to the debate about the nature of nursing itself. Two well-known models of nursing are described below.

Roy's adaptation model of nursing

There is a convention that all nursing models say something about four concepts that are central to nursing: the nature of human beings, the environment, health and nursing. These concepts provide useful headings under which to discuss Roy's model.

The nature of human beings

Roy says that people are biopsychosocial beings. By this, she means that we have biological, psychological and social characteristics. For Roy, the *biological* part of the human being can be expressed as a series of needs (Table 14.1).

The *psychological* element of Roy's discussion of the person draws upon the notion of self-concept. Basically, the self-concept represents the view that each person has a mental picture of him- or herself that influences the ways in which he or she interacts with other people. The first part of the self-concept is known as the 'body image'. Body image refers to the fact that we each hold certain beliefs about our body. Each person considers their body to have a certain shape and particular dimensions. They may also believe it to be attractive or unattractive to other people. Body image disturbance occurs when the person has an inaccurate perception of his or her body, causing him to behave in an unhealthy way. In cases of anorexia nervosa, for instance, people who are extremely thin think of

Table 14.1 Biological needs	
Basic physiological need	Possible associated problem
Exercise and rest	Immobility Hyperactivity Fatigue and insomnia
Nutrition	Malnutrition Nausea and vomiting
Elimination	Constipation Diarrhoea Incontinence
Fluid and electrolytes	Dehydration Oedema Electrolyte imbalance
Oxygen	Oxygen deficit
Circulation	Shock Overload
Regulation of temperature	Fever Hypothermia
Regulation of senses	Sensory deprivation
Regulation of endocrine system	Endocrine imbalance, such as diabetes mellitus

themselves as being obese, and diet to the extent that they become ill and may die. The second part of the self-concept concerns judgements that the person makes about other aspects of himself, such as his worthiness as a human being and the degree of influence he has on the things that happen in his life.

The *social* element of Roy's model has two elements: role function concerns our ability to fulfil various roles that are ascribed to us by society and the way in which this ability might be compromised by illness; interdependence concerns the extent to which we depend on, or are independent of, other people.

The nature of the environment

Roy argues that each person exists in an environment and has to adapt to changes in that environment in order to remain healthy. The range of ways in which we can cope with environmental threats is governed by physical, psychological and social factors, some of which are inborn and others of which are acquired. Perhaps the simplest example of adaptation is the behaviour of the person who adjusts his clothing in response to changes in the external temperature. Our response to a threat such as the death of a loved one is more complex and is at least partially determined by patterns of learning that have occurred earlier in life.

Roy suggests that our responses to threats of all kinds are determined by the nature of the threat itself (which she calls the focal stimulus), by other significant factors in the current environment (contextual stimuli) and by beliefs, attitudes, traits and other features that also have a bearing on our response (residual stimuli). If our response to a stimulus promotes our well-being, it is called an adaptive response. If it does not, it is called a maladaptive response.

The nature of health and the nature of nursing

Health and illness, for Roy, are inevitable dimensions of human life and the concern of professional nurses. The need for nursing care arises when a person is unable to respond in an adaptive way to stimuli that challenge his state of health. Nursing care begins as the nurse assesses the patient, using an approach that explores his physiological needs, self-concept, role function and interdependence, as discussed above. Subsequent nursing actions are designed to promote the person's ability to respond in an adaptive way under each of these headings. If the person's responses are adaptive, the nurse's role is to maintain that response. If the person is not managing to respond in an adaptive way, the nurses might, in extreme cases, perform a particular function on the person's behalf for a period of time. In less extreme cases, the nurse might offer support and education.

Case example 14.2 may help to illuminate the more difficult aspects of Roy's model.

Activities of living model of nursing

Nancy Roper and her colleagues (Roper et al 1981) propose a model of nursing that concentrates on 12 key 'activities of living'. The person's ability to conduct each of these activities can be plotted along a 'dependence–independence continuum'. Levels of independence in the various activities of living are related to the lifespan. A healthy baby, for example, is totally independent with regard to breathing because this is a reflex activity, but does not become independent in the activity of dressing and cleansing until later childhood. As the individual progresses further along the lifespan, there may be a reversal from total independence to dependence in some of the living activities, especially if illness occurs. The activities of living nursing model recognises that rates of development are influenced by individual differences and by circumstance and that, as a consequence, independence levels are also affected.

Categories of activity

Roper et al (1981) suggest that the activities of living fall into three categories: 'preventing', 'comforting' and 'seeking'. Preventing activities are those carried out by the individual to avoid illness and harm, by such means as avoiding

Case study 14.2

Dr Francis Jackson is a 74-year-old retired consultant physician who has suffered a stroke. He lives at home with his wife. The stroke has caused a hemiparesis (a type of partial paralysis) and a number of other problems. His primary nurse, Diane Bailey, assesses Dr Jackson using Roy's framework and makes a number of observations. Read through the assessment, and then answer the questions at the end.

Basic physiological need	Findings on nursing assessment
Exercise and rest	Dr Jackson is able to sit in a chair without support for short periods. He cannot balance when standing and is unable to walk. His affected arm is in a state of flaccid paralysis
Nutrition	Dr Jackson is able to feed himself with his unaffected arm. Food tends to 'pouch' in the cheek on the side of his mouth affected by the stroke. Because of his problem in perception (see below), he leaves food on one side of the plate
Elimination	Dr Jackson is aware of the sensation to micturate and is able to use a bottle if he gets help with his clothing in time
Fluid and electrolytes	Dr Jackson is able to drink without help if fluids are put within his reach
Oxygen	There are no problems here
Circulation	The ankle on the affected side has pitting oedema. The skin to the sacral area has non-blanching erythema
Regulation of temperature	There are no problems here
Regulation of senses	Dr Jackson is unable to perceive one half of his visual field
Regulation of endocrine system	There are no problems here
Psychological needs	
Self-concept: body image	Dr Jackson does not recognise that his affected arm is part of his body. This is shown by his tendency to treat the arm as a distinct object, and his habit of calling it 'Fred'
Self concept: other aspects	No problems are apparent here
Social needs	
Role function	Mrs Jackson says that, in private conversation, her husband constantly remarks about the fact that he is a patient in the hospital where he used to work as a consultant. He refuses to see his former colleagues when they come to visit
Interdependence	Dr Jackson appears to be distressed by the fact that he is dependent upon nursing staff for intimate care

Now work with a colleague to consider the following:

1. Does Roy's assessment framework appear to produce a comprehensive list of Dr Jackson's problems?
2. Discuss the care that a nurse might be able to provide with respect to each part of the assessment.

harmful situations and keeping high standards of personal hygiene. Comforting activities may help to sustain the individual during physical and emotional discomfort and are also employed as diversions during periods of boredom or enforced inactivity. Seeking activities have as their motivating force the tendencies of inquisitiveness and adventure that are very evident in children and which, in the adult, take on the more sophisticated qualities of ambition and enquiry.

Applying the model

A person's degree of independence in the conduct of activities of living may be altered by illness. Nursing interventions are concerned with helping the patient with problems associated with activities of living, through the 'preventing', 'comforting' and 'dependent' components of nursing care.

The preventing component. During the application of this component of nursing, the nurse ensures that the patient's condition is not worsened and that secondary conditions (side-effects) are avoided or reduced. If a patient is confined to bed, the preventing component of nursing would address the problems associated with the prolonged confinement, such as loss of muscle power, pressure sores and respiratory infection. In the home setting, the nurse's ability to help an elderly person to reduce the risks of injury, hypothermia and malnutrition demonstrates the preventing component of nursing.

The comforting component. The aim of this component of nursing is to enable maximum physical, emotional and spiritual comfort to be attained by patients, thus increasing independence as much as possible. Something as simple as the nurse making time to listen to an anxious patient is a good example of how the comforting component can be applied. Providing opportunity for a child in hospital to play with favourite toys, thus diverting attention from the apprehensions associated with his surroundings, is beneficial to both child and nurse. The comforting component of nursing is not concerned with high technology and clinical skills, but with interpersonal relationships and the provision of a personalised service.

The dependent component. Despite the patient's ability to participate in some aspects of the preventing and comforting components of care, there is a component for which the patient is totally dependent upon the nurse. This component of nursing includes all those actions that usually involve special knowledge and skills, many of which will be initiated or prescribed by the doctor in charge of the patient. The administration of drugs, the collection of specimens and the application of diagnostic tests are just some of the procedures that the nurse will perform within the context of the dependent component of nursing.

Interrelationship of the components of nursing action

The preventing, comforting and dependent components of nursing are not carried out as isolated actions. Each impinges upon, or has a consequence for, the others. When administering a drug by injection to a patient, the nurse is not only using her knowledge and skills related to that specific procedure, but is also ensuring that the patient is at ease and reassured. At the same time, the nurse must take precautions to prevent complications or problems arising.

The activities of living model is predominantly a nurse-active one, in which the nurse usually takes the lead role in carrying out preventing and comforting measures, as well as the specific treatments and procedures designed to restore the ability of the patient to carry out his own living activities appropriate to his developmental level of life. Figure 14.1 illustrates the activities of living model of nursing, and Case example 14.3 illustrates the model in action.

THE PROCESS OF NURSING

In order to apply models of nursing to patient care, it is usual to use a problem-solving strategy known as the 'nursing process'. Although many textbooks depict the nursing process as containing four stages, it is, in reality, a cyclical process (Fig. 14.2). As the condition of the patient changes as a result of the nursing care given, so must the care plan be adjusted to meet the new needs of the patient. Table 14.2 details the four stages of the nursing process and suggests appropriate nurse and patient activities at each stage.

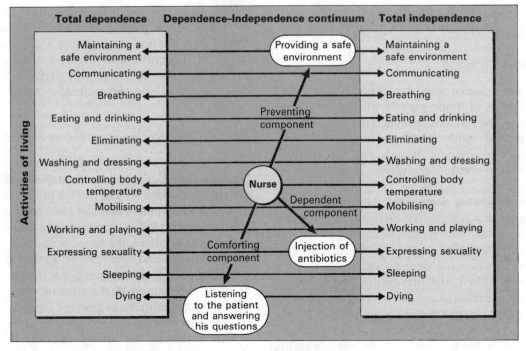

Figure 14.1   Activities of living model of nursing. (After Roper et al 1990.)

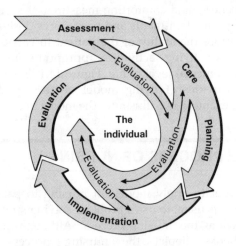

Figure 14.2   The nursing process.

USING THE NURSING PROCESS WITH THE ACTIVITIES OF LIVING MODEL

Assessment

The nurse must carry out those assessment actions relating to observation, interviewing, data collection and analysis, and problem identification. She must do this for each of the activities of living and make judgements about the level of dependence or independence at which the patient can function. Many hospitals and community care services will have documentation designed to assist the nurse with data analysis and presentation. On completion of this assessment, which may in some cases take days, the nurse will built up a profile of the patient's 'normal' life. It is unlikely that the levels of dependence/independence will be the same for each activity. Figure 14.3 represents the type of profile that a nurse may build up during the assessment stage.

Planning

The four stages of the nursing process are not necessarily carried out separately. If a full and comprehensive assessment of the patient takes place over a number of days, planning and implementation of some part of the care programme may take place at the same time. Inevitably, the nature of the patient's illness will,

Case example 14.3 Applying the activities of living nursing model (Contributed by David Howard)

Edith Baker, aged 58, has been admitted to hospital for urgent treatment of a severe urinary tract infection. She is married to George, a bank manager, and enjoys an active social life. She is a member of the local Women's Institute, and she and her husband are committed members of the local Neighbourhood Watch scheme and regular dinner party attenders.

Over the past 3 weeks, Edith has developed frequency and urgency to pass urine during the day and night. She is in constant pain, has a high temperature and has become weak and pessimistic, and is frightened that she is 'losing her faculties'.

Soon after Edith's admission to the ward, the nurse used an activities of living model as the framework for completing an assessment and initial care plan for Edith.

Assessment and nursing care plan

Activity of living	Assessment	Problem	Intervention	Goal
Maintaining a safe environment	Edith is normally able to maintain a safe environment. At the present time, she is easily distracted because of her weakness and constant pain			
Communicating	Edith feels embarrassed and guilty about her condition and blames herself. She has a continuous burning pain in her lower abdomen and perineal area	Anxiety about the condition Burning pain in the lower abdomen and perineal area	Give 1 g of paracetamol, when Edith requests, at 6-hourly intervals according to prescription See Eating and drinking Allow time for discussion	No pain
Breathing	Edith does not suffer from any chronic respiratory or circulatory disorder. She does not normally get unduly breathless			
Eating and drinking	Normally Edith eats a well-balanced diet and drinks approx. 2.5 litres of fluid daily. Her weight of 54.4 kg is within an acceptable range for her height of 1.67 m. Edith attempted to control her symptoms by reducing her fluid intake to approx. 750 ml daily.	Edith is not drinking sufficient fluids to flush bacteria adequately from her bladder	Edith will drink 200 ml of fluid every hour she is awake to produce a daily fluid intake of 2.5–3 litres	To achieve a good urinary output of 1.5–2.0 litres per day
	As her health deteriorated, she also lost her appetite and has not eaten for the past 3 days	Anorexia	Provide Edith with small, nourishing, well-presented meals	Return to normal appetite
Eliminating	Normally Edith has daily bowel movements and no urinary problems. Over the past 3 weeks, she has experienced pain,	Painful and frequent urine micturition	See Communicating and Eating and drinking	Pain-free micturition

(cont'd)

Case example 14.3 (contd)

Activity of living	Assessment	Problem	Intervention	Goal
Eliminating (cont'd)	frequency and urgency to pass urine. She has noticed that her urine has recently become thick and cloudy with an offensive odour			
Washing and dressing	Edith sweats profusely, and because of this she states that she feels dirty as she is permanently wet	Excessive perspiration leading to wet clothing	Allow Edith to bathe/shower when she feels the need Change nightclothes as soon as they become damp	Edith will cater for her own hygiene needs
Controlling body temperature	Edith has a high body temperature of 39.2°C	Pyrexia	Ensure Edith wears light cotton clothing Encourage Edith to drink cold fluids Tepid sponge Edith Record Edith's temperature 4 hourly	Edith's body temperature will return to within normal limits
Mobilising	Normally an active woman with many local interests, Edith now feels weak and finds it difficult to walk very far. She feels 'drained of energy'	Lethargy	See Eating and drinking, Elimination, and Washing and dressing	Normal energy and activity
Working and playing	Because of the frequency and urgency to pass urine, Edith has not been able to socialise or do the shopping. She now feels too weak to even contemplate this	Lethargy	As above	
Expressing sexuality	Edith is normally sexually active. Since the onset of her problems, she and George have slept in separate rooms. This, allied with the pain and worry regarding her urinary problem, has prevented Edith continuing her sexual activity. Because of her tiredness, frequency and pain she has also lost interest in her appearance and dress	Anxiety Unhappiness	Make opportunities for discussion Allow privacy for George and Edith to be alone	
Sleeping	Normally Edith 'sleeps like a log for 7 hours each night'. Since the onset of her problems, she has needed to get up three or four times each night. Once up, the pain makes it difficult for her to go back to sleep. This makes her tired during the day	Poor sleeping	See all other interventions	Normal sleep pattern
Dying	Not applicable			

Table 14.2   Stages of the nursing process

Stage	Sub-division	Activity
Assessment	Data collection Analysis of data Problem identification Nursing diagnosis	Observe patient Interview patient and relatives Measure data Classify data Make judgements Formulate a diagnosis from problem identification
Planning	Goals Priorities Methods of attaining goals Plan of action	Determine between short/medium/long-term goals Justify priorities Explore options for nursing approaches Determine plan based upon the above Agree appropriate nursing model
Implementation	Selection of appropriate interventions Execution of plans	Apply care within the nursing model
Evaluation	Degree of goal achievement Feedback	Determine with patient the amount of progress made Refer back to previous stages

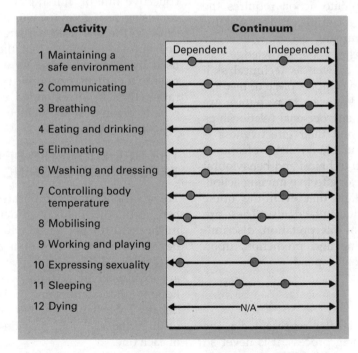

● On admission in a state of acute pain

● 4 days after an appendicectomy

Figure 14.3   Assessment of a 14-year-old girl with acute appendicitis. The profile will change continually as the levels of dependency change.

to a large extent, dictate the balance between assessing, planning and carrying out nursing care. In life-threatening emergencies, the nurse will carry out emergency procedures and leave full assessment and planning until the danger has passed. The actions will have been planned according to the degree of dependence or independence of the patient and will have required the nurse to consider all three nursing components of the model, i.e. 'comforting', 'preventing' and 'dependent'. Specific nursing activities that take place during the planning stage of the process may involve the nurse in distinguishing between short-term and longer-term goals, setting and justifying priorities of care, exploring alternative options to care and, finally, taking the decision to implement the plan.

Implementation

Putting the care plan into action requires the nurse to demonstrate a complex range of skills. An analysis of the nursing action will easily reveal the cognitive aspect (the knowledge that the nurse possesses), as well as technical skill (e.g. being able to use a complex piece of medical equipment). Perhaps less easy to recognise are those skills relating to interpersonal relationships and communication, and their effectiveness is not immediately measurable. Whilst professional knowledge, along with technical and behavioural skills, is a prerequisite for effective nursing action, there are perhaps skills that even the nurse herself may not consciously recognise. These are the intellectual skills of interpretation, discrimination, problem-solving and prediction, upon which most other actions depend.

Evaluation

Although 'evaluation' is often represented as the final stage of the nursing process, it is never so in practice. The nurse should be constantly assessing the information that she may have about the patient's condition and reviewing the total situation. In a formal sense, however, there must be an inbuilt system of measuring the degree to which what has been planned and implemented has been successful. The documentation for preparing an assessment or a care plan should allow also for the outcomes of care to be recorded. Evaluation of nursing care is effective only when it is put to some useful purpose. In terms of the nursing process, it enables the nurse to proceed either to further planning and application of care or, if the planned care has not been effective, to the reassessment of the patient's problems. This demonstrates that the nursing process is indeed cyclical, as depicted in Figure 14.2, above, rather than being a linear activity.

NURSING THEORY

The relationship between concepts, theories, models and nursing practice is often given the collective title of 'nursing theory'. This may be confusing, as it gives the word 'theory' additional sense to the one used earlier. Perhaps it would be helpful to remember that 'theory' is sometimes used in a limited sense, as when it is used to refer to a particular scientific theory, for instance, rather than in an extended or global sense to refer to theoretical knowledge in general.

THE RELATIONSHIP BETWEEN THEORY AND NURSING PRACTICE

This relationship is complicated by the fact that here, as in other fields of academic study, experts in the field do not agree with each other. It is beyond the limitations of a single chapter to resolve the differences between the views that are expressed by various writers, but we can hope to understand some of the issues that they debate. This chapter touches briefly on the work of three theorists and provides a critical review of each one.

Fawcett: nursing models as the necessary basis of nursing practice

The American nursing scholar Jacqueline Fawcett has consistently advocated the use of nursing models as the necessary basis of nursing practice. This account of Fawcett's thinking is based on her paper 'Conceptual models and nursing practice: the reciprocal relationship' (Fawcett 1992). In this paper, Fawcett argues that there is a reciprocal relationship between conceptual models of nursing and nursing practice. It is her view that 'conceptual models inform and transform nursing practice by informing and transforming the way in which nursing practice is understood, and that nursing practice informs and transforms nursing models by informing and transforming the content of the conceptual model'.

For all that Fawcett claims the relationship between models and practice to be a reciprocal one, she makes it clear that, in her view, conceptual models are the essential starting point of the theory–practice relationship. She argues that if practice were the starting point, the boundaries of nursing knowledge would be severely restricted, and professional nursing would be unable to serve as a force for the promotion of world health. Fawcett offers a list of 10 different ways in which conceptual models influence nursing practice (Box 14.1).

> **Box 14.1 How conceptual models influence nursing practice** (From Fawcett 1992)
>
> - Identify standards for nursing practice.
> - Identify the purposes to be fulfilled by nursing practice.
> - Identify clinical problems to be considered by nurses.
> - Identify settings in which nursing practice should occur.
> - Define the legitimate recipients of nursing care.
> - Identify the format and content of the nursing process.
> - Direct the delivery of nursing care.
> - Form the basis for clinical information systems.
> - Form the basis of patient classification systems.

Although Fawcett's belief that nursing models form the basis of nursing practice is clear from her article, she also suggests that nursing practice shapes the content of nursing models. This process of shaping can occur as data from clinical practice, and audits of patient satisfaction and

the quality of care are used to evaluate the credibility of the model.

Fawcett's account of the relationship between conceptual models and nursing practice provokes many important questions. The first of these relates to her view that conceptual models define the purposes to be fulfilled by nursing practice, the range of clinical problems with which nurses should be involved, the setting in which practice should occur and so on (see Box 14.1). This approach ignores the fact that, for the most part, the nursing contribution to health care takes place in partnership with other health professionals, such as doctors and physiotherapists, and is controlled by large organisations that have the power to determine priorities and allocate resources for care. In a system in which medical consultants hold the ultimate responsibility for the admission and discharge of patients, and in which even consultants must respond to organisational priorities, it is unrealistic for individual nurses to expect to have the power to define who is and who is not a legitimate recipient of nursing care, or the setting in which that care will be delivered.

Fawcett's belief that conceptual models of nursing must be given priority in the theory–practice relationship also deserves close scrutiny. We have seen that the function of models is to represent some of the parts of an object or activity of interest. It follows that the function of a conceptual model of nursing is to show the parts of nursing and how they are related (Riehl & Roy 1980). Consequently, a model of nursing must be dependent for its meaning upon the phenomenon of clinical nursing practice, which it claims to *re-present*. For instance, the statement 'Nurses care' will only make sense to a person with a conceptual understanding of nursing and caring, and these concepts must be gained though participation in a society in which nursing and caring already exist. In this sense, models of nursing cannot precede practice but must follow it.

Fawcett's insistence upon the priority of a small number of conceptual models produced by a handful of American theorists can also be criticised for undervaluing and diverting attention away from the insights of clinical practitioners themselves. Fawcett claims that nursing models were devised to move nursing away from ritualistic and task-oriented care. This is a laudable goal, but it is not clear why the views of nursing theorists should be given greater weight than those of the well-educated and experienced clinical practitioner. It is reasonable to argue that a professional nurse who is familiar with clinical research and practice development in her own field, and is responsible for the delivery of care within the confines of a given organisational structure, is better placed to generate clinical strategies for nursing care and to evaluate their effectiveness through research than the author of a nursing model.

Argyris & Schön: theories-in-use

The work of Argyris and Schön proceeds from the assumption that practitioners are guided not so much by conceptual models and schemes imposed from without, but by internally held values and sets of belief.

Chris Argyris and Donald Schön are professors of education who have conducted research into the nature of professional practice. Although Argyris and Schön are not nurses, their insights make a useful contribution to our understanding of the relationship between theory and practice in nursing. Their book 'Theory and Practice: Increasing Professional Effectiveness' (Argyris & Schön 1989) seeks to examine the nature of professional competence and to discover how it is learned or acquired. Argyris and Schön argue that the actions that professionals take in their day-to-day work are guided by theories. These theories, however, are not formal or scientific theories of the kind that Fawcett describes, but are given the special title of 'theories-in-use'. A theory-in-use is a set of interconnected beliefs about people, situations, the nature of professional work, the means by which certain desirable ends may be obtained and many other issues. Theories-in-use represent sets of working assumptions that help the practitioner to decide how to act in various circumstances. Argyris & Schön argue that practitioners are not fully aware of their

theories-in-use, as the latter can only be inferred from observations of behaviour. Furthermore, a practitioner's theory-in-use may actually conflict with the values that he or she claims to hold (or in Argyris & Schön's terminology, the 'espoused theory').

An example may clarify the nature of theory-in-use and espoused theory, and highlight the differences between them. The example is taken from a recent research project that examined the meaning of the quality of life for older people (Draper 1994). A number of nurses were interviewed to discover how they promoted the quality of life of older people in their care. Many of these nurses claimed that it was important to treat older people as individuals. In practical terms, this meant that older people in hospital should be given the opportunity to make choices about the way in which they lived their lives: choices about what time to get out of bed, what to eat at meal times, the selection of clothes to wear, what to watch on the television and so on. The comments of one interviewee, Nurse X, are given below:

Nurse X: I think the most important word I would suggest is an element of choice . . . Choice has got to be the most important thing, I'd say. Choice about everything from when you have a meal, to when you have a wash, to when you get up on a morning, to whether you decide to take some medical advice or not . . . or where you're going to live, everything. From getting up on a morning, to deciding whether you're going to move from your home into an old people's home.

and later:

This man we're talking about, he's had a stroke so all down his left side he's got no movement at all. Now ideally, you should approach him from his left side. You approach him from this side so he's not going to hit you, and see if you can get it done . . . and try to get it done as quickly as possible, really. The more you try to communicate with him the more he's hitting you, and there comes a time when you think, 'Lets get on with it, stop him doing this', and we do it pretty quickly and ask for help, two of us to do him.

It is reasonable to say that this nurse's espoused theory – the set of beliefs that she claims to hold and take as a guiding principle for practice – is that the quality of life of older people in hospital is enhanced if they are given choice. However, other parts of the interview data show that some nurses do not always act in a way that promotes choice, even though this is what they claim to do. It is clear that this nurse's priority is not to promote the quality of the life of her patient but to accomplish the task of washing him as quickly as possible, whatever the cost to his dignity and independence. Perhaps this nurse's theory-in-use runs something like this:

A. Nursing involves creating patient choice, humane treatment and effective communication.
B. Nursing also involves getting through the work as quickly as possible.
C. Where A and B come into conflict, B should always be given priority.

You may be surprised and even rather shocked to learn that there can be such a wide difference between a single practitioner's espoused theory and theory-in-use. In fact, the recognition of this difference represents progress, for the practitioner is now in a position to understand that the actions she takes are in direct conflict with the values that she claims to hold.

It would be unhelpful to suggest that the principal value of the notion of theory-in-use lies in its power to highlight differences between value and action. Theory-in-use also shows us that practitioners are unlike computers; they do not need to be programmed with software in the form of a nursing model before they can act. They already have opinions about the role of nursing, theories about what works and what does not work in a given set of circumstances, and the creative ability to generate and evaluate strategies for care. Theories-in-use may not always be well formulated or articulated, and from time to time they may be erroneous, but then so may be the more formal theories developed by scientists. Practitioner theories are a potent force in nursing care, and they have a contribution to make to nursing scholarship.

As we have seen, Fawcett and Argyris & Schön each approach the theory–practice debate from a different perspective. Fawcett takes a top-down approach, beginning with theory in the form of conceptual models and proceeding to nursing practice. Argyris & Schön, on the other hand, work from the bottom up, beginning with professional practice and then inferring the theories that guide it. The strength of Argyris & Schön's approach lies in its recognition that all practice has an inherent theoretical basis, and its weakness lies in their failure to suggest a way of clarifying the underlying theoretical basis of practice in order to test it and then, if useful, apply it in new settings. Conversely, Fawcett argues that conceptual models are broadly useful, but her approach has been criticised for undervaluing the theoretical insights of the practitioner. In addition to this, neither Fawcett nor Argyris & Schön have much to say about the contribution that can be made to nursing or other professional practice by theoretical knowledge from a broad range of academic disciplines.

Bright: field disciplines

The previous section of the chapter ended with an important question unresolved. How can we preserve the most useful features of the complementary approaches of Fawcett and Argyris & Schön whilst discarding the limitations of each? The task is to retain Argyris & Schön's respect for the perspective of the practitioner, whilst moving beyond the severe limitations of practitioner theory, and to recognise that conceptual models of nursing make a useful contribution in many fields of nursing practice, whilst being properly spectical of some of the extravagant claims that are made about them. The work of Bright (1985) helps us towards this goal.

Bright, who works in the field of adult education, draws upon the work of Hirst (1974) to distinguish between 'forms' of knowledge and 'fields' of knowledge. Disciplines that possess a distinctive body of knowledge that is characterised by its own logical and conceptual structure are known as forms of knowledge. Forms of knowledge include mathematics, religion, philosophy, history, human sciences, natural sciences, and literature and the fine arts. Each form of knowledge may contain a number of distinct disciplines. For instance, natural science encompasses physics, chemistry and biology. Characteristically, forms of knowledge are said to be solely concerned with developing the content of their own domain.

Fields of knowledge, on the other hand, exist in order to accumulate and organise knowledge that is relevant to some specific theoretical or practical activity. They derive their content from one or more disciplines or forms of knowledge, which they then focus, organise and integrate according to their purpose. This does not mean that the content of fields of knowledge is entirely second-hand or derivative, for, in organising it, practitioners may develop their own theoretical insights.

The differences between forms and fields of knowledge are summarised in Table 14.3.

NURSING AS A FIELD DISCIPLINE

Nursing displays many of the characteristics of a practical field discipline. It is an occupation whose members possess an extensive repertoire of practical skills that can be applied to the health-related problems of patient and client groups, and, ultimately, all nursing scholarship is directed towards extending, clarifying and refining these skills. This does not imply that nursing consists of blind technique. The notion of theory-in-use shows us that nursing practice is inherently theoretical. Every nurse is guided in her practice by an interlocking set of beliefs, assumptions, knowledge and values that are acquired during initial professional education and may be refined through experience.

Although theories-in-use exist and are used by practitioners, they are not in themselves a sufficient basis for professional practice. One of the reasons we cannot rely entirely upon theories-in-use to guide nursing practice is that they may not be in the best interests of patients or clients (as was seen in the example given above). Another reason is that they may only relate to certain aspects of professional practice, whilst having nothing to say about other parts. For these and other reasons, nurses need to make use of theoretical knowledge from other sources.

The notion of nursing as a practical field discipline is useful precisely because it enables us to make use of theoretical material from a broad range of sources. In principle, there is no limit to the range of disciplines from which nursing can draw. Your studies will already have shown you that our profession makes use of knowledge from physiology, psychology, sociology, social policy, ethics and many other fields. There are also signs that the contemporary profession is complementing its traditional scientific basis by drawing more deeply upon the arts and humanities. An excellent example of this can be seen in the work of Darbyshire (1994), who encourages his students to enhance their understanding of caring and the experience of illness by drawing upon cultural resources that are available in poetry, literature and music. There is no reason at all why nurses should not enhance their practice by drawing upon resources of this kind, as long as they remember that artistic knowledge, like scientific knowledge, has certain limitations.

The notion of nursing as a practical field discipline is useful, but it is important to be aware of its limitations. Although theoretical knowledge from other disciplines can guide nursing practice, it can never tell us precisely what to do in a given set of clinical circumstances. This is because nursing always takes place in a complex social context. For example, a nurse who has studied philosophy will be familiar with certain principles of ethics. Although these principles will

Table 14.3 Characteristics of 'forms of knowledge' and 'fields of knowledge'

	Forms of knowledge	Fields of knowledge
Origin of knowledge	Internal Intrinsic	External Derived
Nature of knowledge	Distinctive Separate Independent	Composite Interdisciplinary Dependent
Purpose	Elaboration of distinctiveness	Composite accumulation around a particular pursuit
Number	Few	Many

guide her ethical decision-making, they will not dictate what the outcome of these decisions will be, because the circumstances of particular patients must always be taken into account. In the same way, a nurse who has studied the practice of effective communication will be familiar with the principles of breaking bad news to patients, but must adapt and apply them in a slightly different way from case to case.

I do not think it is appropriate for nurses to feel that they must be experts in every field of knowledge. I do not even think it is necessary for individual nurses to have a passing knowledge of all the theoretical fields upon which our profession draws. In fact, it does the nursing profession no good at all for practitioners who only have a passing knowledge of some fields to pretend to be experts. What is appropriate, however, is for some members of our profession to be well educated in each of the major disciplines related to nursing practice. These individuals will then be in a position to bring new knowledge and new perspectives to bear upon the problems of nursing practice.

CONCLUSION: WILL USING NURSING MODELS PROVIDE INDIVIDUALISED CARE?

The advocates of nursing models often emphasise the contribution that models can make to the organisation and delivery of nursing care. They claim, for instance, that nursing models offer strategies for patient assessment. It is less commonly recognised that nursing models are often given a role in the debate about the nature of nursing itself. The very existence of this debate may seem rather unnecessary to the newcomer to the nursing profession who may consider the nature of nursing to be self-evident, but the modern nursing profession is, in fact, the product of decades of social change.

An important theme in the contemporary development of nursing concerns the efforts of some nurses to transform nursing from an occupation that they believe is subservient to the

medical profession into one whose practitioners can claim to be autonomous professionals possessing an independent body of knowledge. An explicit example of this approach can be seen in a paper by the American authors Wald & Leonard (1992), who suggest that nurses have tried and failed to find a theoretical basis for nursing practice in medicine, natural science and the social sciences. They claim that an alternative that has been overlooked is for nurses to develop their own theories, and make the explicit claim that this would enable nursing to become 'an independent discipline in its own right'.

The tendency to use nursing models for political purposes in this way tempts people to make exaggerated claims about what the models are and what can be achieved through their use. There is a tendency for the debate to become polarised, as people either reject models out of hand or claim that their use will sweep away ritualised practice and herald a new dawn of professional autonomy for the nursing profession. The notion of nursing as a field discipline enables us to make a more moderate assessment of the usefulness of nursing models.

The nursing profession should draw upon a range of theoretical disciplines in order to inform its practice, whilst always being aware of the necessity to modify and adapt ideas gained according to the contingencies of clinical practice. In my view, it is useful simply to regard nursing models as case studies of the way in which this can be done. Let us consider the case of Roy's models of nursing as an example. Roy draws upon concepts and theories from a number of disciplines in the natural and social sciences. She makes use of theories of self-concept and body image from psychology, role function from sociology, and a range of concepts from the natural sciences. The implications of these concepts and theories for nursing practice may not be immediately apparent to the nurse who limits herself to the primary literature of that discipline. Indeed, she may have neither the time nor the background knowledge to understand them in their original form. Roy's model of nursing (and other models of nursing) act as bridges between the original sources and clinical nursing practice, showing how the work of various disciplines can give rise to patient assessment tools and strategies for clinical intervention. In this way, the notion of nursing as a field discipline enables us to identify a useful clinical role for nursing models without committing us to some of the more excessive claims of their advocates.

Summary

The boundaries of nursing practice are constantly shifting in response to developments in legislation and changes in the roles of other members of the health care team. For nursing to be able to hold and defend its position as a profession, an understanding of the principles underlying nursing practice needs to be gained.

Historically, nursing has been dominated by the medical profession, but in the 1970s, it began to emphasise the specific role that nursing had to play in the care of patients. As a result of this, new concepts, theories and models of nursing developed as a framework for care. To apply such models to practice, the problem-solving approach of the nursing process, a continuous cycle of assessing, planning, implementing and evaluating, is usually employed.

The complex relationship between models of care and nursing practice is defined as 'nursing theory'. The work of the theorists Fawcett, Argyris & Schön and Bright is described to examine this relationship and consider why nurses alter their practice in various situations. It is suggested that nursing possesses many of the characteristics of a field discipline, with an eclectic approach to the gathering of information.

Thus, the provision of high-quality and individualised patient care demands a framework for applying and developing practice and also the recognition that one's actions should, and will, be influenced by the complex social and environmental context in which the care is provided.

REFERENCES

Argyris C, Schön D 1989 Theory in practice: increasing professional effectiveness. Jossey Bass, San Francisco

Baker D 1978 Attitudes of nurses to care of the elderly. PhD thesis, University of Manchester

Bright B 1985 The content method relationship in the study of adult education. Studies in the education of adults 17(2): 168–183

Darbyshire P 1994 Understanding caring through the arts and humanities: a medical/nursing humanities approach to promoting alternative experiences of thinking and learning. Journal of Advanced Nursing 19(5): 856–863

Draper P 1994 Promoting the quality of life of elderly people in nursing home care: a hermeneutical approach. PhD thesis, University of Hull

Fawcett J 1984 Analysis and evaluation of conceptual models of nursing. F A Davis, Philadelphia

Fawcett J 1992 Conceptual models and nursing practice: the reciprocal relationship. Journal of Advanced Nursing 17(2): 224–228

Hirst P 1974 Knowledge and the curriculum. Routledge & Kegan Paul, London

Melia K 1987 Learning and working: the occupational socialisation of nurses. Tavistock, London

Rafferty A M 1993 Decorous didactics: early explanations in the art and science of caring, circa 1860–90. In: Kitson A (ed) Nursing: art and science, Chapman and Hall, London, pp 48–60

Riehl J, Roy C 1980 Conceptual models for nursing practice. Appleton Century Crofts, New York

Robb B 1967 Sans everything: a case to answer. Nelson, London

Roper N, Logan W, Tierney A 1981 Learning to use the process of nursing. Churchill Livingstone, Edinburgh

Roy C 1981 Theory construction in nursing: an adaptation model. Prentice Hall, Englewood Cliffs, New Jersey

Wald F, Leonard R 1992 Towards development of nursing practice theory. In: Nicoll L (ed.) Perspectives on nursing theory. J B Lippincott, Philadelphia, pp 20–28

15 Research and its application

Pam Smith

CHAPTER CONTENTS

Nursing research is vital in understanding the complex factors associated with health, disease and illness and to devise and evaluate treatment and care. This chapter aims to:

- discuss the concept of research-mindedness
- explore the relevance of research to nursing knowledge and practice
- outline different types of research
- describe the stages of the research process, as a basis for their practical application.

The purpose of learning about research as a nursing student is to become 'research aware', rather than to turn into a fully fledged researcher. Becoming 'research aware' is an important part of becoming 'research minded' and means:

315

- developing the confidence to have ideas and ask questions about nursing
- becoming familiar with research literature, methods and techniques
- being able critically to assess research reports
- being able to incorporate research methods and findings into knowledge and practice.

The Royal College of Nursing (1982) states that research mindedness 'implies a critical and questioning approach to one's work, the desire and ability to find out about the latest research in the area and apply it as appropriate'.

In short, this chapter will help you to achieve competency in your UKCC learning outcome 'to demonstrate an appreciation of research and relevant literature as an aid to practice' (Great Britain Statutory Instrument 1989).

NURSING RESEARCH

HISTORICAL PERSPECTIVE

Research is not new to nursing. Florence Nightingale was a tireless researcher and a passionate statistician, who stressed the importance of accurate observation and skilful questioning in the collection of patient information. Leading questions, she observed, always elicited inaccurate information (Nightingale 1859):

A want of the habit of observing conditions and an inveterate habit of taking averages are each of them equally misleading. There is no more silly or universal question scarcely asked than this, 'Is he better?' Who can have any opinion of any value as to whether the patient is better or worse, excepting the constant medical attendant, or the really observing nurse.

Nightingale's advice to 19th century nurses is still relevant to nursing practice and research today:

The most important practical lesson that can be given to nurses is to teach them what to observe – how to observe – what symptoms indicate improvement, what the reverse – which are of importance – which are of none – which are the evidence of neglect – and of what kind of neglect?

A study undertaken by Doreen Norton over a century later has since been recognised as an important landmark in the development of nursing research. Norton's study investigated problems associated with nursing elderly people and critically examined their care (Norton et al 1962). One important consequence of the study was a revolution in the prevention and treatment of pressure sores. The application of potions such as alcohol, iodine and egg white was replaced by the relief of pressure and the use of a risk assessment 'scale' to identify vulnerable patients.

Another landmark for nursing research was the inquiry into the 'Proper Study of the Nurse', undertaken by the Royal College of Nursing (RCN). This study, which in fact comprised a number of projects, was an example of systematic research undertaken to investigate various aspects of nursing care (McFarlane 1970, Inman 1975). Spencer (1983) has criticised this research as being dominated by a 'medical' approach, yielding statistical, 'objective' results rather than the subjective, 'qualitative' findings more appropriate, in his view, to nursing. However, despite its limitations, the RCN research provided nurses with their first large-scale opportunity to investigate their practice.

In 1972, the Briggs Report (DHSS 1972) made a major impact on the development of nursing research, with the recommendations that nursing should become a research-based profession and that 'a sense of the need for research should become part of the mental equipment of every practising nurse or midwife'. These recommendations were made in the light of evidence that insufficient attention was paid by nursing and midwifery education to research as 'a continuing activity' and a 'prelude to innovation'.

More recently, a Taskforce was set up as part of the Department of Health Research and Development Strategy (Department of Health 1993). The importance of research to nursing was reaffirmed, and the contribution of small-scale projects undertaken as part of educational studies recognised. However, the Taskforce saw these studies as no 'substitute for the generalisable and cumulative research which we would place at the heart of a strategy for advancing research in nursing'. Becoming research aware and research minded will therefore give you insights into not only what makes research 'generalisable and cumulative', but also how it may fit in to your own career plans.

WHAT IS NURSING RESEARCH?

In common with other disciplines, nursing requires research to support both theory and practice. Research expands the profession's knowledge base and supports the development of new techniques. It contributes to the description and explanation of phenomena and provides a forum in which to generate and test ideas. 'Good' research comes from 'good' ideas, rather than from just perfecting one's research techniques (Open University 1979). Research is creative. It demands imagination and constant questioning of the world about us. Nurses should be alert to the unique opportunities for questioning the experiences that are presented to them by their professional circumstances. A researcher in a Boston hospital once told me how one of her projects had arisen (Rempusheski 1987). She was a specialist nurse in the care of the elderly, but, by chance, her office was situated close to the maternity unit. She found that distressed elderly relatives often found their way into her office as they waited anxiously for news of the progress of their premature grandchildren in the special care baby unit. In the 'foreign land' of obstetrics, Rempusheski found a research project about the elderly. There was little in the literature about the involvement of grandparents in family care, especially of their pre-term grandchildren. Rempusheski submitted a research proposal and obtained funding, so that now 'the unknown is in the process of becoming known'. McHaffie (1991) has since published on the topic in Britain.

Hockey (1985) defines nursing research as research into activities that are 'predominantly and appropriately the concern and responsibility of nurses' (Cormack 1991). McFarlane (1980), and other nursing theorists such as Parse (1989) and Watson (1985), sees nursing as both an art and a science, and argues that nursing research cannot be limited to the quantitative approaches adopted by many doctors and criticised by Spencer (1983).

NURSING STEREOTYPES

As part of becoming 'research minded', it is important to begin exploring some of the conflicting stereotypes relating to nursing and research. The popular conception of the nurse as engaged in 'women's work', which involves physical rather than mental labour, is hardly compatible with the notion of research as 'scientific', 'objective', and thus somehow a more masculine, endeavour. Although Salvage began to explode some of these stereotypes in the mid-1980s (Salvage 1985), there remains a persistent view of the medical and nursing hierarchy of the questioning nurse as an anomaly. Questioning still sometimes elicits the response 'You are not here to think, Nurse, but to do' (Hockey 1985).

Hockey (1985) writes that even as a young student nurse she kept a notebook in which she jotted down her ideas:

My first note dated September 1940 relates the elements of a discussion between a ward sister and myself, then a very junior probationer nurse. I was concerned about some patients getting bedsores (the notion of pressure sores was still many light years away) and why others did not: 'It could be the bed linen – it feels like boards but that is the same for all patients'. The ward sister did not seem too pleased. She informed me that I was here to heal the sores not to ask questions about them, and that we were far too busy, and in any case, if we knew the answer there wouldn't be any sores. I wrote: 'We don't know the answer, but shouldn't we?'

Hockey also describes nursing in a fever hospital during the Blitz. Because of the risk of shattering, glass partitions were removed. Surprisingly, there was no subsequent increase in the rate of cross-infection. Hockey asked the sister why this was so, given that the partitions had been seen as vital in preventing the spread of infection. What, therefore, was preventing it now? The reply came that she was tempting providence. 'Keep washing your hands,' Hockey was told, 'Watch and pray. We don't know why not, but we are thankful', Hockey notes in her diary 'We don't know why not, but shouldn't we?' (Hockey 1985).

TYPES OF RESEARCH

SCIENTIFIC DEDUCTIVE RESEARCH

Research has traditionally been seen to be removed from practical matters, such as those described in Hockey's diary. It has been associated with intellectuals and academics, whose pursuit of objective truth is conducted systematically and scientifically under experimental conditions. It is assumed that men are best suited to such endeavours, because women will confound the truth with their subjectivity and intuition (Roberts 1981).

According to Chalmers (1982), many self-styled 'scientific' researchers mistakenly believe that, in order to undertake 'reliable' research, it is necessary to adopt the 'pure' scientific methods used by physicists. These methods, said to be based on 'positivism', consist of careful observation and experiment and are used to collect 'facts', study their relationships and derive laws and theories from them. This 'scientific' style of research, which is used to test hypotheses and theories, is also referred to as 'quantitative' or 'deductive' research, which follows set rules to deduce conclusions from a set of premises.

Because physics so closely matches the popular idea of a pure science, its theories and associated research methods hold high status as dealing in 'hard' facts. In reality, physicists do not take their theories as fixed and unchangeable. Einstein was trying to prove all his life that his original theories were wrong – a process that the philosopher Karl Popper calls the 'falsification' of science. The spirit of scientific research is to falsify results by retesting them.

Modern advances in biology illustrate that the knowledge and techniques used in scientific research are not necessarily 'pure', nor do they produce 'hard' facts. DNA, for example, was only discovered using new techniques from physics, the electron microscope showing that original theories on molecules were wrong. These findings were very important for the advancement of molecular biology. In 'The Double Helix',

Watson, one scientist involved in these discoveries, describes the excitement and competition they felt as they pushed back the frontiers of knowledge (Watson 1980).

More recently, ruthless scientific competition was demonstrated by US medical researchers towards their French counterparts in their bid to be the first to isolate the human immunodeficiency (HIV) virus. Behaviour like this is a salutary reminder that scientists may be motivated by self-interests as well as altruism. The AIDS story, as told by Shilts in 'And the Band Played On' (Shilts 1987) is a powerful account of the interplay between politics and societal values in setting research agendas.

NATURALISTIC INDUCTIVE RESEARCH

The assumptions underlying research in the so-called 'pure' sciences are not necessarily appropriate to research associated with the social sciences, for example the ethnographic methods of participant observation and interviews used by anthropologists and sociologists to produce detailed accounts of social interactions and their associated meanings for different groups of people in their 'natural' settings. This naturalistic research style is referred to as 'qualitative' or 'inductive' research. Moving from particular observations to generalisations, the inductive researcher develops rather than tests theories based on interpretations from the data.

Inductive research is grounded in practice. McFarlane (1977) discusses this notion in the context of nursing as a practice discipline, and in response to the introduction of 'the nursing process' in the UK. The nursing process, in McFarlane's view, provides a means of systematising, recording and analysing nursing practice as a basis for research. The stages of assessment, planning and identification of outcomes constitute 'a form of research to which every nursing practitioner can contribute and only the practitioner can identify the cognitive process by which she arrived at certain actions' (McFarlane 1977). Benner's (1984) research describes these cognitive processes through 'exemplars', which describe how nurses learn, through practice, to become 'experts' able to make highly skilled clinical judgements about their patients. The exemplar and commentary given in Box 15.1 illustrates nursing knowledge as derived from and grounded in practice.

Box 15.1 Inductive reasoning (Reproduced with kind permission from Benner 1984)

Expert nurse

In the beginning, I was writing down all the times the blood pressures were to be taken, and then I thought 'Hey, wait a minute, let me think about this and decide whether I need to take them or not. After all it's not just something I'm supposed to do to make *me* feel better.' So I stop and think, what if I know what someone's blood pressure is? What does that tell me? Do I really need to know it? Especially with some of the postoperative eye patients who have been postop for a couple of days. We are expected to use our judgement as to when to discontinue the vital signs at night. So we carefully study the trends and the patient. Sometimes I substitute close observations so the patient can sleep.

Benner's commentary

In this example the nurse makes a judgement about the relative merits of rest and comfort over the prescribed therapy at a particular time in the patient's illness. There can never be precise scientific guidelines for these decisions because there could never be enough research done to capture the particulars of all situations. The nurse will always need to be able to weigh the important against the unimportant and, given the particular situation, risk choosing in the best interests of the patient.

ACTION RESEARCH

'Action research' is a good example of research that integrates a variety of methods and which is particularly popular among nurses, social workers and teachers. In this approach, the researcher is an active participant working closely with the subjects – identifying problems, implementing solutions and evaluating their effectiveness as part of a cyclical process. Bell (1993) concludes: 'The essentially practical, problem-solving nature of action research makes this approach attractive to practitioner–

researchers who have identified a problem during the course of their work, see the merits of investigating it and, if possible, of improving practice.'

TRIANGULATION

'Triangulation' is the term used to describe the use of a multimethod approach and/or data source to study a given research problem.

'Investigator triangulation' refers to the collection of data by more than one researcher in the same setting. The researcher can be more confident in the findings of a study if the same conclusions are reached by more than one method or investigator and/or through more than one data source. Corner (1991), a nurse researcher, confirms this view. She states that 'the use of triangulation of different methods and types of data in a simple study provides a richer and deeper understanding of the area under investigation than would otherwise be possible'.

THE RESEARCH PROCESS

We have already met the term 'process' in connection with McFarlane's (1977) discussion of the nursing process. The notion of process as 'a movement forward' is easily demonstrated in the four stages of the nursing process:

- assessment
- care planning
- implementation
- evaluation.

In rethinking the nursing process for the 1990s, Marks-Maran (1992) stresses the need for nurses to go beyond the method to define what underpins it. She suggests that nursing's value systems, including holism and the centrality of nurse–patient relationships, are the key. Naturalistic research is closely associated with such values, especially the importance of the relationship between the researcher and the researched.

The term 'process' is also used in the quality assurance literature, where it appears as one of the categories within which quality of care may be evaluated. The American physician Donabedian wrote a paper in the mid-1960s that has since become very influential. He suggested that quality may be evaluated according to the 'structure', 'process' and 'outcomes' of care. By 'process', Donabedian meant the actual content and methods of work used by physicians whilst in contact with patients (Donabedian 1966).

The 'research process' refers to the different steps involved in undertaking a research project. Like any process, its various stages may overlap. The research process consists of identifying a topic, specifying underlying theories, formulating questions, selecting a suitable approach or style, specifying methods and devising a plan to take the study forward.

An important part of the research plan includes the careful consideration of time and financial budgeting, secretarial support and ethical clearance. Time spent resolving organisational, political and ethical issues repays itself with interest over the rest of the study.

The research process can be divided into the following stages.

- Stage 1: Identifying the research topic
- Stage 2: Selecting an appropriate research approach
- Stage 3: Designing the study
- Stage 4: Developing data-collection methods and instruments
- Stage 5: Collecting and recording the data
- Stage 6: Analysing and interpreting the data
- Stage 7: Presenting the research findings.

The following sections outline these stages in the research process in some detail. Boxes within each section suggest questions that the student might pose with respect to each stage when critically evaluating her own and others' research.

STAGE 1: IDENTIFYING THE RESEARCH TOPIC

Ideas for research can derive from everyday experience. When researchers embark on a new project, they usually have a broad idea of what they want to study. They may discuss it with colleagues in order to compile a 'first thoughts' list of questions to help focus the research (Bell 1993). They will also search the literature, to find out what has already been written on the subject. The library is the best place to start: bibliographies, abstracts and indexes help to identify appropriate information quickly. Obtaining this information is referred to as 'information retrieval'.

Ogier (1989) gives some sound advice on searching the literature. First, she suggests clarifying the topic by identifying and listing key words associated with it. For example, when Ogier wanted to find out how the ward sister affected the learning environment for student nurses, she made a list of key words associated with her main research question in the following way (Ogier 1982).

- Sister: charge nurse, head nurse
- Learning: studying, teaching, understanding

Making a list helps to give the researcher some idea of where to start when visiting a library and beginning to look through abstracts, indexes and computerised information. It also makes it easier for the librarian to assist in selecting material. It is helpful to have a 'cut-off' date for searching the literature. Depending on the topic and the amount of information available, this could be as little as 5 or as many as 40 years.

The organised researcher immediately records the details of what she is reading on index cards or in a designated exercise book. The most common referencing systems are the Harvard and the Vancouver (numerical) systems, used in both books and articles, depending on the 'house' style of the publishers (Fig. 15.1).

Relationship between research topic and literature search

The researcher goes back and forth between the literature and the research topic in order to formulate research objectives, questions or hypotheses, and select a suitable approach, style and method. The relationship between the research topic, the developing question and the literature search as described by Cormack (1991) is illustrated in Figure 15.2.

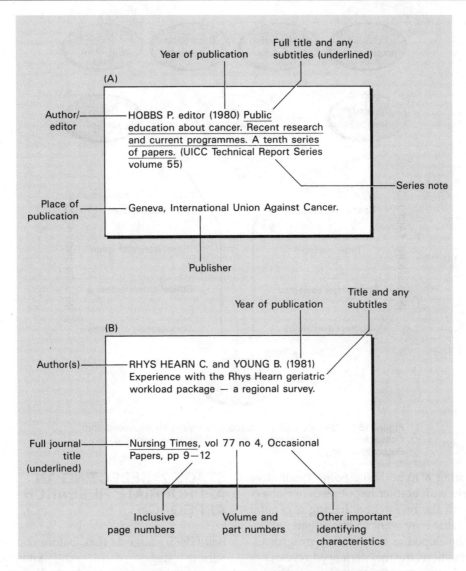

Figure 15.1 The Harvard referencing system. (A) Monograph reference. (B) Journal reference. (Reproduced from Cormack (1984) with the kind permission of Blackwell Scientific Publications Ltd.)

The formulation of the research question and approach should be summarised in a literature review at the beginning of a research report or article; this review should be comprehensive, up-to-date and relevant to the study (Box 15.2).

Formulating objectives, questions and hypotheses

The decision to set up objectives, questions or hypotheses will depend not only on the topic but also on the researcher's favoured research approach. Most experimental studies are geared

---

Box 15.2 **Critical assessment of research: Stage 1**

At the beginning of a research report or article, the research objectives/hypotheses and approach are summarised in a literature review; you will need to assess whether this review is comprehensive, recent and relevant to the study.

Questions to ask are:

- Does the literature review give evidence that the researcher knows her subject?
- Is the literature critically evaluated?
- Is the research problem stated as a hypothesis, as study objectives or as a general area of interest?

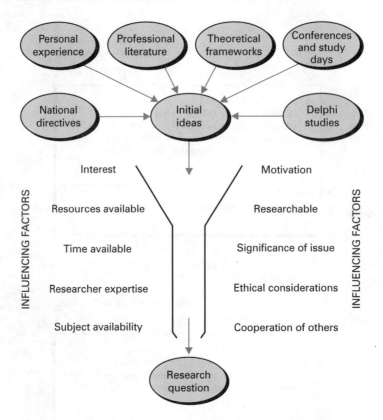

Figure 15.2   Development of a research question. (Reproduced from Cormack (1991) with the kind permission of Blackwell Scientific Publications Ltd.)

towards testing a hypothesis. Some qualitative studies begin with neither hypotheses nor objectives but with the researchers having a general idea about what they want to investigate; hypotheses are developed as the research progresses. Bell (1993) cautions the inexperienced researcher against this unstructured approach and advises, at the very least, 'a precise statement of objectives'.

James, a nurse sociologist, illustrates these difficulties at the beginning of her qualitative research on nursing the dying. Among her field-work notes is the comment, 'One of the problems all during today has been the vast input of possible information and not knowing how to select it.' It was not until James had time to withdraw and reflect on her nursing fieldwork 'that what had been written during it looked as though it had any purpose or explanatory use' (James 1984).

STAGE 2: SELECTING AN APPROPRIATE RESEARCH APPROACH

Bell (1993) suggests that 'before considering the various stages of planning and conducting investigations, researchers need to consider the main features of well-established and well reported styles of research'. These, as discussed in 'Types of research' above, may be classified as either quantitative or qualitative research styles, and depend to some extent on the different disciplines with which they are associated.

In the past, nurse researchers were more likely to adopt quantitative research approaches, possibly because, as Spencer (1983) suggests, these styles were more in keeping with the work of their medical colleagues. However, over the past decade or so, nurse researchers have also begun to embrace qualitative approaches, preferring to see the so-called 'divide' between the two approaches as more of a continuum in which, as Bell (1993) suggests, 'no approach prescribes nor automatically rejects any particular method'. Similarly, Haase and Myers (1988) note that some nurse researchers 'dissatisfied with a forced choice between approaches have advocated combining' qualitative and quantitative methods.

Influencing factors

In the end, a researcher's decision to select a particular research approach depends on a number of factors. It may be that one approach is more suitable to a particular research topic than another, or that the resources available to the researcher, including her own experience and preferences, the availability of a research supervisor (also with particular preferences), time, secretarial support and money all contribute to the final decision.

Take the example of my own research (Smith 1987). I began with the aim of studying the relationship between the quality of the nursing care received by patients and the quality of the ward as a learning environment for student nurses. At first, I set out with a quantitative view of research, in which I wanted to test the hypothesis that the quality of the nursing on the ward would determine whether the learning environment was negative or positive. In research language, what I was trying to 'prove' was that quality of nursing on a ward was directly related to the quality of the learning environment. In other words, the learning environment was dependent on the quality of nursing. This way of posing a research hypothesis is very much in the deductive or quantitative tradition of experimental research, in which hypotheses are 'tested' on the basis of an underlying theory.

However, once I entered the research setting, I quickly realised the impossibility of defining the relationship between quality of nursing and the learning environment in this way. I decided, therefore, to disregard my original strategy in favour of qualitative inductive research. The reason for changing to a qualitative approach

---

> **Box 15.3 Critical assessment of research: Stage 2**
>
> Questions to ask are:
>
> - Does the researcher declare her particular research approach?
> - Is it appropriate to the research topic under study?
> - Are any other factors evident, for example available time, money or expertise, for why the researcher has chosen the particular research approach?
> - Does the researcher make clear a particular theoretical framework underlying the approach?

was because I felt that it was more appropriate to exploring with nurses and patients what quality of nursing and the learning environment meant to them and how they saw the two relating to each other. This approach was very time-consuming, because I decided that, in order to find out about these issues, I needed to work on a variety of shifts and wards in order to talk to nurses and patients. In this way, I was able to allow my data to generate research questions inductively and shape the direction of the research, rather than fit them into a ready-made hypothesis.

Box 15.3 outlines several questions to be asked during the critical assessment of Stage 2 of the research process.

STAGE 3: DESIGNING THE STUDY

The design of a research study depends largely on whether the researcher adopts a quantitative, deductive research approach or a qualitative, inductive one. The most common types of study design are experimental and descriptive. The notion of study design is more applicable to quantitative than to qualitative research.

Quantitative research

Experimental designs

Experimental designs range from the very simple to the very complex. A simple design would be to test the effects of one single variable on another one. In the experimental context, variables are studied in pairs. Each of the paired variables has a separate name: the 'independent' (or 'causal') variable and the 'dependent' variable, which alters as a consequence of the independent variable.

The **randomised controlled trial** (RCT) is the most common example of an experiment used by doctors and familiar to many nurses in the context of drug and product (i.e. clinical) trials. The Department of Health's Research and Development strategy identifies the RCT as one of the most important ways of finding out whether or not treatments are effective. The Cochrane Centre in Oxford has been set up to review trial findings and disseminate them to clinicians and purchasers. In the context of the new market-led health service, this is seen as important in encouraging the use and purchase of 'tried and tested' health care. Nursing treatments have also been reviewed in this way. For example, Cullum, a nurse researcher, undertook a review of the community nursing management of leg ulcers and found the need for more trials to be undertaken to demonstrate their effectiveness (Cullum 1994). Sapsford & Abbott (1992) also point out that 'the logic of experimental design underlies all serious attempts to evaluate policy or practice'.

In order to set up an experiment or trial, the researcher decides, on the basis of logic, which variable is to be independent or dependent within a given experiment. For instance, if the researcher wanted to test whether a particular intervention, i.e. the independent variable (for example the introduction of a new drug, leg ulcer treatment or a counselling session) has affected the patient's recovery, i.e. the dependent variable, she would choose an experimental design for the study, involving a control group and an experimental group. The experimental group is a group of people to whom the experimental treatment (drug or counselling session) is given. The experimental group is compared with the control group, to whom no experimental treatment is given. The researcher studies the effects than each variable has on the other in two randomly selected experimental and control groups. In cross-over designs, the study subjects may also be used as their own controls, receiving different types of interventions at different stages of the study, using a 'cross-over' design. The logic behind this type of design is that more precise results may be obtained by comparing interventions in the same individual rather than across different groups.

The principles of **random selection and matching** are applied to the study's subjects. In random selection, all members of the population under study have an equal chance of being included in the study. 'Matching' refers to ensuring that subjects in the experimental and control groups are as similar as possible on characteristics (e.g. race, age, gender, class and occupation) that one might judge to be important. Any differences observed following the intervention could therefore be deemed to be attributable to the intervention rather than to differences between the two groups. Thus, random selection and matching allows causal inferences to be drawn from the results or outcomes of the intervention (e.g. the speed of recovery).

Webb & Wilson-Barnett chose an experimental design for their study of the relationship between counselling and women undergoing hysterectomy (Webb & Wilson-Barnett 1983). The design of the study is presented in Figure 15.3.

Webb & Wilson-Barnett (1983) added a third or 'placebo' group to their study design. Rather than receiving no intervention at all, as in the case of the control group, the placebo group was involved in a 20-minute conversation. This conversation avoided the topic of recovery, whereas the experimental group received a 20-minute counselling session offering them information and advice to promote recovery.

The reason for introducing a placebo group into a study is two-fold. First, it may help to discount any bias on the part of researcher or patient in their judgement (whether favourable or otherwise) with regard to the experimental intervention. Second, it provides a control for the frequency of spontaneous changes that may occur in the patient independent of the intervention under study. That spontaneous changes can occur during the experimental process is referred to as the 'Hawthorne' effect, because it was first described by researchers undertaking

PRIVATE AND CONFIDENTIAL

WARD LEARNING ENVIRONMENT RATING QUESTIONNAIRE

Ward.. Student ☐   Pupil ☐   Trained nurse ☐
(Please tick)

The following statements are concerned with nurse training in the ward. For each statement please indicate your opinion by placing a tick (✔) in one of the five boxes. There are no right or wrong answers, but please try to avoid the 'uncertain' column unless you really cannot agree or disagree. If you want to clarify or explain your choice, make your comments in the box provided.

Note: The term 'learner' is intended to include both student and pupil nurses. 'Sister' applies equally to charge nurses.

SECTION A (Questions 1 to 3 to be answered by student and pupil nurses only.)	Strongly agree	Agree	Uncertain	Disagree	Strongly disagree	Comments
1. This was a good ward for student/pupil learning.						
2. I am happy with the experience I have had on this ward.						
3. I learnt very much on this ward.						
(Remaining questions to be answered by everyone.)						
4. The number of staff is adequate for the workload.						
5. There is very much to learn on this ward.						
6. There are enough trained nurses in relation to learners and auxiliaries.						
7. The workload does not interfere with teaching or learning.						

Figure 15.3 Extract from Ward Learning Environment Rating Questionnaire. (Reproduced with kind permission from Fretwell 1985.)

studies in a factory of that name. If, however, differences only occur in the experimental group when compared with both the placebo and control groups, researchers are more able to claim that the differences are attributable to the intervention under study (Sapsford & Abbott 1992).

Webb & Wilson-Barnett (1983) also designed their study in such a way as to reduce the risk of the researcher having an effect, thus biasing the outcome of the study. Two researchers were involved. One researcher randomly allocated the patients to one of the three study groups and carried out the intervention (phase 2), whilst another researcher carried out the data collection visits (phases 1 and 3; see Fig. 15.3). Roles were regularly changed so that the researchers were unaware of the group to which the patient had been assigned.

It should be noted that structured interview schedules were used. Scales included a depression inventory, a mood adjective checklist and a self-concept scale.

In this way, the researchers did not have any expectations based on any prior knowledge of the three groups to which the patients were assigned; if they had, this may have influenced the outcome of the interviews and rating scales. For example, had the researchers known that the patients had received the experimental intervention, they might unconsciously have behaved in particular ways (e.g. using an encouraging tone of voice), which might have influenced the results obtained from the interviews and scales. Designing the study in this way helped to reduce the effects of researcher bias.

Trials are said to be 'double blind' when neither researcher nor subject knows which group he has been allocated to. Thus, as both parties are 'blind' to the particular treatment being given to particular patients, it is hoped to reduce what have been described as 'expectancy effects'.

Descriptive study design

The survey is an example of a descriptive study design and is also in the quantitative tradition. The aim of a survey is to obtain information that can be analysed and from which patterns can be extracted (Bell 1993). Information can be gathered in a survey in a variety of ways, including questionnaires, schedules and checklists. It is very important that all the respondents are asked the same questions in the same way. Rating scales of the type used by Webb & Wilson-Barnett (1983) may be devised in order to measure attitudes, beliefs or motivation. The survey primarily aims to collect facts in response to the questions 'What?' 'Where?', 'When?' and 'How?' (Bell 1993). Explanatory surveys that ask the question 'Why?' are sometimes conducted to follow up the information obtained from descriptive surveys.

If the study population is too big for everyone to be included in the survey, respondents will be randomly selected, as in an experimental study. This will help to ensure that the results are representative of the population from which they are drawn.

Study design depends largely on whether the researcher adopts a qualitative or quantitative research approach. For example, had I wanted to test whether a particular intervention (e.g. the introduction of specialised tutorials) had affected the relationship between the quality of nursing and the ward learning environment (Smith 1987), I would have chosen an experimental design for my study. I would have required a control group (ward 1) and an experimental group (ward 2). Each ward population, i.e. patients and nurses, would have had to be randomly selected and then matched, so that causal inferences could be drawn from the outcome measures (e.g. quality of nursing and ward learning) that I had chosen.

Qualitative research

Since qualitative research is concerned with subjective meanings for the participants in naturalistic settings, the principles applied to quantitative research in order to control the research environment are inappropriate. Differences in sampling technique illustrate this point.

Sampling is purposive and theoretical. Qualitative researchers do not seek 'representative' samples, but rather select those individuals with special knowledge or characteristics that will increase their understanding of the study phenomena. The next step is to develop theory from their findings and, where necessary, to collect additional information, through further theoretical sampling of groups and settings.

James (1984) and Melia (1982) both used purposive, or theoretical, sampling to establish their study subjects and settings. James worked on hospital wards and in a hospice in order to study the different ways in which dying patients were nursed. Melia asked for student nurse volunteers from a school of nursing, in order to find out about their experiences of nurse training. In quantitative research traditions, it would not have been acceptable to ask for volunteers to take part in the study: only random sampling would be seen to guarantee that the study sample was representative of the target population. However, for the qualitative researcher who wants to increase her understanding of the research setting, purposive or theoretical sampling is the method of choice. She also believes in declaring her biases and acknowledging her own part in the research setting from the outset. Melia, for example, declares that by actively involving herself with the people she was studying, she was in a much better position to present an 'account of how the participants see the situation or phenomenon in question; the analysis then goes beyond this point when analytical concepts which transcend the meanings of actors are developed' (Melia 1982).

In qualitative research, the steps of the research process are much less distinct than in quantitative research. Study design, development of hypotheses and methods, collection and analysis of data are closely integrated, and for this reason are not described separately.

Feminist perspectives

Qualitative research permits researchers to write themselves into the research and declare their biases. In recent years, feminist researchers have drawn attention to this important issue, particularly in relation to gender.

Many feminists favour qualitative research. Oakley (1981) criticises quantitative research for the way in which it mystifies 'the researcher and the researched as objective instruments of data production' and condemns 'personal involvement as dangerous bias'. For Oakley, who has studied various aspects of women's lives, ranging from housework to childbirth, the use of subjectivity in research is essential to both the collection and production of data (Oakley 1974, 1981). Oakley's favoured method of data collec-

tion is in-depth interviewing, which allows her to develop rapport, and in some instances friendships, with the women studied.

The feminist researchers Stanley & Wise (1983) drew attention to the potential power of the researcher over the researched, as information is extracted without reciprocity or responsibility. These observations are particularly relevant to nursing and health care research, in which nurses and patients can be especially vulnerable to external authority structures. James, for example, was concerned that because she was a participant observer, the nurses would become so used to her being around that they might forget they were the subjects of her research. She decided, therefore, periodically to make outrageous statements to remind people that there was a researcher in their midst (James 1984).

Webb has explicitly introduced feminist perspectives into nursing research. She describes feminist research (Webb 1984) as 'critique' that:

aims specifically to work towards defining alternatives and understanding everyday experience in order to bring about change. Analysis and critique of research methods leads on to analysis and critique in the research context through consciousness raising both for researcher and researched.

In her 1993 update, Webb suggests that 'a shorthand definition [of feminist research] perhaps could be phrased as "research *on* women, *by* women, *for* women". What is distinctive about feminist methodology is its engagement with issues of concern particularly to women and its acceptance of a variety of methods.'

The contribution of feminist perspectives to nursing research is particularly pertinent, given that nursing is a predominantly female occupation, and nurses are involved in traditionally female roles and work activities prescribed by the predominantly male medical profession. Feminist perspectives are committed to making gender and power relations visible in the world about us and in the relationships between researcher and researched.

Until recently, feminist research almost exclusively embraced qualitative approaches. Oakley (1989), in an apparent break with tradition, brought a feminist perspective to the seemingly most explicit of quantitative research approaches, the RCT, in order to study social support in the ante-natal care of 'at-risk' mothers. In a detailed article, she demonstrated how the best of the two approaches could be combined to address sampling accuracy, the selection of appropriate methods, the informed consent of subjects, the formulation of research questions, and the analysis and use of findings from women's perspectives rather than from the dominant male medicoscientific, professional view of the world.

The following example gives an unexpected perspective on sampling accuracy. Citing the case of random allocation of subjects to experimental and control groups, Oakley showed how midwives' intuitive judgements were sometimes in conflict with objective sampling techniques. She put this down to health professionals' ideology, which previous researchers had shown led 'to discriminatory stereotyping of women, based on such characteristics as working class or ethnic minority'. This example is a further illustration of how a feminist approach differed from the more usual 'hands-off' conduction of RCTs. Midwives were responsible for recruiting and randomly sampling the women who attended ante-natal clinic. It was only because Oakley chose to keep in close contact with the midwives that she was able to discuss how they felt about random sampling. In the end, she probably obtained a more accurate sample than she might have done had she not engaged with them.

Box 15.4 outlines questions to be asked in Stage 3 of the research process.

STAGE 4: DEVELOPING DATA-COLLECTION METHODS AND INSTRUMENTS

Quantitative research

The pilot study

In the quantitative research tradition, a pilot study is likely to be conducted when data collection methods and techniques are developed as a

---

Box 15.4 Critical assessment of research: Stage 3

The questions you ask here will depend very much on the underlying approach adopted by the researcher and how it has influenced the study design:

- What is the sample size? How was it selected, and is it representative of the population under study?
- Were there a control group and an experimental group?
- (In qualitative studies) Are the unique issues of sampling of the qualitative study addressed, and are the characteristics of the population outlined?
- Does the researcher write herself into the study and declare her biases?
- Is the statement of the research problem, as hypotheses or objectives, appropriate to the study design and the topic for investigation?

---

prelude to the main study. Common tools include questionnaires and non-participant observation schedules.

One of the reasons for conducting a pilot study is to develop research tools that are reliable (i.e. whose results can be replicated under a variety of conditions) and valid (i.e. they measure what they purport to). This emphasis is seen to be a vital component of pursuing objective scientific proof.

Developing the questionnaire

A common questionnaire design is the Likert scale, in which respondents are asked to rate their responses on a scale of 1 to 4, 5 or 6. One such example is Fretwell's Ward Learning Environment Rating Questionnaire (Fretwell 1985) (Fig. 15.4). This 36-item questionnaire covers different aspects of the learning environment, including ward atmosphere and staff relations, ward teaching, provision of learning opportunities, patient care, anxiety and stress. Nursing students and staff were asked to rate each item as a factor in the ward learning environment on a scale of 1 (strongly disagree) to 5 (strongly agree). The scores were then added together and an average mean score obtained for each aspect of the learning environment and for the ward overall.

Date:

QUALITY PATIENT CARE SCALE

Qualpacs

Patient (name or no.):   Rater (name or no.):

INTERACTIONS RECORD: AM/PM

No.:

Time:

PSYCHOSOCIAL: INDIVIDUAL

Actions directed toward meeting
psychosocial needs of individual patients

ITEM NUMBER	BEST CARE	BETWEEN	AVERAGE CARE	BETWEEN	POOREST CARE	NOT APPLICABLE	NOT OBSERVED	MEAN SCORE
								11—12
1. Patient receives nurse's full attention. — 1								
								13—14
2. Patient is given an opportunity to explain his feelings. — 2								
								15—16
3. Patient is approached in a kind, gentle and friendly manner. — 3								

Figure 15.4 Extract from Wandelt & Ager (1974) 68-item Quality Patient Care Scale. (Reproduced with kind permission of Appleton & Lange.)

Entire textbooks have been written on questionnaire design. The student may find Oppenheim (1992) and Moser & Kalton (1985) especially helpful.

However, there are a few basic rules to observe in designing a questionnaire, such as constructing questions that use language familiar to the respondents and that are free of in-built biases (thus avoiding the 'leading questions' that Florence Nightingale warned against). Cicourel believes that research instruments such as questionnaires allow researchers to devise coding rules and scaling devices to 'transform the structure of social action into quantifiable elements', from their own but not necessarily the respondents' point of view. He gives important advice when he says (Cicourel 1964), 'Operational definitions of sociological concepts [e.g. nursing, quality of care, learning environment] need to be constructed in such a way in order that every-day life experience and conduct is reflected in them.'

Non-participant observation schedules

Similarly, the same basic rules should be followed in constructing observation schedules, such as those for observing quality of nursing (Wandelt & Ager 1974), ward sister activity (Pembrey 1980), ward reporting systems (Lelean 1975) and paediatric ward organisation (Hawthorne 1974). An extract from Wandelt & Ager's Quality Patient Care Scale is given in Figure 15.5.

Qualitative research

Qualitative research approaches are inductive, in that theoretical concepts are developed from the data as they are collected, and analysed as the study progresses. We can see that this approach differs from quantitative, deductive research, in which all the data are collected before analysing them in order to test existing concepts and theories. The qualitative researcher regularly leaves the field to code, reflect on what she has observed and make inferences from the data to guide future fieldwork.

Grounded theory is an example of an integrated, qualitative research approach popular among nurse researchers (Glaser & Strauss 1967). The approach provides a flexible framework for inductive research. Data are collected, coded and analysed, in order to develop conceptual categories and to formulate hypotheses to guide ongoing data collection. Grounded theory shares features with other qualitative approaches, in that data analysis is part and parcel of the research process and begins early on in the study.

Ethnography and **phenomenology** are other examples of qualitative research approaches that have gained in popularity among nurse researchers over the last decade. Ethnography is seen by many nurses as being eminently suitable to the detailed study of small groups within health care settings, because of its attention to culture and meaning. The key method of ethnography is participant observation, through which in-depth descriptive accounts are developed from detailed fieldnotes. Some ethnographers go beyond descriptions to compare their findings with existing social theories (e.g. 'deviance') and also to reflect on how one in-depth study may also reflect what is going on in the outside world. For example, a detailed study of health care reforms among district nurses in one health care setting reflected the wider policy issues taking place at government level (Smith et al 1993). Critical ethographers give back their accounts to the people they have observed to challenge their perspectives and incorporate the participants' views into their findings (Street 1992).

Benner has popularised phenomenology through her writings, including 'From Novice to Expert' referred to above (see Box 15.1). Benner gives credence to the unique nature of the individual and the importance of the 'lived

	Phase 1 5–6 days postoperatively	Phase 2 6–7 days postoperatively	Phase 3 4 months postoperatively
Experimental group	Interview and scales	20-minute advice and information session	interview and scales
Placebo group	Interview and scales	20-minute conversation	Interview and scales
Control group	Interview and scales	No intervention	Interview and scales
Note: Structured interview schedules were used. Scales included a depression inventory, a mood adjective check-list and a self-concept scale.			

Figure 15.5 Diagram of a study by Webb & Wilson-Barnett on the relationship between counselling and recovery from hysterectomy. (Reproduced by kind permission of *Nursing Times*, where this article first appeared on 23 November 1983.)

experience'. Phenomenologists use in-depth interviewing and detailed analysis and commentary of the content.

Each of the above approaches is informed by the social sciences. Grounded theory, for example, was first developed by sociologists, ethnography by anthropologists and phenomenology by philosophers (Thorne 1991). They were formulated by social scientists who were reacting to what they saw as the 'rigidity' of the 'scientific' quantitative approach to research.

Validity and reliability

The validity and reliability of data are integral to qualitative research approaches. Validity is implicit when data are simultaneously collected, handled and analysed to shape ongoing data collection and to develop and confirm evolving theories and concepts. Hall & Stevens (1991) prefer to use the term 'adequacy' rather than validity to evaluate the whole research process from formulation of questions, selection of methods to outcomes that incorporate the participants' perspectives. Reliability (which Hall & Stevens call 'dependability') is ascertained by means of the researcher's in-depth involvement in the field over time and with increasing familiarity, which means she is able to check the accuracy and recurrence of the data in a number of settings and from a number of participants (Field & Morse 1985).

Questions concerning validity and reliability are among those to be asked in Stage 4 of the research process (Box 15.5).

Box 15.5 Critical assessment of research: Stage 4

The questions you ask here will depend very much on the underlying approach adopted by the researcher:

- (In quantitative studies) Was a pilot study carried out? If so, what changes were made to the main study as a result of the pilot?
- Were issues of validity and reliability (including adequacy and dependability) addressed from each perspective?
- (In qualitative studies) Does the researcher present hypotheses, concepts and theories derived from the data?

STAGE 5: COLLECTING AND RECORDING THE DATA

Quantitative research

The most common quantitative means of data collection are questionnaires, semi-structured interviews and non-participant observation; these are developed during the pilot phase of the study. Webb & Wilson-Barnett (1983) (see above), for example, used a variety of these methods, including structured interview schedules, a depression inventory scale, a mood adjective checklist and a self-concept scale. The process of developing such data collection tools is described in the preceding section.

In order for researchers to retrieve their data easily and accurately for analysis and interpretation, it is important that, during data collection, they develop systems to ensure this. In quantitative studies, it is likely that the data are collected and recorded on standardised forms, for example self-administered questionnaires and structured interview schedules.

Qualitative research

As noted above, the most common qualitative research methods include participant observation and in-depth interviewing, to study complex phenomena such as care of the dying and student nurse socialisation.

Participant observation

The classification of the participant observer role is well documented in the literature. The observer's participant role can be seen on a continuum from complete, even covert, in which the subjects are unaware that they are being studied, to non-participant, in which the observer records data from the sidelines. A common compromise is for the researcher to adopt the role of observer-as-participant, in which she is known to be conducting research but participates in the everyday activities of the research setting.

Collins (1984) suggests that full participation is essential if the researcher is to understand the subjects and settings under study. He calls this understanding 'participant comprehension'. My own research (Smith 1987, 1992) aimed to emulate this approach during participant observation on the wards. When observing classroom activities, I was a complete observer, sitting at the back of the room trying to be a 'fly on the wall'.

Melia (1982) applies the participant observer concept to in-depth interviewing. She contends that 'the close involvement of the researcher in the production of the data is as true of the informal interview method of data production as it is of participant observation'. Not only was Melia familiar with the setting from which her subjects came, being a nurse herself, but she also used the interview as a forum through which to interact with them in the production of data.

In qualitative studies, the researcher has to develop ways of recording fieldwork notes during participant observation, such as by keeping index cards to record observations as events take place, for example mealtimes in a day nursery. Interviews are (with the participants' permission) most often tape-recorded. The tapes are then transcribed into typescript form to facilitate analysis of the interview contents.

Box 15.6 outlines questions for Stage 5.

STAGE 6: ANALYSIS AND INTERPRETATION

Data analysis and interpretation is often the most time-consuming phase of the research process. In planning a research project, it is wise to allocate twice as much time for analysis and interpretation as for data collection: if it takes 2 months to collect data, it is likely to take 4 months to analyse and interpret them. Processed data are referred to as 'findings' or 'results'. Methods of data analysis vary according to the underlying research approach.

Quantitative research

In quantitative research, data are analysed numerically once they have been collected. Large-scale surveys and experimental studies require statistical testing of hypotheses. Statistical associations and differences between variables are established, and causal inferences may be made. Tests are used to establish the statistical significance of these associations and differences.

Statistical tests are based on probability theory, and the researcher will need to consult a statistician in order to choose the appropriate test given the size of sample, type of data and questions being asked. Most statistics textbooks include a chart that helps the researcher to select the appropriate tests. In short, the data are manipulated statistically in order to ensure that the results have not occurred by chance. You will usually see this written as '$p < 0.05$' or '$p < 0.01$' beside the results. The p values mean that the probability of the results having occurred by chance is less than 5% or 1% respectively. When the probability of results occurring by chance is greater than 5%, they are usually considered to be 'not significant' ('NS').

The importance of logic in interpreting results cannot be underestimated. Just because a 'significant' result seems to have been obtained does not mean that 'cause' and 'effect' are automatically established. A number of conditions need to be met if causality between variables is to be demonstrated. First and foremost, the researcher must make sure that an accidental link does not bind independent and dependent variables together in a 'spurious' relationship. The sociologist Rosenberg gives a familiar example to illustrate this point. In Sweden, a relationship was found between the number of storks and the number of children born in a

---

Box 15.6 Critical assessment of research: Stage 5

The questions you ask here will depend very much on the underlying approach adopted by the researcher and how it has influenced the choice of method. For both qualitative and quantitative studies:

- What research methods were used?
- Were they justified and explained according to the approach adopted?
- Were they appropriate?
- Were copies of questionnaires, and of interview and observation schedules, available in the report?
- Were methods of recording and retrieving data clearly described?

given area. This finding could be interpreted as meaning that in some way the storks were a 'causal' factor in the number of babies being born. Rosenberg explains: 'The reason for the relationship between number of storks and number of babies is urban–rural location. Most storks are found in rural areas and the rural birth rate is higher than the urban birth rate. . . . Unless one guards against such accidental associations, one is in danger of reaching erroneous and misleading conclusions.'

Using computers

In large-sample surveys, it is likely that the researcher will store data in a computer. This will potentially ease and speed up data analysis. If the sample is small, however, it may be quicker to analyse the data by hand. Data, it should be remembered, are only as good as the operator who enters them into the computer and the logic that inspires decisions about statistical tests. Preparing data for analysis may also be very time-consuming. First, crude data are taken from the questionnaire or interview schedule and coded, ready to be 'punched' into the computer. The data will ideally be inserted into a ready made spreadsheet to create a database. The database can then be used in conjunction with a statistical programme such as SPSS (Statistical Package for the Social Sciences) to analyse the data using summary statistics (e.g. frequencies and average – mean, median and modes) and appropriate statistical significance tests (Jolley 1991).

Truman (1992) defines information technology (IT) as 'the generic term used to describe the processing of information using micro-processor-based electronic equipment' (i.e. computers). The 1970s marked the advent of the computer age, and intensive research and development has ensured a rapidly changing technology. Because of this, computers are constantly being updated. The development of the microchip has meant not only that their design has become much more compact, but that their 'memory', i.e. the amount of information they are able to store on their hard disk at any one time, and the speed with which they can process it, has also increased.

The computer's 'nerve centre' is the central processing unit (CPU), which responds to instructions contained in specially designed programmes or 'software'. A computer system is made up of a number of components, known as 'hardware', represented diagrammatically in Figure 15.6. These include the 'input devices', such as the keyboard, mouse and modem; the 'output devices', including the printer, monitor or visual display unit (VDU) and modem; and

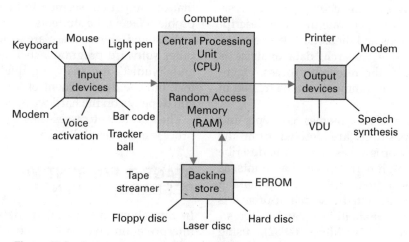

Figure 15.6   A computer system (Truman 1992).

data storage systems – hard disk, floppy disk, laser disk or CD-ROM (compact disc – Read Only Memory).

The most common applications of IT to research, including some of the examples referred to elsewhere, are: word processing; spreadsheets; databases, including CD-ROMs of references and other library information; statistical analysis, using, for example, SPSS; and textual analysis, for example the 'Nudist' and 'Ethnograph' programs. There are many different programs available for each of these applications, and (like computer hardware) they are constantly being updated and developed.

Since large amounts of personal information can be stored on databases, the Data Protection Act was introduced in 1983 to ensure the accuracy and security of the data being stored. Anyone undertaking research using personal records is required to register under the Act with a local Data Protection Officer. This measure helps to ensure that the data are being used for the purposes stated, and to maintain confidentiality and security of the system.

Qualitative research

In qualitative research, analysis takes place alongside data collection. Data are collected, coded and analysed in order that the researcher can decide what future data should be collected, and from where and whom they should be obtained. The process of coding and analysis continues in order to generate in-depth descriptions, interpretations and theoretical perspectives. Thus, in qualitative research, data analysis is part and parcel of the research process. Open-ended questionnaire comments can be treated in a similar way.

In qualitative analysis, themes, concepts and theoretical propositions are derived from the data as the study progresses, in order to describe phenomena through narratives and accounts, as a way of understanding, explaining and making inferences. This integrated research approach is the hallmark of the qualitative research process.

We have seen how Melia (1982), using grounded theory, approached the study of student nurse socialisation and involved herself in the research process and in data production, but how did she produce her findings? The following gives an example of how she derived categories from her data in order to explain the way in which student nurses constructed their world.

Analysis of the interviews yielded six conceptual categories, which Melia used as a framework for presenting substantive issues raised by the students in her study. The categories were as follows: 'learning and working', 'getting the work done', 'learning the rules', 'nursing in the dark', 'just passing through', 'doing nursing' and 'being professional'. From 'nursing in the dark', for example, she derived further categories, which she labelled 'coping with the dark', 'fobbing off the patient' and 'awareness contexts'. 'Awareness contexts' related to confusion about who knew what about patients' diagnoses and treatments, and was a concept first developed by Glaser & Strauss (1965) in a study of dying patients.

Melia illustrated her findings with interview data. She also illustrated the way in which qualitative researchers use concepts described in previous studies to interpret and confirm their findings. Rather than fitting in her data to the exact categories derived by Glaser & Strauss, Melia used their work to 'highlight the uncertainty which surrounds the whole business of student nurses talking with patients. The uncertainty both of their own knowledge and that of the patient seemed to be the crux of the problem facing the students.'

As stated above, there are a number of computer software programs, such as 'Ethnograph' and 'Nudist', for analysing qualitative data as text, but the development of ideas and findings still depends on the hard work of the researcher.

The questions to assess Stage 6 of the research process are given in Box 15.7.

STAGE 7: PRESENTING THE RESEARCH FINDINGS

In our above discussion of data analysis and interpretation, we saw some of the ways in which research findings and results can be

Box 15.8 identifies questions for Stage 7.

Box 15.7 **Critical assessment of research: Stage 6**

Questions to ask are:

- Does the researcher outline a plan for keeping data organised and retrievable from fieldwork observation and interviews?
- Does the researcher clearly explain how the data were prepared for analysis and how they were analysed?
- (In quantitative research) Are the reasons for choosing particular statistical tests given?
- (In quantitative research) Does the researcher include the statistical significance of the results?
- (In qualitative research) Do the findings contribute to theory-building?
- Do the results/findings relate to the original research questions, and does the researcher show evidence of having drawn logical conclusions from the data?

Box 15.8 **Critical assessment of research: Stage 7**

Questions to ask are:

- Is the research clearly presented, both visually and verbally?
- Do the recommendations and applications to practice follow logically from the preceding sections of the report?

ETHICAL ISSUES

Research must always be scrutinised for its ethical implications. In order to protect both subjects and researchers, most hospitals have set up ethics committees. Guidelines for preparing research proposals prior to submission to the ethics committee have been produced by the Royal College of Physicians and the Royal College of Nursing (Royal College of Nursing 1991). The Centre for Nursing and Midwifery Ethics, re-named the European Centre for Professional Ethics and located at the University of East London, was founded to encourage 'a critique of mainsteam biomedical ethics'. It also promotes discussion among practitioners and emphasises the views of patients (Hunt 1991). The Centre produces a *Journal of Nursing Ethics* and has set up a carers' network, called 'Freedom to Care', which supports individuals in speaking out against unethical practices.

presented: qualitative research is presented through words and narratives, quantitative research through numbers and statistical manipulations and perhaps also in tables and graphs.

Researchers may change their style of presentation according to their audience. Melia wrote up her research for two journals: the *Journal of Advanced Nursing* (Melia 1982) and *Nursing Times* (Melia 1983). To the non-researcher, the article in the first journal may appear 'jargonistic', using language that is difficult to understand. In the *Nursing Times* article, the language is much more accessible and easier to understand by the field-level nurse.

The issue of whether the researcher should write in the first or third person is discussed by Webb (1992). The convention in quantitative research has been to maintain objectivity by writing in the third person. In this way, the researcher is seen to be authoritative. Qualitative, and particularly feminist, researchers have preferred to write in the first person. In this way, they are able to write themselves into their research accounts and make their methods and findings more accessible to the reader.

Researchers have a responsibility to disseminate their findings and demonstrate their application to practice. Norton et al's (1962) early research on pressure area care is a case in point (see 'Historical perspectives', above).

Unexpected ethical consequences can result from seemingly 'neutral' theoretical science; for example, the application of theoretical physics to the development of the atom bomb did untold harm and formed no part of Einstein's original intentions.

Unlike obviously intrusive clinical trials, and research practices such as giving placebos rather than treatment or testing drugs with unknown side-effects, qualitative research is often seen as exempt from the need to be scrutinised by an ethics committee. However, the ethical implications of covert research, i.e. research undertaken without the subjects' knowledge, are apparent when findings are reported without the subjects ever having known they were being observed.

Consider, too, the ethical implications of interviews about feelings and emotions, such as those conducted during Brown & Harris' study (1978) of the social origins of women's depression. Such interviews need to be carefully managed so as not to distress the interviewee.

Many ethics committees now expect the researcher to prepare a written consent form, to be signed by the subjects, following a full explanation of events, before the research commences. This is known as informed consent. Any nurse is within her rights to ask to see the consent form before allowing researchers access to patients (see Ch. 12).

RESEARCH AS PART OF NURSING KNOWLEDGE AND PRACTICE

EDUCATION

Most students in institutes of higher education would take it for granted that the knowledge being imparted was research based. However, as we have seen, nursing is a relative newcomer to the world of research. What, then, is research likely to mean for student nurses? In class, teachers may refer to the latest research findings. They will also expect students to undertake a literature review on a given topic as part of written assignments, whether projects or essays. In clinical areas, students may find that trained staff apply research to practice or use it to evaluate care.

There is still some controversy on whether or not there is a discrete body of knowledge that constitutes nursing theory. Some educators and researchers prefer to see nursing as a multi-disciplinary field, drawing on a variety of areas, such as psychology, biology and sociology, for its theoretical underpinning. When I undertook some research into nursing education in the early 1980s, many nurses still used A-level biology as the yardstick by which to measure their knowledge of nursing. Their programme of studies did not offer them any alternative

measure. Even the biological knowledge that they were given was outdated and failed to take account of developments in molecular biology.

The new educational programme for nurses, Project 2000, promises to redefine nursing knowledge in terms of the 'new nursing'. According to Salvage (1990), the 'new nursing' dates back to the 1970s and is linked to an interest in nursing theory associated with the growth of academic nursing, the women's movement challenging male (i.e. doctor) domination and the redefinition of the nurse's unique contribution to healing. Salvage summarises an important element of the 'new nursing' ideology and practice as 'transforming relationships with patients – away from the biomedical model which views medical intervention as the solution to health problems, towards a holistic approach promoting the patient's active participation in care'.

Others, particularly feminists, prefer to see knowledge redefined in nursing's and women's own terms.

PRACTICE

Research is learned by doing as well as by reading what researchers have chosen to record about their methods and results. Physics and psychology students learn research techniques in the laboratory. Nurses learn them in the wards as they observe, measure and question. Thus, as Bond said, 'measurement in nursing is not only the province of those whose orientation leans towards research' (cited in Tierney et al 1988).

As Hockey (1985) and Rempusheski (1987) show us, some of the best research ideas come from everyday practice. Nurses now have a body of knowledge to which they can refer, unlike Hockey, who could only speculate on the cause of pressure sores and the spread of infection.

The advent of the 'new nursing' has been associated with a number of innovations, including primary nursing and the setting up of nursing development units (NDUs). Such units are ideally suited to the development of research and research-based practice. For example, the

NDU at London's Middlesex Hospital, during its 3-year history, undertook a number of research-based initiatives, such as evaluating the quality of nursing following the introduction of primary nursing and a study of the effect on patients and staff when nurses came out of uniform (Bamford & Sparrow 1990, Bamford et al 1990). The reasons for the rise and fall of the unit are discussed in a forthcoming publication by some of its founder members.

Rees (1992), citing Schön, suggests that research skills are closely associated with developing the skills of reflective practice and promoting new ways of seeing, thinking, doing and knowing.

NURSING RESEARCH

Nursing research takes place at a number of different levels. There are those nurses who have studied for higher degrees such as Masters and doctoral degrees. Many of the resulting dissertations and theses can be found in the Steinberg Collection of the Royal College of Nursing library in London. This collection bears witness to the vast range of nursing topics that have been researched over the years. In addition, many nurses have undertaken research-based projects as part of their pre- and post-registration nursing courses. Other nurses have decided that they would like to undertake a research project as part of their job. I knew a clinical nurse specialist who cared for children with long-term tracheostomies. She felt that these families' needs were so special that she wanted to find out more in order to evaluate and perhaps improve the children's care. She did this by interviewing the children's mothers. Her findings helped her to prepare discharge guidelines for the children, which included the allocation of a primary nurse to promote continuity of care, planned home visits prior to discharge, improved community liaison and the preparation of as many people associated with the child as possible to undertake tracheostomy care, rather than relying solely on the mother (Jennings 1989). This study is a good example of applied research undertaken to evaluate and improve practice.

Many nurses still acquire their research experience through working as data collectors with doctors. It is not unusual for them to feel frustrated if they find that nursing and medical values come into conflict. One research nurse, an experienced ward sister, was involved in a two-centre study to investigate palliative treatments of oesophageal cancer. She found herself unable 'objectively' to fill in quality of life scales with the patients. As the patients came back for repeat treatments and clinic attendances, the research nurse got to know them, and a rapport was established. Some patients visibly brightened when they saw her, and she was aware that this, in turn, improved their quality of life scores. In other words, her presence biased the scores of some patients for the better. The doctors found great difficulty in accepting her 'subjective' observations (Grigg & Smith 1989). However, medical research can often be an important starting point for a career as a nurse researcher. Students should watch for medical research being undertaken on their ward; it could be that the person collecting the data is a nurse.

Being 'research-minded'

The content of this chapter has been designed to make nursing students 'research-minded' so that they feel confident enough to ask questions and seek information about the clinical and educational world about them. Choosing a user-friendly textbook is a good starting-point. Everyone has his or her favourite, and I have referred to some of mine throughout this chapter. Reading research reports and being able to evaluate them critically is an important consideration in research-mindedness, since we need to be confident in research findings if we are to apply them to practice. Recently, I asked some of my students, who were experienced clinical nurses and teachers, if they thought that research had changed and improved practice. They immediately referred to pressure area research (Norton et al 1962) and to studies recommending the need to allow more parent involvement in the care of children on paediatric wards (Hawthorne 1974). I hope that during his or her nursing course, the present reader will be able to identify many other examples of how research has improved practice.

Local colleges or NHS Trusts may employ nurse researchers and run research interest groups or journal clubs as part of a research network. The library is always a good place to begin the search. It seems that we have progressed some way from the days when Hockey, as an enquiring probationer nurse, was told to 'watch and pray'. After nearly 50 years, we have a few more answers to our questions but many more remain.

Summary

Until the 1960s, research played only a minor role in the development of nursing practice, education and management. Now, however, it is realised that high-quality care cannot be achieved without challenging previously-held beliefs and practices, and formulating innovative approaches to nursing, teaching and managing. Consequently research now enjoys a higher profile in nursing.

There are many approaches and types of research. This chapter outlines these different types and clarifies the stages of the research process, with examples from the literature. Principles to ensure valid collecting, analysis and interpretation of data are highlighted.

Having worked through this chapter, the reader will be able to criticise and contribute towards research studies, incorporating the results into his or her own practice and improving the quality of patient care as the ultimate goal.

ACKNOWLEDGEMENTS

To all my students at the RCN's Institute of Advanced Nursing Education, London who have responded to and challenged my research assumptions and teaching methods over the past 2 years.

REFERENCES

Bamford O, Sparrow S 1990 Nursing development units: a virtue in uniformity? Nursing Times 86(41): 46–48
Bamford O, Dinean L, Pritchard B, Smith P 1990 Change for the better. Nursing Times 86(23): 28–33
Bell J 1993 Doing your research project: a guide for first time researchers in education and social science, 2nd edn. Open University Press, Buckingham
Benner P 1984 From novice to expert: excellence and power in clinical nursing practice. Addison Wesley, Menlo Park, California
Brown G, Harris T 1978 The social origins of depression in women. Tavistock, London
Chalmers A F 1982 What is this thing called science?, 2nd edn. Open University Press, Milton Keynes
Cicourel A 1964 Fixed choice questionnaires. Method and measurement in sociology. Free Press, New York
Collins H M 1984 Researching spoonbending: concepts and practice of participatory fieldwork. In: Bell C, Roberts H (eds) Social researching: politics, problems, practice. Routledge & Kegan Paul, London, pp 54–69
Cormack D F S (ed.) 1991 The research process in nursing, 2nd edn. Blackwell Scientific, Oxford
Corner J 1991 In search of more complete answers to research questions. Quantitative versus qualitative research methods: is there a way forward? Journal of Advanced Nursing 16(3): 718–727
Cullum N 1994 Leg ulcer treatments: a critical review, parts 1 and 2. Nursing Standard 9(1): 29–33; 9(2): 32–36
Department of Health (1993) Report of the Taskforce on the Strategy in Nursing, Midwifery and Health Visiting. HMSO, London
DHSS 1972 Report of the Committee on Nursing (The Briggs Report). HMSO, London
Donabedian A 1966 Evaluating the quality of medical care. Millbank Memorial Fund Quarterly 44: 166–206
Field P A, Morse J M 1985 Nursing research: the application of qualitative approaches. Croom Helm, London
Fretwell J 1985 Freedom to change. RCN, London
Glaser B G, Strauss A L 1965 Awareness of dying. Aldine, Chicago
Glaser B G, Strauss A L 1967 The discovery of grounded theory. Weidenfeld & Nicolson, London
Great Britain Statutory Instrument (1989) Nurses, Midwives and Health Visitors Training Amendment Rules, Schedule 2, S.I. No. 1456, Rule 18a. HMSO, London
Grigg D, Smith P 1989 Emotional labour, nursing worth and the research process: measuring the quality of life. Paper presented at Royal College of Nursing Research Society Conference, Swansea University, 14–16 April
Haase J E, Myers S T 1988 Reconciling paradigm assumptions of qualitative and quantitative research. Western Journal of Nursing Research 10(2): 128–137
Hall J M, Stevens P E 1991 Rigor in feminist research. Advances in Nursing Science 13(3): 16–29
Hawthorne P 1974 Nurse, I want my mummy! RCN, London
Hockey L 1985 Nursing research: mistakes and misconceptions. Churchill Livingstone, Edinburgh
Hunt G 1991 Can nursing lead care? Nursing Standard 5(25): 18
Inman U 1975 Towards a theory of nursing care. RCN, London
James N 1984 A postscript to nursing. In: Bell C, Roberts H (eds) Social researching: politics, problems, practice. Routledge & Kegan Paul, London, p 137
Jennings P 1989 Tracheostomy care: learning to cope at home. Paediatric Nursing 7(1): 13–15
Jolley J 1991 Using statistics. Computing in practice: information management and technology series. Nursing Times 87(25): 57–59
Lelean S R 1975 Ready for report, nurse? RCN, London

McFarlane J K 1970 The proper study of the nurse. RCN, London

McFarlane J K 1977 Developing a theory of nursing: the relation of theory to practice, education and research. Journal of Advanced Nursing 2: 261–270

McFarlane J K 1980 Nursing as a research-based profession. Nursing Times Occasional Paper 76(13): 57–60

McHaffie H E 1991 Neonatal intensive care units: visiting policies for grandparents. Midwifery 7(3): 122–123; 7(4): 193–203

Marks-Maran D 1992 Rethinking the nursing process. In: Jolley M and Brykczynska G (eds) Nursing care – the challenge to change. Edward Arnold, London, pp 92–95

Melia K 1982 'Tell it as it is': qualitative methodology and nursing research: understanding the student nurse's world. Journal of Advanced Nursing 7: 327–335

Melia K 1983 Students' view of nursing: discussion of method. Nursing Times 79(20): 24–25

Moser C A, Kalton G 1985 Survey methods in social investigations, 2nd edn. Gower, Aldershot

Nightingale F 1859, Republished 1990 Notes on nursing. Churchill Livingstone, Edinburgh

Norton D, McLaren R, Exton-Smith A N 1962, Republished 1975 Investigation of geriatric nursing problems in hospitals. Churchill Livingstone, Edinburgh

Oakley A 1974 The sociology of housework. Martin Robinson, London

Oakley A 1981 Interviewing women: a contradiction in terms. In: Roberts H (ed.) Doing feminist research. Routledge & Kegan Paul, London, p 581

Oakley A 1989 Who's afraid of the RCT? Some dilemmas of the sample method and 'good research practice'. Women and Health 15(4): 25–59

Ogier M 1982 An ideal Sister. RCN, London

Ogier M 1989 Reading research. Scutari Press, London

Open University (The Course Team DE304) 1979 Block 1, Variety in social science research. Introduction to the course and block 1. In: Research methods in education and the social sciences. Open University Press, Milton Keynes, p 3

Oppenheim A N 1992 Questionnaire design and attitude measurement. Heinemann, London

Parse R R 1989 Essentials for practising the art of nursing. Nursing Science Quarterly 2(3): 111

Pembrey S E M 1980 The ward sister: key to nursing. RCN, London

Rees C 1992 Practising research based teaching. Nursing Times 88(2): 55–57

Rempusheski V 1987 Making lemonade out of lemons. Alpha Chi News 10(2): 3

Roberts H (ed.) 1981 Doing feminist research. Routledge & Kegan Paul, London

Rosenberg M 1968 The logic of survey analysis. Basic Books, New York

Royal College of Nursing 1982 Promoting Research Mindedness. RCN, London

Royal College of Nursing 1991 Ethics related to research in nursing. Scutari Press, London

Salvage J 1985 The politics of nursing. Heinemann, London

Salvage J 1990 The theory and practice of the 'new nursing'. Nursing Times Occasional Paper 86(4): 42–45

Sapsford R, Abbott P 1992 Research methods for nurses and the caring professions. Open University Press, Milton Keynes

Shilts R 1987 And the band played on – people, politics and the AIDS epidemic. Viking, New York

Smith P 1987 The relationship between quality of nursing care and the ward as a learning environment: developing a methodology. Journal of Advanced Nursing 12: 413–420

Smith P 1992 The emotional labour of nursing: how nurses care. Methodological Appendix. Macmillan, Basingstoke

Smith P, Mackintosh M, Towers B 1993 Implications of the new NHS contracting system for the district nursing service in one health authority: a pilot study. Journal of Interprofessional Care 7(2): 115–124

Spencer J 1983 Research with a human touch. Nursing Times 79(12): 24–27

Stanley L, Wise S 1983 Breaking out: feminist consciousness and feminist research. Routledge & Kegan Paul, London

Street A F 1992 Inside nursing: a critical ethnography of clinical nursing practice. SUNY, New York

Thorne S E 1991 Methodological orthodoxy in qualitative nursing research: analysis of the issues. Qualitative Health Research 1(2): 178–199

Tierney A, Closs J, Atkinson I et al 1988 On measurement and nursing research. Nursing Times Occasional Paper 84(12): 55–58

Truman A 1992 Information systems in modern nursing. In: Jolley M, Brykczynska G (eds) Nursing care – the challenge to change. Edward Arnold, London, p 140

Wandelt M A, Ager J 1974 Quality patient care scale. Appleton Century Crofts, Norwalk, Connecticut

Watson J 1985 Nursing: the philosophy and science of caring. Little, Brown, Boston

Watson J D 1980 The double helix: a personal account of the discovery of the structure of DNA. Atheneum Paperback, New York

Webb C 1984 Feminist methodology in nursing research. Journal of Advanced Nursing 9: 249–250

Webb C 1992 The use of the first person in academic writing: objectivity, language and getekeeping. Journal of Advanced Nursing 17: 747–752

Webb C 1993 Feminist research: definitions, methodology, methods and evaluation. Journal of Advanced Nursing 18: 416–423

Webb C, Wilson-Barnett J 1983 Hysterectomy: dispelling the myths – 1 & 2. Nursing Times Occasional Paper 79(30): 52–54; 79 (31): 44–46

FURTHER READING

Cobb A K, Hagemaster J D 1987 Ten criteria for evaluating qualitative research proposals. Journal of Nursing Education 26(21): 138–143

Cormack D F S (ed.) 1991 The research process in nursing, 2nd edn. Blackwell Scientific, Oxford

Hawthorne P 1983 Principles of research: a checklist. Nursing Times Occasional Paper 79(35): 41–43

Hockey L 1985 Nursing research – mistakes and misconceptions. Churchill Livingstone, Edinburgh

Polgar S, Thomas S A 1991 Introduction to research in the health sciences, 2nd edn. Churchill Livingstone, Melbourne

16

The professional role of the nurse

Cynthia Gilling

This chapter outlines a foundation for the many aspects that constitute the professional role of the nurse.

It aims to:
- consider nursing's status as a profession
- discuss the interpretation and application of the 16 clauses of the UKCC's Code of Professional Conduct
- describe the role of the statutory bodies, professional organisations and trade unions.

For a greater understanding of the process of professionalisation, the reader must look further at the history of nursing (see Ch. 11), social factors, issues of gender, education and developments in health care. These aspects are constantly changing and influencing nursing as it strives to maintain a professional role in today's society.

CRITERIA FOR PROFESSIONALISM

There is an ongoing debate as to whether nursing is a profession. Many sociologists would label it as a semi-profession, as it does not meet all the criteria usually considered to be the hallmarks of a profession. Blanchfield (1978) itemises the following as the criteria that an occupational group must fulfil in order to be classified as a true profession.

1. Body of knowledge. It must have a specific, research-based body of knowledge.
2. Regulating council. It must have a regulating board or council that defines criteria of admission, educational standards, license to practise and other areas of jurisdiction.
3. Client benefit. Its members must recognise that its practice is for the benefit of the client before that of the professional.
4. Code of conduct. Its relationships with colleagues and clients must be regulated by a code of ethics.
5. Advancement of knowledge. It has a responsibility to advance and extend the body of knowledge on which it is based and enhance the learning of present practitioners.
6. Autonomy and equality. It must have legitimate autonomy and equality of status with other professional groups.

Application of these criteria to nursing

Body of knowledge. The medical profession recognises the fact that it 'borrows' knowledge from other disciplines, such as the biological and behaviourial sciences. For many years, nursing knowledge was derived from medical knowledge, and in some areas this still has to be the case.

However, nursing's own body of knowledge is now growing and is being used to define nursing interventions as distinct from actions that merely follow the medical model (see Ch. 14). Developments in nursing research, particularly in relation to clinical practice, are expanding this body of knowledge (see Ch. 15).

Regulating council. The United Kingdom Central Council for Nursing, Midwifery and Health Visiting (UKCC) meets this criterion by defining professional standards for nursing, and maintaining a register of all those licenced to practise. Educational standards are also outlined in the Nurses Act 1979.

Client benefit. That nursing practice is primarily for the benefit of the client seems an unnecessary statement, but it serves to remind us of the trust a patient puts in the health professional. This trust is accompanied by the patient's confidence in the knowledge and skills of the professional to meet his particular needs to a particular standard. Public recognition and trust are also important in enhancing the image and enabling the practice of nursing. Those who see the fight for professional status as a way of gaining status and financial rewards may not be meeting this criterion.

Code of conduct. A code of conduct is another means of enabling colleagues and patients to have trust in the health professional. Through such a code, the profession is regulated and the public protected. This area is explored in detail later in the chapter.

Advancement of knowledge. The need for a profession to keep up to date with new knowledge and practice would appear to be essential, although it is only recently that the UKCC has considered this as a vital part of professional practice. Recent documents on Post Registration Education and Practice (PREP) advocate that a refresher course be required for all those who have not practised for 5 years or more, as well as evidence, through the keeping of a portfolio, of professional updating, prior to renewal of a licence. Such requirements have been warmly welcomed by the profession. Most nurses are now seeing continuing education as an essential part of their own professional development, and this is enhanced by the many flexible approaches by which members of the profession can maintain their competence (see Clause 3: professional development).

Autonomy and equality. This criterion is the most problematic one and the most difficult for nurses to meet. Autonomy can be described as the freedom to make and act on one's own decisions. Nurses have not, until recently, had the power to be independent and to make decisions. Historically, nursing developed in the shadow of medical practice and within the powerful patriarchal system of the Victorian era. Prevailing attitudes encouraged the devaluation of women, and, as the medical profession developed, it became one of the major producers and enforcers of gender roles in our society. Nurses in the Victorian period were predominantly women and were seen as handmaidens or subordinates to the doctor; the patriarchal element was acted out in the ward situation, and its legacy is still with us today (Gamarnikov 1978).

The strictly defined roles identified in Figure 16.1 endorsed the hierarchial structure in both medicine and nursing, producing communication problems and role conflict within the doctor–nurse–patient triad. Whilst such roles are still to be recognised, particularly in the hospital setting (Jolly & Brykczynska 1993), there are areas in which nursing is gaining more autonomy. Care units such as that at Burford, Oxfordshire, are run by nurses who are responsible for admitting and discharging patients. Developments of a nurse practitioner role in the community, as envisaged in the Cumberledge Report (DHSS 1986), and deliberations by the World Health Organization that see nursing as the key element in improving health (Mahler 1981), all point the

way to a more autonomous practitioner. A more difficult issue concerns the wide range of tasks that nurses undertake and the definition of the nurse's role. This has been brought to a head with the advent of training for health care assistants and reassessment of the nursing skill mix required to care for patients with different needs and dependencies.

In looking at the above criteria, it would appear that nursing can confidently call itself a profession, although in certain areas it is only just fulfilling this role.

THE CODE OF PROFESSIONAL CONDUCT

The first code of ethics for nurses was produced by the International Council of Nurses (ICN) in Brazil in 1953 and was subsequently revised in 1965 and again in 1973. This Code was similar to the one now adhered to in the UK, i.e. the Code of Professional Conduct formulated by the UKCC in 1983 and revised in 1992 (UKCC 1992a).

PURPOSE

The Code of Professional Conduct aims to define and improve professional standards and grows out of a clear background of law, in particular Sections 2(1) and 2(5) of the Nurses, Midwives and Health Visitors Act 1979. The Code makes ethically based statements regarding the value of life, justice, honesty and individual freedom. It therefore assists in safeguarding the public and provides guidance regarding appropriate conduct to the profession. Pyne (1987) states that the code is intended to be:

- One of the main ways by which the council seeks to satisfy the requirement of the law and gives advice to all those on the register on standards of professional conduct.
- a portrait of the kind of practitioner the council believes we need in the profession.
- the backcloth against which allegations of misconduct are judged.
- a weapon with which to fight for improved standards and the elimination of risks in the interest of patients.

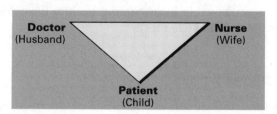

Figure 16.1 The nurse within a patriarchal triad (Gamarnikov 1978).

- an extended definition of accountability for the profession.
- a statement to the profession of the primacy of the patients' interests.

STUDENTS AND THE CODE

Before we turn to its individual clauses, we might consider how the Code of Professional Conduct affects the student nurse. The overall responsibility for a student's actions lies with the qualified member of staff supervising the practice. In reality, however, the supervisor is not able to watch the student every minute of the day. As the student gains more knowledge and experience, she may be able to undertake some aspects of care without being closely supervised. A student is accountable under the common law of negligence. Any action considered as negligent would, of course, take into account the standard of care expected of the student at her stage of training.

The student should, therefore, guard against undertaking care for which adequate instruction has not been received or in which her role is unclear or inappropriate The UKCC has produced a very useful guide for students, which covers many key issues (UKCC 1992). The Code of Professional Conduct is also a guide to the student in developing a professional role.

Registration as a nurse, midwife or health visitor by the UKCC gives the holder the legal right to practise in that specialty. This too, through the UKCC, helps to safeguard the public and the profession. All these points are summarised in the introduction to the Code (Box 16.1).

APPLYING THE CODE

The following sections will take each of the 16 clauses of the UKCC Code of Professional Conduct in turn, considering their interpretation and application. Heywood Jones (1993) provides a number of case studies involving issues of professional conduct and accountability, which make salutory reading for any member of the profession.

Clause 1

Act always in such a manner as to promote and safeguard the interests and well-being of patients.

Chapter 14 illustrates aspects of the relationship between the patient and the nurse, and the need to respect patients as individuals. The chapter develops this theme through the concept of individual care and illustrates the reciprocal nature of the nurse–patient relationship: i.e. the nurse takes on certain responsibilities in the delivery of care in return for the trust and confidence that the patient freely gives.

The move away from routine care to a more individualised approach heightens the awareness of this special relationship and may present the nurse with new difficulties in upholding this part of the Code. For instance, how can a nurse have an equally trusting and warm relationship with every patient, when the nurse, like anyone else, relates better to some people than to others. To illustrate this, nurses often 'categorise' patients, to the detriment of their well-being. For instance, they may refer to patients as 'difficult' or 'awkward', and this will influence their attitudes and relationships and the care they give (see also Chs 2 and 17). Nurses should be able to make better judgements regarding patients through exploring their own values, beliefs and attitudes and by having discussions with peers, seniors and patients on this subject.

Another area of potential uncertainty concerns knowledge and skills related to patient safety. To use equipment in an unsafe manner may be harmful to the patient and result in an accident. Failure to observe the principles of cross-infection may also bring harm. Clause 1 of the UKCC Code calls upon the nurse to 'promote' the well-being of the patient as well as to 'safeguard' it. The nurse's role in promoting healthy lifestyles is described in Chapter 6.

Clause 2

Ensure that no action or omission on your part or within your sphere of influence is detrimental to the interests or safety of patients and clients.

Box 16.1 **UKCC Code of Professional Conduct** (Reproduced with kind permission from UKCC 1992a)

Each registered nurse, midwife and health visitor shall act, at all times, in such a manner as to:

- safeguard and promote the interests of individual patients and clients;
- serve the interests of society;
- justify public trust and confidence and
- uphold and enhance the good standing and reputation of the professions.

As a registered nurse, midwife or health visitor, you are personally accountable for your practice and, in the exercise of your professional accountability, must:

1 act always in such a manner as to promote and safeguard the interest and well-being of patients and clients;

2 ensure that no action or omission on your part, or within your sphere of responsibility, is detrimental to the interests, condition or safety of patients and clients;

3 maintain and improve your professional knowledge and competence;

4 acknowledge any limitations in your knowledge and competence and decline any duties or responsibilities unless able to perform them in a safe and skilled manner;

5 work in an open and co-operative manner with patients, clients and their families, foster their independence and recognise and respect their involvement in the planning and delivery of care;

6 work in a collaborative and co-operative manner with health care professionals and others involved in providing care, and recognise and respect their particular contributions within the care team;

7 recognise and respect the uniqueness and dignity of each patient and client, and respond to their need for care, irrespective of their ethnic origin, religious beliefs, personal attributes, the nature of their health problems or any other factor;

8 report to an appropriate person or authority, at the earliest possible time, any conscientious objection which may be relevant to your professional practice;

9 avoid any abuse of your privileged relationship with patients and clients and of the privileged access allowed to their person, property, residence or workplace;

10 protect all confidential information concerning patients and clients obtained in the course of professional practice and make disclosures only with consent, where required by the order of a court or where you can justify disclosure in the wider public interest;

11 report to an appropriate person or authority, having regard to the physical, psychological and social effects on patients and clients, any circumstances in the environment of care which could jeopardise standards of practice;

12 report to an appropriate person or authority any circumstances in which safe and appropriate care for patients and clients cannot be provided;

13 report to an appropriate person or authority where it appears that the health or safety of colleagues is at risk, as such circumstances may compromise standards of practice and care;

14 assist professional colleagues, in the context of your own knowledge, experience and sphere of responsibility, to develop their professional competence, and assist others in the care team, including informal carers, to contribute safely and to a degree appropriate to their roles;

15 refuse any gift, favour or hospitality from patients or clients currently in your care which might be interpreted as seeking to exert influence to obtain preferential consideration and

16 ensure that your registration status is not used in the promotion of commercial products or services, declare any financial or other interests in relevant organisations providing such goods or services and ensure that your professional judgement is not influenced by any commercial considerations.

**Notice to all Registered Nurses,
Midwives and Health Visitors**

This Code of Professional Conduct for the Nurse, Midwife and Health Visitor is issued to all registered nurses, midwives and health visitors by the United Kingdom Central Council for Nursing, Midwifery and Health Visiting. The Council is the regulatory body responsible for the standards of these professions and it requires members of the professions to practise and conduct themselves within the standards and framework provided by the Code.

Responsibility can be viewed as falling into the following categories:

- legal: relating to the law
- ethical: relating to an informed sense of right or wrong
- moral: relating to society in general
- professional: relating to standards in our work
- contractual: relating to agreements
- personal: relating to how we feel and think about the welfare of others

For the nurse, all these aspects have to be considered, as her prime responsibility is to deliver the highest standard of care to her patients. Crow (1983) suggests that the nurse's responsibility includes four main aspects:

1. Responsibility for all nursing care. This includes delegation to others and confirmation that care is carried out satisfactorily.

2. Responsibility to ensure through research and

evaluation that the care given is effective and safe.

3. Responsibility to deliver care in a caring manner, i.e. with compassion, competence, confidence, conscience and commitment (Roach 1982).

4. Responsibility to deliver care within the framework of agreed moral principles, for instance those reflected in the Code itself.

The fundamental issues that underlie professional responsibility in clinical care (Crow 1983) are:

- total commitment to patients, motivated by an overwhelming desire to deliver care of a high standard
- personal accountability and integrity
- a real desire to ensure that one's knowledge and skill is maintained.

The nurse may on occasion be asked to give an account of her actions – for instance if legal action is taken as a result of an action or omission that was detrimental to a patient. In such circumstances, the nurse's knowledge and experience would be called into question and any written evidence examined. This emphasises the importance of writing down correct, relevant details of the nursing care.

Clause 3

Maintain and improve your professional knowledge and competence.

The UKCC has introduced compulsory updating for all qualified staff (UKCC 1994). There are already numerous and flexible ways of maintaining competence within one's own specialism. Study days, courses and clinical experience will, through the Credit Accumulation and Transfer Scheme (CATS) go towards a diploma or degree. Post-registration programmes are provided by hospitals and by health departments in higher education. They offer study days and courses ranging from orientation of new staff, clinical updating, clinical courses (e.g. renal nursing and community psychiatric nursing) to special-skills based courses (e.g. 'introduction to counselling skills' and 'preparation for management'). A new area being developed is the assessment of the knowledge gained through clinical practice and experience.

Such programmes are designed to meet the needs of the service as well as those of the professional. Some courses may be run on a multidisciplinary basis to enhance understanding and teamwork among health care workers.

Chapter 18 deals with some of the principles of learning and demonstrates the need for the nurse to take a more adult approach to learning in order to become a more reflective practitioner. This, in turn, puts the responsibility for learning with the student.

Clause 4

Acknowledge any limitations in your knowledge and decline any duties or responsibilities unless able to perform them in a safe and skilled manner.

Both students and qualified nurses need to be aware of their limitations in carrying out procedures or giving information. Either of these actions, performed badly, could put a patient in jeopardy. Most methods of competence assessment include a self-assessment component, which helps the learner to explore her limitations. Part of knowing one's limitations is having self-awareness, and this has been a key element in many nursing courses.

Another difficult area, often called the 'extended role', refers to the nurse undertaking procedures usually (in the UK) carried out by a doctor, for example giving intravenous drugs or performing a simple suture. Ward (1991) and Rieu (1994) outline the development of the extended role and explore the areas of accountability and competency. The dangers associated with such procedures, for example damage to the vein or poor scar formation through faulty suturing technique, could be used by patients as examples of negligence. The UKCC's document on The Scope of Professional Practice (1992b) is a position statement on the issue of extended role. It stresses that accountability rests firmly with the registered nurse. The document sets out six principles:

9. The registered nurse, midwife or health visitor:

   9.1 must be satisfied that each aspect of practice is directed to meeting the needs and serving the interests of the patient;

   9.2 must endeavour always to achieve, maintain and develop knowledge, skill and competence to respond to those needs and interests;

   9.3 must honestly acknowledge any limits of personal knowledge and skill and take steps to remedy any relevant deficits in order effectively and appropriately to meet the needs of patients and clients;

   9.4 must ensure that any enlargement or adjustment of the scope of professional practice must be achieved without compromising or fragmenting existing aspects of professional practice and care and that the requirements of the Council's Code of Professional Conduct are satisfied throughout the whole area of practice;

   9.5 must recognise and honour the direct or indirect personal accountability borne for all aspects of professional practice and

   9.6 must, in serving the interests of patients and clients and the wider interests of society, avoid any inappropriate delegation to others which compromises those interests.

This area of practice has recently undergone further debate with the issuing of The Greenhalgh Report (1994), in response to the government's proposal to reduce junior doctors' hours.

Clause 5

Work in an open and co-operative manner with patients, clients and their families, foster their independence and recognise and respect their involvement in the planning and delivery of care.

This clause emphasises the importance of involving patients in their own care. The Patient's Charter (1992) details patients' rights and includes the concept of the named nurse. Combined with primary nursing (see Ch. 12), this should lead to greater patient/client involvement and continuity of care.

Clause 6

Work in a collaborative and co-operative manner with health care professionals and others involved in providing care, and recognise and respect their particular contributions within the care team.

Many people with specialist knowledge and skills contribute to the care of the patient. The doctor, nurse, physiotherapist, occupational therapist, speech therapist and others form what is often referred to as a 'health care team'. This collaboration works well when each team member respects the others' knowledge and skills and considers the patient's welfare to be the prime objective.

'Collaboration' does not always have to mean 'acquiescence', and the nurse should feel able to contribute on an equal basis with other colleagues. Nurses who have extended their knowledge and experience in a particular field will feel more confident in challenging and contributing to the decision-making process (Question 16.1). Small units, such as intensive care, renal therapy or palliative care, work well through team collaboration. Perhaps teamwork is also easier in such units because objectives are clearer and more easily defined.

Question 16.1

The doctor states that a certain patient should be discharged (his bed is required for another patient). The occupational therapist feels that the patient is not ready to cope on his own. How would you, as the nurse, contribute to a solution?

Clause 7

Recognise and respect the uniqueness and dignity of each patient and client and respond to their need for care, irrespective of their ethnic origin, religious beliefs, personal attributes, the nature of their health problems or any other factor.

It is quite easy to forget this aspect of the Code even though we live in a multiracial, multicultural society. Mares et al (1985) found a distinct lack of input into the nursing and medical curricula on these very issues. This deficiency is lessening, partly due to the great increase in the non-European, non-Christian population in the UK, and partly through an increased awareness of the nature of different customs and beliefs through the media and the introduction of equal opportunities legislation. There are many textbooks and pamphlets now available to help staff and patients understand different religions and have more insight into customs and rituals. Having more knowledge assists the nurse not only to respect the patient's beliefs but also to recognise the associated rituals and customs. Particularly distressing to some bereaved families is the failure to observe certain customs and beliefs surrounding death. Many hospitals give guidance on this, and it is usually possible to seek advice from the hospital Chaplain or an official of the particular religious group concerned (Question 16.2). (See also Clause 8 regarding particular health problems.)

Question 16.2

Sister asks you to prepare Mr Shah, who is a practising Muslim, for surgery. Mr Shah insists that he must get out of bed to pray to Mecca several times a day and that he will not undress for a female nurse. Mr Shah is second on the operating list and you need to give him his premedication in half an hour. How would you uphold Mr Shah's wishes and have him prepared for his operation in time?

Clause 8

Report to an appropriate person or authority, at the earliest possible time, any conscientious objection which may be relevant to your professional practice.

The law does not provide a basic right for a practitioner to register a conscientious objection to participation in care and/or treatment except with respect to the termination of pregnancy under the terms of Section 4 of the Abortion Act 1967 and the Human Fertilisation and Embryology Act 1990. It is therefore advisable for students or trained staff to check with nurse managers of operating theatres and gynaecology day wards on the extent to which nursing staff are involved in abortion procedures. They can then decide whether to exercise this right or to seek employment elsewhere.

There may also be other times when a nurse may question her participation in certain forms of treatment, for example electroconvulsive ther-

apy (ECT) or resuscitation of the elderly. If this is the case, the nurse should consider carefully why she objects to such forms of treatment and discuss this with senior staff in good time, so that, if appropriate, arrangements can be made for others to care for the patient during the treatment.

Refusal to give treatment on professional rather than conscientious grounds calls for a different approach. An example might be when a nurse feels that a drug should not be given, although it is due, because the patient's condition has changed. If the nurse then decides not to administer the drug, she must record carefully the reasons for this decision, discuss the issue with the prescribing doctor and request a visit to the patient. Following this discussion, if the nurse still feels that the doctor was wrong, she should confirm again to the doctor, in writing, why she decided not to give the drug.

It is not acceptable under the Code of Conduct to refuse to care for patients with acquired immune deficiency syndrome (AIDS) or who are HIV-positive. There is no difference between caring for these patients and caring for any other patient who is suffering from an infectious disease (e.g. open tuberculosis, gastroenteritis or methicillin-resistant staphylococcus infection) as long as the principles underlying infection control are observed. The UKCC (1989) states: 'To seek to be so selective is to demonstrate unacceptable conduct. The UKCC expects the practitioner to adopt a non-judgemental approach in the exercise of their caring role.' In January 1991, a registered nurse was removed from the register for refusing to care for a patient with AIDS (Question 16.3).

Question 16.3

You are asked to look after a patient whilst he is having ECT. You have been observing and talking to Mr Brown for the last 4 weeks since his last treatment and feel that there is an improvement in his depressive state, and you are personally against the use of such treatment. How would you solve this problem to the benefit of Mr Brown?

Clause 9

Avoid any abuse of your privileged relationship with patients and clients and of the privileged access allowed to their person, property, residence or workplace.

The relationship built up between a nurse and the patient is very different from normal relationships: as Burnard & Chapman (1993) state, it is in fact unique. It is different from normal social relationships because the nurse cannot choose the patient, nor the patient the nurse. The patient may be different from the nurse in age, culture and religion, and may have little in common with her socially. Yet the nurse is expected quickly to gain a rapport with the patient and put him at ease. Not only does the nurse have to forge this relationship, but at the same time she must also perform intimate care that in normal social/ethical circumstances would not be acceptable. In the case of the mentally ill, the nurse listens to detailed accounts of very personal feelings and actions. Such situations put the nurse in a privileged position because the patient is demonstrating his trust in the nurse at a time when he is at his most vulnerable. It is therefore the nurse's duty to treat the patient's disclosures with the utmost confidentiality. This includes not discussing one patient with another and not discussing nursing details in public places, such as restaurants or when travelling in public transport, where one might be overheard.

A nurse may have access to the patient's property in hospital or in the home. If patients' property is left in the hospital for safe-keeping, local procedures must be adhered to in detailing every item, be it jewellery, money or clothing. The same applies to any items used in personal care kept on or in the patient's locker.

Just as they cannot choose their patients, nurses cannot choose which homes they visit. Consequently, they may come across, in their work, standards and ways of life that are very different from their own and which go against their own values and beliefs. Unless the situation is such as to endanger the health of the individual, such issues should not be discussed either with the patient or with anyone else.

The occupational nurse who cares for patients within their work setting has a particular role to play and one in which the importance of confidentiality must be emphasised. This is particularly so in relation to management. The question may arise of whether certain information regarding an employee's health status should be divulged, particularly if it has a bearing on work performance. This is for the occupational nurse to judge; such decisions are usually discussed with the employee before the minimum details are relayed to one manager in confidence.

Clause 10

Protect all confidential information concerning patients and clients obtained in the course of professional practice and make disclosure only with consent, where required by the order of a court or where you can justify disclosure in the wider public interest.

The respect by nurses of confidential information has always been stressed but has been emphasised with the Data Protection Act 1984. Confidentiality, as already discussed in Clause 9, implies a trusting relationship, but there may be exceptional circumstances, as the Code states, in which 'disclosure is required by law ... or is necessary in the public interest'. However, situations do arise in which an appropriate course of action is not clear. Examples of such dilemmas are given in Box 16.2 (see also Question 16.4).

Question 16.4

What action would you take in the situations outlined in Box 16.2?

The most important part of this clause is its emphasis on confidentiality as the right of the patient. Although the document on the elaboration of the clause states that the ultimate decision to disclose information is that of the practitioner and that this decision cannot be delegated, it does not prevent the very real need to discuss the situation first with other practitioners or professional bodies (Box 16.3).

> **Box 16.2 Examples of cases considered by the UKCC Confidentiality Committee** (UKCC 1987)
>
> A Sister in a psychiatric day hospital found a patient in possession of large quantities of controlled drugs that he could not have obtained legally.
>
> A Health Visitor was told by one child that another child was being sexually abused.
>
> Accident and emergency department nursing staff found that an unconscious patient they were treating had a gun on his person.
>
> Nurses working in the community were instructed by their managers to give researchers direct access to confidential information in respect of patients, but knew that the consent of these patients had not been sought.

> **Box 16.3 Questions to pose when deciding matters of confidentiality** (Reproduced with kind permission of *Nursing Times* from Lee 1987)
>
> 1. Has the information really been received in confidence?
> 2. Why not ask the patient whether he will waive the confidentiality?
> 3. If that is not possible or desirable (for example, if you think it will upset the patient unnecessarily), what do you think the patient would say if asked?
> 4. Is there any other way of dealing with the problem without breaking confidentiality?
> 5. Even if the patient wants the confidentiality protected is there any overriding reason to disclose information, for example, of serious danger to others, or child abuse?
> 6. How will disclosure affect your relationship with this patient, his relationship with other medical staff and other patients' trust in the profession?
> 7. On balance, should the patient's prima facie right to confidentiality be defeated by another right, for example, the right of a child not to be abused, the right of somebody else not to be infected with the HIV virus?
>
> Such questions will also help in deciding whether the problem is really one of confidentiality.

One area that always comes to mind in connection with the issue of confidentiality is, of course, that of patients' personal records. Problems arise from the number of people who may have legitimate access to notes, i.e. not just doctors and nurses but also paramedical staff and, of course, students. Students are sometimes required to use patient information for assignments; in such cases, care must be taken to protect the identity of the patient and to ensure that notes are not left lying around in public places where access cannot be monitored.

Clause 11

Report to an appropriate person or authority, having regard to the physical, psychological and social effects on patients and clients, any circumstances in the environment of care which could jeopardise standards of practice.

This clause and the next have implications of a political and ethical nature and point to the fact that it is really not possible to separate the private and personal from the public and political (Clay 1987). These clauses raise the question of acting upon conscience – something that is often more easily said than done.

The most vulnerable groups of patients are the mentally ill and include older people and people with learning disability. Such patients cannot readily articulate physical and mental abuse, lack of privacy or a want of social stimulation (Question 16.5). Individualised care, the change in the role of those working with the mentally ill from custodian to a more therapeutic function and specific courses in caring for older people have done much to improve standards. Standards of care and principles of nursing practice are now being based more on research than on conventional practice. Research can guide our judgements on when standards are reduced; moreover, without documented evidence, a complaint may be ignored or dismissed.

The environment of care embraces not only safe nursing practice and the physical surroundings, but also the atmosphere of the ward

Question 16.5

What action would you take if you were contributing to the care of patients who were mentally ill and resident in the community but were not being accepted by the local population?

Activity 16.2

During a practice placement, make a note of changes that could be made to enhance the environment. These may vary from devising a more comfortable seating arrangement in a GP's waiting room to creating a more homely atmosphere in the day-room of an elderly care ward.

or department (Activity 16.2). This will have an effect on the patient's physical and mental state and on his capacity to get better.

Adequacy of resources is certainly a political issue in these days of financial restraint. Too often, new surgical techniques or complex medical investigations are introduced without any consideration of the extra workload they create for the staff involved. Current staffing levels are frequently deemed adequate to accommodate these developments when, in reality, extra staff are required. Before putting a case forward for additional staff, it is the duty of the nurse to have knowledge of the resources available and to question first whether or not these are being used effectively and efficiently. Nursing costs are among the highest expenditure in the NHS and, when resources are strained, are the first to be questioned. They therefore frequently have to be justified. Recent developments in the area of quality of care will also be a useful tool in measuring standards of nursing care (see Ch. 10).

Clause 12

Report to an appropriate person or authority any circumstances in which safe and appropriate care for patients cannot be provided.

Clause 12 ties in with Clause 6 in its emphasis on respecting and working in a collaborative and cooperative way with other health care workers. The purpose of the NHS is to care for others, but it sometimes fails to acknowledge the stress it creates for its employees. This may be due partly to it being such a large organisation (the largest employer in Europe) and partly to the traditional view of medical and nursing staff as being

(unaccountably) different from other people in their ability to cope with anything and everything that comes along.

There is now more recognition of nurses as individuals and of the fact that they have different capacities to cope with different workloads and pressures. Many hospitals have created support groups in areas of clinical care such as intensive care and accident and emergency. These are usually multidisciplinary and help in explaining issues and coping with problems as a team. What is stressful to one person may not be to another, and joint problem-solving will go a long way towards reducing the pressures of colleagues.

Managers need to recognise that they are breaking this clause of the Code of Conduct when they leave second-level nurses and students to cope with heavy workloads without sufficient supervision. This results in mistakes being made and standards being reduced. If adequate cover cannot be provided, admissions should be reduced, and if staffing problems cannot be surmounted, the ward should be closed.

Clause 13

Report to an appropriate person or authority where it appears that the health or safety of colleagues is at risk, as such circumstances may compromise standards of practice and care.

This new clause emphasises the role of the Professional Conduct Committee in recognising that a registered practitioner's misconduct may be due to ill health. The clause urges both practitioners and managers to recognise early on if standards are being reduced owing to ill health and to take action before lowering of standards or misconduct occurs.

Clause 14

Assist professional colleagues, in the context of your own knowledge, experience and sphere of responsibility, to develop their professional competence, and assist others in the care team, including formal carers, to contribute safely and to a degree appropriate to their roles.

It is often said that after the initial introduction into nursing, students take on the teaching role of introducing nursing skills to the next new intake of students. This continues and increases with the individual's level of knowledge, experience and authority. Hence the sister/charge nurse role has always contained a teaching element. With the development of a more individual approach to learning, students are involved in identifying their own learning needs against identified objectives. It is usually the senior staff who have made the greatest contribution in developing the clinical competence of students and the newly qualified. Using their experience and knowledge, senior staff can contribute to the development of nursing practice through the setting of policies and standards and through the implementation of research. However, in order to achieve this, they must keep up to date with developments in the profession and within their sphere of practice.

This clause is emphasised through the concept of 'preceptorship' for the newly qualified nurse, and of clinical supervision and its contribution to developing nursing practice (Faugier & Butterworth 1994).

Clause 15

Refuse any gifts, favour or hospitality from patients or clients currently in your care which might be interpreted as seeking to exert influence to obtain preferential consideration.

Many patients naturally wish to express their gratitude for the care and attention they have received in hospital and offer gifts or money to staff. As this clause implies, accepting favours or hospitality could be interpreted by the patient as a promise of preferential consideration. Most hospitals have local policies regarding gifts, particularly if they involve money. In most cases, gifts go into a general fund to help with extras for patients and staff that cannot be provided through the usual channels.

Care should also be taken when accepting gifts from pharmaceutical companies that they are not a means of seeking preference in the purchase of their products against those of another (Question 16.6).

Question 16.6

What would you say to a patient who offered you money or an expensive present?

Clause 16

Ensure that your registration status is not used in the promotion of commercial products or services, declare any financial or other interests in relevant organisations providing such goods or services and ensure that your professional judgement is not influenced by any commercial considerations.

It is inadvisable to use a professional qualification in a commercial context as it may cast doubt upon the independence of professional judgement, on which patients rely. Advertising is in fact a form of propaganda and seeks to influence people to buy certain products. Firms seek to use nurses in their advertisement of products because nurses are seen by the public to have a high level of knowledge and reliable judgement. For a nurse to recommend just one product, over many others, is not advisable.

The UKCC has produced a guidance booklet for this clause, which describes commercial contexts in which using professional qualification is permissible (UKCC 1985). For example, a nurse who owns a nursing home may use her qualifications in advertising the business (Question 16.7).

Question 16.7

1. You are a nurse currently working as a sales representative for a pharmaceutical firm. Would it be permissible to use your nursing qualifications on your business card?
2. You assist with making a video on patient care and your name appears on the credits. Can it be followed by your registration status?

THE ROLE OF THE STATUTORY BODIES

THE UKCC

The Nurses, Midwives and Health Visitors Act 1979 provided for the establishment of the UKCC, which replaced six previous statutory bodies representing the nursing, midwifery and health visiting professions in England, Scotland, Wales and Northern Ireland. By the terms of the Act, the UKCC also took on responsibility for the organisations concerned with post-registration clinical practice, i.e the Joint Board of Clinical Nursing Studies for England and Wales, and the Committee for Clinical Nursing Studies for Scotland.

The principle functions of the UKCC set out in Section 2 of the Act are:

(1) The principal functions of the central Council shall be to establish and improve standards of training and professional conduct for nurses, midwives and health visitors.

(2) The Council shall ensure that the standards of training they establish are such as to meet any Community obligation of the United Kingdom.

(3) The Council shall by means of rules determine the conditions of a person being admitted to training, and the kind and standard of training to be undertaken, with a view to registration.

(4) The rules may also make provision with respect to the kind and standard of further training available to persons who are already registered.

(5) The powers of the Council shall include that of providing, in such manner as it thinks fit, advice for nurses, midwives and health visitors on standards of professional conduct.

(6) In the discharge of its functions the Council shall have proper regard for the interests of all groups within the professions, including those with minority representation.

Each of these functions will now be considered in turn.

Improving standards of training

The UKCC initiated the proposals set out in 'Project 2000: A New Preparation for Practice' (UKCC 1986). This document followed a number of working papers relating to the reform of nursing education and training. Areas of dis-

cussion included the number of nursing levels needed, manpower and costing. The UKCC proposals also used previous reports on nursing education, for example the Briggs Report (DHSS 1972). The case for change, as urged by the 'Project 2000' document, was based on three general concerns:

- changing patterns of health care
- potential recruitment/manpower difficulties
- the need to update education and training.

Changing patterns of health care. That health care patterns are changing is obvious. There are now fewer acute hospitals, and more care is required in the community for the very young, the elderly and those with problems for which there is no immediate cure, such as drug abuse, AIDS and other chronic conditions.

Recruitment and manpower. The predictions were that, in the mid-1990s, there would be fewer 18-year-olds leaving school. This group of school leavers (particularly females) has always been the main source of recruitment into nursing. There are also many more attractive careers, other than nursing, for women than there were 20 years ago.

Education. Nursing training had always been of the apprenticeship type and had low academic status, owing to the small amount of time spent in a formal educational setting. In addition to this, changing shift patterns, increased hours of work and a higher turnover of patients led to a reduction of supervision and teaching for students on the wards. Moreover, students were counted as part of the nursing establishment: wards and departments relied heavily on them to take responsibility for giving nursing care. New groups of students were reorientated to practice settings at frequent intervals (sometimes every 8 weeks), and staffing levels were seriously reduced if students were not recruited or dropped out. Research shows that 70–80% of care is given by unqualified staff (i.e. mainly by students). This means that students were often left unsupervised and were expected to take on responsibilities for which they had not been prepared.

Outside the profession, the previous qualification of Registered Nurse had little more value than an A-level, making further advancement difficult. Student nurses did not have the time to explore in greater depth curriculum subjects such as sociology and psychology.

Meeting EC guidelines

Planning health care for the future involves bringing educational standards into line with European Community directives. Already, general students have to undertake particular experiences (maternity, mental health and community nursing) to be permitted to practise in Europe, and this requirement is being extended to *all* students.

Admission conditions

The UKCC has set up a 'live' register for first- and second-level nurses (Box 16.4), and is responsible for determining what theoretical and

---

Box 16.4 **Qualifications included in the UKCC Register: Parts of the UKCC Professional Register**

Part 1	First-level nurses trained in general nursing
Part 2	Second-level nurses trained in general nursing (England and Wales)
Part 3	First-level nurses trained in the nursing of persons suffering from mental illness
Part 4	Second-level nurses trained in the nursing of persons suffering from mental illness (England and Wales)
Part 5	First-level nurses trained in the nursing of persons suffering from mental handicap
Part 6	Second-level nurses trained in the nursing of persons suffering from mental handicap (England and Wales)
Part 7	Second-level nurses (Scotland and Northern Ireland)
Part 8	Nurses trained in the nursing of sick children
Part 9	Nurses trained in the nursing of persons suffering from fever
Part 10	Midwives
Part 11	Health visitors
Part 12	First-level nurses trained in adult nursing*
Part 13	First-level nurses trained in mental health nursing*
Part 14	First-level nurses trained in mental handicap nursing*
Part 15	First-level nurses trained in chidlren's nursing*

*Diploma in Higher Education in Nursing (Project 2000)

First-level nurses (3 years preparation)
Second-level nurses (2 years preparation)

---

practical preparation is required at each level. It is then the role of the National Boards to translate these standards into more detailed course regulations and curriculum guidelines. First- and second-level nurses can all now use the title of Registered Nurse (RN). The level and branch of practice will be indicated elsewhere, for example in a curriculum vitae. Nurses applying from overseas must demonstrate that their programmes of preparation meet the same criteria. There is often variation in nursing programmes, and applicants are required to undertake a satisfactory period of adaptation before applying for registration. Length of experience since qualifying and other criteria may be considered before admission to courses leading to qualification beyond first or second level.

Further training

The need for continuing education was discussed in 'Clause 3: professional development'.

Standards of professional conduct

The question of standards puts a great responsibility on the UKCC, which ensures that standards are met and maintained through its Professional Conduct Committee, composed of Council members. How the Committee functions is outlined in Figure 16.2.

Minority groups within the profession

With the majority being Registered General Nurses, smaller groups like Occupational Health Nurses are sometimes forgotten. Regulations concerning the election of members of the profession to the statutory bodies and the required numbers from each of the specialisms are aimed at assisting the UKCC to ensure that all subgroups within the profession are adequately represented.

THE NATIONAL BOARDS

The Nurses, Midwives and Health Visitors Act 1979 and 1992 requires that England, Wales, Scotland and Northern Ireland shall each have a

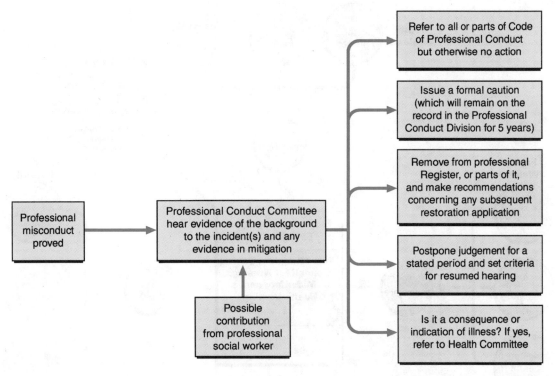

Figure 16.2 Review procedures of the UKCC Professional Conduct Committee (Pyne 1984, review 1993).

National Board for nursing, midwifery and health visiting. These are corporate bodies with the following functions:

- to provide or arrange for others to provide, at institutions approved by the Board:
  - courses of training with a view to enabling persons to qualify for registration as nurses, midwives or health visitors or for the recording of additional qualifications
  - courses of further training for those already registered

- to ensure that such courses meet the requirements of the Central Council (UKCC) as to their content and standard
- to hold or arrange for others to hold such examinations as are necessary to enable persons to satisfy requirements for registration or to obtain additional qualifications
- to discharge their functions subject to and in accordance with any applicable rule of the

Council and have proper regard for the interests of all groups within the profession, including those with minority representation.

The National Boards, therefore, have a major executive function with respect to all that is involved in education, training and examinations. With the changes in the NHS, the National Boards no longer handle the funds for education. These have been devolved to the Regional Health Authorities, who will contract with local education providers.

The National Boards and the UKCC

With the 1992 Nurses, Midwives and Health Visitors Act, the UKCC became the elected body and the National Boards much smaller in membership, the majority of members being appointed by government ministers. The new relationship between the Boards and the UKCC is illustrated in Figure 16.3, which shows the four National

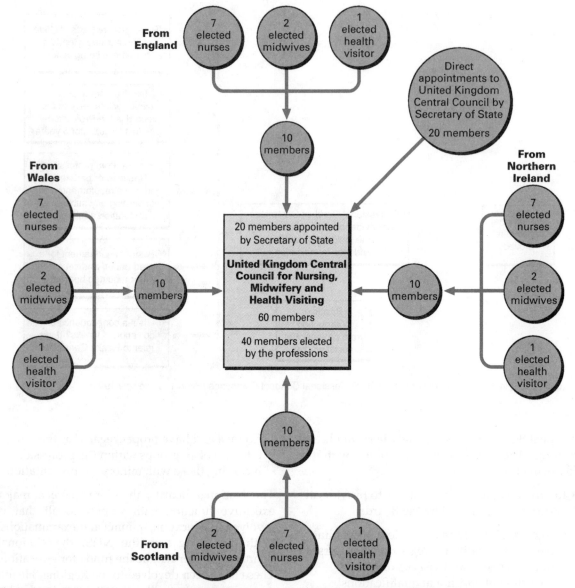

Figure 16.3   Relationships between the National Boards and the UKCC as at 1993 (after Rowden 1984).

Boards and the numbers representing the professions.

Having a central representative body has enabled the nursing profession in the UK to speak with one voice on matters of concern and to initiate constructive reforms such as the establishment of a 'live' Register, Project 2000 and the requirement of regular updating of all practitioners.

PROFESSIONAL ORGANISATIONS AND TRADE UNIONS

Of the many professional organisations and trade unions that represent NHS employees only two will be mentioned here:

• the Royal College of Nursing (RCN)

• Unison: previously the Confederation of Health Service Employees (COHSE), the National Union of Public Employees (NUPE) and the National Association of Local Government Officers (NALGO).

THE ROYAL COLLEGE OF NURSING (RCN)

Developments since 1916

The RCN was founded in 1916 and, initially, pressed for registration of all nurses. Its aims are, as in the beginning, to promote the science and art of nursing and to advance nursing as a profession. Membership is open only to nurses and students, and men were not admitted until 1960. However, some men within nursing sought to pursue their professional aims through the Society of Registered Male Nurses, rather than by the more traditional trade union route. The RCN balloted members on issues of affiliation with the Trades Union Congress (TUC), but the majority voted against; thus it became a non-affiliated trade union in 1977. Another pending issue is to consider whether or not the RCN should admit nursing auxiliaries and health care assistants.

Benefits of membership

In the past 20 years, the RCN has become more proactive in matters of pay, conditions and standards in the NHS. Membership, now at 303 000, provides a comprehensive indemnity insurance scheme, which helps members found guilty of professional negligence. This is particularly attractive to members in view of the movement within the profession for more autonomy, and given that those practising in the community, for example community psychiatric nurses, often do so independently.

Other activities

The RCN supports its own Institute of Advanced Nursing, with a range of academic and professional courses and an extensive library. It is now affiliated to the University of Manchester.

The RCN also provides the opportunity for specialist nurses to share their knowledge and experience through official forums and committees.

UNISON

In July 1993, as indicated above, three fomer unions – COHSE, NUPE and NALGO – combined to form Unison, making it the largest union in the TUC, with 1.4 million members. Of these, 455 000 are health workers, and there is a special nursing section. Unison recruits and represents all types of nursing staff, and all nurse members are protected by an indemnity insurance. It is also expanding its Specialist Advisory Groups (SAGs) to reflect fully the scope of expertise within the membership, for example in HIV/AIDS and the care of older people and those with learning difficulties. More groups are being considered, including one for Project 2000 students. Thirteen Unison nurses sit on the current UKCC (Cohen 1994).

JOINING AN ORGANISATION

Students and qualified staff should seek information regarding these and other organisations before deciding to join a particular group. Such a decision should take into account the individual's priorities and should include an assessment of which organisation may be able to offer more than another. Issues to consider are whether or not a branch of the organisation is well represented in the working area, its track record for negotiating better pay and conditions of service, and its support for individual members over grievances, professional issues, standards in the NHS and so forth.

THE INTERNATIONAL SETTING

THE EUROPEAN COMMUNITY

Legislation within nursing in the UK is required to change in line with EC policy. The UKCC has a representative from its Council on the Advisory

Committee on Training of Nurses in the European Community. It also has a representative on the comparable committee for midwifery. Discussion has been taking place with the EC for some time on 'sectional directives' for psychiatric nurses and, more recently, paediatric nurses.

THE INTERNATIONAL COUNCIL OF NURSES (ICN)

The ICN was founded in 1900 by Mrs Bedford Fenwick, then Matron of St Bartholomew's Hospital in London (Hector 1973). The Council has gone from strength to strength, particularly in the last 30 years. Every member country provides from its national organisation (in the UK, the RCN) a nurse (usually its President) to serve on the Council of National Representatives, which determines the policies of the International Council of Nurses. The headquarters of the ICN are in Geneva. Here it links with the World Health Organization and publishes the *International Nursing Review*. The ICN Congress is now held every 4 years, attended by thousands of nurses from all over the world. Recent Congresses have been held in Japan, Mexico, the USA, Korea and, in 1993, Spain.

Summary

Is nursing a profession? It is considered by many to be a semi-profession, meeting most, but not all, of the generally accepted criteria for professionalism. However, nursing fulfils all the criteria suggested by Blanchfield (1978) for a profession – a body of knowledge, a regulating council, client benefit, a code of conduct, advancement of knowledge and, increasingly, autonomy and equality.

The UKCC's Code of Professional Conduct aims to define and improve professional standards. In this chapter, its 16 clauses are scrutinised with respect to their interpretation and application to nursing practice.

The UKCC's other functions include standards for admission to the professional Register, meeting EC guidelines and regulating standards of conduct. The National Boards for Nursing, Midwifery and Health Visiting, the UK professional organisations and trade unions, and international bodies are also important in regulating and directing the profession.

The professionalisation of nursing is an exciting area, and the effect of recent political events will undoubtedly contribute to its continued future development.

REFERENCES

Abortion Act 1967 HMSO, London
Blanchfield J R 1978 Cited in: Pyne R 1981 Professional discipline in nursing: theory and practice. Blackwell Scientific, Oxford
Burnard P, Chapman C 1993 Professional and ethical issues in nursing, a code of professional conduct, 2nd edn. Scutari Press, London
Clay T 1987 Nurses: power and politics. Heinemann, London
Cohen P 1994 Stately union. Nursing Times 90(9)
Crow R 1983 Professional responsibility. Nursing Times 79 (1)
Data Protection Act 1984 HMSO, London
DHSS and Scottish Home and Health Department 1972 The Report of the Committee on Nursing (The Briggs Report). HMSO, London
DHSS 1986 Neighbourhood nursing: a focus for care. Report on the Community Nursing Review (The Cumberlege Report). HMSO, London
Faugier J, Butterworth T 1994 Clinical supervision – a position paper. School of Nursing Studies, University of Manchester
Gamarnikov E 1978 Sexual division of labour: the case in nursing. In: Kuhn A, Wople A M Feminism and materialism. Routledge and Kegan Paul, London
Greenhalgh and Co Ltd 1994 The interface between junior doctors and nurses – a research study for the DoH. Greenhalgh and Co Ltd Management Consultant, Macclesfield, Cheshire
Hector W 1973 The work of Mrs Bedford Fenwick and the rise of professional nursing. RCN, London
Human Fertilisation and Embryology Act 1990 HMSO, London
Jolly M, Brykczynska G 1993 Nursing – its hidden agendas. Edward Arnold, London
Jones I Heywood 1990 The Nurse Code – a practical approach to the Code of Professional Conduct for Nurses, Midwives and Health Visitors. Macmillan, Basingstoke
Lee S 1987 Do you want to know a secret? Nursing Times 83 (42)
Mahler H 1981 The meaning of 'Health for all by the year 2000'. World Health Forum 2(1): 5–22
Mares P, Henley A, Baxter C 1985 Health care in multiracial Britain. London Health Education Council and National Extension College Trust, Cambridge
Pyne R 1987 The professional duty to shout. Nursing Times 83(42)
Rieu S 1994 Error and trial: the extended role dilemma. British Journal of Nursing 3(4)
Roach M S 1982 Caring: a framework for nursing ethics. Programme and abstracts, First International Congress on Nursing Law and Ethics, Jerusalem
Rowden R 1984 Managing nursing – a practical introduction to management for nurses. Baillière Tindall, London
UKCC 1985 Advertising by registered nurses, midwives and health visitors (an elaboration of clause 14 of the Code of Professional Conduct). UKCC, London
UKCC 1986 Project 2000: a new preparation for practice. UKCC, London
UKCC 1987 Confidentiality: an elaboration of clause 9 and the 2nd edition of the UKCC's Code of Professional Conduct. UKCC, London

UKCC 1992a Code of Professional Conduct, 3rd edn. UKCC, London

UKCC 1992b The scope of professional practice. UKCC, London

UKCC 1992c A guide for students of nursing and midwifery. UKCC, London

UKCC 1994 The future of professional practice – the Council's Standards for Education and Practice following Registration. UKCC, London

Ward R 1991 The extended role of the nurse: a review. Nursing Times 6(11)

FURTHER READING

Alleyne J, Papadopoulos I, Tilki M 1994 Antiracism within trans cultural nurse education. British Journal of Nursing 3(2)

Carlisle D 1991 To tell or not to tell. Nursing Times 87(16)

Casteldine G 1992 What is a registered nurse? British Journal of Nursing 1(8)

Caseldine G 1994 The role of the nurse in the 21st century. British Journal of Nursing 3(12)

Department of Health 1992 Report of the Committee of inquiry into complaints about Ashworth Hospital. HMSO, London

Department of Health 1994 The challenge for nursing and midwifery in the 21st century (The Heathrow Debate). DoH, London

Dimond B 1989 Accountability in a legal context. Nursing Standard 3(49): 29–31

Hunt G 1991 Professional accountability. Nursing Standard 6(4)

Hunt G 1995 Whistleblowing in the health service, accountability, law and professional practice. Edward Arnold, London

Hunt G, Wainwright P 1994 Expanding the role of the nurse – the scope of professional practice. Blackwell Scientific, Oxford

Mangan P 1994 Registered approval. Nursing Times 90(7)

Melia K M 1987 Learning and working – the occupational socialization of nurses. Tavistock, London

Murphy K, Macleod Clark J 1993 Nurses' experiences of caring for ethnic minority clients. Journal of Advanced Nursing 18: 442–450

National Health Service Management Executive 1990 Ministerial Group on Junior Doctors Hours – Heads of Agreement. NHSME, London

Nurses, Midwives and Health Visitors Act 1979 HMSO, London

Pyne R 1984 Managing the profession. In: Rowden R (ed.) Managing nursing. Baillière Tindall, London

Pyne R 1991 Accountability. Nursing Times 87(3)

Pyne R 1992 Professional discipline in nursing, midwifery and health visiting. Blackwell, Oxford

Pyne R 1994 Empowerment through use of the Code of Conduct. British Journal of Nursing 3(12)

Salvage J 1985 The politics of nursing. Heinemann, London

Salvage J 1988 Professionalisation – or struggle for survival: a consideration of current proposals for the reform of nursing in the UK. Journal of Advanced Nursing 13: 515–519

Stockwell F 1972 The unpopular patient. RCN, London

Thompson J, Melia K, Boyd K 1994 Nursing ethics. Churchill Livingstone, Edinburgh

UKCC 1986, revised 1991 A midwife's Code of Practice. UKCC, London

UKCC 1989 Exercising accountability: a framework to assist nurses, midwives and health visitors to consider ethical aspects of professional practice. UKCC, London

Vousden M 1987 Top secret code. Nursing Times 83(42)

Wright S 1991 Nursing development. Nursing Standard 5(38)

Young B, Dimond B 1994 If something had gone wrong. British Journal of Nursing 1(9)

17 The nurse as communicator

Roger B Ellis   Andrew M Betts

Underlying the development of a therapeutic relationship is communication between the nurse and the patient. This chapter aims to:

- **consider what is meant by communication, in spoken, written and non-verbal forms**
- **describe a model of the person as an individual and relate personal interaction to this**
- **examine the concepts and principles of counselling**
- **discuss how the skills of effective communication between nurse and patient can be developed.**

It has become commonplace to say that nursing has shifted its emphasis from the treatment of illness in a patient to the treatment of the patient as a person who happens to be ill. The implication of this shift is that both nurse and patient are now seen as people who bring their full humanity to their relationship, the quality of which contributes significantly to the therapeutic effectiveness of any treatment the patient receives. This can be both reassuring and daunting for a nurse: reassuring, because *all* personal resources, and not only the competence achieved as a direct result of training, are relevant to her professional role; daunting, because there is no opting out of recognising the relevance of the nurse's whole personality and behaviour to the treatment of a patient.

As nursing, by definition, takes place in the presence of others, it is possible to perceive it as essentially an interpersonal process. If one accepts this perspective, the effectiveness of any nurse will be largely determined by her competence and sensitivity as a communicator.

Many of the ideas introduced in this chapter are examined in greater depth in Ellis et al (1995).

COMMUNICATION: WHAT IS IT?

Human beings have a basic drive to relate to one another, which is expressed through communication. When two or more people are together they cannot help but communicate (Watzlawick et al 1968). It is difficult to imagine strangers on a train sitting together for any length of time without some form of communication taking place between them, even if no one speaks. Smiling is a communication, as is not smiling. In other words, all behaviour has message value, even when this in not consciously intended.

Communication has three fundamental components, all of which are necessary for it to live up to its name; these are the sender, the receiver and the message, as shown in Figure 17.1. Because of the power of human language, it is easy to equate the message with words and overlook other ways in which we communicate, for example with our bodies, with posture, with gestures, and with tone of voice and intonation. This non-verbal communication (NVC) is often of a more primitive and unconscious kind than is verbal communication, and powerfully modifies the meaning of words. Other species use sound, colour, smell, ritualistic movements, chemical markers and other means to transfer information from one member to another. Scientists are constantly discovering how complex and subtle are communication systems in the lowliest of species, and how necessary these are for survival.

Shortcomings of both intimate and work relationships are often similar, centring around poor communication: not being listened to, not knowing what is going on, not being valued for one's individual self, not being taken into account. Statements such as 'We live in the same house but we just don't communicate' or 'No one tells me anything around here' suggest the feelings of anger, frustration and even helplessness that are aroused by poor communication. They also show that sending a message is not, in itself, communication. The message has to be received and understood by the receiver for communication to take place. Perhaps it is not surprising that dissatisfaction with communication in the NHS has been consistently highlighted by users of the service (Gerard et al 1980, Ley 1988).

It follows from these general remarks that a nurse is expected to take seriously the communication aspects of her work and to develop professional communication skills alongside more obvious practical competence. A nurse works within a web of relationships, each of which is able to affect the others in subtle ways.

The nurse's relationships

Figure 17.2 gives a general picture of the variety of relationships that a nurse is likely to have.

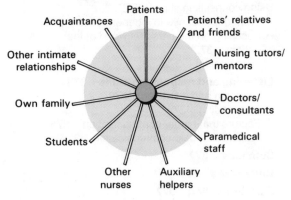

Figure 17.2   A web of relationships.

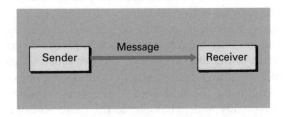

Figure 17.1   The three components of communication.

The nurse's relationships with such a wide range of people give rise to a need for the sensitive use of a variety of communication styles, depending on the context and position of the other person or persons involved. Young children have normally not acquired the capacity to make the subtle judgements needed to adopt appropriate ways of communicating in different circumstances. Such naivety is charming in children but less so in adult professionals.

How can these various types of communication be described? Consider the dimensions of communication identified in Figure 17.3. Any communication is likely to be biased towards one end of each dimension, depending on the context and the people involved. For example, a doctor who says, 'And this patient's blood pressure?' is likely to expect an answer of objective information rather than an expression of personal feelings about the patient's treatment. A nurse's question 'How are you?' to a patient is likely to carry a different weight from the same words addressed to an old friend.

Personal flexibility

Some people are flexible in their use of different communication styles and manage to respond to different contexts in an appropriate way. Others find it difficult to adjust so that, for example, they always talk impersonally and factually even when an expression of feelings and subjective views is of pressing importance. Another person might be emotional and subjective when a cool look at the facts is what is really needed. The multifaceted role of the nurse within a complex social context necessitates nurses' flexibility in matching the appropriate communication to the individual(s) and the set of circumstances.

The way in which we communicate can be seen as dependent on our whole personality. Certainly, what is communicated between two people is a product of the interaction of the three basic components: sender, receiver and message. A patient who is asked the question 'How are you?' by two different nurses might pick up quite different meanings. From one, it might be an empty phrase, said perhaps whilst the nurse was attending to something else. From the other, it might be a genuine empathic enquiry into the patient's thoughts and feelings at the time. Which message is received will depend on the patient processing all of the information available. The judgement about the meaning of that information will depend on the patient's own expectations and personality. All three components are involved in the actual communication received by the patient. Many problems occur in communication because of a mismatch between the sender's intention and the reading of that intention by the receiver.

Channels of communication

We have noted that when we communicate with each other, we do so not only with the verbal message sent, but also by virtue of the context of that message. Information passes along various channels of communication, namely:

- lexical content – *what* is said
- non-lexical content – *how* it is said: intonation, pitch
- NVC – actions, gestures, body language, touch and eye contact.

In face-to-face communication, all three channels are open and carrying information. When all three give a consistent message, the receiver is likely to receive the message at face value as being sincere. When there are inconsistencies, NVC is normally taken to be more reliable than the words spoken (Case example 17.1). This is summed up in the cliché, 'Actions speak louder than words.' We commonly hear people say: 'It's not so much *what* he said, it's *how* he said it' or 'Even though she's tough with you, you know she really cares.'

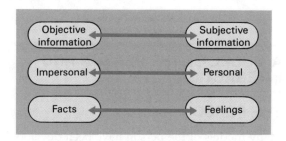

Figure 17.3 Dimensions of communication.

Case example 17.1 Incongruence in communication

As David prepared to leave the acute psychiatric ward where he had spent the past 4 weeks, everything that he said to the staff nurse suggested that he was confident about managing his life after his discharge home. Despite David's words, the staff nurse sensed that, far from being confident, David was actually apprehensive about leaving the ward. The staff nurse was unsure of her basis for this perception, but when she was asked by a colleague to justify her assessment, she realised what she had observed. David had avoided eye contact by looking down at the floor, he was hesitant in packing his belongings and, as he turned to leave, his shoulders dropped slightly and he adopted a heavy posture as he walked away. It was the non-verbal communication that reflected his true feelings, and David was later given the opportunity to talk about his fears and address the issues involved before being discharged.

The subtlety of human communication arises from the interplay of these various channels. The capacity to be ironic or sarcastic, or to mean the opposite of what is said, depends on the exploitation of this rich resource in human communication.

Modes of communication

Not all communication is face-to-face with all channels open. Consider the variety of communication modes that a nurse might use in the course of a day's work:

- rules
- memos
- letters
- reports
- information technology
- phone calls
- face-to-face contact.

She might refer to written rules of procedure or safety regulations that are impersonal and faceless, because they are sent from 'the authorities' to a generalised person of no particular identity. A memo can have personal or impersonal qualities, depending on whether it is sent from one person to another or is of a general nature. A report is a more formalised method of information-sharing and may be written to selected individuals or for general access. A letter is more commonly a communication between two individuals, the writer having in mind a particular person when it is written. Letters can, of course, also be generalised and public. Information technology is increasingly being used in all walks at life as a method of communication. This may take the form of direct messages, such as electronic mailing systems, or data files that are accessible to others. A telephone call allows for the immediate interaction that is missing from the written word, so that the message is not only in *what* is being said but also in *how* it is said. If a telephone message is written down, it is reduced to the verbal channel only, this losing the meaning carried by the other channels. Only in face-to-face contact are all channels open. That is why, when important matters are being discussed, there is no substitute for face-to-face meetings. Lovers have always known this!

Different modes for different uses

Everyday experience shows that we gradually learn the subtleties of each mode of communication and use them to suit our purposes. Making a complaint about faulty goods, for example, is most easily done for some people by writing a letter, so that the complainer is in sole charge of the language used. Another person might prefer the fuller contact of a telephone call but avoid face-to-face encounter. All of this points to the complexity of human communication. Several models have been produced to attempt to describe this complexity one of which is outlined below.

A MODEL OF THE PERSON AND INTERACTION

THE PERSON

Many models of the person have been developed in a wide variety of human contexts: philosophical, sociological, political, religious, economic, psychological and scientific. The assumptions that these models make about human beings reflect the specific purposes for which the models were designed. This is equally true of the concepts put forward in this chapter, which have the needs of a particular audience – nurses in training – in mind.

Body and personality

Each individual is both a body and a personality. The body (**soma**) is directly accessible to our senses, whilst the personality (**psyche**) is less accessible but nonetheless real, as was discussed in Chapter 2. In our culture, historically rooted in the dualism of mind and body, it is easy to think of these aspects as separate, even though the fully functioning individual is both all the time. The word 'psychosomatic' recognises both the common division and the unity of both aspects of the person.

Exterior and interior worlds

Similar to the soma–psyche distinction is the idea that a person lives simultaneously in two worlds; the exterior world of objects and people, and the interior world of feelings and thoughts. Some people focus their attention and energy on what is outside themselves, others on their inner experience, but most of us are aware that both worlds need attending to, in differing degrees at different times, and that they interact.

The conscious and unconscious mind

Another distinction is between the conscious and unconscious aspects of the psyche. Put simply, the conscious mind is aware that it knows; the unconscious is not aware that it knows. Sigmund Freud was the first to study the unconscious mind seriously and has greatly enriched our understanding of human nature, although many of his views are still controversial. The common experience of not knowing why we do things, or of saying things contrary to our conscious wishes, suggests the working of the unconscious mind as, of course, do dreams.

Relating

A baby cannot survive without someone relating to him. His body is made out of the bodies of his closest relatives. His capacity to be fully human in an emotional sense is realised through relationships with others. As the child matures, this external relating gradually becomes internalised, so that the quality of his earliest relationships with others profoundly affects the way in which he relates to himself. In turn, this inner world of relating is projected onto the outside world (see Ch. 2), affecting the way he relates to other people. It is helpful for a nurse to be aware of this basic pattern of relating and of how the present is built on the past.

The human need to relate remains fundamental and universal. It does not go away with time or maturity. Its very intensity and permanence gives rise to the multifarious ways in which it is expressed – in love, in sex, in marriage, in friendship, in social activities, in sport, in religion – and is the glue that holds families, communities and nations together. It can also be suppressed or hated. Nevertheless, the 'Me – You' issues of life never go away; they determine our happiness and sense of fulfilment.

The way in which a nurse relates to a patient affects both of them physically and emotionally. The significance of this has tended to be denied in the past, when the 'Don't get involved' attitude prevailed. This denial often went hand in hand with an unwillingness to examine the motives that sustained nurses in their jobs and a reluctance to acknowledge the real distress experienced as a result of their human involvement with patients (Menzies 1960).

The way an individual's internal world affects how he relates to other people was studied by Eric Berne in America (Berne 1961, 1968) and developed into a framework that he called transactional analysis.

TRANSACTIONAL ANALYSIS
Three ego states

According to Berne, a person's internal world is made up of interacting states that determine feelings and behaviour at any given moment. He called these sub-personalities 'ego states'. The whole person is made up of three ego states, Parent, Adult and Child, as shown in Figure 17.4.

The ego states explained

The Parent ego state is the one that internally criticises but also supports and nurtures. The Child ego state is the one that receives the criticism or nurturing: it can be delightfully spontaneous and free but can also be fretful and aggressive. The Adult takes in information objectively, processes it and makes decisions that are thought out and adapted to the demands of the outside world.

Imagine yourself walking past a shoe shop when a stunning pair of shoes catches your eye. The internal exchange between the three ego states might be something like:

Child: Oh, I'd *love* them. I'd look great in those.
Parent: You know you don't need them. You've got enough already.
Adult: I could reserve them, have another look another day and see whether I still feel the same.

Your decision of whether or not to buy the shoes will be the result of an internal dialogue, with arguments put for and against, just as if three separate people were arguing and struggling for dominance. If the Child dominates, you will buy them anyway, regardless of what 'anyone else' says, because you want them. If the Parent dominates, you may feel hurt that your Child did not get its way – or you might feel superior for doing the 'right' thing. If the Adult prevails, you are likely to think that you have given yourself wise counsel.

In a nursing setting, a patient about to receive an injection might behave towards the nurse in quite different ways within a short space of time,

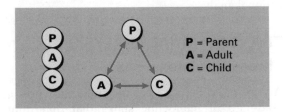

Figure 17.4 Three ego states.

depending on which ego state the behaviour derives from: 'I know I've got to have this and it's for my own good (Adult), but please don't hurt me! (Child) ... You did it much better last time (Parent).'

Ego states in one individual

It is worth emphasising that all people have all ego states regardless of age: the Child is not outgrown as a person matures, and the Parent and Adult are apparent in young children. The Child and Parent ego states are based on experience in the past, often the distant past, so that they can sometimes appear to be archaic and inappropriate. The Parent state can be full of injunctions such as 'Be nice', 'Tell the truth', 'Work hard', 'Don't be stupid' and 'Look after yourself'. These are likely to have come (or to be imagined to have come) from early learning, from our real parents or from someone else in authority along the way. They are like tape-recordings that cannot be erased and which are triggered by certain events, feelings or behaviour in the present. The Child ego state is made up of the characteristic thoughts, feelings and behaviour of our childhood; in this state, we can still be as impulsive, demanding, sulky, charming or flirtatious as we were in our early years. The Adult state has the capacity to be affected more by experience and learning than are the other two, so that it is more likely to be up to date and relevant.

There is no one state that is 'better' than another. Sometimes a person is dominated by one particular state; for example, the unpredictable, impulsive person, careless with time and money, may be dominated by the Child. The person who wants to stop others having fun and finds it difficult to be spontaneous is likely to be dominated by the critical Parent. The cool individual whose head rules his heart and who is sensible to the point of being irritating may be Adult dominated.

A harmonious, fully-functioning self is one in which all three states are freely available to interact and play their part, so that we, as individuals, can respond appropriately to any situation. Figure 17.5 shows how the three ego states interact in response to different demands.

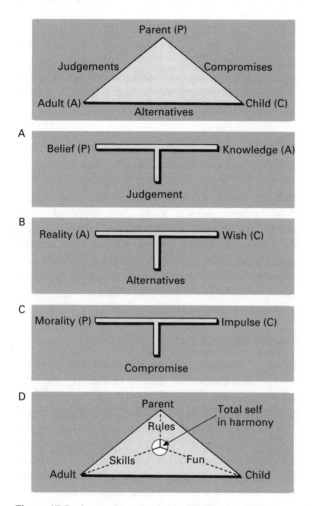

Figure 17.5 Interacting ego states. (**A**) Parent–adult collaboration. (**B**) Adult–child collaboration. (**C**) Parent–child collaboration. (**D**) Parent–adult–child collaboration.

Self-awareness

Before we explore further Berne's ideas on how people interact, we might consider for a moment the role of self-awareness. The Greek injunction on the temple of Delphi, 'Know Thyself', points to the central importance given in human wisdom to self-awareness. The teaching 'Love your neighbour as yourself' has its equivalent in many religions and points to an ancient understanding that how one relates to others and how one relates to oneself are directly linked. If a person is harsh with himself, never offering himself mercy or the benefit of a doubt, he is likely to treat others in the same basic way, even though he may try not to. Our capacity to care for others is linked to our capacity to care for ourselves. Any gain in self-awareness and self-knowledge, although it is more immediately for the benefit of the individual, must inevitably find its way into relationships with other people.

The importance of self-awareness for nurses

Carl Rogers (1974) suggested that those who are motivated towards helping others have a lifetime job ahead of them in terms of stretching and developing their personal growth. Self-awareness is particularly important for those in the caring professions because an understanding of why we should want to care for other people as a paid job helps us to do the job more effectively. We could all probably cite cases of carers who seem to be the last people to know that their efforts produce a negative effect and who seem to be getting more out of 'caring' than do the persons receiving that 'care'. It is an occupational hazard that we can be tempted to think that we can care for others *more* than for ourselves and, in extreme cases, *instead* of for ourselves. A community nurse, for example, may be over-conscientious in caring for others and try to meet their endless demands to the point at which her own health breaks down. She may be unaware that such behaviour may be motivated by a need to feel significant and appreciated and to have others depend on her. Therefore, to have some insight into what needs of our own are being met by taking care of others can make a significant contribution towards the quality of the care we offer.

A general principle can be stated here: a nurse's capacity to listen, care for and communicate effectively with another person is related to her capacity to do those things for herself. That is why a focus on the patient as a person *necessarily* implies a focus on the nurse-in-training as a person.

Interaction

Eric Berne uses the structural model of the person (the three ego states) to analyse communication between people. He refers to the smallest unit of communication as a 'transaction', of which there are three types:

- complementary
- crossed
- ulterior.

Complementary transactions

In complementary transactions, the vectors of the transactions are parallel. In Type I, the same ego state dominates in each person: Parent speaks to Parent, Adult to Adult, and Child to Child, as shown in Figure 17.6.

In Type 2, the vectors are still parallel but originate in one ego state and are directed at a different ego state. Thus, for example, Child speaks to Parent and Parent to Child, as in Figure 17.7.

Both of these types of transaction are called 'complementary' because the second person accepts the terms of the transaction as implicity defined by the first person and responds in a complementary way: 'If you ask me a straight question, I'll give you a straight answer' (Type 1, A–A); 'If you speak to me like a child, I'll treat you like a parent' (Type 2, C–P).

Crossed transactions

Here the vectors are not parallel, but crossed, as shown in Figure 17.8. In this example, the first person sends the message as Adult to Adult. The second person does not respond in a complementary way but 'crosses' by responding as Parent to Child. Such crossed transactions usually result in communication breakdown and remain unproductive until negotiation takes place to make them complementary.

Another example is given in Figure 17.9.

Ulterior transactions

Ulterior transactions are the most complicated and have the essential quality of bearing multiple messages, one straightforward and apparent at surface level, the other implied at a deeper level.

The first type of ulterior transaction is the angular transaction involving three ego states, as illustrated in Figure 17.10. In this example, the nurse might pick up an ulterior message from 'I'm not sure whether anyone here could

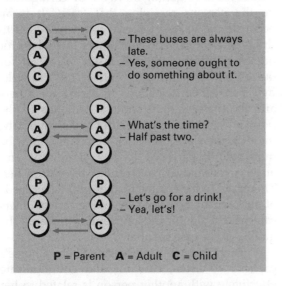

P = Parent   A = Adult   C = Child

Figure 17.6   Complementary transactions, Type 1.

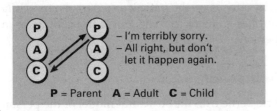

P = Parent   A = Adult   C = Child

Figure 17.7   Complementary transactions, Type 2.

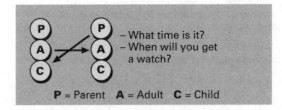

P = Parent   A = Adult   C = Child

Figure 17.8   Crossed transactions.

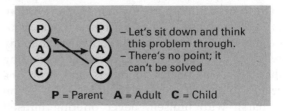

P = Parent   A = Adult   C = Child

Figure 17.9   Another crossed transaction.

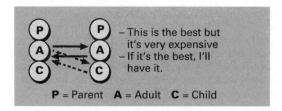

Figure 17.10   Angular transaction.

do it', which might be received (and be intended to be received) as 'You are not really good enough for the job.' This may produce an inner reaction of 'So, you think I'm not up to it. I'll show you.' This inner processing may in turn result in the response 'I know I can do it. Give me a chance.'

A second type of ulterior transaction is the duplex type involving four ego states, as shown in Figure 17.11. In this example, the transaction appears to be on one level (A–A) but psychologically the message is at another level. Both people may understand this; otherwise, there may be misunderstanding because the important message is implied, rather than explicit. An employee may, for example, be apparently giving factual information to a boss, but she may also, and more importantly, be seeking approval for her efforts or showing how exhausted she is.

In general, both ulterior and crossed transactions can add subtlety to communication in intimate relationships – but they can also reduce the effectiveness of communication at work and can undermine relationships: 'He says one thing but means another'; 'I never know where I am with her.' We ourselves may be unaware of the

'mixed messages' we give in ulterior transactions with others, hence the emphasis given earlier to the need for self-awareness if we are to be more effective in our communication with others.

Transactions in health care

The example in Box 17.1 illustrates a subtle but significant contrast in communication styles. Although the first example is grounded in a caring attitude, it takes responsibility away from the client. In transactional analysis terms, it is a Parent–Child interaction. The contrasting example is an Adult–Adult interaction, as the carer respects the autonomy of the client but still shows her genuine concern.

The traditional hierarchy of a hospital may well encourage Parent–Child-type transactions at different levels in the hierarchy, for example doctor–sister or sister–nurse. This style of communication tends to be built into nursing culture and can therefore easily be passed on to the nurse–patient relationship. The current emphasis on community care gives more autonomy to the individual nurse and thus has implications for the type and style of communication within management hierarchies. The fuller use of a nurse's resources as a whole person in a more

---

Box 17.1 Transactions in health care

Karen is a 25-year-old woman with learning disabilities. The carers at her residential home who know her well realise that she is capable of making decisions for herself (although it takes a while for her to do so). Compare the two interactions below. The former involves a carer who does not know Karen, and the latter a carer who knows her well and recognises her potential for autonomy.

Example 1.   Well Karen, we are organising a shopping trip with a few of the residents, and I thought it would be a chance for you to get some new clothes so that you will look smart for your visitors at the weekend.

Example 2.   Karen, some of the residents are going into town to buy a few things. I wondered whether there was anything you needed or whether you would like to come with us.

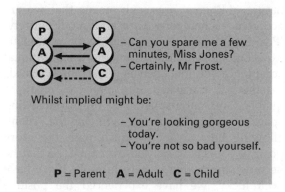

Figure 17.11   Duplex transaction.

open, person-centred approach to patients implies a shift away from a Parent–Child style of relating to a more Adult–Adult style. This shift has implications for *all* relationships in an institution, including the way in which staff treat one another.

AN INTRODUCTION TO COUNSELLING

WHAT IS COUNSELLING?

Counselling is a professional activity in its own right, and it may be more appropriate in the nursing context to think of a nurse using counselling *skills* rather than being a counsellor to her patients. Consider the basic situation shown in Figure 17.12. Each person brings his or her internal world and outward behaviour into a common space in which the counselling work is carried out. This can happen only if the space is protected from intrusion or distraction and the two people are engaging with each other in a voluntary way. In nursing, the word 'counselling' has been linked to disciplinary procedures, and it is important to extract it from such a context and place it within the general framework of supportive one-to-one contact between people.

The basic aim of counselling is to help an individual help himself. The British Association for Counselling makes the following comments on the nature of counselling in its leaflet, 'Code of Ethics and Practice for Counsellors' (British Association for Counselling 1992):

The overall aim of counselling is to provide an opportunity for the client to work towards living in a more satisfying and resourceful way ... Counselling may be concerned with developmental issues,

addressing and resolving specific problems, making decisions, coping with crisis, developing personal insight and knowledge, working through feelings of inner conflict or improving relationships with others. The counsellor's role is to facilitate the client's work in ways which respect the client's values, personal resources and capacity for self-determination.

Requirements for effective counselling

Carl Rogers (1974) has suggested that for counselling to be effective, three core conditions are necessary: trust, respect and empathy. Without trust in the capacity of the client to help himself, the counsellor is joining forces with those who would keep the client exactly where he is. Respect for the client is linked to trust. It suggests that the individual rights, beliefs and resources of the client are respected for what they are, without judgement. Showing empathy involves attempting to experience the world as the client experiences it, without implying that it should change.

Unconditional positive regard

Rogers summarises these conditions in the concept of 'unconditional positive regard', which he believes is the most helpful basic attitude and approach to a client. In his view, there should be no conditions laid down by the counsellor for his or her acceptance and care for the client. So often we are brought up to believe that we will be accepted if we are good, successful and pleasant, and rejected if we are bad, unsuccessful and unpleasant. The 'unconditional' nature of Rogers' approach means that we are accepted – whatever we are, and in our entirety. 'Positive regard' is an attitude of optimistic expectation, stemming from the unconditional acceptance of the person. The three words together, if translated into practice, create a quality and atmosphere in the 'counselling space' that facilitates growth in the client, allowing him to get in touch with the more positive aspects of his self over time, so that he becomes more able to help himself. If we have been lucky, we have experienced the positive effect of someone else who is benign, who believes in us, who accepts us and who is on our side.

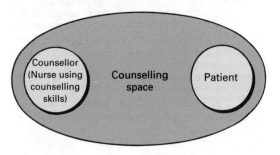

Figure 17.12 The basic counselling situation.

Such experience releases the potential in us, which otherwise may have remained dormant and unrealised.

HOW DOES COUNSELLING FIT IN TO NURSING?

Counselling is one of a number of strategies that one person can use in order to try to be helpful to another. A summary of these various strategies is given in Box 17.2.

A nurse is likely to be called on to use any or all of these strategies in the course of a working day. In moving from 'taking action' to 'supporting', the basis of the helping relationship changes by degrees from 'helper in control' to 'patient in control'. The issue of where the balance of control lies between helper and patient distinguishes one strategy from another and gives each its own special characteristics.

Clearly, a good deal of a nurse's role involves taking action on behalf of the patient and advising him. Referral on to others is also common, as are teaching and informing. Nurses are currently encouraged to use a whole range of helping strategies, including those in which the patient can exert a certain degree of control over what is happening. That is why counselling and support skills have become the focus of attention recently.

None of these skills is better than another. The versatile, skilled nurse will be able to judge which approach is appropriate, according to the needs of the patient at the time (Case example 17.2).

Case example 17.2 Effective communications are adaptable

Simon is an experienced nurse on a children's ward. He is the mentor for a student nurse who is on a short placement. As a component of the student's work is connected with a communication and interpersonal skills module, the student is required to observe and write up nurse–patient interactions.

What impresses the student about Simon is his versatility as a communicator. At one point he demonstrates a rapport with a 6-year-old girl, and at another he listens attentively to the concerns of a visiting parent. The student notices that Simon matches his intervention to the individual in a seemingly effortless manner. He recognises when it is appropriate to give advice or information to patients and relatives, and also when it is more appropriate to encourage self-disclosure and emotional expression through the effective use of counselling skills.

The student reflects on the crucial importance of developing the ability to be adaptable and intentional in nursing interactions. She wonders whether she herself will ever be able to achieve Simon's level of competence, judgement and confidence.

Box 17.2 Strategies for helping: adapted from the NICEC (National Institute for Careers Education and Counselling) model

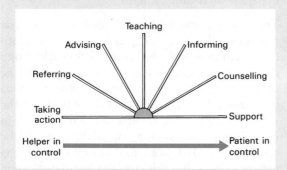

Taking action: Implies that the helper is working on behalf of the individual: 'Sit there. I'll get it for you.

Referring: Takes place when a client is presenting difficulties

beyond the extent of the helper's skills. Referral is an underlying resource that needs to be available irrespective of other strategies.

Advising: Gives the individual information through suggestion, e.g. 'I think it would be useful if you were to...'.

Teaching: Manages learning so that the individual might gain knowledge or necessary skills needed to achieve his goals: 'Let me show you how to...'.

Informing: Provides data without suggesting how such data should be used: 'Here is the bus timetable'.

Counselling: Works with the internal world of the individual; deals with feelings as well as thoughts; addresses conflict.

Supporting: Involves 'being there' for someone who is moving towards accepting the reality of a situation and who is not seeking any direct help.

USING COUNSELLING SKILLS

The goal of counselling is to enable people to be in closer touch with their own resources so that they can move towards greater freedom, autonomy and independence. It assumes that any conflict or anxiety arising within the personal world of the individual can only be dealt with using the resources within that person. An individual may ask for help or advice from another person but until such assistance is actually accepted, it cannot be used for self-help.

From dependence to independence

The paradox that is central to counselling stems from the basic human need to relate, the theme throughout this chapter. It is out of relating to another person that the individual is able to develop a surer sense of 'I, myself' – a common outcome of successful counselling. The individual can have no clear sense of identity without relating to others, just as he can have no real independence without having had, at some time, the experience of dependence.

Focusing on the personal world of the patient

The focus is on the person and his personal world, especially his feelings. The nurse needs to listen, think, imagine and feel in the counselling space between herself and the patient, so that she gets as good an idea as possible of what it is like to be that person, as he is, in the present. This empathy has a 'with you' quality about it, which goes beyond intellectual understanding and sympathy, concentrating as it does on 'being there' with and for the patient rather than 'doing something' for him. It enables the nurse to 'hold' a patient's fears and anxieties, without being tempted to try to give answers or solutions. The following exchange illustrates the quality of interaction referred to here:

Patient: *Why* did this happen to me?
Nurse: (*Silence, then:*) It's difficult to understand.
Patient: But why *me*?
Nurse: (*Silence, then:*) I can see how angry you feel.

Patient: That's not much use, is it?
Nurse: (*Quietly accepting the expressed feelings.*)

This kind of exchange allows for an acceptance of the patient's feelings (unhappiness and anger in this case) rather than brushing them aside, retaliating or referring to people who are worse off.

Commitment

All this requires of the counsellor a commitment to the patient – to his well-being and best interests. A word such as 'commitment' can sound heavy and serious, but it describes quality rather than quantity. Such real human contact can happen over a few seconds of time or over a much longer period. The counsellor is available and open, rather than distant or insincere. It immediately becomes clear that such a commitment involves the resources of the inner private world of the counsellor, as well as skills and knowledge. It necessarily involves a willingness to be affected emotionally by the patient and to be somewhat vulnerable (which is often confused with being weak), but it also involves a certain toughness and resilience. It hardly helps the client if the counsellor is overwhelmed by the feelings that are expressed and becomes *too* involved, so losing the objectivity that is also needed. There is an optimum 'therapeutic distance' between counsellor and patient that allows the best possible counselling to take place.

Implications of commitment

This commitment to the patient also implies that the counsellor is willing to suspend the gratification of personal needs should they come into conflict with those of the patient. Naturally, the counsellor has a need to relate to others, just as the patient does, and she would not be doing the work of counselling if there were no reward in it. However, within the counselling space, the counsellor is dedicated to concentrating on the patient's needs. It is this combination of dedication and abstinence by the counsellor that gives the counselling space its unique quality and distinguishes it from other forms of human contact.

Effects of commitment

The patient's experienced of committed attention and concern from another person, even for a short time, has been found to be effective and therapeutic. If, for example, I know that I have a space in another person's mind dedicated to me, that helps me to be surer about my own value, my own existence and my own resources. Counsellors often meet individuals who feel they have never, to their knowledge, received the complete, undivided attention of any other person, even for a few minutes, at any time in their lives.

The counsellor's need for growth

Counselling involves yet another form of commitment: the counsellor's commitment of continual self-exploration, growth and development. Greater self-awareness nearly always results in an individual being clearer about what feelings and thoughts originate from his internal world, in contrast to what has originated from other people. Such clarity makes personal responsibility more realistic. In the counsellor's case, it helps to put a boundary around her own experience so that it is less likely to interfere with her work with the patient.

LISTENING AND RESPONDING SKILLS

This section draws on what has been said before about the importance of approaching patients as individuals, about forms of interaction between persons and about the principles of counselling. What are now examined are the *skills* of communication, i.e. what a nurse might actually do and how she might behave with another person, in practical rather than theoretical terms. It has been noted that a nurse might be called on to make contact with several categories of people during the course of a day: doctors, patients, fellow nurses, relatives. The focus in what follows is the particular relationship and communication between a nurse and patient. It is assumed that the nurse regards relating to the patient as part of the patient's total care.

The context in which an interaction takes place affects its content and quality. This seems obvious when gross differences are considered, such as the difference between talking to someone in a bar as opposed to in his own home, but more subtle differences may be overlooked, for example the contrast between a ward in a hospital and a day room: a move from one to the other may be beneficial. Community workers may complain that the television set is left on during home visits, but they also find it difficult to suggest that it be turned off.

Certain features of the setting may militate against effective communication. The principles that are urged here are for nurses to be sensitive to the ways in which the setting affects any interaction, and for them to endeavour to make the most strategic use out of what are often far from ideal settings.

Listening and attending

To listen to someone with attention and commitment is a caring response that is all too rare. It is the basis of all effective communication on a one-to-one basis and requires hard work on the part of the listener. This work involves much more than accurate recording of what is said. It involves making accurate perceptions through several senses, looking for patterns and checking creative ideas against new information. It also requires flexibility and a willingness to give up preconceptions about the person in the face of the evidence.

Silence

The possibility of silence is often referred to with anxiety by those wishing to help others. Paradoxically, the capacity to be comfortable with silence is often a good indicator of listening skill. It normally means that the listener is able to contain her own anxiety (if any) and to concentrate on the other person. The rush to 'help' another person with words or gestures is often misplaced and can have its roots in our attempt to deal with our own feelings of awkwardness. An acceptance of silence, on the other hand, can be an eloquent recognition of the patient's need for someone to *be* there rather than for something to be *done*.

Encouraging

Some people, who are able to talk freely about their ideas and feelings, need only the slightest encouragement to explore these further. This encouragement may be given by a 'Mm' or 'Aha', a nod or smile, depending on the listener's own conversational style. Other people will falter without such feedback, needing reassurance before they continue talking. Some seem to need no encouragement at all, but a compulsive way of talking may indicate that real relating is difficult for the patient and may cover painful feelings.

The way in which the listener listens is communicated by both non-verbal and verbal signals. Posture, eye contact, position, gestures and distance from the patient all carry messages about the listeners's degree of interest and attention.

Responding

Reflecting

To reflect back to a patient what has just been heard may initially seem a strange way of responding, but it is surprising how facilitating it can be. It gives clear feedback that what has been said has been received and understood. It lets the patient know that any implied message (often about feelings) that has not been directly expressed has also been understood. The patient's question 'How long will I be in here, nurse?' may have several layers of meaning behind it. The nurse's answer, if she has successfully decoded these layers, will reflect back something of the underlying feelings as well as giving a direct answer to the question. This response might be: 'It's normally about three days ... You seem a bit concerned about it.'

Paraphrasing

Another responding skill is that of paraphrasing. This goes beyond reflecting back the content of what has been said and allows for some personal interpretation and imaginative input on the part of the listener. It can often be helpful to use an image that catches the emotional force of the message: 'It's as though you feel trapped, with no way out.' The patient may accept the image and elaborate further or may wish to modify it in some way to make it more suitable.

Summarising

Summarising what has been said after a suitable interval serves a similar purpose, i.e. consolidating information and verifying whether or not the sense the listener has made of it coincides with the intended message: 'Let me see if I've got this right. What you seem to be saying is ...'. For the patient to hear what he has just been saying in summary form from somebody else can be reassuring and give space for more reflection before he goes on.

Asking open questions

Asking open rather than closed questions, as in 'Can you say a little more about how you felt when ...', rather than 'Did you feel angry when ...', can help the patient to explore his experience. The first form of question makes a demand on the patient to examine experience and to express it in his own language. The second invites a yes/no response, which is less exploratory and potentially less useful to the patient. Often students on counselling skills courses will start by assuming that asking a lot of questions of the individual will somehow help understanding. Such questioning may be a way of coping with the uncomfortable feeling of being unskilled by *doing* lots of things verbally. The idea that a timely open question indicates more skill in communication than do a large number of closed questions is difficult for the relative novice to accept.

Factors that hinder communication

Many writers list the thoughts, feelings and behaviour that are likely to reduce the effectiveness of one-to-one communication. Hopson & Scally (1982) have produce such a list, addressing both the sender and the receiver of messages: this is given in Box 17.3. It summarises and makes concrete those factors that hinder communication and illustrates in a negative form the more general principles given before.

Factors that help communication

As well as a list of negative factors to avoid if possible, a list of positive suggestions may be helpful. Porritt (1990) gives a 'how to respond' list for someone deliberately using the skills of reflective listening. She refers to what a person is actually saying as 'the message' and the possible underlying meaning as the 'music'. She urges nurses to be sensitive to the 'music of the message'. Her list is given in Box 17.4.

The imaginary dialogue in Case example 17.3 between a practice nurse and a patient acts as a summary and a practical application of the identified areas in this section.

Box 17.3 Negative aspects of communications (Reproduced from Hopson & Scally (1982) with kind permission from Lifeskills Communications Ltd.)

Effectiveness of communication will be impaired if the *sender*:

- does not maintain eye contact
- assumes the receiver feels the same as the sender about the exchange
- imposes ideas to the exclusion of others. Unless there is a balance, and exchange, listening is likely to be short-lived. People who don't listen themselves are unlikely to find others receptive
- uses irritants. Certain words are 'loaded' and using them will immediately create resentment and barriers. Addressing somebody as 'Dearie' or 'Sonny' can ensure that little is heard after that
- forgets that though the topic she is talking about is the focal point of the exchange, she is also saying something about herself when she speaks
- assumes that the person hears *exactly* what the sender wishes to convey
- uses inappropriate language which the other person does not understand or is uncomfortable with
- mumbles, fidgets or otherwise distracts with mannerisms
- fails to check what the receiver has heard or makes this check sound like an examination.

The *receiver* can reduce the effectiveness of a communication by:

- jumping to conclusions. Making up her mind what the sender is going to say before it is said and reacting prematurely.
- changing the subject, deflecting the point the sender is trying to make
- interrupting or talking too much
- thinking of the question she wants to ask next rather than concentrating on what the sender is saying
- latching on to minor details while ignoring the main points
- switching off or ignoring what is said
- seeking to score over the other person: competing rather than cooperating will mean the receiver listens with her own interests in mind
- failing to ask for clarification and concreteness
- failing to check out assumptions; not summarising what she has heard
- not recognising, or responding to, the level of the sender's message, e.g. being flippant when the sender is attempting to say something serious
- pretending to understand
- being judgemental of what the sender is saying
- being defensive rather than open
- being unaware of any discrepancy between verbal and non-verbal messages, e.g. 'I'm not worried' said in an anxious way.

Box 17.4 How to respond using reflective listening skills (Reproduced with kind permission from Porritt 1990)

- Recognise the cues and clues that others send which alert you to their strong feeling state.
- Attempt not to hook to the content by defending or justifying yourself or by giving information.
- Look for the music of the message by attending to non-verbal and verbal cues –the metacommunication.
- Put into your own words the music of the message you are picking up from the sender and reflect this back as simply as possible, in a non-judgemental empathic way.
- Stay with the other person and what they bring to the interaction.
- Banish your own thoughts, fantasies, and experiences from your mind as much as possible and attend to the other person's experience.
- Give sufficient and appropriate eye contact.

- Reflect back what you hear from the other person; it is preferable to go only as deep as the person is willing; *do not push* beyond where the person is ready to go.
- Realise that reflective listening is a useful skill for recognising, clarifying and understanding problems or obstacles but that other skills may also be required.
- Use other skills, such as asking questions, giving information, remaining silent, passively listening, making a statement of reality, or bringing attention to incongruence and what it means, when reflecting back the music of messages. Once a problem is clarified choices for problem-solving and decision making are elicited. No skill stands totally alone. However, when it is the other person's obstacle an effective listener will find herself using reflective listening responses far more frequently than other responses.

Case example 17.3 A dialogue

The GP has referred Mr White to the practice nurse. Mr White has been under pressure at work over the past 18 months, resulting in a series of minor ailments and conflict within his relationships with his family. The GP thought that the nurse might be able to help with stress management strategies. The following dialogue is an extract from the interaction.

Practice nurse	How has this increased pressure affected you? (**Open question**)
Mr White	The worst part is that I feel tired all the time. When I get home in the evenings, I don't feel like communicating with my family. All I want to do is go to sleep. I used to be so full of life, but now I'm not much company.
Practice nurse	It's as if your batteries are run down and you have nothing left at the end of the day. (**Paraphrase – repeating back the core message in her own words**)
Mr White	Yes, but I feel so bad about it. I don't like what I'm doing, but I can't seem to stop it. It's not my family's fault, and I feel guilty about the way I treat them.
Practice nurse	So it's like you feel powerless but you still blame yourself for what is happening. (**Reflection of feelings**)
Mr White	I suppose it's like I'm putting my job before them. I'm sure my children see it that way ... it's like a battle between work, and what's expected of me there, and my family ...
Practice nurse	Mm, mm. (**Minimal encouragement**)
Mr White	It's such a difficult balance. If I slack off at work, I run the risk of losing my job, and that would be of no use to my family. If I don't, my family and my health suffer ...
Practice nurse	(**Remains silent for some time – she can sense that the silence is far from empty**)
Mr White	It's like a no-win situation ... I can't think how things could be improved.
Practice nurse	So far you have talked about the difficulty of balancing work and home life, of how exhausting your lifestyle is at the moment, and of how little control you seem to have over changing things. You seem to feel stuck and pessimistic about finding any solution. Is that how you see things? (**Summarising the main points that have been brought up and checking her understanding is accurate**)

Summary

With the increasing recognition of the patient as a person who happens to be ill, the therapeutic interaction is now being viewed as a human, personal relationship between two people, the quality of which significantly affects any treatment interventions.

The communication process has three components – the sender, the receiver and the message – and for communication to take place, the message must be not only received but also understood. The style of the interaction will be influenced by personality, but the nurse must be encouraged to be flexible to the needs and communication style of her patients, colleagues and family, in order to strengthen her relationships with them.

According to Berne, the personal internal world is composed of 'ego states', sub-personalities that determine feelings and behaviour. This chapter explores these and considers the effect they may have on personal interactions, emphasising the nurse's need for self-awareness to optimise the results of her communications.

As the nurse becomes more aware of and practised in communication techniques, she will become more adept in using counselling skills with her patients, enabling them better to use their own resources in the move towards independence. Underlying this are listening and responding skills, which need to be learnt and developed.

The nurse who is developing the quality of interaction within the work setting is one who has realised both the importance of communication skills and their place in professional effectiveness.

REFERENCES

Berne E 1961 Transactional analysis in psychotherapy. Souvenir Press, London
Berne E 1968 Games people play. Penguin, Harmondsworth
British Association for Counselling 1992 Code of ethics and practice for counsellors. BAC Office, Rugby
Ellis R, Gates R, Kenworthy N 1995 Interpersonal communication in nursing theory and practice. Churchill Livingstone, Edinburgh
Gerrad B, Boniface W, Love B 1980 Interpersonal skills for health professionals. Reston Publishing, Reston
Hopson B, Scally M 1982 Lifeskills teaching programme. Lifeskills Associates, Leeds
Ley P 1988 Communication with patients. Croom Helm, London
Menzies I 1960 The functioning of social systems as a defence against anxiety. Tavistock, London
Porritt L 1990 Interaction strategies, 2nd edn. Churchill Livingstone, Melbourne
Rogers C 1974 On becoming a person, 4th edn. Constable, London
Watzlawick P, Beavin J, Jackson D 1968 Pragmatics of human communication. Faber, London

FURTHER READING

Faulkner A 1992 Effective interaction with patients. Churchill Livingstone, Edinburgh
Pease A 1981 Body language. Sheldon Press, London
Porritt L 1990 Interaction strategies, 2nd edn. Churchill Livingstone, Melbourne
Rissman A 1975 Trilog. In: Klein M (ed.) Lives people live. John Wiley & Sons, Chichester
Stewart I, Joines V 1987 TA today. Lifespace Publishing, Nottingham

18

The nurse as educator

Mary Watkins   Peter Janitsch   Gillian McEwing

There is increasing recognition that the nursing role includes promoting health and teaching individuals how to maximise their independence when they are ill or disabled. This chapter focuses on the nurse as educator, and aims to cover four themes:

- **aims and target population**
- **learning**
- **teaching**
- **application in clinical practice.**

AIMS AND TARGET POPULATION

WHO GOALS

In its document 'Health for All' the World Health Organization (WHO) defined goals for health care within Europe (World Health Organization 1985); some of these are listed in Table 18.1. It may be useful to consider how nurses can assist the partial achievement of these aims. Is it possible, for example, to eliminate rubella, with

Table 18.1 Some minimum targets for health in Europe by the year 2000

Target change	Disease/problem
Elimination	Measles, polio, rubella, neonatal tetanus, diphtheria, congenital syphilis
15% reduction	Mortality from cardiovascular diseases in under-65s
15% reduction	Mortality from cancer in under-65s
25% reduction	Mortality from accidents (traffic/home/work)
50% reduction	Differences in health between groups (e.g. ethnic)
25% reduction	Prescription of hypnotics and sedatives by reason of mental illness
10% reduction	Mental handicap
50% reduction	Tooth loss
25% reduction	Unwanted pregnancy in under-20s
Reverse trend	Suicide and parasuicide

its associated complications in pregnant women and resultant births of severely handicapped children, by the year 2000? If so, how?

The WHO report suggests that there is a need to promote healthy behaviour, to discourage unhealthy behaviour and to 'add years to life', 'health to life' and 'life to years'. The last aim may appear esoteric but it is extremely important. Few individuals would wish to live longer if this merely meant existing, but if an extended lifespan can be accompanied by an enhanced quality of life, much will have been achieved.

There is clearly a great challenge in 'educating the public' if the WHO goals for health are to be reached. While this job is not exclusively the responsibility of nurses, they make up the greatest percentage of manpower within the NHS and must make a significant contribution to the task.

'HEALTH OF THE NATION' TARGETS

In 1993, the Department of Health for England and Wales produced a document entitled 'The Health of the Nation'. This detailed minimum targets for health to be achieved by the year 2000. Particular emphasis was placed on coronary heart disease and stroke, cancers, mental illness, sexual health and the prevention of accidents (Box 18.1). Clearly, these targets reflect those of the minimum targets defined by the WHO for Europe, as identified in Table 18.1.

COUNCIL OF EUROPE GOALS

A Council of Europe document (1980) identifies the need for all patients to be active participants in their own treatment, in accordance with the belief that the self-help capacities of patients can make an important contribution to both health protection and rehabilitation. The same report suggests that there needs to be a shift away from an emphasis on patient *compliance* with treatment towards an emphasis on *cooperation* between patients and health care workers. If patients are to be equal partners with health care professionals, it is essential that they are given sufficient information regarding:

Box 18.1 The 'Health of the Nation' targets

Coronary heart disease and stroke

A1 To reduce the death rate for coronary heart disease in people under 65 by at least 40% by the year 2000 (from 58 per 100 000 population in 1990 to no more than 35 per 100 000).

A2 To reduce the death rate for coronary heart disease in people aged 65–74 by at least 30% by the year 2000 (from 884 per 100 000 population in 1990 to no more than 619 per 100 000).

A3 To reduce mean systolic blood pressure in the adult population by at least 5 mmHg by the year 2005.

Cancers

B1 To reduce death rate for breast cancer in the population invited for screening by at least 25% by the year 2000 (from 96.3 per 100 000 population in 1990 to no more than 72.2 per 100 000).

B2 To reduce the incidence of invasive cervical cancer by at least 20% by the year 2000 (from 15 per 100 000 population in 1986 to no more than 12 per 100 000).

B3 To reduce the smoking prevalence among 11–15-year-olds by at least 33% by 1994 (from about 8% in 1988 to less than 6%).

Mental illness

C1 To improve significantly the health and social functioning of mentally ill people.

C2 To reduce the overall suicide rate (including undetermined deaths) by at least 15% by the year 2000 (from 11.0 per 100 000 population in 1990 to no more than 9.4 per 100 000).

C3 To reduce the suicide rate (including undetermined deaths) of severely mentally ill people by at least 33% by the year 2000 (from the estimate of 15% in 1990 to no more than 10%).

HIV/AIDS and sexual health

D1 To reduce the incidence of gonorrhea among men and women aged 15–64 by at least 20% by 1995 (from 61 new cases per 100 000 population in 1990 to no more than 49 new cases per 100 000).

D2 To reduce the percentage of injecting drug misusers who report sharing injecting equipment in the previous four weeks by at least 50% by 1997, and by at least a further 50% by the year 2000 (from 20% in 1990 to no more than 10% by 1997 and no more than 5% by the year 2000).

D3 To reduce the rate of conceptions among the under 16s by at least 50% by the year 2000 (from 9.5 per 1000 girls aged 13–15 in 1989 to no more than 4.8 per 1000).

Accidents

E1 To reduce the death rate for accidents among children aged under 15 by at least 33% by the year 2005 (from 6.6 per 100 000 population in 1990 to no more than 4.4 per 100 000).

E2 To reduce the death rate for accidents among young people aged 15–24 by at least 25% by the year 2005 (from 24.0 per 100 000 population in 1990 to no more than 18.0 per 100 000).

E3 To reduce the death rate for accidents among people aged 65 and over by at least 33% by the year 2005 (from 55.8 per 100 000 population in 1990 to no more than 37.4 per 100 000).

• ways of promoting health
• the causes and prevention of illness/disease
• the nature of any illness/disease relevant to them as individuals
• ways of treating illness/disease relevant to them as individuals.

THE TARGET POPULATION

The nurse's role as educator has been defined with regard to three key client groups (Council of Europe 1980):

• healthy people
• people at risk of illness
• sick people.

These groups may appear to be separate entities, but the dividing lines between them are, in fact, rarely clear. For example, an occupational health nurse giving information regarding 'stress management' to a group of apparently healthy employees in a large firm, may, as a result of questions from the target group, move into giving advice to a person who identifies himself as 'at risk' of developing an alcohol problem.

Promoting health involves health education. As health promotion is the subject of Chapter 6, it is not discussed in detail here, except with regard to patients who are at risk of developing illness or who have been diagnosed as having a specific disease. Figure 18.1 indicates the aim of education provided by nurses to these two groups.

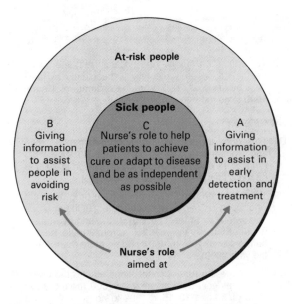

Figure 18.1 The nurse's teaching roles with sick and at-risk populations.

Patients at risk

The at-risk group of women who attend breast screening clinics to ensure early detection of malignancy are usually taught by the nurse in the clinic how to conduct self-examination of their breasts to identify future changes. If this in turn leads to early detection and successful treatment, the nurse's teaching can be considered successful, her role being that of A in Figure 18.1.

The link between stress and heart disease may be a factor that the practice nurse chooses to emphasise when conducting health screening of at-risk patients. She may give patients copies of leaflets that indicate ways of reducing stress, or refer them to popular texts describing ways of coping with stress.

These examples clearly illustrate that there is only a fine line between health education and patient teaching. It is rarely useful to be pedantic about terms, but far more constructive to identify those areas in which nurses can usefully educate patients to reduce their risk of disease.

Sick people

The nurse's teaching is not always successful in helping patients to achieve a cure, particularly when progressive disease is present. This should not be used as a reason to discount the value of patient education in such situations. Henderson (1960) defines the unique function of the nurse as being:

to assist the individual, sick or well, in the performance of those activities contributing to health or its recovery (or to a peaceful death) that he would perform unaided if he had the necessary strength, will or knowledge. And to do this in such a way as to help him gain independence as rapidly as possible.

This definition illustrates that nurses who teach a dying patient how to position himself to reduce breathlessness are undertaking as important an intervention as are those who teach diabetic patients to self-medicate.

Other health care workers

In addition to teaching patients, the qualified nurse has a responsibility to educate other health care workers. The Department of Health (1989) states that students prepared under a syllabus that involves both common foundation and branch programmes shall, on completion of their course, be able to assume the responsibility and accountability that registration confers for 'the assignment of appropriate duties to others and the supervision, teaching and monitoring of assigned duties'.

The first-level nurse is required to be competent at teaching other health care workers how safely to conduct delegated care. This will involve educating student nurses and health care assistants. However, when qualified nurses return to practice after a period of absence or change their sphere of practice, they may need guidance from another qualified nurse.

Relatives

It may sometimes be necessary to teach a particular skill or piece of knowledge to patients' relatives to enable them to conduct care in the absence of a trained nurse. To achieve the goals outlined, it is necessary to understand the principles of learning and of teaching.

LEARNING

INFLUENCING FACTORS

Each individual will be subject to factors that can inhibit or promote the learning process (Quinn 1988). It is useful to think of these in terms of:

- intrinsic factors: those from within the person
- extrinsic stimuli: those which impinge on the individual from both society and the environment.

This section focuses on patient learning, although its principles apply to any teacher–student relationship. When planning individualised nursing care that involves achieving goals related to the patient's 'learning', it is useful to consider the list in Box 18.2, adapted from the Council of Europe paper (1980) on patient participation in care.

The recognition of promoting factors that can assist a patient in the learning process is necessary to maximise their use when planning a teaching programme. Similarly, the nurse needs to identify those factors that inhibit learning and try to find ways of overcoming them. Consideration should be given to both intrinsic and extrinsic factors.

Box 18.2 Factors that may affect the patient's learning (Adapted from Council of Europe 1980)

Intrinsic factors

- level of anxiety
- level of motivation to learn
- ability to learn in terms of level of intelligence
- sensory impairment which may affect learning, e.g. poor vision, hearing
- physical disabilities which may interfere with dexterity
- personal characteristics, e.g. philosophy of life
- attitude towards illness

Extrinsic factors

- family attitude in encouraging individual to achieve self-care
- financial factors: increased salary or reduced allowance
- cultural factors, including over-protection, negative life expectancy

---

Intrinsic factors

Anxiety

Anxiety can inhibit learning. If, for example, a patient is very anxious following a stroke and says that he does not want to learn to walk again because it is too risky, the nurse must try to find out the cause of the anxiety. It may be that, with reassurance and physical assistance to prevent a fall, the patient's anxiety can be sufficiently alleviated for him to attempt walking.

Motivation

If a patient is well motivated to learn and has a positive attitude to his illness or handicap (perceiving it as a challenge), the teaching plan should be organised in such a way that he is stretched to his maximum capacity. The more reluctant patient may find it helpful to use the simple technique of 'force field analysis' at this stage. This involves listing the positive and negative outcomes that may result from the patient learning (in our example) to walk again (Fig. 18.2). The list should be constructed in conjunction with the patient so that he is actively participating in the exercise. Positive benefits clearly outweighing negative ones is often enough of a motivator for the patient to enter into a learning programme. When the reverse occurs and the negative outcomes exceed the position, it can be extremely difficult to motivate an individual.

Level of intelligence

Nurses need to be aware of the patient's level of intelligence to plan an individualised and appropriate teaching programme. For example, the highly intelligent patient may study the theory of a particular illness to a level of understanding beyond that which the nurse herself has. In this instance, the nurse may be taught by the patient, rather than vice versa. Conversely, patients with learning difficulties may need special help with learning simple skills.

Sensory/physical impairment

If a patient has difficulty hearing, seeing or feeling, this can severely affect the learning

---

Resisting forces for change

Possible negative outcomes, as perceived by the patient:

- more would be expected of the patient
- may fall and hurt himself
- may be painful
- wife may expect too much independence
- may loose sickness benefits but be unable to return to current well-paid job

---

Driving forces for change

Possible positive outcomes, as perceived by the patient:

- freedom to move unaided
- could make a cup of tea
- less for wife to do
- could get back to work of some kind

Figure 18.2 Force field analysis. The nurse and patient together identify and write down all the positive outcomes that the patient would enjoy on learning to walk again. Similarly, they identify all the inhibiting factors that are preventing the patient from walking, together with the negative outcomes of not learning to walk again. When exploring the types and strengths of the driving and resisting forces, it is often easier to attempt to reduce or weaken the resisting forces than to increase or intensify the driving forces.

process. A thorough assessment should enable the nurse to identify individual patients' problems in these spheres. Nurse and patient can then collaborate to find a way around the difficulties identified. It may be impossible for a person with a hearing deficit to learn how to use a hearing aid, without the nurse first having to fit the aid and explain how it was done. Similarly, a client who has lost feeling in her fingers may need to be told by colour which side of a flange should be fitted to her colostomy stoma, rather than by feeling for the smooth and rough sides.

Personal attitudes

The school nurse trying to educate a group of 14-year-olds about 'healthy eating' may be faced with a challenge if the group's 'normal diet' consists of fast foods with high animal fat content,

and none of their family members or relatives have suffered heart disease. Conversely, if a group member has personal experience of a parent suffering a myocardial infarction that has been partly attributable to diet, this may become a major motivating factor in the group accepting the education offered.

The greatest asset or inhibitor to learning can be the individual's attitude to the process. Whilst attitudes to disease can be difficult to change, patients will sometimes, through the mastery of knowledge and skills, alter their attitudes to disease as they gain more authority and control over their situation. Further reading on attitude change may help the student nurse to recognise the complexity of this subject, which is examined in more detail in Chapter 6.

Extrinsic factors

Family attitude

Family involvement can increase a patient's motivation to learn. Orem (1985), a nursing theorist, believes that patients have a responsibility to maintain their own health by extending their self-care functions as necessary. She states that, if an individual is unable to do this, the next logical care-giver is an immediate family member or close friend. A nurse may find that if a patient's relative accepts responsibility for undertaking a task, such as colostomy bag changing, this may in turn motivate the patient to take on the task himself. In other families, it may be better for the spouse or other relative to undertake the task on the patient's behalf. Either solution should be acceptable to the nurse as long as the family are happy with the outcome.

Financial factors

Some patients and their families can be financially better off whilst in receipt of sickness benefits and related allowances than if the sick person were enabled to become more independent and lose his right to the benefits. Such a situation can inhibit learning and present the nurse with a difficult situation. At the opposite end of the spectrum, an individual earning a good salary may not be motivated to learn how a change in job may prevent a second myocardial infarction if it seems likely to lead to short-term financial difficulties.

Cultural factors

Cultural factors may prevent an individual from being motivated to acquire increased independence. For example, a mother may say that her son suffering from epilepsy need not learn how to use a school bus because she drives him to school. The mother may be over-protective and dread her son having a fit in public, as epilepsy is seen in her culture to be a 'mental illness'. The nurse will have to encourage the mother to learn and understand the true nature of epilepsy before attempting to teach the son greater independence.

The patient's right to choose

The influencing factors that promote or inhibit patients' learning have been discussed (see also Activity 18.1), but it should also be borne in mind that learning new lifestyles and health behaviours can have negative outcomes for individuals as well as positive ones. If patients are perceived as individuals who have a right to decline health care and choose the way in which they cope with disability or illness, the nurse should not feel guilty if her intervention is declined. It may be necessary for the patient and nurse to agree not to proceed with a teaching programme. A psychiatric nurse's perception on the patient's education may also be useful to consider at this stage.

Peplau (1968) acknowledges that the nurse has an important role in educating the patient with a view to facilitating development and growth, but reminds nurses that, ultimately, only the patient can change himself. This viewpoint is supported by Orem (1985), who recognises that it is difficult to teach a patient if he lacks the motivation to learn new knowledge or skills.

Overcoming patient difficulties

Although patients must be given the right to refuse interventions, the nurse needs to be able to recognise the difference between the person

Activity 18.1

Identify two factors that you would consider in order to optimise learning when planning a teaching programme for:

- a patient in his own home
- a group of 20 adolescents in a school
- a patient in an institutional setting.

who has made an informed choice to refuse help and the one who needs additional assistance to overcome difficulties in order to learn. Whilst illness and hospitalisation are extremely stressful and anxiety-provoking (Wilson-Barnett 1986), there are ways of assisting patients to overcome anxiety and stress. Relaxation therapy and the provision of specific information are common methods used. Case Examples 18.1 and 18.2 illustrate how two patients who needed to be taught to change colostomy bags required different educational approaches (see also Activity 18.2).

Case example 18.1

Mrs Smith, aged 46, had recently had a hemicolectomy and formation of temporary colostomy. She told the nurse that she did not want to learn to change her colostomy bag because the district nurse could come and do it on a daily basis until an operation to close the stoma was performed.

Following discussion, the nurse identified that Mrs Smith was highly anxious, not only about the colostomy, but also about life in general. Mrs Smith agreed to try learning a relaxation technique, because she thought this might help her in everyday life, particularly as a friend had found yoga helpful.

The nurse used a relaxation audiotape because Mrs Smith identified that she learned well through music and hearing. Over a period of 3 days, Mrs Smith learned to relax by lying in a comfortable position, breathing in time to the tape and imagining herself in a garden full of spring flowers (the latter visualisation being her response to the tapes suggestion to 'imagine you are in an environment that you would find relaxing'). Subsequently, Mrs Smith stated that she would be willing to try to change her colostomy bag immediately after a period of relaxation therapy. She acknowledged that it would be more convenient to be able to do it herself than have to rely on the district nurse.

Case example 18.2

Mr Wilson, aged 35, was in exactly the same situation as Mrs Smith (Case example 18.1). He, too, expressed the opinion that there was no point in learning how to change his colostomy bag as it was only temporary and the district nurse could do it for him. On further questioning, the nurse established that Mr Wilson was really worried about one specific point. He wanted to know what would happen if his bowels moved when he was in the process of a bag change, as he feared making a terrible mess.

At this stage, the nurse responded by giving specific information, about both the likelihood of this happening and how to cope if it did, including the idea of always having a large square of cotton wool available when changing the bag. In this way, the nurse took the occasion to discuss what was important to the patient – an opportunity often missed (Macleod Clark 1983). She gave information that provided reassurance about the limits of the threat, correcting the patient's distortion of the magnitude of the problem. This kind of intervention, Ray (1982) believes, assists in helping patients to cope, because it gives an 'illusion of control' by providing a realistic perspective on the threatened event, while enabling the patient to think through how he would act if the event occurred.

Following this very practical information-giving session, Mr Wilson agreed 'to have a go' at changing his bag, as long as the nurse stayed with him throughout the process.

LEARNING STYLES

It is well recognised that individuals have different learning styles, and that in most instances students are able accurately to predict the method that will best help them learn (de Tornyay & Thompson 1982).

There are four main learning modes, and, for many individuals, learning is enhanced by using a combination of two or more of these.

The four learning modes

1. *Seeing*. This mode concentrates on visual representation and pictorial materials. Videos, television, posters, cartoons, photographs and flow charts can be powerful tools in assisting people to assimilate knowledge if their identified learning mode is 'seeing'.

Activity 18.2

List three methods for teaching stress reduction to individual patients.

2. *Reading* involves using printed materials such as charts, pamphlets, handouts and textbooks.

3. *Listening*. The person whose learning mode is identified as 'listening' will respond best to the spoken word, the most common examples being the use of one-to-one verbal teaching sessions or the group lecture/seminar.

4. *Manipulating*. Many individuals find the 'manipulation' mode of learning constructive, particularly when being taught a manual skill. This mode would involve a person in practising with real or simulated items or preparing their own 'package' on a particular subject.

To take a simple example, the nurse who is skilled at injection administration but has never given an oil-based, slow-release major tranquilliser may be told that extra pressure will be needed in order to give the substance efficiently, in comparison to less viscous fluids. More significant learning may occur, however, when she actually experiences administrating the fluid.

Some individuals assimilate information most quickly through the manipulation mode, and this may be facilitated by providing self-directed learning materials such as workbooks and computer-aided learning packages, which allow the user to work out answers for himself and check these against model answers.

The role of the nurse

An important role of the nurse is to identify with the patient the methods of learning he prefers and then to use appropriate tools for teaching. In this way, the nurse is most likely to assist the patient in reaching stated objectives of learning.

TEACHING

CONSIDERATIONS IN PLANNING

There are four important questions to consider when planning any teaching:

1. What is the aim of the teaching in terms of participant outcome?
2. How much time will be available?
3. How many people will be in the group to be taught?
4. What technology is available for use in the teaching session?

Aims

The aims determined will be those of the patient and the structure of the nursing process will be used to formulate the patient's expected outcomes (McFarlane & Castledine 1982). Sometimes it will be necessary to write down goals for a patient's relative or friend. The nurse may also wish to record clear goals to be achieved by nursing students or health care assistants through clinical teaching.

Time

Once the nurse has decided the objectives to be achieved by the patient as a result of instruction, it is important to relate these to the time available. If time is short, it may be necessary to reduce the number of objectives in any given session in order that the patient has sufficient time to master them. In addition, it is vital to break down large items, such as teaching a patient who has had an arm amputated how to dress unaided, into small, readily achievable objectives, so that he is able to measure his progress and maintain sufficient motivation to work towards the long-term goal (McFarlane & Castledine 1982). It may be helpful in teaching those who learn through the 'seeing' mode to consider the graph in Figure 18.3.

The time axis in Figure 18.3 extends only to 60 minutes because research demonstrates that few

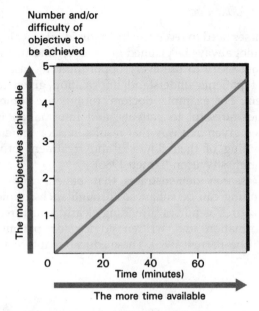

Figure 18.3 The relationship between the time available to teach and the number of objectives that can be met.

individuals can concentrate for any longer than an hour in an educational environment, whilst most people will be ready for a break after 40 minutes, with attention reducing after 20 minutes, particularly if the mode of delivery is a formal lecture (Bligh 1972). Generally speaking, the more difficult the objective to be achieved, the less information one should expect to be absorbed in any session or series of sessions.

Size of group

Teaching can be conducted both on an individual basis and in groups. The nature of the topic to be taught will often guide the nurse in her selection of approach; for example, when teaching a patient how to fit an artificial limb, the group method would be unacceptable in terms of patient privacy and dignity. Conversely, when teaching exercise skills in a cardiac rehabilitation programme, the encouragement and support from other group members can be an important factor in motivating individuals (Howard & Erlanger 1983).

Individual teaching

Nurses need to recognise that individual teaching cannot always be planned in advance, and that it is necessary to use every opportunity to ensure that patients understand information given to them. For example, doctors' rounds are sometimes stressful to patients, and information is often given in a way that results in poor understanding of their illnesses and treatment programmes (Wilson-Barnett 1986).

Research demonstrates that patient understanding can be enhanced through such simple measures as nurses providing clearly structured information and written advice for patients (Wilson-Barnett 1986). These educative interventions can be conducted in any nursing environment, from the anaesthetic room to the patient's own home, to support the information provided by the doctor.

Technology

When planning any teaching, the nurse must identify the equipment available to assist in the task and use it appropriately in relation to the size of the group (Fig. 18.4).

A session should always be rehearsed prior to its first delivery to check that the content fits the time available and to test audiovisual aids for clarity and accuracy.

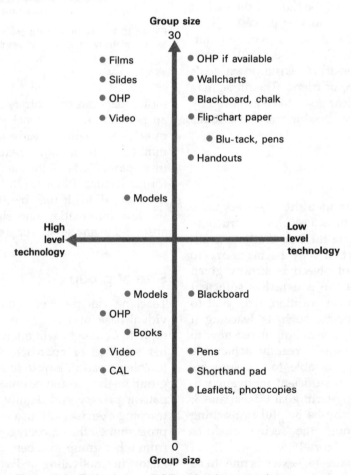

Figure 18.4   Technology availability related to group size.

Audiovisual aids

Once these are selected, it is important that any necessary planning and preparation is done. For example, videotapes borrowed from drug companies will have to be ordered at least 2 weeks in advance.

Simple tools

Explaining the nature of an operation to a single patient in a ward may require only a shorthand notebook and two coloured pens, making preparation time short. These simple tools will enable the nurse to draw a diagram, or write pertinent phrases to illustrate main points. The page can then be torn off and given to the patient for reference.

The overhead projector (OHP)

The OHP is a popular medium for teaching groups, and many hospital wards and health centres own their own. Portable machines are also available. When preparing slides for use on the projector, it is important to produce sufficiently large letters or diagrams and to use only two or three colours: a multicolour approach can be distracting.

IMPARTING KNOWLEDGE

Knowledge is associated with the cognitive domain and involves the learner in using his intellectual ability to recall and remember information (Redman 1984).

Assessing existing knowledge

The nurse planning to teach a patient or group about a specific subject should organise the session in such a way that she first discovers the extent of the target group's knowledge of the topic. It is then possible to build on that knowledge and to correct misinformation. Pertinent points should be made particularly clear; this may involve explaining in detail or extrapolating specific information from a handout or video.

Language level

It is necessary to communicate with individuals in a language that they understand, using terminology that is appropriate to their level of understanding. This must also be considered when conducting health education programmes on a larger scale.

There is a cautionary tale concerning an occasion when this did not occur. In 1987, a leaflet designed to tell people about HIV and AIDS was delivered to each household in Great Britain. The leaflet, printed in English, had an iceberg on the front and the initials A, I, D, S in capital letters. It is reported that at least one elderly man, whose first language was Welsh, took the leaflet to his local Post Office to claim his heating allowance.

Feedback

At the end of the session, the nurse can question the group to receive feedback on the learning that has taken place. It is then still possible to repeat information and/or to correct misunderstanding.

Repetition

Patient anxiety will often hamper learning; this can be overcome to some extent by imparting small pieces of information at any one time and not overloading the receiver. People forget information over time, but repetition at regular intervals may help overcome this.

TEACHING A PRACTICAL SKILL

A skill has been defined as 'a learned ability to bring about a predetermined result with maximum certainty and minimum time and effort' (Fitts & Posner 1967). Acquiring a practical skill involves more than physical actions. The reason for applying the skill, together with knowledge of potential problems and hazards, are essential. The acquisition of a skill generally follows a smooth curve when plotted against time and the number of trials (Quinn 1988); the more frequently a skill is practised, the more proficient individuals become. These principles are the same whether the skill is taught to a student nurse or to a patient.

Preparation

Three steps are involved in the process of skills teaching preparation:

- formulating objectives
- conducting skills analysis
- assessing the existing level of knowledge or skill.

Formulating objectives

Predetermined objectives, if over-prescriptive, may restrict the scope of teaching, but educational theory still favours the setting of broad learning and teaching objectives, providing the teacher appreciates that unintended objectives sometimes occur (Redman 1984). The learning of unintended objectives can be both good and bad: good, in that the learner may acquire knowledge and/or skills in addition to what was anticipated, and bad, in that a negative, unintended outcome may be learnt. For example, if the teacher provides inadequate explanation regarding the reasons for conducting a skill in a certain manner, the student may assume that she can achieve the same end without going through all the steps. If the skill of changing a catheter bag was taught without explaining the need for cleanliness, the learner might believe it was quicker to conduct without handwashing, thus acquiring an 'unintended learning objective'.

Objectives assist in directing teaching – especially if they are expressed by means of verbs that describe the expected student outcome. Examples of useful words to consider when formulating objectives include: 'identify', 'list', 'recall', 'recognise', 'state', 'describe' and 'demonstrate', as these verbs are unambiguous and give clear direction to the task (Redman 1984).

Once the main objectives in the teaching of a skill have been identified, an analysis of the skill needs to be conducted.

Skills analysis

Conducting a skills analysis involves identifying the steps and sequences used in performing the skills. Examples of breaking down a skill in this way are given in 'Clinical practice: two examples'.

Assessing existing abilities

Once the steps involved in the skill are identified, it is necessary to establish whether the learner can already perform any part of the skill competently. This will preclude unnecessary teaching and allow the existing skills of the learner to be used to best effect.

The teaching session

Explaining underlying principles

There is a danger in teaching people a practical skill without conveying the underlying knowledge relevant to the behaviour. The patient may be unable to *adapt* the skill if he does not know the essential principles involved, as when the technique of cleansing and dressing wounds, but not the principles of asepsis, is taught to a patient.

Demonstration

The skill should initially be demonstrated at normal speed so that the patient can identify the 'finished product'. The following steps should be taken to facilitate the learning process:

1. Write down the sequence of the parts of the skills to act as a checklist for the patient. (Skills analysis will be useful at this stage.)
2. Demonstrate the skill slowly, step by step.
3. Using feedback, verify the patient's understanding and clarify as necessary.

Practice

Following the demonstration, it is essential provide a period of supervised practice as soon as possible. Adequate time must be made available for all patients to become proficient at the skill. Because individuals learn at different speeds, allowances should be made for this at the planning stage.

The nurse needs to provide a psychologically safe environment for learning, so that embarrassment is not caused when mistakes are made. Encouraging and motivating the patient using verbal rather than physical guidance is preferred, as the latter can cause confusion (Quinn 1988). Physical guidance may sometimes be necessary when teaching skills to children or to people with learning difficulties. Complex skills are best taught and practised as a whole, while less complex skills can be practised part by part more successfully.

Once the patient can perform the skill without hesitation, it is essential to continue to reinforce it by intermittent repetition, otherwise the ease with which the skill is performed will decrease over time (Redman 1984).

Activity 18.3

Describe the four learning modes and list three types of teaching that may promote learning in each mode.

CLINICAL PRACTICE: TWO EXAMPLES

This section outlines examples of the nurse acting as educator in clinical practice. Nurse teachers who are closely involved with the relevant clinical specialities described have contributed these studies, which clearly illustrate the diversity of approaches required to meet individual patients' needs. The first example involves teaching a skill to a child and parent, the second involves teaching a skill to an adult who has a learning difficulty.

TEACHING SELF-ADMINISTRATION OF INSULIN TO A CHILD WITH DIABETES

Diabetes mellitus is a serious disease, especially in children, and requires lifelong management. It may take several weeks for the family to accept the implications of the diagnosis and to learn the techniques necessary to maintain stable glucose levels. It is generally accepted that the best person for the daily management of diabetes is the patient, and the nurse may decide to use the 'self-care' model of nursing to teach the child how best to manage his condition. A child's age and stage of development will dictate the degree of his dependency on his parents.

The self-care model of nursing described by Orem (1985) is based on the premise that people are usually self-reliant, responsible individuals capable of meeting their own self-care needs and willing to take responsibility for their dependants. In some instances, patients or their relatives may lack the necessary skill or knowledge to meet their health care needs. In such cases, Orem (1985) suggests, nursing intervention should aim to extend the patient's ability using one or more of the following methods:

- acting for or doing for the patient
- guiding the patient
- supporting him physically or psychologically
- teaching him
- providing an environment that promotes the learning of new skills.

Assessing readiness to learn

The nurse must be able to assess the readiness of the child and his parents to learn. She must then decide, on an individual basis, who in the family unit will be primarily responsible for managing the disease.

The child's ability to perform self-care will be influenced by his physical development and psychological state, while the parents' ability will be influenced by psychological, sociocultural and educational factors. Parents and child will be more motivated to learn the skill of injection administration once they understand the nature of diabetes.

Understanding the disease

The nurse will teach the child and his family about the nature of diabetes and how stability can be maintained. Teaching must be at a level that is understandable to the family, and the environment must provide sufficient psychological support to make learning effective. The nurse may use audiovisual aids to assist in the educational process; these might include explanatory leaflets produced by the British Diabetic Association, some of which are specifically designed for children.

Learning the skill of injecting

When the family understand the nature of diabetes and the action of insulin, and appreciate the need for accuracy when drawing up the dosage, they can proceed to learning the specific skill of injection.

Diabetic children require at least one and frequently two injections every day, making it essential for the parents and child to learn the task. Parents are often more anxious than is the child, and much patience and reassurance is required. Every encouragement should be given for the child to administer his own insulin. Where the child does not self-administer the injection, his involvement in drawing up the insulin should be encouraged.

Equipment such as injector guns and pen injectors can be used to assist in the self-administration of insulin by children.

Using multidose pen injectors the child primes the injector, dials the dose of insulin required and by pushing the button the correct dose of insulin is administered. Some children use pen injectors while at school and use the standard syringe and needle under parental supervision at home (Swift 1995).

Even when these alternative devices are to be used the child and parent are usually taught the syringe and needle method initially to ensure they are competent using the standard equipment.

Teaching the skill

All the necessary equipment should first be assembled: insulin syringe/needle, insulin bottle, cotton wool and alcohol.

The task can be divided into two major parts:

- drawing up the insulin into the syringe
- injecting the insulin (Boxes 18.3 and 18.4).

Involving the child

The first injection can be traumatic for both the child and the parents. The degree of involvement of the child may vary, and it may take a

---

Box 18.3 Drawing up insulin

1. Wash and dry the hands.
2. Check the label on the insulin bottle for strength and expiry date.
3. Wipe the top of the bottle with cotton wool soaked in some alcohol.
4. Remove the sheath and draw into the syringe approximately the same volume of air as insulin dose required. This prevents a vacuum developing in the bottle.
5. Insert the needle through the rubber cap of the bottle and inject in the air.
6. Invert the bottle and ensure the needle is well below the surface.
7. Maintain this position and, with the needle vertical, withdraw the plunger, allowing insulin to flow into the barrel. Continue until there is slightly more insulin than is required.
8. Tap the syringe barrel to help air bubbles to rise and collect at the top.
9. Depress the plunger to inject back any air, and adjust the plunger again to measure the correct dose.
10. Withdraw the needle from the bottle and replace the needle sheath.

Box 18.4 Safely injecting a child with insulin

1. The child should be correctly seated, comfortable and within easy reach of the equipment.
2. Select and expose the injection site.
3. Hold the syringe firmly, like a dart or a pencil.
4. With the thumb and forefinger of the other hand, pinch up a fold of skin.
5. Quickly insert the needle at 90° into the side of the skin fold to a depth of 1 cm.
6. Hold the syringe with one hand, and use the thumb to depress the plunger gently, injecting all the contents.
7. Slowly withdraw the needle, stretching the skin as the needle comes out to prevent leakage of insulin.
8. Dispose of and/or safely store the equipment.

little time for him to be able to insert the needle through his skin. In the early stages, the child should be encouraged to do what he feels able to do. The nurse needs to avoid rushing the child, but must be aware that progressing too slowly can allow fears to develop.

Teaching the child and his parents the skill of administering insulin follows the theory of teaching any skill described by Fitts & Posner (1967). The nurse should demonstrate the complete skill at the normal speed, and then the skill should be broken down into chains of stimulus–response units. The parent or child should then perform some or all of the steps under supervision as the nurse gives praise and guidance. As confidence develops, parents and child will perform more, and eventually all, of the steps involved. Speed and agility will increase and the need for prompting will disappear. At this stage, the parents and/or child will be able to perform the task unaided.

TEACHING A SKILL TO A PERSON WITH SEVERE LEARNING DIFFICULTIES

Roger Jones, aged 24, lives in a residential home with two other people who, like himself, have severe learning difficulties. Mr Jones is currently unemployed and is in receipt of benefits. He attends a local work training centre, and it is hoped that this will eventually help him find paid employment.

Aim

As an individual with learning difficulties, Mr Jones belongs to a group of people who are socially devalued, but as he acquires new skills, his competence will be enhanced. Since society values people who are competent, the more skills Mr Jones learns, the more he will be seen by others (and himself) as a valued person, and be able to integrate and participate in the life of the community (O'Brien 1986).

The process of 'social role valorisation', previously known as 'normalisation' (Wolfensberger & Glenn 1986), is an accepted method by which Mr Jones may be assisted to attain valued social roles.

In addition, a structure will be required within this framework to explore Mr Jones' real needs as an individual; these may be wider than learning how to perform isolated skills.

Shared action planning

Shared action planning is a suitable strategy for this purpose. It takes as its starting point the idea that any plans for Mr Jones' future belong to him, and that he will share these (if he wishes) with those who work with him. The immediate person with whom Mr Jones might like to share planning for the future would probably be someone who has a close relationship with him, in this care, his 'keyworker'. This relationship between Mr Jones and his keyworker is at the heart of the process; developing such a relationship is, therefore, the first essential step.

Once a relationship based on mutual trust and respect has been established, Mr Jones and his keyworker can begin to assess some of the areas that Mr Jones would like to develop.

The Bereweeke skill teaching system for adults

The nurse may find that the Bereweeke system (Felce et al 1986) provides a useful guide for assessment and for planning skills teaching. The assessment package within this system looks at 'component skills', 'self-care and household skills', 'language skills', 'socialisation skills' and 'number skills', whilst the teaching system provides a method for planning teaching for individuals with learning difficulties. The following example illustrates how this package can be used.

Assessment

Mr Jones and his keyworker have agreed to assess his self-care skills. They go about this by setting tasks for Mr Jones to perform and then identifying what, if any, degree of help he requires successfully to accomplish them. This task analysis is used, for example, to assess Mr Jones' ability in putting on his coat before going out. Mr Jones puts his left arm through the left sleeve, his right arm through the right sleeve, and successfully adjusts the coat on his shoulders. He fails, however, to button the coat. The keyworker reminds Mr Jones to fasten his buttons. What happens next will depend on Mr Jones' response. If he fastens the buttons correctly, he will have completed the task of putting on his coat successfully. An immediate 'Well done!' will act as a social reinforcer, raising Mr Jones' self-esteem and motivating him to do it again.

If, however, Mr Jones does not fasten his buttons on request, the keyworker repeats the instruction (verbal prompt). If this fails to elicit a response, the keyworker immediately shows Mr Jones what to do, by pointing at the button and buttonhole and repeating the request (verbal prompt and gestural prompt). If, again, this fails to elicit the correct response, the keyworker immediately takes Mr Jones hands and physically helps him to fasten his buttons. This must always be followed by strong social reinforcement, such as by saying 'Well done!' on completion.

The keyworker here goes through a set sequence:

1. Initial request (prompt).
2. Verbal prompt.
3. Gestural prompt.
4. Physical prompt.

In this case, the written assessment would state: 'Mr Jones can put on his coat but needs a physical prompt to fasten his buttons.'

Activity 18.4

Conduct a skills analysis of a task that you may have to teach to another person.

Establishing priorities

Once a number of Mr Jones's skills have been assessed, a discussion should take place between Mr Jones, the keyworker and his supervisor to determine which skills are priorities for teaching. There are numerous criteria for deciding this, but one very useful approach is to ask the question 'Of the skills Mr Jones needs to learn, which ones will provide him with the greatest opportunities for fuller integration and participation in the life of the community, such that further learning opportunities become available?'

It may be decided that, in order to enable Mr Jones to achieve his personally defined goal of going out more in the evening, being able to put his coat on unaided would be a valuable step. Assuming that everyone involved agrees, this aim will become part of the shared action plan that is concerned with his skill teaching. The keyworker should inform other health care workers of the programme, to ensure that continuity of care is achieved. Each time Mr Jones needs to put on his coat, the person working with him will go through the sequence of initial request, verbal prompt, gestural prompt and physical prompt.

As Mr Jones becomes more competent, he will no longer need the physical prompt. (Three consecutive successful attempts are usually enough to indicate a skill has been mastered.) It will then be recorded that 'Mr Jones can put his coat on but needs a gestural prompt to fasten his buttons.'

The teaching programme will continue, gradually reducing the prompts, until Mr Jones no longer needs to be reminded about fastening his buttons, but fastens them automatically. Success would be measured by a noticeable increase in Mr Jones' independence and competence, highlighted through thorough record-keeping.

This teaching method is based on simple behavioural techniques. People working with individuals with learning difficulties can acquire those techniques through such training materials as 'Skills Teaching Education Programme Planning' (Chamberlain et al 1985).

Mr Jones, as he learns how to put on his coat independently, is treated as a valued person by being invited to set his own goals and being helped to achieve them through 'shared action planning'. These are valued means to the valued ends of seeing himself, and being seen by others, as more competent. This is but one facet of the process of achieving a valued social role.

EFFECTIVENESS OF THE NURSE AS EDUCATOR

There is increasing interest in measuring the effectiveness of the nurse's role as educator in terms of patient outcomes. This is very exciting, for it is by measuring the outcome of nursing interventions that useful theory will develop to guide practitioners in selecting the most appropriate actions for given situations (Bloch 1975). A sample of recently reported projects is presented here to illustrate developments in the field of patient teaching with respect to the two areas of:

- patient compliance with treatment
- patient skills teaching.

These topics relate to all spheres of nursing practice in both hospital and community settings, although the examples referred to have been examined in only one particular branch of nursing.

PATIENT COMPLIANCE WITH TREATMENT

It has been demonstrated that a relationship exists between the degree of the patient's understanding of his particular disease and treatment and his compliance with treatment regimens (Council of Europe 1980, Brearley 1990).

Compliance with prescribed medication is often erratic but research demonstrates that, when they are given the following written information, patients show improved adherence (Goldberg 1980):

- Name of drugs.
- Purpose of medication.
- Dosage schedule.
- Side-effects.
- Special considerations.
- When to notify doctors.
- Summary.

A written plan

Some patients may find it helpful to have a simple plan outlining the medication regimen expected; a particularly clear one, which includes the use of symbols for patients who cannot read, has been developed by Gooch (1990).

Following any illness, it is sometimes necessary to restrict activities, and patients report a preference for being given precise information rather than vague suggestions regarding what they can and cannot do (Wilson-Barnett 1981). The nurse might usefully provide a list of activities a patient can expect to perform during the first week of returning home following an operation, for example a hernia repair. The list should then be extended, specifically stating when other activities may be resumed. Following a caesarian section, the author was told by the physiotherapist not to lift anything heavier than her baby for 3 months. This information was sufficiently simple to remember, but written guidance was also welcomed with respect to post-natal exercises. To encourage compliance with treatment programmes, nurses need to know their individual patients well so that they can decide what information can be given verbally and what should be written down.

Psychiatric patients

While the principles of providing written information, together with one-to-one and group teaching, are reported to improve adherence to treatment regimens, problems can and do arise with both the unmotivated and the psychiatrically ill patient (Council of Europe 1980).

Miller (1983) reports that while psychiatric nurses perceive teaching as an integral part of their role, it is often conducted on an informal level, rather than being made explicit. Miller's sample was small but representative, in that nurses working in long-term mental hospitals, the community and general hospital psychiatric units were included.

Although integration of teaching into many nursing actions is essential, problems may occur when teaching is not made explicit to the recipient. People suffering from psychiatric illness may require clear guidelines regarding medication, the reduction of stress or ways of recognising relapse. If nurses make the teaching of these issues explicit by defining outcomes and checking the extent of patients' learning outcomes, in terms of patient compliance and self-care, may improve.

Pollock's (1989) recent study of community psychiatric nurses indicates that, owing to 'labelling', nurses are still encouraging dependence in psychiatric patients, rather than promoting independence by educating them about their disease. Pollock believes that one way to remedy this situation would be to teach community psychiatric nurses to use a behavioural model of care.

It is important to stress that this deficit in effective teaching is not restricted to psychiatric nurses. Macleod Clard (1983) reports that general nurses frequently miss opportunities for one-to-one education. However, general nursing has historically been more task-orientated than has been the case in mental health nursing, which perhaps explains the latter's informal approach to teaching patients about their illnesses and treatments.

PATIENT SKILLS TEACHING: CURRENT DEVELOPMENTS

A major part of this chapter has been devoted to demonstrating well-researched methods by which nurses can teach patients skills. It is important to recognise that, increasingly, skills that were regarded solely as the province of the nurse are now being taught to patients and their families.

Self-care

An example of such a skill is intermittent self-catheterisation, which helps to prevent long-term complications associated with chronic retention (McSweeney 1990). Competent patients can self-catheterise in their own homes as and when necessary, without needing to contact a professional for assistance.

Activity 18.5

Plan a teaching programme for a group of eight patients in a particular age group who are at risk of developing a named health-related problem.

Care by parent

A 'care by parent' scheme for children in hospital involved parents passing nasogastric tubes and conducting chest percussion and postural drainage, all skills taught by nurses (Clearly 1989). The children in the project spent less time alone than did the average child in hospital, received care from familiar people and cried less than others, demonstrating a positive patient outcome.

The vast majority of the carers reported that if their child were readmitted, they would wish to be involved again, although one single mother felt the responsibility should be with the nurse.

Individual preference

Not all patients will feel able to become such active partners in their own care, and personal preference should be assessed on an individual basis. Brearley (1990) believes that factors such as 'disease severity, available social support and age' affect individual preference in this area.

Towards patient-led health care

This brief discussion has demonstrated that the nurse's role as educator can help to improve patient outcomes. The next logical step would be to involve patients in the critical evaluation of the effectiveness of the health care professional (Brownlea 1987). When this occurs, the stage will be set for a consumer-led health service to emerge.

Summary

The process of nursing, which involves assessing, planning, implementing and evaluating the outcomes of individualised care in a participatory relationship with patients (see Ch. 14) is closely aligned with the process of adult education.

In some instances, patient education may be more powerful in groups than on a one-to-one basis, given the positive effects of peer pressure on learning. The nurse's role in education is made much easier when patients are motivated to learn. Sometimes nurses will have to assist individuals in moving towards a state of readiness to learn when this is being obstructed by pain, anxiety or depression. All teaching conducted by nurses should be evaluated by means of patient feedback, which enables the nurse not only to deduce what has been learned and to observe resultant changes in behaviour, but also to correct any misunderstandings promptly.

REFERENCES

Bligh D 1972 What's the use of lectures? Penguin, Harmondsworth

Bloch D 1975 Evaluation of nursing care in terms of process and outcome: issues in research and quality assurance. Nursing Research 24(4): 256–263

Brearley S 1990 Patient participation: the literature. Scutari Press, London

Brownlea A 1987 Participation: myths, realities and prognosis. Social Science and Medicine 25(6): 605–614

Chamberlain P, Eysenk A, Hill P, Wallis J 1985 Skills teaching education programme planning. British Association for Behavioural Psychotherapy. STEP Publications, Southsea

Clearly J 1989 The care-by-parent scheme: an innovation in the hospital care of child patients. In: Seedhouse D, Crigg A (eds) Changing ideas in health care. John Wiley, Chichester, pp 77–98

Council of Europe: European Public Health Committee 1980 The patient as an active participant in his own treatment: final report. Council of Europe, Strasbourg

Department of Health (1989) UK Statutory Instrument. Nurses, midwives and health visitors approval. Order No. 1456 Amendment 2. HMSO, London

de Tornyay R, Thompson M A 1982 Strategies for teaching nurse education. John Wiley, New York

Felce D, Jenkins J, De Kock U, Mansell J 1986 The Bereweeke Skill Teaching System for Adults. NFER, Nelson

Fitts P, Posner M 1967 Human performance. Prentice-Hall, New Jersey

Goldberg S 1980 Doing it yourself: a guide to writing patient literature. Nursing Administration Quarterly 4(2): 30–33

Gooch J 1990 Medication to take home. In: Professional nurse: patient education plus. Austen Cornish, London pp 106–107

Henderson V 1960 Basic principles of nursing care. International Council of Nurses, Geneva

Howard J, Erlanger H 1983 Teaching methods for coronary patients. In: Wilson-Barnett J (ed.) Patient teaching. Churchill Livingstone, Edinburgh, p 56–80

McFarlane J, Castledine G 1982 A guide to the practice of nursing using the nursing process. Mosby, London

Macleod Clark J 1983 Nurse–patient communication: an analysis of conversations from surgical wards. In: Wilson-Barnett J (ed.) Nursing research: studies in patient care. John Wiley, Chichester, pp 25–26

McSweeney P 1990 Self-catheterisation. In: Professional nurse: patient education plus. Austen Cornish, London, pp 91–93

Miller G E 1983 Teaching psychiatric patients. In: Wilson-Barnett J (ed.) Patient teaching. Churchill Livingstone, Edinburgh, pp 129–152

O'Brien J 1986 A guide to personal futures planning. In: Bellamy Q T, Wilcox B (eds) A comprehensive guide to the activities catalogue on alternative curriculum for youth and adults with severe disabilities. Paul H Brookes, Baltimore

Orem D E 1985 Nursing: concepts of practice, 3rd edn. McGraw-Hill, New York

Peplau H E 1968 Psychotherapeutic strategies. Perspectives in Psychiatric Care 6(6): 264–289

Pollock L C 1989 Community psychiatric nursing: myths and reality. Scutari Press, London

Quinn F M 1988 The principles and practice of nurse education. Croom Helm, London

Ray C 1982 The surgical patient: psychological stress and coping resources. In: Eisser J R (ed.) Social psychology and behavioural medicine. John Wiley, Chichester, pp 483–507

Redman B K 1984 The process of patient education. C V Mosby, St Louis

Swift P G 1995 Insulin: types and regimens. In: Kelnar C (ed.) Childhood and adolescent diabetes. Chapman and Hall, London, Ch. 17

Wilson-Barnett J 1981 Looking down the road to recovery. Nursing Mirror (May 27): 30–33

Wilson-Barnett J 1986 Reducing stress in hospital. In: Tierney A J (ed.) Clinical nursing practice. Churchill Livingstone, Edinburgh, pp 1–20

Wolfensberger W, Glenn L 1986 Programme analysis of service systems: a method for the quantitative evaluation of human services. NIMR, Toronto

World Health Organization 1985 Health for All. WHO, Geneva

FURTHER READING

Beck A T, Emery G 1985 Anxiety disorders and phobias: a cognitive perspective. Basic Books, New York

Coutts L, Hardy L 1985 Teaching for health. Churchill Livingstone, Edinburgh

Jacobsen E 1933 Progressive relaxation. University of Chicago Press, Chicago

Lang P J 1969 The mechanics of desensitization and the

laboratory study of fear. In: Franks C M (ed.) Behaviour therapy: appraisal and status. McGraw-Hill, New York

Mahoney M J 1980 Abnormal psychology: perspectives on human variance. Harper & Row, San Francisco

Marks I M 1978 Living with fear. McGraw-Hill, New York

Marks I M 1981 Cure and care of neuroses: theory and practice of behavioural psychotherapy. John Wiley, Chichester

Meichenbaum D, Cameron R 1983 Stress innoculation training: towards a general paradigm for training coping skills. In: Meichenbaum D, Jaremko M (eds) Stress reduction and prevention. Plenum, New York

Norton C 1986 Nursing for continence. Beaconsfield, Beaconsfield, Bucks

Powell T J, Enright S J 1990 Anxiety and stress management. Routledge, London

Richards D, McDonald R 1990 Behavioural psychotherapy: a handbook for nurses. Heinemann, Oxford

Rogers J 1977 Adult learning, 2nd edn. Open University Press, Milton Keynes

Salkovskis P M 1988 Hyperventilation and anxiety. Current Opinion in Psychiatry 1: 76–82

Watts N 1990 Handbook of clinical teaching. Churchill Livingstone, Edinburgh

19

Care of the dying and bereaved

Eva Garland   Gillian Pharaoh   Alison Barnes

At some point in her career, the nurse will be faced with the prospect of dealing with a dying person, his relatives and friends. To enable her to give the best possible care and deal with her own reactions, this chapter aims to:

- provide an understanding of the development of attitudes towards, and care of, the dying
- explore the emotions encountered in adjusting to the prospect of one's own or another's death
- consider the physical, emotional and spiritual needs of the dying person
- examine the concepts of, and feelings involved in, bereavement, loss and grief
- draw attention to the stress produced by nursing the dying.

INTRODUCTION

The process of dying is part of living, and nurses can help the dying person only if they are willing to get involved in the situation as it happens. Each individual's journey to death is a very personal and intimate experience. It is affected by a whole range of different issues, cultural and religious, as well as by the environment and family structure in which the individual exists. It is important to remember that peoples' previous experience of death will often colour their own expectations. If they have seen somebody suffering a painful death, they themselves will probably expect the same.

During the time surrounding death, the nurse should be able to provide skilled support to meet the emotional, spiritual and physical needs of the dying person, the family and other members of their social group. The smallest things may assume great significance, and meticulous attention to minute detail is essential. There should also be recognition of, and support to meet, the needs of colleagues who are involved in caring for the dying.

Not all death is expected or timely. The families and loved ones of those who have died suddenly (e.g. stillborn and cot-death babies, suicides and victims of trauma or myocardial infarction) require special consideration. Nurses must develop the resources to comfort the bereaved, bear the sorrow of grieving and help people to face death with dignity.

Above all, the aim should be to develop mutual understanding between the patient, the relatives and professionals, so that fear and anxiety disappear.

Causes of death

Life expectancy in the UK has increased over the twentieth century, in common with most other advanced industrial societies. In 1991, life expectancy for men was 73.2 years and for women 78.2 years. These changes can be attributed to improvements in standards of living, primarily through hygiene and nutrition.

Such improvements have led to changes in the nature and pattern of disease. Acute diseases now rarely have fatal outcomes, and the primary causes of death are chronic degenerative diseases of the respiratory and circulatory systems. This has caused an increase in the average age of death to beyond retirement age, when people

Table 19.1	The main causes of death in England and Wales in 1993 (OPCS data)		
		Male (%)	Female (%)
Diseases of the circulatory system		44	45
Malignant neoplasm		27	22
Diseases of the respiratory system		15	16
Injury and poisoning		3	2
Remainder		11	15

have fulfilled their parental responsibilities, so the social impact of death has lessened.

Advances in medical knowledge and medical technology have, for the most part, been to the advantage of the health care of patients. Today, relieving the suffering and saving the lives of the critically ill is often feasible. For example, premature babies or those born with serious disabilities, who would in the past have died at birth, are now being 'saved' in special care baby units. Table 19.1 gives details of the main causes of death in England and Wales.

HISTORY OF CARE OF THE DYING

In any society, *where* death takes place and *how* it is handled reflects societal values and priorities. Changes in the typical place of death over the twentieth century reflect broader social movements, whether death takes place in an institution or in the home, demonstrating the changing family and occupational structures, and increased geographical and social mobility.

The history of the care of the dying is diverse. The professions of medicine and nursing have traditionally regarded death as failure, but the evolution of the modern hospice movement since 1970, as well as major changes in the NHS, has contributed to a change in the perception of care provided for dying people. Hospices have, however, been in existence for many centuries; records show that, as far back as the 4th century, Christians were welcomed on their journeys to holy sites in 'hospices'. This name was used for premises where care was available for those who became sick whilst on a pilgrimage. The name 'hospice' referring to a place that specialised in services for the care of the dying was first used in Lyons, France, in 1942.

In previous centuries, most people died at home, but since the 1960s, particularly in urban areas, people have looked to hospitals as the place to die. This increasing tendency was expected to continue, but recent social policy changes seem to have reversed the trend. In recent years, research has shown that, with adequate support, the majority of people would prefer to die at home (Townsend et al 1990). With extended families to support patients, they could also expect to be cared for at home, but now people are living longer, and the carer is often elderly, or the dying patient may even be living alone. However, according to the Patient's Charter, all patients should be given the choice of where they prefer to die.

Most people die in NHS hospitals in a variety of settings. This may be on the ward, or in the accident and emergency, intensive care, theatre or even maternity unit. In 1986, approximately 22% of hospital beds were occupied by terminally ill patients; therefore, looking after the dying person is an important part of the work of nursing staff in hospitals, and the ways in which the nurses define and perform this work has an important effect on the experience of dying patients and their families.

Nurses working in NHS hospitals have very different experiences of death. If they work in a maternity or intensive care unit, or on an acute surgical ward, they may experience unexpected deaths that are often traumatic. This may also involve younger patients, whose death it is often more difficult to accept. Since the control of infectious diseases, sudden deaths affecting younger people are usually caused by accidents on the road, at work or in the home, while for older people sudden deaths are caused by heart attacks or strokes.

DEVELOPMENT OF THE PALLIATIVE CARE AND HOSPICE MOVEMENT

Palliative care is defined by the World Health Organization as 'the active total care of patients whose disease no longer responds to curative treatment and for whom the goal must be the best quality of life for them and their families'.

Palliative care is now a distinct specialty in both medical and nursing disciplines. It focuses on controlling pain and other symptoms, and enhancing the life that remains. It encompasses the physical, psychological, social and spiritual aspects of care, enabling people to live out their lives with dignity.

The development of palliative care is practically synonymous with the development of the modern hospice movement and has traditionally concentrated on people with cancer. However, there are many other diagnoses (e.g. motor neurone disease and AIDS) for which the death process may be prolonged and where patients could benefit from palliative care. Despite the dedication of nursing and medical staff in acute hospitals, the experience of many patients and their relatives is unsatisfactory. This is mainly because there is general shortage of people trained in the care of the dying, and because the facilities for privacy and to accommodate families are not available.

During the period from World War II to the 1960s, the word 'death' was seldom used; euphemisms, such as 'passed over' or 'expired', were preferred. Active, strenuous, 'high-tech' or heroic treatments were preferred. Gradually, the climate of opinion began to change; people began to question the application of all-out life-saving techniques in every situation and began to consider the quality of life. The decision of when to stop curative treatment and start palliative care is usually a medical one, but with the multidisciplinary approach to care, nurses are increasingly involved.

Acceptance of the need for training in palliative care

In 1851, The Cancer Hospital in London (now known as the Royal Marsden) was established by Dr William Marsden exclusively to treat people with cancer and was the venue for many developments in treatment. Later, in the 20th century, it became the centre for the development of the specialisation of oncology nursing in the UK, also having a strong international influence.

In the 19th century, the role of both doctors and nurses was seen as one of prolonging life, at almost any cost, by the amazing life-saving techniques that were being developed. This presented them with a very difficult moral and ethical dilemma, as prolonging existence in this way often led to patients living lives of poor quality. At the first International Conference in Cancer Nursing held in London in September 1978, Robert Tiffany, the subsequent chairman, gave a paper on the delivery of nursing care that highlighted this dilemma and the changing role of the cancer nurse, including the need for additional training. In 1984, a specialist group of palliative care nurses formed the Palliative Care Nurses Group. However, the medical profession did not recognise the speciality of palliative medicine until the late 1980s.

The principles of palliative care for cancer patients are now widely accepted and seen as applicable for a wide range of people with terminal illness other than just cancer.

The modern hospice movement

The foundation of the modern hospice movement is often attributed to the work of Dame Cicely Saunders and the establishment in 1967 of St Christopher's Hospice in Sydenham, England.

Dame Cicely, who began her career as a nurse before moving on to become a social worker and then undertaking medical training, spent many years researching pain, symptom control and planning for the special needs of the dying.

Another major contribution to the modern hospice movement was the establishment of the charity the Marie Curie Memorial Foundation. Established in 1948 and known today as Marie Curie Cancer Care, it is still the largest single provider of voluntary hospice beds in the UK, and through its 5000 Marie Curie nurses, provides a 'hospice at home' service for cancer patients in their own homes. Another provider of palliative services for the dying is the Cancer Relief Macmillan Fund.

The philosophy of hospice care has spread, crossing political and religious boundaries, to more than 60 countries. Yet, although hospices and palliative care units are to be found in almost every country in the Western World, the vast majority of people in the Third World have no access to such services.

Still the biggest provider of care for the dying, the NHS maintains hospice beds within its hospitals. As the number of specialist nursing and medical posts in palliative care increases, there is greater awareness of the specialty and, of course, of the needs of the dying person.

The most recent trend against long-term care in acute hospitals will probably mean that there will be a rise in the number of deaths occurring in nursing homes and at home, where care is provided by the primary health care team, with additional help available from specialist (Marie Curie and Macmillan) nurses and, most importantly, the family.

FACING THE POSSIBILITY OF DEATH

For much of this century, people in our society have tended to shy away from the subject of death. While the subject no longer has the same taboo, many patients still experience problems in getting people around them to talk openly about their impending death. Many patients find relief when at last they are given the opportunity to talk freely about the probability that they are dying. Many gain comfort from this knowledge, and it is clearly unkind to withhold the information from them. There is, however, a need for caution, as some people may react adversely. Discussing death with somebody who is dying demands great sensitivity; a tentative exploratory approach is necessary.

The decision of whether to tell or not to tell was traditionally the prerogative of the doctor, but patients often find nurses easier to talk to, which may leave the nurse in a very difficult situation. Greater cooperation and the recognition of the multidisciplinary teamwork approach to patient care and individual accountability has ameliorated this problem.

It is important, therefore, sensitively to assess the patient's wishes, to listen to the family, who will often have strong views, and then, within the multidisciplinary team, to decide who is the best person to break the news.

ADJUSTING TO THE PROSPECT OF DEATH

Nobody who is fit and healthy wants to die, and even seriously ill people often want to prolong their life. No matter what age a person might be, the shift from health to grave illness is a difficult one.

The following stages of adjustment are based on the findings of Kubler-Ross (1969), who observed a large number of dying people. She divided the process of facing death into five stages:

- denial
- anger
- bargaining
- depression
- acceptance.

It is important to remember that these stages do not necessarily follow a sequence but may well overlap and are sometimes almost undetected. It is important to recognise that patterns vary, and that people facing death ebb and flow in their experience of these reactions to the threat of death.

Denial

Denial is thought to be a means of protecting oneself until one is able to absorb the full impact of the problem. Some people tend to ignore or deny crises that threaten their equilibrium. During a fatal illness, this evasion of the truth sometimes reveals itself as the individual's conviction that a remedy will be found to the dilemma, the experts will be proved wrong and he will survive.

In order to establish to what extent the dying person grasps his situation, it is necessary to find out what he knows already. However, there is a great controversy over the actual extent of the awareness that the dying person has about the nearness of the end. Without direct reference to it, by the person or by onlookers, this is difficult to assess.

Anger

Anger often accompanies illness, perhaps the most common reason being the individual's sense that he has lost control over his life. We spend so much time demonstrating that we have control over our lives and what happens to us, but serious illness does not occur of our own choosing, and it follows its own course. The anger that this provokes sometimes seems to be directed at care-givers and loved ones (Kubler-Ross 1969):

The more energetic and alive the nurse is, the more anger she is likely to evoke in the patient who has been told he is incurable and terminal. In this stage he is not angry at the nurse, but at the attributes that she represents – vitality, freedom and purpose – which he has lost or is about to lose.

Families and friends need to be aware of the reason for such anger, otherwise it can become heartbreaking for them to witness their loved ones behaving in uncharacteristic ways.

Bargaining

Bargaining with others, especially God, can be interpreted as warfare between hope and despair. Here the person may be accepting the reality of the threat of death in a small way, rather than being overtaken by it. Often this stage is a result of a battle between the reality of the situation and the fading survival strategies of the past.

Struggle, as shock and disbelief begin to cloud the picture, is another stage associated with dying. This may be a most distressing response to witness, especially if the person who fears death struggles vainly against the inevitable. There is, however, the consolation that the person has not surrendered to the desolation of terminal illness, but has retained hope and refuses to give in. This may provide a source of comfort to the relatives and others as they try to come to terms with the death.

Depression

The suffering and the sadness that the seriously ill person experiences are sometimes overlooked, as it is easy to assume that features of depression, such a loss of pleasure, interest and gratitude, are part and parcel of the illness. This can be a false assumption, since other people who are seriously ill but have a reasonable chance of recovery do not experience or express the same degree of sadness.

Acceptance

Acceptance of and resignation to death are seen as appropriate and as allowing peace of mind when death is inevitable. Struggle has no benefit at this time and is abandoned. Often the individual is less troubled about leaving life than onlookers are about letting him go.

ATTITUDES TOWARDS DEATH

An important aspect of death is that it forces people to separate, and morbid fears are likely to occur at the prospect of the imposed and unsought-for parting. Although we would like to prevent death, we are also inclined to regard ourselves as powerful creatures with resources and potentials that make death senseless. Except when we deny the evidence of our mortality, we have the foreknowledge that one day we must die. In our struggle against death, we can attempt to defer it, or deny that death is final as far as this world is concerned. We often hold notions of the rights and wrongs of life and death, as when we feel cheated by an 'untimely' death.

The dying person watches the realisation of separation dawn upon those around him. Often the best therapy for family and close friends comes from the dying person. The relatives are helped by the dying person to face the reality of their own sense of loss, which is natural and proper.

Mixed emotions

Giving love and care without due results can give rise to a sense of loss of control over circumstances. During the practical aspects of care, the carer may be busy doing many things for the person and may have been appreciated and valued. However, as the person deteriorates, a strong element of disappointment may arise. As the final period is entered and the disease

takes over, feelings of powerlessness and failure may grow. There is a possibility of self-reproach and withdrawal from the person because of the emotion already expended in vain.

Fear of death

Death may be expected or unexpected, anticipated or sudden. It is not uncommon for many people, including Christians, to have a fear of death. Theorists would remind us that it is not so much death that one fears as the process of dying itself. If dying is regarded as suffering, it generally arouses fear. When people are questioned on how they would choose to die, the universal wish is for a quick, painless, peaceful departure from this world. Most would wish to die quickly in order to avoid suffering. To pass away during sleep would be acceptable, providing that there had been a period of saying one's goodbyes.

Fear of the dead

This fear includes many misgivings concerning death, particularly with regard to dead bodies and spirits, and is less straightforward than is the fear of dying. The dead provoke a range of strong but mixed emotions, and there is often a paradoxical association of feelings, for example reverence and disgust, or sadness and relief. The mixture of feelings is not only experienced by the individual involved with the death but is also reflected in patterns of social life, i.e. its taboos and rituals.

These feelings often reflect the conflict within childhood responses to death. They may be macabre, matter-of-fact or intensely apprehensive. For children and adults, the change from the living person they have known to a lifeless body can be a shocking and perplexing event.

Changed relationships

It comes as a surprise to many that death exposes the breakdown of relationships and the hostility that sometimes exist in families. An embarrassing situation often occurs when contact is renewed between family members visiting the dying person or attending the funeral. Those in conflict with others will find it much more difficult to understand what their feelings, whether of anger, guilt or relief, really are.

Prolonging life

To what extent and by what means to prolong life is a vexed question. Most people will want to live for as long as is reasonably possible. The doctor has to assume final responsibility and must take some very hard decisions when the person's incurable illness is nearing its end. He may have to decide what palliative treatments to repeat or to discontinue on the basis of whether or not they can contribute any further to the patient's quality of life.

MEETING THE NEEDS OF THE DYING PERSON

PHYSICAL NEEDS

Many terminally ill people experience a sequence of physiological events that relate specifically to the process of dying. When the doctors responsible for the patient confess that nothing more can be done to reverse the process of his illness, palliative care begins.

Drugs are not the only means of alleviating physical discomfort. A number of other expedients may have beneficial effects in reducing the more distressing symptoms of the disease, even though these measures may not prolong life.

In terminal illness, the individual's quality of life fluctuates, and it is important that frequent assessments are made for the optimum treatment and care. Nurses spend more time with the patient, so are in a key position to monitor symptoms and ensure that appropriate treatment is given. The following are just some of the major physical problems that can affect the dying person.

Pain

The pain experienced by the dying person is a major concern of the palliative care movement. Pain is the experience that many people naturally fear will be the awful accompaniment to their terminal illness, but while pain may well be an integral part of some incurable diseases, it is by no means inevitable. An armoury of analgesic drugs is available to doctors in the UK; a painful death should therefore not be necessary. (See Ch. 5 for detailed information about pain control and management.)

Nausea and vomiting

Nausea and vomiting can make the dying person feel miserable and exhausted. Vomiting may be the manifestation of many different diseases and occurs frequently when the kidneys or liver are beginning to falter in their function. Anti-emetics and adjustment of diet may be appropriate; mouthwashes and an immediate change of linen will be required.

If there is an obstruction high up in the alimentary tract, swallowing may be interfered with to such an extent that food and sometimes liquids cannot be tolerated (dysphagia). Surgery or the insertion of a tube into the oesophagus, or directly into the stomach, may be the only means of relieving the symptoms.

Anorexia

A general lack of interest in food, and subsequent weight loss and debilitation, is a common problem for the dying person. The nurse is often able to encourage eating and drinking by preparing, or making available, special meals in response to the person's expressed desires. Encouraging family members to bring special meals or drinks is also important.

Debilitation and immobility

General weakness often occurs as death approaches, and strength fades in the limbs. Pressure on the extremities at this time seems to trouble the dying person. Various measures can be taken to relieve the weight of bedclothes and thus reduce the discomfort. Gentle exercising of the limbs may be possible, and prevention of pressure sores should be an important aim of the nurse.

Thirst and sore mouth

Jobbins et al (1992) found that distressing oral dryness affected more then three-quarters of their study group. The cause can be the drug regimens but is more commonly oral candidiasis (85%). Denture problems are also often common following the wasting of terminal illness.

Nurses are able to help by ensuring good oral hygiene and observation of symptoms. Giving drinks, mouthwashes and lemon drops may all help to provide relief and help to stimulate the production of saliva.

Changes in appearance

These may be considerable, for example extreme loss of weight, sudden gross puffiness in the face, or ascites, resulting in a large and heavy abdomen. There may be loss or thinning of the hair, or changes in its colour and condition; looking in the mirror will be a constant reminder of the illness. Physical debility alters the way someone walks, the clothes worn, the whole way that life is played out. It also alters the way in which one is treated by strangers, colleagues and family. Extreme sensitivity is required of nurses and carers, and negotiation with the dying person about what to wear and other aspects of personal appearance can be very rewarding.

Insomnia

This can be a major problem and is often listed as one of the main causes of distress. A number of people have a particular dislike of the dark and usually appreciate the provision of a dimmed light at night. A few treasured belongings, such as photographs or a special pillow, help the patient to feel more at home and in touch with reality. It has been customary in this country to move patients who are dying in hospital to a single side ward. Such a move should be discussed, if possible, with the patient and his relatives. Some patients will gain comfort and support from other patients in the ward and from seeing what is going on, whilst others may welcome more privacy. The temperature and

noise levels of the environment may need adjusting, and physical comfort is vital.

Terminal restlessness

Sometimes the causes of restlessness are difficult to define, but it is important that it is recognised by nurses. There have been occasions where people who wished to die at home have been restless and taken by ambulance to hospital, where they immediately died – all because the nurse did not recognise terminal restlessness.

EMOTIONAL NEEDS

The relief of physical suffering has traditionally been the primary aim of palliative care. Gradually, as expertise in controlling or relieving the physical symptoms of disease has increased to the point at which patients may be expected to be almost pain-free, there are feelings of failure if they have to suffer symptoms such as vomiting or breathlessness for any length of time. Having achieved this level of symptom control, carers are often faced with a new problem. No longer overwhelmed by pain and other symptoms, patients become more aware of the emotional and spiritual distress that often accompanies dying. They are free to contemplate what they are losing, and few can do this with equilibrium.

Companionship

Dying people may feel very alone and alienated. Their world becomes small, in both the physical and social sense, and they often see literally only one room for much of the time. Often a dying person, even with a group of chatting friends and relatives, can appear quite isolated. The dying person needs to know that those around him are still interested in him and respect him. Even though he and his work colleagues may know that his working life has come to an end, he needs to know that the personal ties remain. If this is not evident, the person then feels that he has been discarded and is already forgotten; he is left with the impression that he is already regarded as dead.

Talking

Talking with the dying is so difficult that the student nurse might be led to question the value of her exchanges with terminally ill patients. However, it should be remembered that, apart from promoting and enriching the relationship between the participants, conversation carries with it several vital benefits (Buckman 1988):

1. Talking is the most revealing and specific way of communicating.
2. Talking helps to ease distress, guilt and fear. Sensitive listening does not demand answers or solutions but encourages the person to clarify his position.
3. Pent-up thoughts will eventually become destructive, and bottled-up feelings may well surge up and overwhelm the person.

Listening

The purpose of sensitive listening is to understand as fully as possible what the other person is experiencing. Sensitive and accurate listening may seem easy, but it is in reality very difficult, and professionals are often no better at it than anyone else. However, rather than becoming discouraged, we can all become more aware, responsive and sensitive listeners by observing a number of guidelines. For example, if the patient is a quiet and private type of person, he may never talk freely and share his feelings; here the important principle is to accept what he offers as the best he can do.

Completing 'unfinished business'

Day by day, most people do and say things they would like to change or retract. At the end of a life, there is often an urgency to make amends, to tie up loose ends, to say something that has been held back for many years. Sometimes it is easier to talk these things through with a stranger or the nurse. There may be nothing to say that can resolve an issue, nothing the nurse can make better, but there are many occasions when the nurse is able to help. What the nurse cannot do is to make assumptions: what the patient *feels* must be accepted by the person listening to him.

SPIRITUAL NEEDS

It is beyond the scope of this chapter to cover, in detail, all of the special religious requirements that may occur in caring for the dying and, probably more significantly, following death and in caring for the bereaved. In providing holistic care, the spiritual needs of the person are as important as are the physical and emotional needs; they often assume greater importance than normal for the dying person.

For some people, help lies with a representative of one of the religious denominations or faiths, but spiritual needs are not synonymous with religious needs, and even someone with a strong faith is not necessarily at peace with himself. Many people do not have a defined faith or belong to a definite group; they may feel great sadness and spiritual pain and be searching for some comfort at the end of their life. The nurse cannot be expected to be the only person who can facilitate the expression of that pain.

The nurse can however, listen, support any request and simply offer non-judgemental empathy. It is never appropriate to push one's own belief system, but it is always possible to support the patient in his own personal search or conclusions. Nevertheless, it is essential to recognise that the special requirements of an individual's religion must be acknowledged during illness and death. Some of these requirements are outlined briefly in Box 19.1.

AT THE TIME OF DEATH

If the individual's family and friends have not accepted the inevitability of his death, they will be ill-prepared to face the actual event. There is a real risk that the person will become isolated and set apart from his friends at the precise time that he most needs their support and confirmation that he will not be forgotten. In today's culture, the major reasons for the dying person becoming isolated are that:

- we expect most people to die in a hospital, hospice or nursing home

---

Box 19.1 Religious requirements during illness and death

Christians. If the dying person is Christian, it is important that he has access to a Minister who can explore with him his thoughts and beliefs and give reassurance. Upon death, the appropriate minister or priest should be contacted in order to be involved in the practical arrangements for the funeral and burial or cremation.

Jews. If the deceased is Jewish, the body is attended by members of the Jewish community and no mutilation of the body is allowed, except where there is a legal requirement for a post mortem. The funeral usually occurs within 24 hours, and cremation is forbidden.

Muslims. The next of kin will want to arrange certain preparations for the body before burial, which is required to be done as quickly as possible. It is necessary, if at all possible, to avoid a post mortem. Some members of the Muslim faith express their emotions freely when a relative dies.

Sikhs. Sikhs show antipathy towards the idea of a post mortem. Certain preparations of the body are made before the act of cremation; for example, the body is washed and dressed in special clothes.

Hindus. If a Hindu person is dying in hospital, relatives may request to bring money and clothes for him to touch before being distributed to the needy. After death, the relatives will wish to attend to the body before its removal from the hospital. If a post mortem is unavoidable, they will be anxious that all organs are returned to the body before cremation.

Buddhists. On the death of a Buddhist, it is vital that a Buddhist priest, preferably of the same school of Buddhism as the deceased, is informed as soon as possible. The body should ideally remain untouched until the priest arrives.

Chinese. Only Muslim Chinese have objections to post mortems. The position and economic situation of the family will influence the rites performed. In some cases, the body may be clothed in traditional Chinese clothing.

Baha'is. Baha'is may not be cremated or embalmed. The actual requirements upon death can be obtained from the Local Assembly of the Baha'is in the area.

- we depend largely on experts to provide care during serious illness
- as a society, we place more emphasis on health than on illness.

Whilst these attitudes and assumptions are not necessarily wrong, they tend to make it difficult for the dying person to receive total care, which includes support from family and friends at the time of death. People seldom want to be left alone to die, and they should, if possible, have someone with them when the time comes. Finally, it is important to remember that the last sense to go as the person drifts into unconsciousness is hearing. Comfort is surely provided by continuing to speak to him in appropriate ways.

PRACTICAL ARRANGEMENTS AND LAST OFFICES

The fact that death has occurred must be certified. Relatives should be allowed to remain at the bedside for a little while. Any special requests of the relatives should be granted if at all possible; this may include other relatives viewing the body.

Often the relatives will have had an anxious time of visiting their loved one and watching the process of dying. The death, when it occurs, may nonetheless seem sudden and relatives may well be in a state of shock. The nurse should make sure that relatives are fit to leave when they prepare to go home. A quiet room or a special unit for bereaved relatives should be available. A cup of tea or coffee and an opportunity to talk and receive counselling should be offered.

Arrangements for the registration of the death need to be explained, with sensitivity, to relatives. Writing down key points may be helpful as relatives often find it difficult to concentrate at this time. If there is property to be collected by the relatives, this should be carefully managed, since these articles represent what remains of the deceased.

When the relatives have left, the body is attended to according to hospital policy, which will include addressing any cultural and religious requirements.

THE FUNERAL

In practice, undertakers are very helpful, and any special arrangements can be agreed between the family, the undertaker and the religious official. It is important that the relatives have the support and involvement of family and friends through to the funeral and beyond. One can expect disbelief and numbness to protect the bereaved and help them to cope well up to and during the funeral; after the funeral, more acute reactions may be felt.

BEREAVEMENT

The grief of near relatives who are bereaved is natural, since death is final and the loved one will never be restored on earth. Loss is at the heart of bereavement.

Feelings of grief may start long before the death of a patient. Relatives and patients have to get used to the idea of a shortened life expectancy, uncertainty and often a great deal of worry and concern.

It is important for nurses to have an understanding of the stages of bereavement in order to be able to help not only patients' carers, but also their own families and friends, recognising when grief is within normal bounds and being able to identify when specialist help is needed.

Whenever a person dies, whether in a hospital, a hospice or at home, the initial reaction of those present can have a lasting effect. A kind comment from a nurse or friend – 'We will miss Fred, he always had something cheerful to say' – may leave a lasting impression for the bereaved relative, a positive memory for the time of death. Spending time on ensuring that relatives know how to register the death and make all the necessary arrangements is time well spent, as the bereaved are very vulnerable at this time and may be stunned and confused.

LOSS

The restoration and healing following bereavement includes acknowledging the sense of loss and then gradually adjusting to it. The loss is real, and the empty room, the extra chair at the table, the absence of the familiar voice are the evidence of it.

No one sustains loss of any magnitude without being deeply affected. Being hurt in this way often gives rise simultaneously to two very powerful emotions: anger and grief. 'Why me?'

is often the predominant question. A bereaved person, years after the death of a loved one, may still be having an inner battle between self and God, or with whomever is thought to have been responsible for the death.

The bereaved person has 'lost' a part of himself – that part which was represented and developed through a relationship with the deceased person. For example, if a child dies, the part of the bereaved that was a parent dies too. If a partner dies, that part of self which existed only in the presence of the partner dies. Moreover, the bereaved person may also lose some very important practical things, such as some of his income and some of his social life. The most radical change will be to lose the identity of a married person and be referred to as a 'widower' or 'widow'. However, there is more to bereavement than grief for the actual loss of the person. When a special person dies, a gap is left somewhere in the emotions, a gap which, according to some theorists, is never really filled.

Special types of loss

Sudden deaths, such as accidents or heart attacks, are likely to be more difficult to grieve over (Parkes 1975). The sense of unreality of the death may be more marked, with a longer period of numbness and nightmare visions of what happened. Often there is a strong feeling of guilt: 'If only I had been there'. There is much more likely to be unfinished business or unresolved matters: 'If only I had not quarrelled'. There is often also the need to blame somebody. If a sudden death involves legal proceedings, which usually take time, the grief is once again delayed, stopping the family from adjusting to the loss.

Suicide is particularly difficult to adjust to. Not only are there the problems of a sudden death, but there is also the stigma associated with suicide, making it more difficult to talk about. Survivors often feel rejected and guilty because they were unable to prevent the death.

Miscarriages and abortions have their own problems. Worries about the future are common, with the danger of wanting to conceive quickly before the current loss has been mourned. There is a strong temptation to try and forget about the loss too soon, before the grief is fully resolved.

GRIEF

Grieving is essentially the work of letting go and saying goodbye. Theories differ as to what grief achieves, but it is often described as the survivor releasing his attachment to the deceased and learning to make attachments with other people in the future. Grieving is the normal and expected response to loss, and a lack of grieving gives rise to suggestions of an abnormal psychology.

There are vast cultural variations within different societies, but basically all societies have strong lines of responsibility running through their laws and traditions. A family's private grief may be interfered with by the requirements of the law, particularly where an inquest and post mortem are necessary.

A major bereavement is a bewildering experience, and a combination of many losses over a number of years can make bereavement through death exceptionally traumatic. We should never underestimate the impact of a bereavement or deny anyone the right to grieve.

Manifestations of grief

The description and classification of grief used here is based mainly on the work of Parkes (1972) and Stedeford (1987), who make a complex subject manageable. The typical manifestations of grief immediately following death are given below (see also Box 19.2).

Numbness. The recently bereaved person may feel very little of anything concerning the death. Although he accepts the fact of what has happened, he goes through the motions of normal living and of doing what needs to be done. This period may last for hours or a week or two.

Disbelief. This is another common reaction in the early period of a few hours or days; it is as though the news has not registered. However, when the protective nature of this reaction has done its job, the truth gradually sinks in. This process can take months.

> Box 19.2 **Manifestations of grief** (Lindemann 1944, Parkes 1986)
>
> *Feelings*
>
> | | | |
> |---|---|---|
> | Shock | Anger | Yearning |
> | Guilt and self-reproach | Anxiety | Emancipation |
> | Loneliness | Fatigue | Numbness |
> | Helplessness | Sadness | Relief |
>
> *Physical sensations*
>
> | | |
> |---|---|
> | Hollowness in the stomach | Tightness in the chest |
> | Tightness in the throat | Breathlessness |
> | Weakness of the muscles | Lack of energy |
> | Dry mouth | Sense of unreality |
>
> *Thoughts*
>
> | | |
> |---|---|
> | Disbelief | Confusion |
> | Preoccupation | Sense of presence |
> | Hallucinations | |
>
> *Behaviours*
>
> | | |
> |---|---|
> | Sleep disturbance | Appetite disturbance |
> | Absent-mindedness | Social withdrawal |
> | Dreams of the deceased | Searching |
> | Sighing | Crying |
> | Irritability | Restlessness |
> | Difficulty with decision-making | |
>
> Visiting or carrying objects as a reminder of the deceased

In the more acute cases of grief the reactions are more powerful and pervasive:

The urge to cry out loudly, so expressing powerful emotions, is often reported by the bereaved person. Unfortunately, our society prefers a more silent and controlled reaction to bereavement.

Searching. The loss of a loved one often leads to a sensation of searching for the person who has died. This can be a distressing side of grief, since the individual knows that it is futile, yet still goes to a room or some other place to no avail.

Anger. Anger is usually related to a sense of outrage at the 'stealing away' of something valuable. Symbolically, this represents the loss of hope for the future. This anger may be directed at the carers who had looked after the dying person or at the deceased person himself.

Guilt. Bereavement often causes the individual to review over and over again in his mind the events that preceded death. In the process of this, he recalls something done or left undone that hurt or upset the deceased.

When a person becomes seriously ill, guilt seems to be all-pervasive, and it can be most destructive. It is such a common emotion because our society tends to assume that someone is to blame for every catastrophe. No one should feel guilty about surviving the deceased, but should seek to continue a meaningful life.

Guilt stirs up memories of failure and conflicts, things left unfinished, words spoken that are regretted, and the longing for the impossible opportunity to explain and ask for forgiveness. When guilt and anger remain unresolved, they may leave an opening for a more debilitating state of depression.

Children can be deeply affected by grief. They have been robbed of a parent or sibling and are capable of responding with anger and guilt. The need to help the children deal with their own grief adds to the weight of a bereaved parent's burden. If children do not get help with anger and guilt, these emotions may possibly surface in the form of restlessness, learning difficulties, truancy, vandalism or withdrawal and depression.

Anxiety. A prominent feature of acute grief, anxiety is part of the alarm response to the loss, and a result of insecurity following the disruption to the routine of life that prevailed before the loved one died. The way forward is to provide a new routine without the deceased.

Agitation. This experience is partly the result of the urge to search for the deceased and the attempt to reduce the number of things that act as reminders of the deceased. The person who is agitated is almost unable to settle down to useful activity.

Pining. As the awareness of the loss increases, a feeling of longing for the deceased grows in intensity. This may reach the point of overwhelming sorrow that lasts for minutes to an hour or more. Messages of sympathy from well-meaning people do not help, but pining does abate with the passage of time.

Bodily responses. The physical responses that accompany grief mainly involve the disturbance of the autonomic nervous system, which operates in fear situations (the 'fight or flight' response). Examples include loss of appetite, sleep disturbance, weight loss, restlessness, fatigue, breathlessness, palpitations and hypochondriasis.

Feeling the presence of the deceased is not uncommon in the early stages of bereavement. It may even provide comfort and a means of being able to 'talk' with the deceased, as it were.

Feeling hurt. Saying goodbye to a close person is painful because the close ties with that person met emotional needs. We form only a few close relationships and when we lose them, it hurts a great deal. Grieving normally helps to reduce this hurt. It is understandable to interpret bereavement as a precipitating factor in depression.

Abnormal grief. Grief is a normal process, and the majority of people cope without needing professional help. Nurses can help bereaved families by identifying those people who are most at risk of having difficulty with their bereavement. (Box 19.3).

HELPING THE BEREAVED

Just as different people cope with dying in different ways, so bereaved people have their own unique ways of coping with the loss experienced.

EXPRESSING FEELINGS

In a society that equates death with failure, we need to provide bereaved carers with the 'space' to express their feelings of failure and loss. We must then encourage them to come to terms with the loss and understand that they have not failed the deceased. Addressing the needs of carers is a great challenge, simply because we are never quite prepared for the impact of the death. To some carers, the death of the loved one will come as a relief, especially if he has died peacefully, surrounded by the love of the family and friends.

Whether the death has been anticipated or sudden, the bereaved are never fully prepared. It is relatively common for most people to experience a traumatic family bereavement when it is least expected. For them, it is as though the bottom has fallen out of their world. Worst of all, there are no quick and easy answers to why

---

Box 19.3 Factors indicating 'high risk' for abnormal grief resolution (Parkes 1990, Worden 1991)

1. *A severe reaction to the loss.* The manifestation of severe distress anger or self-reproach.
2. *An ambivalent relationship.* Where the individuals involved had ambivalent feelings toward each other, often with unexpressed hostility or in situations when the relationship was highly dependent.
3. *Circumstances surrounding the death.* Sudden deaths where there was less than 2 weeks to adjust to the loss, and unnatural deaths, such as suicide or murder, or when confirmation of the death is uncertain and the body never found.
4. *Previous unresolved grief.* One of the complications of bereavement is unresolved grief, and when a subsequent death occurs, it is much harder for the bereaved person to adjust.
5. *Multiple life crisis.* If the bereaved person has many additional problems or losses to cope with, this may inhibit normal grief resolution.
6. *Personality factors.* People with a strong self-concept

are usually better able to cope with crisis situations, including bereavement, by using their own coping mechanisms more appropriately.

7. *Low socioeconomic status.* Although this was found to be a factor in the early period in the study of Parkes and Weiss (1983), grief resolution had returned to normal after 2 years for those in the low socioeconomic group.
8. *Poor social support.* Those who have a close family and supportive friends cope better with bereavement. At risk would be those individuals who have recently moved house or whose family live at a distance. Probably as important as the amount of support an individual has is his or her perception of that support. Those who perceived themselves to be unsupported had more problems with their bereavement.
9. *Age.* Young adults have more difficulty adjusting to bereavement than do older individuals.

---

such a thing should have happened. Often the bereaved feel as though they have been tried and tested beyond the point of endurance, yet they must hold on to something.

In a society uneasy about death, whether sudden or expected, we need to provide the opportunity for bereaved people to voice their feelings; only then can they start to pick up the pieces and begin to restructure their lives.

Bereavement counselling

A mistake that is commonly made by nurses engaged in bereavement counselling is to think that encouraging the bereaved person to cry is always beneficial. The absence of crying is not a reliable indicator of the denial of grief, as grieving comes in many different guises (Llewellyn and Trent 1987).

The following steps are features of effective bereavement counselling, although they need not necessarily be performed in this order:

• Helping the bereaved to acknowledge the loss by talking about it. Through this, the bereaved person begins the business of making sense of a world without the deceased.

• Providing by one's physical presence a form of emotional support. For a limited period, the bereaved person may be dependent on the nurse as someone to 'be there' and to confide in.

• Listening and accepting whatever feelings of guilt, self-reproach or anger the bereaved may express. Often the bereaved person may refer to unresolved arguments and disagreements, or, more dramatically, blame himself as a contributor to the death.

• Reintegrating and reinvolving the bereaved person within the community. Obviously, this has to be done at the person's own pace and with much support.

In summary, the contribution of the nurse in counselling a bereaved person is to offer acceptance, understanding of the grief and encouragement. A very clear description of how the counsellor might help has been provided by Parkes (1972).

Among the attributes of the counsellor should be respect and interest. By drawing on the counsellor's understanding of his suffering, the bereaved person may begin to extend compassion and forgiveness towards himself. He may discover unexpected abilities to cope, and from this discovery derive further strength to rebuild a full and meaningful life.

Charitable organisations for the bereaved

It is useful for nurses to identify support groups and services available locally. Some of the national support organisations are listed at the end of the chapter.

THE STRESS OF NURSING THE DYING

Deaths that occur within a short time scale are somewhat easier for hospital staff to cope with than are slower deaths. Sudden deaths most often occur in emergency and intensive care situations, where the extent of the threat to life quickly becomes apparent. However, most deaths in hospitals are not of this type, and these present a greater emotional challenge to doctors and nurses by creating problems associated with the awareness, denial and disclosure of dying.

It is important to remember that most, if not all, carers do not know how best to help the dying person. This is not a question of the carer's failings and inadequacies, but is simply a reflection of the fact that dying and bereavement are very powerful and challenging forces that can, and usually do, tear people apart, isolating and dividing individuals from family and friends, and producing feelings of embarrassment and confusion.

The nurse's first encounter with death will be crucial in determining her future attitudes. Witnessing death for the first time in her professional career may well inspire the rise of feelings and emotions otherwise hidden and awaken the memory of personal losses. Although the nurse may have little or no control over the events that take place, she can take control of how she views them, dispensing with automatic feelings of embarrassment and fear in order to be able to offer care and counsel to the dying and the bereaved.

The dying person will look for help and counsel to the nurse, who cannot shirk her responsibility to provide this support. It is both a duty and a privilege to share in the care of the dying and the bereaved, and nurses must do all they can to prepare themselves for this task.

As part of a multidisciplinary team, the nurse should not attempt to deal with the issues surrounding death by herself, but should take advantage of the people and facilities around her that can provide supervision and support. In particular, she should seek the guidance of others who are more experienced.

Emotional involvement

Coping with another person's despair is one of the most difficult aspects of supporting a dying person, and it is often this aspect of care that costs the nurse most in terms of emotional effort. Strong emotions may be aroused in the care of the dying, ranging from sympathy and sadness, pain and disbelief, to optimism and hope. Professional and other carers may refuse to face the fact that they can get angry, irritated or frustrated. This can be serious, as such negative reactions, if they are not expressed, may never be fully resolved. It is important for carers to find a way of acknowledging, identifying and accepting such reactions.

Support networks for nurses

Having supported a dying patient and his family as well as her own colleagues, the nurse may need to talk through this difficult time in a supportive environment. Some hospitals have arrangements for trained counsellors, often chaplains or psychologists, to be on hand for nurses working in palliative care to talk to in complete confidence.

Support groups are of great value to nurses working with the terminally ill. Nurses can also support one another more informally simply by offering their time to distressed colleagues so that they can talk or cry during or after a particularly distressing event.

Summary

The inevitable process of dying is complex and traumatic, both for the dying person and his family, and for the nurse and her colleagues. To better enable the nurse to cope with her own reactions and support others involved, an understanding of the process is vital. Especially demanding are unexpected deaths and those in special circumstances, for example involving young children.

Today, the nurse may encounter a dying patient in a variety of settings, from hospital wards to hospices, and often the patient's own home. Flexibility, sensitivity and specialist training are needed to cope with the wide range of physical, emotional and spiritual needs encountered.

Adjusting to the prospect of one's own death has been described as being composed of several stages, from initial denial to final acceptance, although not necessarily in a predicatable sequence. The nurse must recognise and support these, as well as dealing with the feelings of fear, guilt and sadness of the patient's family and friends, both before death, and afterwards, during the course of bereavement and grief. In doing this, she can identify those having difficulty with bereavement and help them to resolve their grief.

Death is an inevitable fact of life, something that none of us can avoid. While grief is the penalty for loving someone, it can be for some, with support, an opportunity for eventual growth.

REFERENCES

Buckman R 1988 I don't know what to say. Papermac, London
Department of Health 1992 The patients' charter. HMSO, London
Jobbins J 1992 Oral and dental disease in terminally ill cancer patients. British Medical Journal 304: 1612
Kubler-Ross E 1969 On death and dying. Tavistock, London
Lindemann 1944 Symptomatology and management of acute grief. American Journal of Psychology 101: 14178
Llewellyn S, Trent D 1987 Nursing in the community: psychology in action. The British Psychological Society/Methuen, London
Parkes C M 1972 Bereavement: studies of grief in adult life. Pelican, London
Parkes C M 1975 Determinants of outcome following bereavement. Omega 6(14): 303–323
Parkes C M, Weiss R S 1983 Recovery from bereavement. Basic Books, New York
Parkes C M 1990 Risk factors in bereavement: implications for the prevention and treatment of pathological grief. Psychiatric Annals 20(6): 308–313
Stedeford A 1987 Bereavement. Medicine International 2(43): 1779–1785
Townsend et al 1990 Terminal cancer care and patients' preference for place of death. British Medical Journal 301: 1
Worden J W 1991 Grief counselling and grief therapy. Tavistock Routledge, London
World Health Organization 1990 Cancer pain relief and palliative care-technical report Series 804. WHO, Geneva

FURTHER READING

Caire D (ed.) 1993 The future for palliative care. Open University Press, Milton Keynes
Charles-Edwards A 1982 The nursing care of the dying patient. Beconsfield Publishers, Bucks
David J 1995 Cancer care. Chapman & Hall, London
Goldman A 1994 Care of the dying child. Oxford University Press, Oxford
Green J 1994 Dying with dignity, Books I and II. Nursing Times Publications, London

USEFUL ADDRESSES

The Compassionate Friends (for bereaved parents)
53 North Street
Bedminster
Bristol   BS3 1EN
Tel: 0117 953 9639

CRUSE (for widowed people and their children)
CRUSE House
126 Sheen Road
Richmond
Surrey   TW9 1UR
Tel: 0181-940 4818

The Foundation for the Study of Infant Deaths (SIDS) (for cot deaths)
35 Belgrave Square
London   SW1X 8QB
Tel: 0171-235 1721

National Association of Widows
54–57 Allison Street
Digbeth, Birmingham B5 5TH

The Stillbirth and Neonatal Death Society
26 Portland Place
London W1N 4DE
Tel: 0171 436 5881 (Helpline)

4

An introduction to the main client groups

During the Common Foundation Programme (CFP) students should obtain a basic introduction to all client groups and should gain an insight into each group's special needs.

Following the CFP students will progress to the further study of a particular patient group. This section of the book helps to prepare students for the further studies that lie ahead.

20 Adults

Jane Hodges

Adult nursing is one of the four branches of study after the common foundation programme. This chapter aims to:

- define adult nursing, the population it encompasses and where it takes place
- investigate the changing patterns of disease over the twentieth and into the twenty-first century
- examine the needs of the main adult care groups and the role of the nurse in meeting these
- discuss some current issues affecting adult nursing.

ADULT NURSING: WHAT IS IT?

Nurses who care for people over 16 years of age are those caring for adults. This comprises the largest group of nurses in practice. Within this group are nurses in a wide variety of specialties and specialisms, for example those working in operating theatre departments, nurses working in medical, surgical and care of the elderly areas,

417

nurses in critical care, and those in health centres and the community.

The general public and many in the nursing profession equate adult nursing with 'general' nursing. This has changed since the implementation of the new diploma level nursing courses (Project 2000). The basic registration courses were previously in general nursing (Registered General Nurse; RGN), nursing the mentally ill (Registered Mental Nurse; RMN) and nursing people with learning disabilities (Registered Nurse for the Mentally Handicapped), which were all largely hospital-based. With the new course, following a common foundation programme, it is subdivided into four branches of adult, child, learning disabilities and mental health nursing, the latter two specialties encompassing care across the lifespan. The major difference from the old training programme is that, on qualification, all nurses (whatever the branch) will be able to work either in hospital or in the community. Nurses working with sick children previously undertook a course combined with the RGN qualification or a post-registration qualification, as becoming an RGN was a prerequisite to becoming a Registered Sick Childrens Nurse (RSCN).

Nurses caring for adults in a variety of settings will all have undergone the same initial pre-registration educational course. Subsequently, nurses may work in critical care areas, caring for young people with injuries following road traffic accidents, or with elderly people with chronic health deficiencies, those with gender-specific health-related concerns, or those with socially-related problems affecting health.

Nurses working in adult care are primarily seen as those preventing ill-health and assisting people to recover from disease. In adult care, the nurse has the complex role of giving care, acting as an educator, supporter and facilitator of patients, relatives and friends in a variety of situations, both in hospital and in the community.

Who are 'adults'?

Within the health care system, the definition of an adult is not an easy one. As previously stated, the age of 16 years is when an individual may give consent and is also seen as when a person may leave home and live independently. Again, it is the age at which one may marry, although with parental consent, and, equally, the age at which medical treatment may be given with the individual's consent. Nonetheless, in other respects, except for driving, the legal age of maturity commences with one's eighteenth birthday. In hospital and institutions, in the absence of an adolescent unit, young people of any age over 13 or 14 years may be cared for in adult wards, even though this may be less than desirable for their individual development.

At the other end of the lifespan continuum, adulthood may continue past the individual's eighth or ninth decade. Those in the adult client group will normally have health problems of a mainly physical nature, requiring either medical management, by way of drugs or other therapeutic means, or surgical removal, repair or replacement of tissues or organs.

Adults today will be seeking and receiving care in a variety of settings, ranging from health centres to hospitals, clinics or even the clients' own homes. In some instances, the care will be continuous, from an institution, for example a hospital, to the community, for example the client's home, whilst the client is being enabled to recover independence or achieve reduced dependency. Those adults in hospital will be requiring support in their sick role. The nurse will be involved in providing psychological support, as well as meeting individuals' physical needs in what, for most, is the acute phase of their illness. Adults requiring terminal care will receive this also in a variety of settings – hospitals, hospices or their own homes – receiving ongoing care until their death.

As human beings, adults are seen in the context of their social environment and are therefore seldom isolated from others – family, close relatives, partners, friends, colleagues, neighbours and acquaintances. Any period of altered health will inevitably lead to practical and emotional consequences for anyone involved with the individual.

During any period of altered health, help may be required from a variety of professionals, such as doctors, nurses, social workers and therapists.

In today's world, individuals are also seeking alternatives, either to combine with or complement traditional care, or to replace it. Nurses will provide liaison and advice in their role as advocate and educator.

Where does care take place?

Thus care takes place in any setting where individuals have health care needs. Acute and investigative care generally occurs in a hospital setting, although following the Community Care Act (1989) and the development of increased GP financial independence, more investigative work occurs in the community. Ongoing and continuous care may take place in hospital, health centres and the community setting or be contracted to facilities within the private sector. The majority of individuals with health care problems receive most of their care within their own homes.

CHANGING PATTERNS OF DISEASE

Disease patterns have altered over the 20th century, although, in the latter part of the century, diseases more associated with the Victorian era, for example tuberculosis, remain present in today's society. The advent of antibiotics changed the pattern of illness, leading causes of death now being cancers and disorders affecting the cardiovascular system, rather than infectious diseases. Changes in disease patterns and the importance of epidemiology in mapping cause and effect of disease are discussed in Ch. 8. Additionally, newly recognised diseases such as human immunodeficiency virus (HIV) infection and acquired immune deficiency syndrome (AIDS), documented since 1982, have become evident in the adult population.

Case example 20.1 illustrates how the treatment of tuberculosis has changed since the 1940s. In 1948, nursing care would have addressed the problems of a patient confined to bed. Specific care following partial removal of the lung would have included the insertion of special drainage tubes into the chest wall to allow the rest of the lung to re-expand. A long rehabilitation period would then have followed. In the 1990s, treatment is by drug therapy, the patient often not

Case example 20.1 Changing patterns of care

A tuberculosis patient in 1948

Jonathan Coleman, a 26-year-old steelworker, is married and has two young children. He has been admitted to a sanatorium some 15–20 miles away from his home and rather isolated after a diagnosis of tuberculosis of the lung. His chest X-ray (CXR) shows the bacillus active in the lung tissue, which may result in Jonathan having surgery to remove a large part of his lung. He will probably require care within the sanatorium for 6 months and ongoing care for 2 years. During the 6 months, he will be lucky to see his family once a fortnight; initially, in fact, he will not see his children at all.

A tuberculosis patient in 1990

John Coleman, a 45-year-old steelworker, is married and has two grown children who have left home. He reported to his GP complaining of night sweats and a productive cough. A CXR was taken and his sputum sent for culture and sensitivity. The CXR showed a possible active lesion in the lung, and the sputum culture was positive for the tubercle bacillus. John is being given a course of antitubercular drugs by his GP and is off work and at home for 6 weeks, or until his sputum shows no active tubercle bacillus. His CXR 6 months later will show a minute scar on the lung tissue but no impairment of respiratory function.

entering hospital for treatment and care. The community services would be involved, providing follow-up care, informing contacts about the disease and its prevention and offering immunisation as required.

Like disease patterns, patterns for care have also changed over time. There have been, and continue to be, considerable advances in science and technology affecting health care provision. High-tech areas, such as operating theatres, are unrecognisable from those of 20 years ago. Cardiac surgery is now an everyday occurrence, with organ transplantations being performed more frequently in a wider variety of health care settings. Equally, the development of prosthetic surgery (e.g. hip replacement) has benefited many, reducing the amount of pain and increasing individuals' mobility. Additionally, those individuals unable to have children but wishing to so do are now benefiting from research in this area. All these advances have affected the role of the nurse caring for adults across the care settings. Present policies for care provision mean shorter acute hospital admissions, with longer periods of convalescence in the community.

POPULATION TRENDS – THE FUTURE REQUIREMENTS FOR CARE

The Department of Health (DoH) uses information from the Central Statistics Office 1991 to predict the requirement for the future. Figure 20.1 and Table 20.1 show these predictors for selected age groups until early into the 21st century. The trend appears to be stability in the number of 16-year-olds, but a steady rise for the middle-aged and elderly in the population by the year 2000 and beyond. The increase in those over 80 years of age will have a marked effect on adult nursing in the future, with a requirement for more elderly care. This will especially affect today's student nurses.

Additionally, the DoH uses other statistical information to predict future health care needs. These include social trends, such as:

- measures of health, for example infant mortality
- death rates by age and sex
- the incidence of infectious diseases

- social habits, for example alcohol consumption and sexual behaviour
- the prevalence of accidents
- the practice of preventive medicine
- the use of the health services themselves.

These changes in potential care needs will have an effect on the settings in which care takes place. Equally, availability of public and private monies will influence the availability of services for adult care.

Hospitals

Traditionally, the hospital was seen as the main setting for adult care, although there are now proportionately fewer beds for the increasing population. Reasons for this have been discussed in Chapter 9.

Outpatients departments

The outpatients department is where large numbers of patients are seen. People are referred by their GP, or following hospital discharge from a ward or from the accident and emergency department. For many, outpatients is their only contact with the hospital service. From this department, patients may be admitted to the hospital for investigations, medical treatment or surgery.

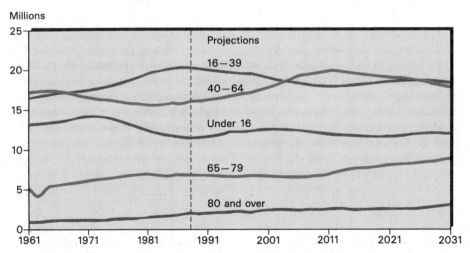

Figure 20.1 UK population by selected age bands 1961–2031. (Reproduced with kind permission from Central Statistics Office 1991.)

Table 20.1 Age and sex structure of the population of the UK 1951–2025, in millions (Reproduced with kind permission from Central Statistics Office 1991)

	Under 16	16–39	40–64	65–79	80 and over	All ages
Mid-year estimates						
1951			15.9	4.8	0.7	50.3
1961	13.1	16.6	16.9	5.2	1.0	52.8
1971	14.3	17.5	16.7	6.1	1.3	55.9
1981	12.5	19.7	15.7	6.9	1.6	56.4
1986	11.7	20.6	15.8	6.8	1.8	56.8
1989	11.5	20.4	16.3	6.9	2.1	57.2
Males	5.9	10.3	8.1	3.0	0.6	27.9
Females	5.6	10.1	8.2	3.9	1.4	29.3
*Mid-year projection**						
1991	11.7	20.2	16.5	6.9	2.2	57.5
1996	12.5	19.8	17.0	6.8	2.4	58.5
2001	12.8	19.2	18.0	6.7	2.5	59.2
2006	12.6	18.4	19.4	6.6	2.6	59.6
2011	12.1	18.1	20.2	7.0	2.7	60.0
2025	12.1	18.6	19.0	8.5	2.9	61.1
Males	6.2	9.5	9.5	3.9	1.1	30.2
Females	5.9	9.1	9.5	4.6	1.8	30.9

*1988-based projections

Outpatients departments are themselves sometimes used for minor treatments, such as the application of plaster of Paris or minor, planned surgical procedures. The number of qualified nurses in outpatients departments is generally diminishing, the routine work being delegated to unqualified support workers. Highly technical and skilled nursing interventions are carried out by qualified nurses, also providing specialist skills such as, for example, ophthalmic testing for visual fields, stoma and mastectomy care and counselling.

The community

The majority of individuals requiring assistance are cared for in the community. Monitoring visits by studying GPs', community nurses' and health visitors' records demonstrates an increase in workload. Much care in the community is given by thousands of unqualified informal carers, such as wives, husbands, sons, daughters, friends and neighbours. These carers manage to care for individuals with little in the way of physical, emotional or financial support.

Adult branch students will work with qualified community nurses during their common foundation and branch programmes. The new registered nurse specialising in adult nursing is eligible, on qualification, to practise in both hospital and community settings.

Health centres

Health centres now provide considerably more care since the advent of GP fundholding. They have become more sophisticated and provide a wide variety of services, for example 'well woman', 'well man', diabetic and asthma clinics. Additionally, some have facilities for investigative and minor surgical procedures. In some areas, health centres are increasingly caring for people who would previously have had to visit their local outpatient departments. Health centres now often have their own qualified nursing staff working alongside other professionals. Practice nurses within health centres have usually taken a specialist post-registration course in community care following their initial pre-registration programme.

Day centres

Day centres may be provided by local authorities, health services or voluntary services and provide a facility that meets a variety of local needs. For the older adult, these day centres may enhance community life and provide amenities for care or rehabilitation, sometimes with the help of a visiting nurse. Day centres can also provide for the more infirm who require assistance in meeting daily health care needs. In this way, they assist the informal carers caring for people in their own homes. They can also provide valuable support for the mentally ill or those with learning disabilities adjusting to life in the community.

Occupational health care

Occupational health care is another setting for adult care within the working environment. Nurses have usually undertaken a post-registration qualification in occupational health nursing. The needs of the individual in the workplace and what is required of the nurse will differ according to the working environment. Workers in mining or the oil industry have needs very different from those of the person working with a word processor or on an assembly line. The role of an occupational health care nurse includes health promotion, the prevention of accidents and the monitoring of industrial diseases.

Private care

Some adults choose to take out insurance to enable them to use private care. In some instances, this is offered by their employers. Private care generally gives greater flexibility in planning admission times, possibly also with shorter waiting lists. However, most private care is for uncomplicated medical and surgical problems. Some private health companies have expanded their services to provide health screening, sports injury clinics and physiotherapy services.

Residential and nursing homes are available for those older adults who can no longer care for themselves. Some of these homes are run by charities and voluntary organisations. Such services are discussed in more detail in Chapter 9.

ADULT CARE GROUPS

As already stated, those ranging from adolescents to the elderly will be receiving care as adults. This care is usually considered under medical specialisms that take place in both hospital and community settings. These care groups are individuals:

- with a medical problem
- with a surgical problem
- requiring critical care
- with infections
- requiring rehabilitation
- requiring elderly care.

Students of the adult branch will gain experience with most of these client groups. Within each of the above care groups, further specialisms have developed as a result of advances in techniques and medical knowledge. There are indeed specialisms within specialisms: asthma specialists within respiratory medicine, plastic surgeons specialising in hand surgery, or diabetes specialists among those interested in endocrinology. Elderly people may be cared for by a specialist in gerontology or by any one of the specialists caring for all adults. Nursing the older adult is, in itself, a specialty within adult nursing.

MEDICAL NURSING

Individuals may be admitted as acute emergencies or following initial investigations as an outpatient. Medical nursing generally takes place in hospital, although many people in the community require the skills of the nurse. These are focused on effective communication and close observations for signs of pain, breathlessness, abnormal body temperature, altered colour, mental distress and so on. In certain extreme circumstances, life-saving interventions, such as cardiopulmonary resuscitation, may be required of the nurse.

Specific nursing care for specific conditions cannot be covered completely in this chapter, but the reader may refer to the case examples as illustrations of the type of nursing care that may be required.

Patients with cardiovascular and respiratory disorders

Many individuals with medical problems have heart and lung disorders. Breathlessness and chest pain are common symptoms associated with coronary thrombosis (or myocardial infarction). This may be mild, the chest pain being referred to as angina (pain from the heart muscle caused by inadequate blood supply from the coronary arteries) and may radiate to the left arm. A severe coronary thrombosis may block one of the coronary vessels supplying the heart muscle, thus depriving it of oxygen and nutrients. An area of the myocardium becomes ineffective and is destroyed (infarcted). The care of a patient who has suffered a myocardial infarction is described in Case example 20.2.

Problems with the lungs may be associated with heart failure, but are more commonly associated with chronic obstructive airways disease or asthma. Both these conditions are associated with air pollution, including smoking. Another contributory factor is the damp climate found in the northern hemisphere. To a lesser extent, chronic bronchitis is considered an occupational hazard for those working in mines and dusty atmospheres. Figure 20.2 illustrates the rise in the death rate in England and Wales owing to the influenza epidemic in 1989–90. Many of those who died were diagnosed as having chronic bronchitis and therefore had a reduced ability to cope with a virulent infection. Those with respiratory problems have difficulty breathing, with consequent damage to the lung tissues. Case example 20.3 describes the care of a young person with an acute asthmatic attack.

Patients with musculoskeletal disorders

One of the most common medical disorders

Case example 20.2 Care of the patient following myocardial infarction

Ted, a 42-year-old chemical engineer, is married with two teenage children. He enjoys the occasional game of squash, is a little overweight and smokes. Whilst doing some alterations to the house, he collapsed, complaining of severe chest pain. His wife rang for the GP and an ambulance, and Ted was subsequently admitted to the local coronary care unit (CCU).

The nurse will be involved in Ted's care in the CCU or later in the medical ward. In the CCU, the nurse will encourage Ted to rest (giving him psychological support), in order to reduce his cardiac activity. She will monitor the administration of analgesics, antiarrhythmics, vasodilators and other drugs, usually via an intravenous cannula.

Observations will include monitoring the electrocardiogram (ECG), noting any arrhythmias, and taking pulse and blood pressure readings. The nurse should be competent to observe for signs of shock, recognise an impending cardiac arrest and, if required, initiate cardiopulmonary resuscitation.

The nurse's role will also include ensuring that Ted is free from pain. She should be aware of his basic nursing needs and any anxieties he has in relation to his condition. The patient's fears should be discussed openly, and he should be given information and reassurance. This aspect of the nursing role will be continued on the medical ward as Ted begins to adapt to a new lifestyle. In this phase of treatment, the nurse will be involved in educating and encouraging him to adopt healthy eating patterns, to reduce or stop smoking, and to exercise regularly once recovery is complete.

affecting the musculoskeletal system is rheumatoid arthritis. Sufferers are cared for in the community but, in acute phases, may be admitted to a medical ward if there is no special rheumatology unit. Although many of these patients are elderly, rheumatoid arthritis can also afflict younger age groups and can have a significant impact on social and work life. Here the role of the nurse is not just one of acute intervention, but also one of providing understanding and support as the individual learns to cope with pain and progressive immobility. The nurse requires a detailed knowledge of joint anatomy and physiology, a clear understanding of the immune system and technical skills in joint management. The nurse should also be able to work in a team with other professionals involved in the care of people with 'rheumatoid' disease.

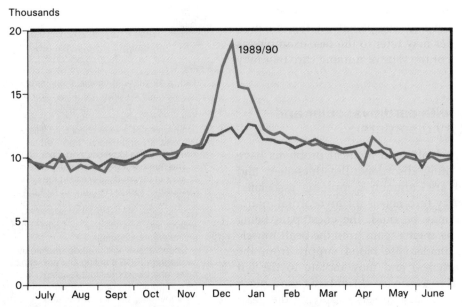

Figure 20.2 Deaths (people aged 1 year or over) mid-1988–89 and mid-1989–90, England and Wales, showing the 1989–90 peak due to influenza. (Reproduced with kind permission from Central Statistics Office 1991.)

Case example 20.3 Care of the patient during an acute asthmatic attack

Simon, aged 14, was admitted to the ward at 10.00 p.m. He had a history of asthma since he was a little boy, but controlled the condition well using an inhaler. He was accompanied by his mother, who was a nurse, but has not practised for some time. Skin tests showed that Simon is allergic to the house dust mite. He looked anxious and pale and was having great difficulty in getting his breath. The houseman immediately gave intravenous hydrocortisone to reduce bronchial inflammation and thereby ease breathing.

The nurse's role in Simon's care will initially be to sit with him and his mother, giving them calm reassurance while the drug takes effect. Later on, by talking to the mother, the nurse may assess her understanding of her son's allergy and determine whether she has taken all possible steps to reduce Simon's contact with house dust mites.

Patients with endocrinological disorders

The endocrine disorder seen most commonly by the nurse in the medical area is diabetes mellitus. The individual with undiagnosed or uncontrolled diabetes may be admitted as an emergency, having fallen into a coma. A person with diagnosed diabetes may be admitted for an assessment to be made regarding the type and amount of insulin required. Increasingly, 'routine' diabetes care is taking place in the community, specialist nurses liaising with the GP and the consultant at the health centre. The nurse has the opportunity, both in hospital and in the community, to advise the patient on the self-care required to minimise the number and extent of complications.

Established diabetics may be admitted following the occurrence of an infection or as a result of acute problems caused by a miscalculation in diet, insulin intake and energy usage. Case example 20.4 provides an example of nursing care for a person with diabetes.

Patients with infectious diseases

Prior to the development of antibiotics and immunisation programmes, special hospitals, known as fever or isolation hospitals, were built to provide treatment for people with infectious diseases. There was also a 2-year nurse training

Case example 20.4 Care of the patient with newly diagnosed diabetes mellitis

Jean, 32, has just returned from a camping holiday with her husband and two small children. Whilst on holiday, she became thirsty and rather tired but attributed this to the hot weather. Her husband returned from his first day back at work to find her slumped in a chair, unconscious. She was admitted to the accident and emergency department of the local hospital, where diabetes mellitus was diagnosed. She was then transferred to the ward for treatment. Following an intravenous infusion of dextrose and insulin, she soon felt much better.

Initially, the nurse's role will be to monitor Jean's blood and urine glucose levels by taking blood samples and testing the urine. Care of the intravenous infusion, with the addition of glucose, will need to be carefully regulated. As Jean recovers, the nurse will need to explain how to adjust to living with diabetes. Jean will need to know how to administer her own injections, how to care for herself with respect to diet, weight and likely infections, and what to do when she has had insufficient glucose or insulin.

programme specifically designed to prepare nurses to care for people with a variety of these diseases, for example poliomyelitis, scarlet fever, whooping cough and tuberculosis. Today, a few of these units survive with modern facilities, but district hospitals can generally provide limited specialist facilities for those individuals presenting with lethal and little known viral infections, such as Marburg disease.

Nurses today are likely to encounter two highly infectious diseases: hepatitis B and HIV infection. The number of people carrying these infections is not fully known as, for ethical reasons, no national screening programme has been carried out. The increasing incidence of AIDS and HIV infection (Fig. 20.3) has had a great effect on society. Table 20.2 gives the number of cases reported during the 1990s in the UK and shows an overall increase. The number of people dying from AIDS has decreased owing to early treatment with Zidovudine, which appears to postpone the development of full-blown AIDS if given early following diagnosis. Its advantages, especially for later use, have, however, been questioned. Substantial DoH funding has been devoted to supporting AIDS and HIV prevention and care services, which are a priority area in the 1990s for all Regional Health Authorities.

HIV/AIDS was initially seen as a condition affecting the homosexual community, but its increasing occurrence in the heterosexual community has aroused public awareness. People with HIV/AIDS have often been treated like

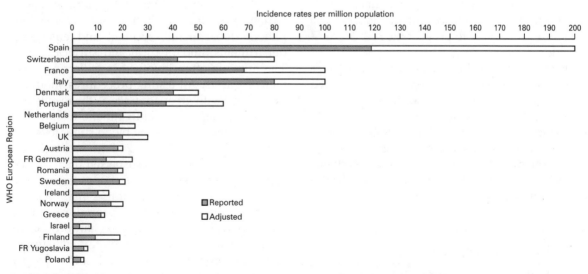

Figure 20.3 The AIDS incidence rates per million population in 1994, together with adjustments for reporting delays, in the 20 countries of the WHO European Region with the highest cumulative number of cases.

Table 20.2   Yearly trend in reports of HIV-1 infected persons:[1] Geographical area of reporting laboratories[2], United Kingdom to end March 1995. (From: PHLS AIDS Centre, Communicable Disease Surveillance Centre and Scottish Centre for Infection & Environmental Health. Unpublished Quarterly Surveillance Tables No 27, March 1995

Country and Region	Number of reports each year					
	1990	1991	1992	1993	1994	1995*
ENGLAND						
Northern & Yorkshire	87	72	105	62	92	28
Trent	83	41	78	86	57	28
Anglia & Oxford	58	90	100	104	93	26
North Thames	1119	1331	1125	1236	1244	389
South Thames	353	479	448	431	416	229
South & Western	97	99	116	72	148	56
West Midlands	92	65	89	80	72	17
North Western	92	93	161	107	81	22
WALES	67	33	46	38	45	8
NORTHERN IRELAND	12	15	17	12	7	8
SCOTLAND	138	161	143	162	155	50
TOTAL UK	2198	2479	2428	2390	2410	861
Isle of Man/Channel Islands	2	3	1	–	7	3

1. Newly confirmed tests of HIV-1 antibody positive persons reported to CDSC and SCIEH.
2. 412 laboratories sent anti HIV positive reports to CDSC or SCIEH.
*1st quarter only

lepers – a step back into the past – probably owing to the ignorance of the population (including nurses). Children who are HIV-positive have been banned from school and not allowed to play with their friends. In health care institutions, including acute hospitals, some employee groups, some nurses included, have demanded that HIV-positive patients be identified on all occasions. For a variety of reasons, this action is not practicable, and therefore nurses must practise standard procedures to prevent the risk of cross-infection.

Health care workers who are themselves known to be HIV-positive are sometimes treated uncaringly. Considerable resources have been expended to try to educate health care workers in caring for people with HIV/AIDS. There is, however, continuing evidence of ignorance and bias in the care of HIV-positive and AIDS clients among nurses and others working in the health care setting (Akinsanya & Rouse 1991).

TESTS, EXAMINATIONS AND THE ROLE OF THE NURSE

A medical diagnosis is made not only on the basis of readily apparent signs or symptoms, but also on the evidence of various physiological tests and examinations. Here, a knowledge of basic science helps the student to understand the reasons for certain tests and the significance of their results. The student nurse can put patients undergoing tests and examinations at ease, and explain both what to expect and the reasons for the investigations.

Tests and examinations take place in a wide variety of settings, including GP surgeries, outpatient departments, accident and emergency departments, and medical and surgical wards. The nurse is often involved in collecting specimens for tests. All testing procedures should be carried out with great accuracy as the results may determine diagnosis and treatment. Examples of such tests include a fasting blood sugar level in a patient with diabetes, a 24-hour collection of urine from a patient with suspected renal disease, or a collection of sputum specimens for bacteriological examination. The nurse may also be involved with more invasive procedures. In this case, she will be required to explain procedures to the patient and to provide comfort and support whilst the procedure, for example a liver biopsy, lumbar puncture, colonscopy or endoscopy, is being carried out by a doctor or technician.

The pathology department

The student will soon become familiar with the role of the pathology department. There are subdivisions within the department, such as chemical pathology (biochemistry), where analysis of blood and other body fluids can assess whether the components are within normal limits for the individual's age group. Biochemical testing may include measurement or analysis of any of the following:

- blood electrolyte levels (e.g. potassium, sodium, chloride and ammonium salts) to assess homeostasis
- blood urea levels as an indication of liver and kidney function
- blood levels of liver enzymes as an indicator of liver function
- blood levels of particular hormones to check the activity of the endocrine glands (e.g. in thyrotoxicosis)
- cardiac enzymes to check for damage to heart muscle
- cerebrospinal fluid to measure electrolyte levels and to check for infection (e.g. in meningitis).

The bacteriology department is concerned with the identification of micro-organisms (bacteria, viruses, yeasts, etc.) in the body as well as with controlling infection within hospitals. Specimens for the bacteriology department may include:

- urine
- faeces
- sputum
- swabs from wounds
- blood

and any other relevant body fluid to check for infection and to determine which antibiotics may be successful in fighting the disease.

Specimens will be sent from doctors' surgeries and health centres, as well as from inpatients on hospital wards.

SURGICAL NURSING

Surgical nursing is a rapidly changing area of care, with new techniques and technology reducing the trauma to the individual and therefore decreasing the amount of time required in hospital.

Some patients are admitted to surgical wards in the event of an emergency (e.g. acute appendicitis); others will be admitted from the waiting list (e.g. for varicose vein removal). Patients undergoing some operations previously with admission times of 10–14 days (e.g. removal of gallstones) can now expect to be discharged in 24–48 hours thanks to advances in surgical techniques and technology, for example keyhole surgery. This type of surgery is now increasingly available, reducing the need for major invasive techniques; examples are laparoscopic cholecystectomy and arthroscopic meniscectomy. Other patients can now be admitted for day surgery, for example for cataract removal, which previously warranted a 1–2 week admission.

These changes have resulted in a role change for both hospital and community nurses. For the hospital nurse, the high 'turnover' of people in the surgical ward means that the care will almost always be for 'high-dependency' patients, a great number of whom will require specialised nursing care. The nurse is therefore less able to build up a rapport with her patients. Conversely, the community nurse will have more 'dependent' patients in their own homes. This also has an effect on the family and friends of people following surgery.

Day surgery

Some of the types of operation being carried out as day cases include:

- minor ear, nose and throat operations, for example removal of nasal polyps
- minor gynaecological operations and investigations, for example dilation and curettage of the uterus (D&C) for heavy menstrual loss, ovarian cystectomy and tubal ligation (female sterilisation)
- herniorrhaphy – a simple hernia repair
- meniscectomy – removal of cartilages from the knee joint
- arthroscopy – an investigation, often carried out under local anaesthetic, of the structure of

- a joint (usually a major joint like the knee or elbow) to check for abnormality, lesions or inflammation
- abdominal surgery, for example laparoscopic cholecystectomy
- laser treatment, for example lithotripsy (shattering of stones, for instance in the kidney).

Common aspects of surgical nursing

General surgical nursing

Nurses working in surgical care have a vital role in preparing the patient, both physically and psychologically, for the impending operation, and for maintaining the person's safety throughout the procedure and following surgery. This includes offering emotional care, as well as supplying skilled and well-informed technical care (e.g. applying dressings, monitoring fluid balance and providing appropriate pain relief).

The most common operations encountered by the nurse on the surgical ward are abdominal or rectal. Among women, lumpectomy or mastec- tomy following a diagnosis of breast cancer is most common, this being the most common malignancy in women. It is estimated that one in 12 women in the UK will develop breast cancer at some stage of their lives (Cancer Research Campaign 1991). For this reason, women are advised to self-examine for breast abnormalities and to seek early advice. For men, prostate surgery is common for a variety of prostatic problems causing bladder outflow obstruction, resulting in difficulty in voiding urine. Some surgery can have a devastating effect upon the patient, especially when it results in a changed body image, as all the examples above show, or if a stoma is made. Case examples 20.5 and 20.6 give some indication of the role that the nurse caring for the adult plays for those having major surgery.

Orthopaedic nursing

Many orthopaedic injuries, such as minor fractures and soft tissue injuries, are dealt with in the

Case example 20.5 Care of the patient following mastectomy

Juliette is a 45-year-old nurse manager of a busy surgical unit. Having been a capable and innovative ward sister for a number of years at the same hospital, she is well respected by junior and senior staff. Following the discovery of a lump in her breast, a diagnosis of cancer is confirmed, and Juliette has been advised by the surgeon that a mastectomy is indicated. Juliette lives alone but has a number of friends.

If there is no specialist nurse available to help mastectomy patients, the nurse on the ward will fulfil this function. In any event, nursing intervention will include discussing with Juliette her hopes and fears and her reaction to taking on the role of a patient. This may include some consideration of the ways in which being in familiar surroundings is or is not a comfort. Involvement of a close friend in these conversations could be suggested.

Post-operatively, the nurse will be responsible for care of the drainage tube and the wound. At this time, she will need to be aware of Juliette's possible reaction to the scar and to a change in body image. The nurse should know what is available in the way of appliances and clothes for women who have had a mastectomy.

Case example 20.6 Care of the patient with a colostomy

John, a 45-year-old solicitor, is married and has two teenage children. He was diagnosed as having cancer of the rectum, and, in view of the pathology report, it was considered that the best treatment for him would be an abdominoperineal resection of the rectum, resulting in a permanent colostomy. The operation was successful, and John was soon discharged home. In the hospital, there was no stoma care nurse. The nurses seemed very busy, so he was reluctant to ask questions regarding caring for the colostomy.

The community nurse will need to show John how to attach his appliance and care for the skin surrounding the colostomy. Advice on diet should help to regulate the action of the colostomy so that John can confidently go out in public. He will need to know how to dispose of both the contents and the bag at home and in public places. He may be anxious about odour and should be advised on special deodorants. He may also wonder whether he can play sports and whether his sex life will be affected. The nurse will need to be able to assess and discuss such fears, and help John to regain sufficient confidence to enjoy sports and resume sexual relations with his wife. Helping the patient to regain confidence in these and other areas is perhaps the most important and rewarding aspect of stoma care nursing.

accident and emergency department, where there is usually a fracture clinic, and many nurses have become proficient in the making of plaster casts. This is a matter of some skill; plaster of Paris must hold the bone firmly enough to allow healing and regeneration, whilst not being so tight as to restrict the patient's circulation. Adult branch students are very likely to spend time in the accident and emergency/fracture clinic and/or the orthopaedic operating theatre, where there will be the opportunity to learn how to apply and care for plaster of Paris.

Patterns of treatment for orthopaedic patients have changed greatly since the 1980s. Newer designs of prosthesis, especially for the hip, have encouraged earlier mobilisation following hip replacement for fractured neck of femur or osteoarthritis. The use of surgical pins for the treatment of fractured femurs (for people following motoring or sporting injuries) has reduced the time spent in traction and therefore made possible greater freedom of movement, early mobilisation and a reduction in the length of stay in hospital. Here again, community nurses will have more dependent people in their care.

The operating theatre and the role of the nurse

In the pre-operative phase, the ward nursing staff ensure that patients are hygienically prepared and dressed in a theatre gown. The individual's consent for surgery form is completed and checked to confirm that it has been signed by the patient. Other important pre-operative procedures are carried out as indicated on a checklist that must be satisfactorily completed prior to the operation. A pre-medication is usually given to make the patient drowsy and to dry his mouth of any secretions.

The patient, on arriving in the operating theatre, is checked by the anaesthetic nurse, who is responsible for seeing the patient prior to the administration of the anaesthetic in order to explain what will happen and provide psychological support to allay any underlying anxieties. The nurse will remain with the patient until he is handed over to the care of the theatre nurse. The anaesthetic nurse will again be with the patient on his return from the theatre as he awakes after the operation. Recovery from anaesthetic is usually quiet and uneventful, but the patient requires constant monitoring and supervision from a qualified anaesthetic nurse.

Other nurses in the operating theatre department assist during the surgery, their prime responsibility being for the patient's safety. They also assist the surgeon, check swabs, anticipate the need for extra instruments, sutures and lotions, and ensure the correct positioning of the individual to avoid injury or damage whilst he is unable to fend for himself.

CRITICAL CARE NURSING

Critical care nursing usually takes place in specialised units, some of which are purpose-built, some of which stand alone within a hospital complex and others of which are incorporated in the main general hospital. The units include:

- intensive therapy units (ITUs)
- coronary care units (CCUs)
- spinal injury units
- burns units
- renal units
- neurosurgical units
- accident and emergency units.

Critical care nursing is that required by individuals both admitted as emergencies and transferred following major surgery or treatments. These units have high technical resources and specially trained staff to provide specialist care to patients and relatives during this critical time.

Nurses working in such units require specialist skills, including the ability to make quick decisions in life-threatening situations. They additionally require a high level of knowledge of physiology, psychology and sociology in order to judge patients' reactions to any given emergency. In dealing with the intricate equipment and in coping with critical situations, it is easy for the nurse to forget the patient as an individual, and that the immediate family are also affected. Researchers have considered the specific needs of patients in such situations, as well as the support required for nurses and other health care professionals working in such stressful

Case example 20.7 Critical care nursing of a tracheostomy patient (Contributed by Pamela Taylor)

Anthony, a 38-year-old builder's labourer, fell 30 ft from some scaffolding, sustaining multiple fractures and a subdural haematoma. Initially, he was intubated and attached to a ventilator so that his respiratory function could be monitored. After 1 week, he was breathing spontaneously, but as access to his chest was still required to remove secretions, a tracheostomy was performed.

Some of the main aspects of Anthony's care related to the tracheostomy. He still required oxygen; this was humidified and supplied through an adaptor set connected to the tracheostomy tube. Regular suction was required to remove secretions. Anthony initially produced large amounts of infected secretions, which were greenish in colour and very tenacious. The observations of the nurse were critical at all times. Anthony's neurological and chest condition improved following a course of antibiotics; subsequently, the tracheostomy tube was changed. As his blood oxygen levels began to improve, he no longer required oxygen. When Anthony's swallowing reflex returned, he was tempted with fluids and a little soft diet. As this was successful, his tracheostomy tube was closed off for short periods until he was finally breathing on his own.

In Anthony's case, the physical nursing care required initially took priority over psychological and social care. Care was concentrated on establishing and sustaining respiration. Correct administration of oxygen and knowledge of the nursing skills required in caring for a tracheostomy were essential. The nursing model chosen to guide care reflected this priority in needs.

areas (Melia 1977). Case example 20.7 describes a possible scenario in critical care nursing.

It is usual for nurses working in critical care areas to undertake further specialist education in both the personal and technical aspects of their work. In every situation the 'adult nurse' should consider the personalised care needed for the very ill person and his immediate family.

Rehabilitation nursing

Adults

Those within the adult care group who require rehabilitation range from the young person severely injured in a road traffic accident to the older person recovering from a cerebrovascular accident (stroke). Some hospitals have specific rehabilitation wards that concentrate facilities and staff (including doctors, physiotherapists, speech and occupational therapists and social workers) in encouraging patients to achieve maximum independence in the activities of living.

The adult nurse working in rehabilitation requires wide-ranging skills. Improved aids and heightened public recognition of the needs of the disabled person make this an interesting and challenging area of care. The nurse is very much part of the team helping the individual regain mobility and independence, and is often the only continuing link with all the involved professionals and others who are giving care.

Experts in the area of rehabilitation believe that this begins as soon as the patient is admitted, initially to prevent complications (such as pressure sores, joint stiffness and nutritional deficits) and subsequently to promote active recovery. Most adults requiring health care need some form of rehabilitation to recover 'normal' levels of activity, but specialist units exist to help those more severely disabled. Case example 20.8 is an illustration of a younger individual requiring rehabilitation.

The Elderly

Older patients who need rehabilitation vary in their requirements. Help may be required

Case example 20.8   Rehabilitation of the patient with severe head injury

Tim is a 24-year-old computer programmer who was admitted to the intensive care unit following a road traffic accident in which he sustained severe head injuries. After 6 weeks, he has been transferred to the rehabilitation ward. At this stage, Tim is still relatively immobile, but is continent and has begun to eat a soft diet. He initiates some movement with his left side and understands everything that is said to him. However, he is dysphasic (unable to speak), which obviously makes him very frustrated.

In contrast to that of the patient in Case example 20.7, the focus of Tim's care has shifted away from basic physical needs. The nurse's role will now be to help him as he regains independence in self-care, recovers communicative skills and addresses his psychological and social needs.

following illness or to prevent general deterioration by keeping the mind and body active in leading a more purposeful and meaningful life. One of the common causes of acute disability in elderly people is cerebrovascular accident (stroke). The rehabilitation of those affected by a stroke presents one of the major and most complex challenges to adult branch nurses (Case example 20.9).

Case example 20.9 Care of the dysphasic stroke patient

Joseph is 75 years old. He has been married for 30 years, has two children and two grandchildren, and is now retired from self-employment as a carpenter. He was diagnosed 10 days ago as having had a cerebrovascular accident, which has left him with weakness in his left arm and difficulty in speaking. He is finding communicating very frustrating. His wife says that he is an extremely private and independent person. Unfortunately, he now finds himself unable to eat, drink or attend to his toilet needs without assistance.

The nurse's role will be to help Joseph to regain some degree of independence in the activities of daily living. In planning a programme of care with him, the nurse can take the opportunity to establish a communication system with Joseph, for example a keywords board with which he can indicate his needs. Enhancing the patient's ability to communicate is arguably the most important and challenging aspect of caring for stroke victims, and one in which patience is paramount. Time and gentleness are required to give Joseph long enough to gesticulate and make sounds; the temptation to speak for him or to make swift assumptions about what he wants must be resisted. The patient must never be treated like a child or like someone who is incapable of understanding. He will be desperately frustrated and anguished and must be given time to express himself. He requires everything that is best in nursing.

Terminal care nursing

Students nurses will be involved in caring for people of all ages who are dying. This terminal care requires a nurse who can communicate empathetically and who can relate to all health care professionals caring for dying patients and their families, whether this be at home, in hospital or in a hospice. Terminally ill people frequently have a fear of pain and discomfort, which can be relieved by careful management and liaison between health care professionals. The nurse needs to relate to the individual's relatives and friends, who will also be affected by the nature of the process (see Ch. 19).

COMMUNITY CARE

It is recognised that hospital care is extremely expensive and is not always cost-effective. Accordingly, and as recommended by the Cumberlege Report (Department of Health 1986), resources and the emphasis of care have been shifting to the community setting. Following the Community Care Act (1989) the number of clients being cared for in the community is therefore rising, and the demand for more community nurses increasing.

The nurse working in the community needs to be skilled in offering care and must be able to make decisions without the support system found in the acute hospital setting. Patients are being discharged home earlier from these acute settings, and, as Case example 20.10 shows, the nurse is then required to liaise with other professionals in the community. Nurses working in hospitals have a responsibility to ensure safe discharge from an acute setting to the community, so discharge planning and liaison between the professionals involved is of paramount importance.

Practice nurses are also found within health centres and GP surgeries, functioning as part of the primary health care team. These nurses may also have a role in running their own clinics, dealing with, for example:

- asthma
- diabetes
- hypertension

and liaising with the other staff to provide a total local service to the community. Part of the role of all nurses is to provide health promotion towards a fitter Britain by advocacy, empowerment and community participation (Department of Health 1990). Those working in the community are in an ideal position to use such approaches.

Case example 20.10 Care in the community

Sylvia, who is 82 years old, suffered a fracture to the neck of her left femur whilst out shopping with Fred, her 84-year-old husband. She was admitted to hospital as an emergency and underwent a total hip replacement.

Two weeks after the operation, she was due to be discharged home to Fred's care. Fred is not as nimble as he used to be, and before the accident Sylvia undertook all of the domestic chores, including cooking, cleaning and washing for them both. They live in a three-bedroom, two-storey terraced house. Before breaking her leg, Sylvia was able to climb the stairs quite easily, which is important because their only toilet is upstairs in the bathroom. She now has restricted movement, which, hopefully, should improve over the next few months.

Their only child, Doreen, lives some 80 miles away. She herself is a widowed grandmother who suffers from arthritis and does not drive, so visits to her parents are infrequent. The Social Services department was informed of Sylvia's admission and was able to begin plans for her discharge. These have included involving the occupational therapist and the community nurse in a joint visit to Fred to assess the facilities available for Sylvia on her

return home. This assessment will include discussions with Fred about facilities, including the assistance and equipment that may be available to help Sylvia to achieve a level of activity enabling them to remain in the home where they have lived for most of their married life.

The community nurse's care plan will be in part based on the joint assessment of the home situation and Sylvia's current ability. Depending on her level of mobility, it may be necessary to move a bed downstairs, along with a commode, to enable Sylvia to carry out her usual activities of living. If she is mobile enough, and has sufficient confidence, it may be realistic to provide a commode downstairs with Sylvia sleeping upstairs and using the bathroom as usual and only using the stairs in the morning and evening, gradually increasing the frequency of this as she progresses. A care assistant may be provided by the Social Services department to help Sylvia in and out of the bath; this help may extend to assisting with shopping and the preparation of meals, depending upon local policies. The community nurse may wish to liaise with others and to monitor the family situation, gradually withdrawing as independence is regained.

CURRENT ISSUES AND DEVELOPMENTS WITHIN ADULT NURSING

GROWING PUBLIC AWARENESS OF ENTITLEMENT

The general public has a growing awareness of their rights in relation to all aspects of health care. People are now less inclined to accept excuses when a service is below standard; individuals are more likely to question unsatisfactory situations and demand remedial action. This awareness will continue to grow, and the Patients' Charter, introduced in 1991, will ensure that all health care professionals work towards maintaining the individual's rights. There is increasing confidence in using established systems to ensure that rights are upheld and maintained. This aspect is explained in more detail in Chapter 13. Aspects of the UKCC Code of Conduct help to guide nurses to ensure individuals' rights to high-quality care.

The nurse is frequently the first person to be confronted with a complaint and must be sure that the client is provided with the right information on how to pursue the matter.

PRIMARY NURSING: A NAMED NURSE

The policy set out in the Patient's Charter of assigning a named nurse to each individual patient to coordinate care is already causing considerable debate within the profession and is being implemented by managers and individual nurses. Nursing care within the hospital has to be adapted to the increased rate of occupancy on the acute wards. The reduced turn-round time after surgery will require nurses in the community to adapt their care accordingly. All nurses involved in the patient's care must ensure that they do not feel that they are on a medical conveyor belt, however abbreviated the hospital stay. Maintaining standards of personalised, individual care in the face of changes in health care policy presents a major challenge to the nurse.

DEVELOPMENTS IN CARE FOR THE ELDERLY

More attention is now being paid to the specific care required by elderly patients (Wright 1988). Pioneering work in this area of practice, carried out at Burford Hospital in Oxford and at the Oxford Nursing Development Unit, has shown a new way forward (Pearson 1988).

Elderly patients may be admitted to either medical or surgical wards for assessment. These patients often present with multiple pathology, for example diabetes with hypertension and anaemia. New techniques in anaesthesia and a reduction in operating times have enabled more elderly patients to undergo anaesthesia without undue risk.

An increasing number of elderly people are now living to their late 80s and into their 90s. At this stage, the body is frail and sight may be failing; reading and watching television may not be possible, and nights may run into days. Some individuals feel at this age that they are a burden to society and see little point in living. Thus, the very elderly perhaps have different needs from those who are 10 years younger and able to be a little more active. Specialist nurses can adapt programmes of care to meet the needs of each age group. All students will spend time working with elderly patients and should take every opportunity to discover the creative and exciting programmes of care that have made caring for the older person such a rewarding area of nursing.

FUTURE TRENDS IN ADULT CARE

The UK has an ageing population. The incidence of chronic illness will increase at the same time as the number of the supporting younger population decreases. These trends will lead to ever-increasing demands on the health care system, and it is important for nurses to become involved in planning for the change in health care provision that will inevitably come.

As discussed earlier, these changes will lead to an increase in care in the community (Department of Health 1986, Community Care Act 1990). The nurse practitioner will need the skills to meet the needs of people in the community and to assist in meeting the 'Health of the Nation' targets (1989). The government has set targets for quality of care in both institutional and community settings, as laid down by the White Paper 'Caring for People' (Department of Health 1990) and the 'Patient's Charter' (Department of Health 1991). Nurses will therefore need to maintain and develop criteria for care for people in need of assistance, which must reflect that the nurse is working with other members of the health care team.

Summary

The greatest number of nurses in practice care for adults – those who are over 16 years of age – although this branch of care encompasses many different specialties and sub-specialties. In all of these areas, however, the nurse's role will be one of preventing ill-health and assisting in the recovery from disease, acting as an educator, supporter and facilitator of both patients and their families, and meeting their physical and psychological needs in the context of their personal environment.

Care of adults takes place in a variety of settings, ranging from hospitals and health centres to the patient's own home, and encompasses a wide age range, from the teenager to the person in his 90s. The nurse must indeed be flexible to cope with all the different situations.

The main adult care groups are those requiring medical nursing, surgical nursing, critical care and infection nursing, rehabilitation and elderly care, and these are introduced in the text.

The nurse caring for adults will also need to be aware of several areas of current concern, for example the public awareness of entitlement, primary nursing and developments in care of the elderly.

The wide variety of patient needs and the rapid changes in the context of health care make care of adults a challenging and satisfying branch of nursing.

REFERENCES

Akinsanya J, Rouse P 1991 Who will care? A survey of the knowledge and attitudes of hospital nurses to people with AIDS. Health and Social Work Research Centre, Anglia Polytechnic, Chelmsford, Essex
Central Statistics Office 1991 Social trends 21, 1991 edn. Governmental Statistical Service. HMSO, London
Department of Health 1986 Neighbourhood nursing: a focus for care (Report of the Community Nursing Review; The Cumberlege Report). HMSO, London

Department of Health 1990 On the state of the public health for the year of 1990. HMSO, London

Department of Health 1991 The patient's charter: raising the standard. HMSO, London

Department of Health 1992 Health of the nation: a strategy for health in England. Command Paper 1986. HMSO, London

Melia K H 1977 The intensive care unit: a stress situation. Nursing Times Occasional Paper 73 (5): 17–20

Pearson A 1988 Primary nursing: nursing in the Burford and Oxford Development Units. Chapman & Hall, London

Wright S 1988 Nursing the older patient. Harper & Row, London

FURTHER READING

Alexander M F, Fawcett J N, Runciman P J (eds) 1994 Nursing Practice: hospital and home – the adult. Churchill Livingstone, Edinburgh

Boore R P, Champion R, Ferguson M C (eds) 1987 Nursing the physically ill adult: a textbook of medical–surgical nursing. Churchill Livingstone, Edinburgh

Brunner L, Suddarth D S 1990 Lippincott manual of medical–surgical nursing. Harper & Row, London

Ehrenfield M, Cheifetz F R 1990 Cardiac nurses: coping with stress. Journal of Advanced Nursing 15: 1002–1008

Fromant P 1988 Coping with stress: helping each other. Nursing Times 84 (36):

Game C, Anderson R, Kidd J 1989 Medical–surgical nursing. Churchill Livingstone, Melbourne

Lewis K S 1987 Successful living with chronic illness. Avery, New York

Long B C, Phipps W J, Cassmeyer V (eds) 1995 Adult nursing: a nursing process approach. Mosby, London

McHenry C 1991 Silent suffering. Nursing Times 87(46): 21

National Association of Theatre Nurses 1983 Code of Practice

Orem D E 1985 Nursing concepts of practice. McGraw Hill, New York

Trevelyan J, Dawson D, West R 1989 Thorson's guide to medical tests. Thorson's, Wellingborough

Walsh M 1990 Accident and emergency nursing: a new approach. Heinemann, London

Wright S 1989 Changing nursing practice. Edward Arnold, London

21

Children

Sally Huband

There are currently 15 million children and adolescents under the age of 19 years in the UK. These young people have the right to be given appropriate care so that they may achieve their full potential; any health deficit must be identified and, where possible, eliminated or minimised. This chapter aims to:

- outline the developmental stages of childhood and adolescence
- discuss patterns of childhood illness and the principles of providing health care for this special group of patients
- examine the role of the sick children's nurse, both in hospital and in the community, considering also the nurse's particular input to the care of adolescents and of children with special needs.

We are guilty of many errors and many faults, but our worst crime is abandoning the children, neglecting the fountain of life. Many of the things we need can wait. The child cannot.
Right now is the time his bones are being formed, his blood is being made and his senses are being developed.
To him we cannot answer 'Tomorrow'.
His name is 'Today'.

Gabriela Mistral (Nobel Prize-winning poet from Chile)

So starts an excellent little book 'My Name is Today' by David Morley and Hermione Lovel. The book is described as an illustrated discussion of child health, society and poverty in less developed countries. The book has much to offer health professionals in the UK who are concerned with maximising the health and potential of children. It is an apt reminder that poverty is the single largest cause of ill-health, and that access to primary health and preventive medicine are crucial factors in improving the quality of children's lives, wherever they reside.

CHILDREN AND ADOLESCENTS

Most literature concerned with the health needs of children will categorise them into age groups for clarification and specific features.

Pre-natal period

The period from conception to birth is further subdivided into:

- embryonic – from conception to 8 weeks of development
- foetal – from 8 weeks to birth.

The outcome of this period depends on the health and well-being of the mother, and is a crucial factor in determining the health of the new-born baby.

The infant or baby

This stage lasts from birth to 12 months of age. It also has a subdivision, the neonatal period, when most major congenital abnormalities become apparent, which is the time from birth to 28 days old. Inherited disorders such as cystic fibrosis or sickle cell anaemia may not manifest themselves until later in the first year of life.

These classifications are important when discussing mortality and morbidity factors in childhood. The peri-natal mortality rate refers to the mortality rate of the infant in utero, during birth and during the neonatal period. The infant mortality rate refers to the mortality rate during the first year of life.

During this period, which is a period of rapid motor, emotional and social development, the child is totally dependent on the carer.

Early childhood

Early childhood is the time from 1 to 5 years of age. The period is further subdivided into:

- the toddler – 1 to 3 years of age
- the pre-school child – 3 to 5 years.

Over this time the child continues to develop rapidly. During the toddler period, he will learn to master the gross motor skills of walking and running. Language development is constant, progressing from single words to simple sentences. The child is still very dependent on his main carer but begins to develop some independence and will test this out by challenging authority. He is also learning social skills of feeding himself, dressing himself and becoming toilet trained. Play is a crucial factor in assisting the child to attain these skills, but at this stage play is usually solitary or parallel, when he plays alongside other children, but not with them.

During the pre-school years, many children will attend play groups or nursery schools. They will be learning to spend time away from their main carer and to make friends of their own age. Their play becomes more interactive, and they will begin to follow simple rules. These rules are, however, often adapted to meet the needs of the players. Play is creative and imaginative, and children do not need expensive toys to facilitate their play.

School-age child, or middle childhood

This period is from 5 to 11 or 12 years of age.

During this time, the child learns to become increasingly independent. Cognitive development is rapid, and the child spends much of his time either at school or with his friends. He has to learn the social skills that enable him to relate to his peer group and to adults other than his immediate family. Play will often involve others and require rules that cannot be changed to suit the individual. Children have to learn to be good losers, and they begin to realise that life is not always fair. They are also learning the difference between right and wrong, and will develop a moral conscience.

Adolescence, or later childhood

This is sometimes divided into the pre-pubertal stage and adolescence, and covers the period from 11 or 12 until 18 years old.

The age of onset of puberty varies considerably, and this variation can itself cause much distress to individual children. The child has to adjust to a rapidly changing physique and learn to cope with the emotional turmoil that often accompanies this stage. The transition from child to adult has not been assisted by the complexity of the law in the UK, which gives different messages to young people as to their status as adults. For instance:

• A boy can join the armed forces, with his parents' consent, at the age of 16, but he cannot vote until he is 18.
• Boys and girls can marry at 16, with their parents' consent, but they cannot buy an alcoholic drink in a pub until they are 18 years old.

Many parents find the adolescent years the most challenging of all. At this stage there may be a breakdown in communication that is often to do with the confusion of the adolescent as he struggles to establish his own identity. He may act as a child one minute and an adult the next. The parent may also be unsure of how to give the adolescent the freedom to develop his own personality and identity, yet protect him from the perceived dangers of drugs, alcohol and crime. Society tends to have a very negative approach to the teenager and adolescent, which is not usually justified. In some societies there is a 'rite of passage' which enables the child to gain acceptance as an adult at a specific time on a specific day. This may lessen the confusion over the expectations and roles of the individual child.

 Activity 21.1

Sit down with some friends and ask them to write down as many words or phrases that they can think of associated with 'teenager' or 'adolescent'.

As a group, go through these and identify the ones that give positive messages and the ones that give negative ones. You will probably find that most of the messages are negative.

Ask the group how they saw their own adolescence. What ages do they think covered their own adolescence? Were they happy during this time? Were they easy as adolescents? What were the major difficulties they faced? Do they think they are now fully adult? It may be useful to ask them to check with their parents whether they have the same perception of their adolescence as their parents do.

HISTORICAL PERSPECTIVES OF CHILDHOOD

Children during the 19th century were valued more for their economic contribution to the family economics than for themselves. The same picture is seen in the developing countries today. A child in a developing country will start work at about the age of 7 years, helping with the care of the animals. By the time he is 15 years old, he will have repaid his family for the investment they have made in him (Morley & Lovel 1986). During the Industrial Revolution, children in the UK were exploited, working long hours for minimal wages, in the same way that children in developing countries still are. The fate of poor children, who were employed in the cotton mills, the mines or as chimney sweeps, has been well documented by popular novelists such as

Charles Dickens. Only relatively recently have children become valued for their intrinsic worth.

However the UK remains an adult-orientated society, compared with some of the continental countries that are more child centred. In January 1995, the United Nations (UN), following an audit on children's rights in Britain, found the British government to be failing children in almost every aspect of their lives. It is not only government policies that often fail children: architects design housing estates with few facilities for children, restaurants often fail to provide suitable seating or meals, and parents with small children will struggle on and off public transport without help.

 Activity 21.2

Visit your local town and observe adults and small children in their day-to-day activities.

- Is the housing suitable for families with small children? Do some families live in high rise blocks, and, if so, where is the play area?
- Can families reach play areas without crossing busy main roads?
- Do children have to play in the streets?
- Observe families at bus stops – is there any help for the parent with small children and shopping when getting on and off?
- How tolerant are other adults of small children?
- Are the local shops and restaurants geared towards small children?
- What are the toilet facilities like?
- Spend half a day in town with a small child and see how you fare – what would you like to change?

Compare facilities for and attitudes to small children in this country and in a more child-centred country, such as France, Italy or Spain. If you have not visited one yourself, ask a friend who has.

CHANGES IN PATTERNS OF CHILDREN'S HEALTH AND ILLNESS SINCE THE 19TH CENTURY

Children's health has improved dramatically over the past 100 years. This is mainly due to changes in social conditions and public health measures, such as the availability of clean water, disposal of sewage, changes in agriculture and an im-provement in transport systems that has led to better nutrition. In England and Wales, the infant mortality rate (IMR) stood at 150 per thousand live births in 1900. This had fallen to 50 per thousand in 1943, and currently stands at 7.4 per thousand (Office of Population Censuses and Surveys 1989, 1991). In addition, in the 1850s, a further 40 children per thousand died between the ages of 1 and 19. In 1990, the mortality rate of the 1–19-year-olds stood at 0.03% of the population of that age group (Office of Population Censuses and Surveys 1991). Children died from malnutrition and infectious and diarrhoeal diseases, a similar pattern to that found in developing countries today. Diseases such as tuberculosis and rheumatic fever were common. Polio led to many children being crippled for life. Although these diseases have not been eradicated, they are rare, with the exception of tuberculosis, which is still a problem in some areas of the UK.

Current mortality and morbidity

Child mortality has fallen steadily and continues to fall. However, poverty remains a significant factor as a cause of death and ill-health. The overall IMR is currently 7.4 per thousand live births: that for social class I is 6 per thousand, whereas that for social class V is 10 per thousand (Office of Population Censuses and Surveys 1992).

During the neonatal period, the most common causes of death are prematurity, congenital abnormalities and respiratory disease. One in every 20 live babies is born with an abnormality, 50% of which are classified as major abnormalities. The most common cause of death between the ages of 1 month and 1 year is sudden infant death syndrome (SIDS). Following the government's 'Back to Sleep' campaign, there was a fall of 46% in the numbers of deaths between January and June 1992 (Office of Population Censuses and Surveys 1992). The campaign encouraged mothers to nurse their infants on their backs, to avoid smoking, to breastfeed and to ensure that the babies did not become overheated.

Although many diseases in children have decreased over the past years, some are on the increase, the most significant rise being in the number of children presenting with asthma. One in every 7 children now suffers from asthma, an increase of 9.4% from 1964 to 1989 (Ninan & Russell, 1992). Diabetes in children is also becoming more common. In 1956, the incidence in 10–11-year-olds was 10 per 100 000; by 1968, this had risen to 60 cases per 100 000 and in 1980, to 180 per 100 000. (Nabarro 1988). Children's wards are also admitting significant numbers of children with cancer and leukaemia. The prognosis has improved significantly, but many children require periods in hospital for treatment. Genetic disorders are another significant cause of childhood morbidity. The gene responsible for cystic fibrosis was discovered in the 1980s. Cystic fibrosis is the most common serious inherited disease, 1 in 20 of the population carrying the defective gene and the condition having an incidence of 1 in 2000 births. Children affected with cystic fibrosis also have an improved prognosis nowadays, but most of them will require a stay in hospital to treat their respiratory infections or improve their nutritional status.

Children and accidents

After the age of 1 year, the most common cause of death for all age groups is accidents. Not only are they a significant cause of death, but they can also result in permanent disability.

About 700 children die each year from accidents, and a further 2 million attend an accident and emergency department (Levene 1992). The developmental age of the child is often a factor in determining the type of accident. Young children are usually being cared for at home, and therefore suffer accidents that occur within the home, such as poisonings, burns and scalds, and falls. As the child gets older, he is exposed to a wider environment, and the most common cause of death is that of the child pedestrian who is involved in a traffic accident. The prevention of accidents to children has been targeted in the government report 'Health of the Nation' (Department of Health 1992). The aim is to reduce the number of deaths in the under-15s by at least one third by the year 2000.

CHANGES IN THE PROVISION OF HEALTH CARE FOR CHILDREN

Prior to the 19th century, sick children were kept at home with their families. It was recognised that separating them from their mothers was detrimental to their psychological well-being, and admission to adult hospitals ran the risk of cross-infection.

However, in the mid-19th century the first children's hospital, Great Ormond Street, was founded by Dr Charles West. This was quickly followed by the foundation of children's hospitals in Brighton and Manchester. The number of children admitted to hospital increased, and many hospitals allocated specific wards for the care of children. Provision for parents to stay or visit their sick child was not, however, made. Children were separated from their parents, often for long periods, with only minimal visiting hours. It was felt that parental visiting only upset the child, and that children would settle more quickly without contact with their parents. In fever hospitals, it was common for children to be nursed in single rooms, by nurses wearing gowns and masks, and to have no contact with their parents until they were fit for discharge.

It was only gradually that it was recognised that children were suffering as a result of this deprivation of parental comfort. The Platt Report in 1959, the work of John Bowlby and other psychologists, and the formation of the pressure group the National Association for the Welfare of Children in Hospital (NAWCH) led to changes in the way in which children were treated. Further reports, such as the Court Report (DHSS 1976) emphasised that, wherever possible, children should be treated at home and that hospital admissions should be kept short. The volume of day surgery increased, and the report 'Just for the Day' (NAWCH 1991) emphasised the need for children to have specific facilities available to them.

WORKING TOWARDS A SEAMLESS SERVICE

Recent reports have emphasised the need for children and families, whether they are in the community or in hospital, to receive continuity of care. In 1991, the British Paediatric Association published a report 'Towards a Combined Health Service', the main conclusions of which were as follows:

1. When children are well they need a service that:

- enables their parents and families to protect them from disease and environmental hazards and to promote their good health
- is performed by professionals who are sensitive to the special needs of children of all ages
- provides counselling for parents and young people appropriate to their understanding, sensitivities, background and culture
- acts to create a safe, healthy environment

2. When they are ill, children need a service that:

- ensures that their parents know when to seek help and how to find it
- provides 24-hour access in emergencies
- supports parents in their care of their children
- is provided by staff who are trained in the care of children of all ages
- provides hospital care according to Department of Health guidance.

The report advocated that hospital and community services for children should be combined and managed together. Although there has been much support, the implementation is less easy, as hospitals and community services are often managed by different NHS Trusts. Further reports on current services include 'Bridging the Gaps', produced in 1993 by Caring for Children in the Health Services, and 'Children First', a study of hospital services published in 1993 by the Audit Commission. This latter report suggested that there were six key areas that should underpin children's hospital services:

1. Child- and family-centred care.
2. Specially skilled staff.
3. Separate facilities.
4. Effective treatments.
5. Appropriate hospitalisation.
6. Strategic commissioning.

The need for a seamless service is illustrated by the following case example.

Case example 21.1

Lucy is 3 weeks old and is seen by her health visitor at home. The health visitor is concerned that Lucy weighs less than she did at birth. She asks Lucy's mother to bring her to the surgery the following day to be seen by the GP. The GP takes a history from Lucy's mother and then examines the baby. He is not satisfied with her condition and rings the local hosptial to arrange admission. Lucy is admitted to the local hospital under the care of a paediatrician. Her mother is able to be resident with her, and all investigations and treatment are explained to her. Lucy is found to have a chronic condition, which means that she will need careful monitoring. She is discharged from hospital after 2 weeks, and a letter is sent to her GP. The liaison health visitor, who works in the hospital, contacts Lucy's own health visitor and asks her to visit the family the next day, as Lucy's mother is still quite apprehensive. Lucy is followed up regularly by the health visitor and GP and also attends the hospital for outpatient appointments with the paediatrician. Following each outpatient appointment, a letter is sent to the GP outlining the treatment that Lucy is receiving. Lucy's mother knows that she can telephone the surgery and make an appointment to see her GP if she is worried about the baby.

CHILDREN'S NURSING

Children's nursing has seen major developments since the 1960s and paediatric nurses can be proud of their record in being in the forefront of humanising hospitals. Children's wards have been among the first to encourage free visiting for relatives and to ensure that children are able to wear their own clothes whilst in hospital. Most paediatric units have abolished the wearing of caps by nurses, and, in some units, traditional uniforms are being discarded in favour of less threatening outfits, which are likely to be more familiar to young children.

These changes have been introduced as paediatric nurses have continued to explain that 'children are not small adults' and have physical, psychological and social needs different from those of adults. Paediatric philosophies of care have been affected by the work of major psychologists and also by major reports, such as the Platt Report (Ministry of Health 1959) and the Court Report (DHSS 1976). They have also been influenced by the list of Children's Rights drawn up by the United Nations in 1987 and finally adopted by the British government in 1991 (Box 21.1).

Box 21.1 United Nations Declaration of the Rights of the Child (abbreviated)

1. The right to equality, regardless of race, colour, religion, sex or nationality.
2. The right to healthy mental and physical development.
3. The right to a name and nationality.
4. The right to sufficient food, housing and medical care.
5. The right to special care if handicapped.
6. The right to love, understanding and care.
7. The right to free education, play and recreation.
8. The right to immediate aid in the event of disasters and emergencies.
9. The right to protection from cruelty, neglect and exploitation.
10. The right to protection from persecution and to an upbringing in the spirit of worldwide brotherhood and peace.

The National Association for the Welfare of Children in Hospital (which is now Action for Sick Children) has also worked with professionals to improve the care and facilities for children in hospital. In 1985, it produced a charter for children in hospital (Box 21.2), which has now been adopted in many European countries.

THE ROLE OF THE CHILDREN'S NURSE

Children who require health care have the right to have their parents with them at all times,

---

Box 21.2 NAWCH Charter for Children in Hospital

1. Children shall be admitted to hospital only if the care they require cannot be equally well provided at home or on a day basis.
2. Children in hospital shall have the right to have their parents with them at all times provided that this is in the best interests of the child. Accommodation should therefore be offered to all parents, and they should be helped and encouraged to stay. In order to share in the care of their child, parents should be fully informed about ward routine and their active participation encouraged.
3. Children and/ or parents shall have the right to information appropriate to age and understanding.
4. Children and/or parents shall have the right to informed participation in all decisions involving their health care. Every child shall be protected from unnecessary medical treatment and steps taken to mitigate physical or emotional distress.
5. Children shall be treated with tact and understanding and at all times their privacy shall be respected.
6. Children shall enjoy the care of appropriately trained staff, fully aware of the physical and emotional needs of each age group.
7. Children shall be able to wear their own clothes and have their own personal possessions.
8. Children shall be cared for with other children of the same age group.
9. Children shall be in an environment furnished and equipped to meet their requirements, and which conforms to recognised standards of safety and supervision.
10. Children shall have full opportunity for play, recreation and education suited to their age and condition.

---

unless it is not in their best interests. Paediatric nursing care is therefore family centred, and the paediatric nurse needs to work with the whole family in order to meet the needs of the sick child. Children are dependent on adults even when they are well, and parents can be encouraged to give the day-to-day care that they would give their child at home. In addition, parents can be taught by the paediatric nurse to give more specialised care. The complexity of care that the parents give should be decided by the parents and the nurse together. Initially, the parents might require teaching in specific areas and then support from the nurse in giving the care. The benefits of the parents remaining the main carer are that:

- the child is likely to feel more secure when cared for by a familiar person
- the parents can contribute to the well-being of the child and can support him when he needs them most
- the parents' ability to undertake much of the care can contribute to an early discharge for the child.

This approach has led to the development of paediatric models of care.

Paediatric nursing models

Most nursing models have been written with adults in mind and, in their pure form, are unsuited to caring for children. The unique relationship between the nurse, the parent and the child needs to be acknowledged in order for the care to be appropriately planned and implemented. The parent should also be involved in the evaluation of the care, and, if the child is old enough, he will also be involved in this evaluation.

Casey (1988) has developed a paediatric nursing model that centres around the partnership of the child and his family with the paediatric nurse. (Fig. 21.1). This model can be used in conjunction with other nursing models, making them more applicable to paediatric nursing. The model is flexible and enables the relationship between the nurse and family to be adjusted according to the nursing needs of the sick child and the proficiency of the parents as carers.

Primary nursing for children

Primary nursing is in its infancy but has much to recommend it for paediatric nursing. Research has demonstrated the benefits of the continuity afforded by this approach (Spitz & Wolf 1946, Ainsworth & Bell 1970, Bowlby 1971). Any model of nursing that reduces the trauma of hospitalisation for the child is to be recommended. Primary nursing is also consistent with the Patient's Charter and the concept of the named nurse.

The children's nurse will need to have the knowledge, skills and attitudes to care for children in a variety of settings. Some of these are illustrated in Case example 21.2.

Paediatric nursing can therefore be seen to be a *partnership* between the nurse and the parent. The parents should be encouraged to be involved as much as they wish but must never be unsupported. The nurse is responsible and accountable for the care given. When the parent is not able or does not wish to be involved, the nurse takes over the parental role and is responsible for the provision of the physical and psychological care of the child. She is responsible for seeing that all his needs are met, and will liaise with other health professionals to meet his play and educational requirements.

CARING FOR CHILDREN IN THE COMMUNITY

Parents are responsible for the care of their children, and members of the primary health care team work with families to maximise the health of all children.

The health visitor

The health visitor is responsible, in conjunction with the GP, for monitoring growth, carrying out developmental assessments and encouraging families to have their children immunised. The health visitor also has a key role in health

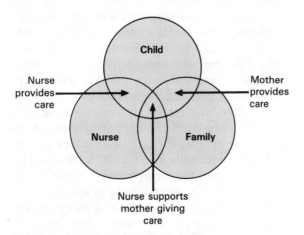

Fig. 21.1 A family-centred model of care

Case example 21.2

Emma was born with an imperforate anus and went to theatre at the age of 24 hours for the formation of a colostomy, which she will need until she is old enough to have special surgery. She is Simon and Jane's first baby and is being cared for on the neonatal unit. Jane wished to breastfeed Emma but needed help to get feeding established, as, to begin with, Emma had an intravenous infusion. Both Simon and Jane were initially frightened of caring for Emma's colostomy.

In the initial stages, the paediatric nurse needed to be able to observe Emma closely, as she had had an anaesthetic and could have developed respiratory problems. Because of her age, she is vulnerable to cold and infection. There could also be problems with the colostomy, and the nurse needed to observe the stoma closely to ensure that there was a good blood supply. Babies have small circulating blood volumes, so the nurse needed to observe the intravenous infusion closely to ensure that Emma received the correct amount of fluid. The nurse therefore needs to have *special skills related to paediatric nursing*. She also needs to understand the anxiety felt by Simon and Jane and support them during the time that they are in hospital, thus being a *counsellor* to the parents.

When Emma was first admitted, a junior doctor made several attempts to site an intravenous infusion. Emma became very distressed and, after the third attempt, the nurse intervened and suggested that the doctor get some assistance. Post-operatively, the nurse is aware that Emma is in pain; however she has not been prescribed any analgesia as the anaesthetist feels that the dangers of using analgesia for neonates outweigh the benefits. The paediatric nurse contacts the surgical registrar, who does prescribe for pain relief. The paediatric nurse is here acting as an *advocate*.

When Emma has made progress, the nurse teaches Jane how to breastfeed and how to give normal baby care. As Jane becomes more confident, the nurse teaches her how to change the colostomy bag. The nurse is acting as a *teacher*.

Prior to Emma's discharge, the nurse will contact the paediatric community nurse, who will visit the ward and develop a relationship with the family prior to discharge. She will ensure that there is continuity of care and that Jane does not feel unsupported when she first gets home. The ward nurse will also contact Emma's health visitor, so that she is prepared for the discharge. In this way, the nurse is acting as a *liaison* between the hospital and the community.

After discharge, the parents will need to know where they can obtain colostomy bags, and they have also asked to meet other parents with babies with a similar condition. The paediatric nurse thus acts as a *resource advisor*.

promotion and early identification of problems within the family. She is in a prime position to work with parents to reduce the numbers of accidents occurring to children.

Paediatric community nursing

Although it has long been recognised that children should not be admitted to hospital unless they are unable to be cared for in the community (Ministry of Health 1959, DHSS 1976), the growth of paediatric community nursing has been slow. Most sick children are cared for in the community by their parents, and they are often able to give all the care that is required, without any help from nurses. However, children have been and are being admitted to hospital because there is insufficient specialist nursing support for their parents within the community, and their discharge from hospital has sometimes been delayed because of this lack of support.

The climate is changing, and there has been a welcome increase in the numbers of paediatric community nursing teams around the country. In 1993, there were 52 general and 124 specialist services (Tatman & Woodroffe 1993).

The way in which the paediatric community nursing service is organised and managed differs in different areas of the country. In some areas, the nurses come under community managers; in others, they are attached to the acute hospital services. Some paediatric nurses are employed to work with a special category of child, for example with asthma or cancer. There are also some specialist neonatal community nurses who support parents in caring for their babies on discharge from hospital, some of whom require fairly intensive care. They may be oxygen-dependent or have a tracheotomy. In other areas, there are teams of paediatric community nurses who are more general in their approach, although they may develop special interests.

It seems likely that the growth in paediatric community nursing services will continue. The length of time that the child branch student nurse will be able to spend working with sick children in the community will depend on the number of paediatric community nurses who are employed in that area. As the demand for the service increases and the benefits become apparent, the numbers of teams should increase and the child branch student nurse may be able to spend more time working with them.

The following case example illustrates the role of the community nurse.

Case example 21.3

Martin is a paediatric community nurse attached to a children's unit. James, one of the children for whom Martin is currently caring, is aged 18 months and has been diagnosed as having diabetes mellitus.

He was initially stabilised in hospital on insulin twice daily. His mother was taught to give his injections but was still quite apprehensive when James was discharged after 3 days. She is also having problems, as James helps himself to biscuits and cakes from the other children's plates if she is not watchful. She is also finding it very traumatic to have to monitor James' blood sugar.

Martin's role is to support and advise James' mother as she comes to terms with his condition. He is monitoring James' blood sugars and is able to contact the doctor should there be a need to alter the dose of insulin. James' mother requires extra support when he develops a viral infection and refuses to eat; Martin is then able to increase his visiting to the family to prevent James being admitted to hospital.

School Health Service

The School Health Service was established following a report in 1904 that identified the importance of health in childhood as a prerequisite for health in adult life (British Paediatric Association 1993). The role of the service is to monitor and promote the health of school children and to identify ill-health, disability and problems of development and behaviour. The British Paediatric Association report, 'Health Services for School Age Children', found that:

- 9.6% of children under the age of 15 have an illness chronically reducing their functional capacity
- 5% of school entrants, 8% of 7-year-olds and 12% of 11-year-olds have a significant visual impairment
- 5–10% of school entrants have a significant degree of hearing impairment
- 20% of primary and secondary age children have emotional and behavioural problems. These problems are severe enough to be disabling in 2.1% of all children up to the age of 16 years.

These figures illustrate a significant degree of disability affecting school-age children. If children are to attain their full potential, it is necessary for these disabilities to be identified and for the child to be given the appropriate help.

The school nurse

School nurses were recognised as being of prime importance in identifying children with problems and also in helping to achieve 'Health of the Nation' targets in accident prevention and improvement in nutrition. Increasing numbers of children are diagnosed as asthmatic, there is an increase in the number of children with diabetes, and there are also more children with special needs who are attending normal schools. Children with chronic health problems should be encouraged to live as normal a life as possible, including attending school. School staff may need extra support in order to cope with these children, and the school nurse is in an excellent position to provide this support.

PAEDIATRIC NURSING IN HOSPITAL

There are currently approximately 15 million children and adolescents under the age of 19 in the UK. Approximately 10% of all children under the age of 5 years were admitted to hospital at least once in 1990 (Office of Population Censuses and Surveys 1992). Apart from those children who are admitted to hospital for one or more nights, a large number will attend outpatient departments, and each year it is estimated that one child in four will attend an accident and emergency department, accounting for almost 4 million children (British Paediatric Association 1988). The length of time that children stay in hospital has declined rapidly over the past few years. In 1974, the average hospital stay for a child in England and Wales was 7.4 days for children between the ages of 0 and 4 years, and 5.9 days for those between 5 and 14 years old. By 1985, this had fallen to 4.8 days for 0–4-year-olds, and to 4.1 days for 5–14-year-olds. There has since (1988/89) been a further decline to 3.7 days and 3.8 days respectively (Office of Population Censuses and Surveys 1990).

Most children who are admitted to hospital will be cared for in a children's ward in a district general hospital. Children's wards are geared to the needs of children, with open visiting, resident mother accommodation and facilities for play and schooling. However, too many children, particularly those requiring ENT treatment or ophthalmic surgery, are still cared for in adult wards without these special facilities. In 1993, the Audit Commission found that 55% of outpatient departments and 43% of accident and emergency departments in 174 health authorities and NHS Trusts did not have designated paediatric areas. As children comprise about one-quarter of all attendances in accident and emergency departments, this remains an area of concern. Although many people recognise that adolescents have special needs, there are still very few hospitals that provide separate facilities for them. Many will be cared for in adult wards, often with a high percentage of elderly patients. Those adolescents who are cared for in paediatric wards often find that the facilities are geared for the younger child.

Staffing of children's wards

The concept of children's nurses is not new. Nursing's professional Register, set up in 1919 under the Registration Act, contained a supplementary part comprising the names of nurses trained in the nursing of sick children (Abel-Smith 1960). However, it has taken far longer to persuade managers that children have the right to be nursed by appropriately qualified nurses. In 1959, the Platt Report (Ministry of Health 1959) stated that children had the right to be nursed by people who had a special training and both understood and tolerated their behaviour. In the 1970s, some paediatric wards still had sisters who had no formal paediatric training but had gained experience 'on the job'. There have been problems in training sufficient numbers of paediatric nurses to enable children to be nursed by suitably qualified staff, but there has also been a lack of motivation among some managers in ensuring that they appoint nurses with the right experience. In 1988, the ENB recognised the problems and, in a directive, stated that by 1995 student nurses caring for children, in whatever setting, must at all times be supervised by a nurse with a paediatric qualification. The publication 'Welfare of Children and Young People in Hospital' (Department of Health 1991) also made recommendations concerning the staffing of children's units (Box 21.3).

Box 21.3 Recommendations for the staffing of children's units

District and provider hospitals are advised to take account of the following standards:

- There are at least two Registered Sick Children's Nurses (or nurses who have completed the child branch of Project 2000) on duty **24 hours a day** in all hospital children's departments and wards.
- There is a RSCN available 24 hours a day to advise on the **nursing of children in other departments** – e.g. the intensive care unit, the A&E department, outpatients.
- There should be sufficient RSCNs to **supervise the training of student nurses**.

In 1993, the Audit Commission published 'Children First: A Study of Hospital Services', the staffing of children's wards and departments forming part of the study. The Audit Commission found that:

Despite having RSCNs on their establishment, most wards are at times during the day staffed with only one RSCN, or occasionally none at all. The situation at night is even worse, with almost 50% of wards failing to meet the DOH standard on any shift.

The commission recommended that managers should try to attract more RSCNs back to children's nursing, that there should be an increase in the training of children's nurses, and that there should be the employment of a RSCN above ward sister level.

The staffing of children's wards was once more the centre of attention following the murder of four children and attempted murder of nine more by the nurse Beverley Allitt in 1991. The subsequent inquiry into the tragedy, headed by Sir Cecil Clothier, resulted in the report 'The Allitt Inquiry' (Department of Health 1994). There were 13 recommendations made by the team, one stating:

we recommend that the Department of Health should take steps to ensure that its guide 'Welfare of Children and young People in Hospital' is more closely observed.

One of the factors that enabled Allitt to assault the children was the lack of paediatric nurses and the poor supervision in the ward. The number of paediatric nurses is increasing, and there is more recognition that children have the right to be cared for by appropriately qualified nurses.

NEONATAL AND PAEDIATRIC INTENSIVE CARE UNITS

Approximately 10% of all newborn babies need to be cared for in special care baby units for a period of time. This may be because they are premature or light for dates (a baby who is below the 10th percentile for his gestation), or because there have been problems before or during the birth. About 2% of newborns need even more intensive treatment and will need to be transferred to a unit that can provide total life support, which, unfortunately, sometimes means that baby and mother have to be cared for some distance from their home.

Some sick children will also need intensive care. The larger paediatric units are able to provide separate facilities for this, especially if the hospital is a regional unit providing a specialised service, such as cardiac surgery. However, it is still not uncommon for children requiring intensive care to be nursed in adult intensive care units (Case example 21.4).

Case example 21.4

Thomas, aged 5, has been knocked down by a car whilst he was playing with his friends in the road. He is admitted to the intensive care unit of the district general hospital with severe head injuries and a fractured femur. The unit has six beds, five of which are occupied by adults. Thomas is too ill to be admitted to the children's ward, which has facilities for high dependency nursing but not intensive care. The unit manager is aware that Thomas has special needs relating to his age group and arranges with the manager of the children's ward that a children's nurse should be transferred to the unit to care for Thomas. The nurse will work with the staff of the unit to ensure that Thomas gets the specialised nursing care he requires in relation to both his physical and psychological needs. After 7 days, Thomas' condition has stabilised and he is transferred to the children's ward.

DAY SURGERY FOR CHILDREN

Many of the children who require surgery can be offered day surgery, which is becoming increasingly popular. However, the standard of care is not always satisfactory. The report, Caring for Children in the Health Services 1991 recommended a checklist based on the 12 quality standards (Box 21.4) which should be followed in order to provide a well-planned day care service for the children and their families.

SPECIAL NEEDS OF ADOLESCENTS REQUIRING HEALTH CARE

In 1990, NAWCH published a document 'Setting Standards for Adolescents in Hospitals'. Sadly, few units or hospitals are able to comply with these, and adolescents remain the forgotten age group. Many people will not accept that there are sufficient numbers of adolescents requiring hospital treatment to justify separate facilities. This is usually because the adolescents are scattered among a variety of adult medical and surgical wards and paediatric wards. The method of clustering admissions by age group often does not identify the numbers of adolescents who would benefit from a special unit, as the groups are 0–4 years, 5–15 years and 16–19 years.

1. Are the three stages of provision planned in an integrated manner; pre-admission; day of admission including handover to the general practitioner; aftercare at home?

2. Is preparation offered to both child and parent both before and during the day of admission?

3. Does the written information for parents clearly outline their responsibilities prior to and following the admission and opportunities for their participation on the day; and is it written in a way that all parents can understand?

4. Is there a specific area designated for day patients separate from that for inpatients who are acutely ill?

5. Are children treated and nursed separately from adults?

6. Are identified staff specifically designated to the day case area?

7. Are medical, nursing and other staff trained for, and skilled in, the care of children and their families?

8. Are the organisation and delivery of patient care planned specifically for day patients so that every child is likely to be discharged within the day?

9. Do the building, equipment and furnishings comply with safety standards for children?

10. Is the environment homely and does it include areas for play and other activities for children and young people?

11. Is essential documentation, including communication with the primary and/or community services, completed before the child goes home?

12. Are there nurses, trained in the care of sick children, available to provide support in the home?

Adolescents have needs different from those of both adults and small children. They are learning to adapt to a different body image, which can make them very self-conscious and also very threatened by anything that may affect their appearance. They identify strongly with their peer group and need their support and contact. Adolescents need privacy, but also the ability to socialise with their peers and interact in as near normal a setting as can be organised. Some may be facing important exams and therefore need the space to study, uninterrupted by ward routines. The different needs of the adolescent were recognised in the publication 'Welfare of Children and Young People in Hospital' (Department of Health 1991), which recommended that the adolescent should have separate facilities, where there could be privacy, a flexibility of regime, independence, and space for socialising, hobbies, homework or just to be alone.

Activity 21.3

With two or three friends, consider how many adolescents you have nursed in both adult and paediatric wards who would have benefited from an adolescent unit.

Bearing in mind the needs of the adolescent, design a unit that would cater for young people between the ages of 12 and 16. Consider the following:

- the number of beds per room
- toilet and washing facilities
- visiting restrictions (if any)
- common rooms, with, for example TV and video, billiard table and areas to study
- the skill mix of the unit: adult branch nurses, child branch nurses, mental health branch nurses
- the uniform of the staff (if any).

OTHER ASPECTS OF CHILDREN'S NURSING

Children with special needs

All children have needs, which are normally met by the parents in cooperation with local authorities and health and education services. Children sometimes also have 'special needs'. The Children Act (1989) focused on children in need; under Section 17 (10) of the Act, a child is defined as being in need if:

a) he is unlikely to achieve or maintain, or to have the opportunity of achieving or maintaining a reasonable standard of health or development without the provision for him of services by a local authority.
b) his health or development is likely to be significantly impaired, or further impaired, without the provision for him of such services.
c) he is disabled.

Section 17 (11) of the Act explains that a child is disabled 'if he is blind, deaf or dumb or suffers from mental disorder of any kind or is substantially and permanently handicapped by illness, injury or congenital deformity or such other disability as may be prescribed.' In the terms of the Act, 'Development means physical, intellectual, emotional, social or behavioural development. Health means physical or mental health.'

Children with special needs may be hospitalised for a variety of reasons, for example with an acute illness or for surgery. Some children may be admitted because they are failing to thrive at home, a period in hospital being used to ensure that there is no organic cause.

Children who have been abused also sometimes require hospitalisation. If the child requires immediate protection, he may be admitted to a paediatric ward whilst the social worker arranges foster care, and sometimes his injuries will necessitate hospitalisation. These children are often emotionally damaged and require patience and understanding. They may distrust all adults or have particular fears or phobias.

Mental health problems in children

The Mental Health Foundation estimates that 2 million children are likely to be suffering from emotional problems. This accounts for almost one-quarter of all children who attend GP surgeries, but only a few will be identified as having a problem. Facilities for children and adolescents with mental health problems are poor. They are often admitted to children's wards, but it is questionable whether this is the right place for them. Many different types of problem are seen, some of which are more obviously due to an emotional problem, for example attempted suicide or anorexia, and some of which may present as a physical problem, such as soiling or abdominal pain, for which no physical cause can be found.

The child with a disability

It is estimated that 3% of all children between the ages of 0 and 15 years are suffering from a disability (Bone & Meltzer 1989). The disability survey relied on parental response to questionnaires. Most disabled children live at home with their parents, and the survey found that, of the 11% of children with the most severe handicaps in the 5–15 year age group, only 1 in 20 was living in an institution.

This move away from institutional care is undoubtedly of benefit to the child but is not without its burdens on the family. The child with a disability may incur higher costs for the family, not all of which are offset by the State benefits that are available. Smyth & Robus (1989) found that disabled children and their families had fewer resources and poorer living conditions than did other families. Apart from the economic cost, there is often a psychological cost. It may be difficult for families to find people who are willing to babysit if one of the children has a serious disability. The family may not be able to go on outings and holidays, and the siblings, as well as the parents, may suffer. Increasing attention is being paid to the needs of the carers, and there are opportunities in some areas for parents to be offered respite care. The disabled child may be admitted to a unit for a short period to give the rest of the family a break. In some areas, special babysitting services are being set up, and the family can set up a relationship with one particular person. The advantage of such services is that the specific needs of the child can be matched with the experience of the babysitter.

Children's nurses are likely to be involved in caring for disabled children in the community and in hospital, and should therefore gain some experience in this area during the child branch programme.

Terminally ill children

The death rate in children is, fortunately, low. However, it is likely that the children's nurse will come into contact with terminally ill children at some time. If the parents wish, it is usually possible for the dying child to be cared for at home, and, with the growth in paediatric community nursing services, this is becoming increasingly common. In order to support the child and family at this time, the nurse will need to have some understanding of the child's concept of death, which is related to his developmental stage.

The death of a child is always hard to face, as it seems to contravene the normal laws of nature. Parents are expected to die before their children, and parents who lose a child will often feel guilty, as if there were some way in which they could have prevented this happening: 'The first duty of a parent is that your child should survive and therefore you have failed' (Davies 1980). The nurse will need to support the parents and child, and may also find herself grieving for the child who is dying. Helping parents through the terminal illness of their child brings some sense of satisfaction if the nurse is able to befriend and support the family.

Child protection and child abuse

All children's nurses, whether they are employed in the community or within hospitals, have a role to play in child protection. It was only in the 1960s that child abuse was recognised as a problem, although it has been occurring throughout history. Charles Dickens documented many such instances, but these were not seen as abusive in the social climate of that era. The inquiry into the death of Maria Colwell in 1973 alerted professionals to the flaws in the system that enabled a child of 7 to be abused over several months and finally killed.

Since that time there has been increasing interest and concern, with several enquiries and reports. In the 1980s, there was an increasing recognition, previously an undiscussed suspicion, that significant numbers of children were being sexually abused by their families or carers. The new openness was mainly due to adults who had been abused as children having the courage to speak out and tell their stories. In the past, children who were being abused had often tried to tell someone of their experiences but had not been believed. In October 1986, the Freephone telephone line 'Childline' was formed following a survey into child abuse. Children can now talk about their experiences with a volunteer, who is in the position to give the child advice on how to handle the situation.

A more recent development has been enquiries into the abuse of children with disabilities, who are among the most vulnerable yet are sometimes unable to communicate. Their abuse may have been continuing for some time before it is uncovered.

Child abuse is currently divided into four categories (Box 21.5).

Box 21.5 The categories of child abuse

1. *Physical abuse*. The child may present with bruises, weals, fractures, burns or other signs of injury that have not resulted from an accident.
2. *Emotional abuse*. There may be no signs of physical abuse, but the child may be deprived of normal warm parenting and may suffer a significant degree of psychological damage.
3. *Neglect*. The child may suffer from malnutrition or cold. He may present as failing to thrive and may be dirty and neglected in appearance.
4. *Sexual abuse*. Kempe & Kempe (1978) defined sexual abuse as:

the involvement of dependent, developmentally immature children and adolescents in sexual activities that they do not fully comprehend, to which they are unable to give informed consent, or that violate the social taboos of family life

---

At-risk register

Children who are deemed at risk of abuse can be placed on the 'At-risk' register. This was introduced following the death of Maria Colwell to ensure that the name of any child suspected of having been abused would be on a register, so that if there were further suspicion, professionals could identify any previous incidents.

Health authorities and NHS Trusts have a responsibility to develop policies and procedures for dealing with cases of suspected child abuse, and the children's nurse must be fully aware of the policies and procedures that should be followed if there is any suspicion of abuse or if she is caring for a child who has been abused.

THE CHILDREN ACT

The Children Act (1989) is the most important recent piece of legislation affecting children. The Act has implications for many aspects of child care, in particular for child protection. The Act emphasises that children have rights, and that parental rights depend on parental responsibility. The Act acknowledges that there are times when the rights of children overrule the rights of the parents to make all the decisions pertaining to their care.

The children's nurse should be aware of all the potential signs and symptoms of child abuse and should be seen as one of the team that is responsible for child protection. She should also be aware of her role as an advocate for the child and accept the responsibility for acting as an advocate, even in the rare cases when this may lead to action that contravenes the wishes of the parents.

One of the ways in which children's nurses may be involved in child protection is shown in the following case example.

Case example 21.5

Jenny is employed as a school nurse attached to a primary school. She is seeing all the children aged 7–8 years for a routine vision test and general health check. She is concerned about Andrew, who had not previously had any problems. His mother has reported that he has recently started soiling, and his class teacher has said that his behaviour is deteriorataing and that he is very disruptive in class. Jenny uses the time she has with Andrew to gain his confidence and try to find out whether he has any current problems. During the course of the interview, Jenny learns from Andrew that he is being sexually abused by an uncle who visits the home. He is scared to talk to his parents about this. Jenny is able to reassure Andrew and support him during further investigations. He is enabled to talk to his parents, who are horrified at his story. Social services are involved, and his uncle is later arrested.

THE FUTURE OF CHILDREN'S NURSING

Children's nursing is alive and well as a specialty, and paediatric nurses have a responsibility to ensure that it remains so. Children have a right to be nursed by appropriately qualified nurses, be this at home or in hospital. Technological advances and shorter stays in hospital now mean that the children who are in hospital are likely to be acutely ill.

There are already courses that enable paediatric nurses to specialise in specific areas of nursing; these include the:

- paediatric renal course
- paediatric intensive care course
- paediatric cardiothoracic course
- paediatric oncology course
- intensive care of the newborn course
- child and adolescent psychiatric course.

In the future, it is likely that more modular courses will be developed, enabling the children's nurse to select a module that will enhance her nursing practice.

The role of the children's nurse in the community is likely to expand, involving more teams and more specialists, so that fewer children are admitted to hospital, more are offered day care and the length of hospital stay is shortened further.

Nurses who belong to the Royal College of Nursing can join their Society of Paediatric Nurses at no extra cost. In addition, there is membership of the Association of British Paediatric Nurses. Both are professional organisations that offer support to the children's nurse and work to promote the cause of children's nursing and high quality services for children.

Summary

When considering health care, it must be remembered that children are not, as was until recently believed, just 'small adults'. Each different age, from newborn to adolescent, is associated with particular physical, psychological and social needs. As, in many cases, the child is not able fully to articulate these needs, the nurse must be aware of the underlying developmental stage and tailor her nursing care to meet both explicit and implicit requirements.

In order for care to be pertinent, special children's wards or areas are recommended, with facilities for play, study and rest, which should be staffed by nurses trained in the care of sick children. However, the ideal is achieved in only a small proportion of establishments.

The sick children's nurse must remember that she is a partner in care with the child's parents and family, and should teach and support them, both in hospital and in the community. Parents of hospitalised children should be encouraged to be resident, and all parents should be helped to give as much care as they feel able.

Such provision of specialised care for sick children and adolescents will promote a speedier recovery and smooth the course of illness.

REFERENCES

Abel-Smith B 1960 A history of the nursing profession. Heinemann Educational, London

Ainsworth M D S, Bell S M 1970 Attachment, exploration and separation illustrated by the behaviour of one-year-olds in a strange situation. Child Development 41: 49–67

Audit Commission 1993 Children first: a study of hospital services. HMSO, London

Bone M, Meltzer H 1989 The prevalence of disability among children. OPCS Surveys of Disability in Great Britain, Report 3. HMSO, London

Bowlby J 1971 Attachment and loss, vol. 1. Penguin, Harmondsworth

British Paediatric Association 1988 Joint Statement of children's attendances at accident and emergency departments. BPA, London

British Paediatric Association 1991 Towards a combined child health service. BPA, London

British Paediatric Association 1993 Health services for school age children. Consultation Report of the Joint Working Party. BPA, London

Caring for Children in the Health Services 1991 Just for the day. NAWCH, London

Caring for Children in the Health Services 1993 Bridging the gaps. Action for Sick Children, London

Casey A 1988 A partnership with child and family. Senior Nurse 8(4): 8–9

Children Act 1989 HMSO, London

Davies J 1980 A parent's reaction (Audio tape). Churchill Livingstone, London

Department of Health 1991 Welfare of children and young people in hospital. HMSO, London

Department of Health 1992 The Health of the Nation. A strategy for health in England. HMSO, London

Department of Health 1994 The Allitt Inquiry. HMSO, London

DHSS 1976 Fit for the future: the report of the committee on child health services (The Court Report). HMSO, London

English National Board for Nursing, Midwifery and Health Visiting 1988 Supervision of students gaining nursing experience in children's wards, Circular 1988/53/RMHLV. ENB, London

Kempe R S, Kempe C H 1978 Child abuse. Fontana, London

Levene S 1992 Play it safe: the complete guide to child accident prevention. BBC Books, London

Ministry of Health 1959 The Welfare of Children in Hospital. Report of Central Health Services Council (The Platt Report). HMSO, London

Morley D, Lovel H 1986 My name is Today. Macmillan, London

Nabarro J D N 1988 Diabetes in the United Kingdom: some facts and figures. Diabetic Medicine 5: 816–822

National Association for the Welfare of Children in Hospital 1985 Charter. NAWCH, London

National Association for the Welfare of Children in Hospital 1990 Setting standards for adolescents. NAWCH, London

Ninan T, Russell G 1992 Respiratory symptoms and atopy in Aberdeen schoolchildren: evidence from 2 surveys 25 years apart. British Medical Journal 304: 873–875

Office of Population Censuses and Surveys 1989 Mortality statistics; surveillance (time trends). DH1/19. HMSO, London

Office of Population Censuses and Surveys 1990 Hospital in patient enquiry. MB4. HMSO, London

Office of Population Censuses and Surveys 1991 Mortality statistics (cause). DH2/17. HMSO, London

Office of Population Censuses and Surveys 1992 Mortality statistics: perinatal and infant. DH3. HMSO, London

Smyth M, Robus N 1989 The financial circumstances of families with disabled children living in private households. OPCS Surveys of Disability in Great Britain, Report 5. HMSO, London

Spitz R A, Wolf K M 1946 Anaclytic depression: the psychoanalytic study of a child 2: 313–342

Tatman M, Woodroffe C 1993 Paediatric home care in the UK. Archives of Disease in Childhood 69: 677–680

United Nations Convention 1987 The United Nations Convention on the Rights of the Child. HMSO, London

FURTHER READING

Allen N 1992 Making sense of the Children Act 1989: a guide for the social and welfare services, 2nd edn. Longman, Essex

Bee H 1992 The developing child, 6th edn. Harper Collins, New York

English National Board for Nursing, Midwifery and Health Visiting 1994 The nursing of children. A resource guide. ENB, London

Pringle M 1986 The needs of children, 3rd edn. Hutchinson, London

Sylva K, Lunt I 1989 Child development: a first course, 6th edn. Blackwell, Oxford

Whaley L, Wong D 1991 Nursing care of infants and children, 4th edn. CV Mosby, St Louis, Missouri

22 Learning disability

Bob Gates

This chapter provides a broad overview of learning disability for common foundation programme nursing students. Clearly, it is not possible for such an overview to provide anything other than a thumb-nail sketch of the many issues that could be discussed.

The aims of this chapter are to:
- explore the range of definitions and accepted criteria of learning disability, both historically and currently
- review the sociological and psychological approaches to understanding learning disability
- outline the prevalence and causes of learning disability
- discuss the role of the learning disability nurse and the importance of care-planning.

DEFINING LEARNING DISABILITY

Students who intend to pursue the learning disability branch or other students who may be interested in pursuing some aspects of further study should seek out the references and suggestions for further reading supplied at the end of the chapter.

It has been estimated that there are 110 000 people with severe learning disability and more than 350 000 with a mild learning disability in England (Gostin 1985). This represents a significant section of society that is entitled to access the resource of a skilled specialist nurse practitioner, who is able to meet their health needs. Health, as defined by Beck et al (1988) includes dimensions of being such as biological, educational, spiritual, cultural and social. Indeed, they have stated that:

Holistic health philosophy includes a primary focus on health promotion, or health as a positive process, rather than the absence of disease, it is a dynamic active process of continual striving to reach one's own balance and highest potential. Health involves working towards optimal functioning in all areas. The process varies among people and even within individuals as they move among people and even within individuals as they move from one situation and life stage to another, and is contingent on personal needs, imbalances and individual perceptions of reality.

The role of the learning disability nurse in enabling the person with a learning disability to reach his own 'balance and highest potential' is vitally important to the health of this segment of society. This issue will be explored below, in the sections that deal with the differing theoretical approaches to learning disability and the role of the nurse. It might be helpful to commence this chapter with a brief exploration of what learning disability means, and then attempt to define it, which is much easier to propose than to achieve. Understanding any concept, idea or phenomenon requires access to an adequate and meaningful language that operationalises a body of knowledge – and learning disability is no exception. Herein lies a problem, because the term 'learning disability' means many different things to many different people.

It may have been the case that the reader of Case example 22.1 has found some difficulty in deciding whether or not Lucy has a learning disability. How one decides whether an individual has a learning disability is, in fact, quite complex.

Case example 22.1

Lucy was born in 1967, following a normal pregnancy and labour. She was the youngest of three sisters. It soon became apparent to the family that Lucy was not reaching the normal developmental milestones. At this time, Lucy was referred to a paediatrician at the local general hospital, who diagnosed her as suffering from a mild mental handicap. The paediatrician advised the parents to 'take her home, give her plenty of love but do not expect too much from her'. During her childhood, Lucy found it difficult to mix well with other children. Her slowness and the distinctive delay in her speech caused much teasing and bullying. Her parents decided that it would be better for Lucy if she were to attend a 'special school'. Lucy thrived in this environment; she learnt to read and write, and was able to undertake basic calculations in mathematics. At 16 years of age, Lucy attended a boarding school for 2 years, where she took a simple catering course that was designed to prepare her for future employment.

However, when Lucy returned home, numerous problems arose. She had become a confident, assertive young woman. Her mother still wanted the 'old' Lucy. Her mother encouraged Lucy to stay in her room to do jigsaw puzzles, colour picture books and play her collection of pop tapes. Soon Lucy developed aggressive outbursts that escalated over a period of time into vicious attacks on members of her family. Her mother sought the advice of their GP, who referred them to a community learning disability team. After a series of visits from a community learning disability nurse, Lucy articulated a desire to leave home. With the reluctant support of her parents, Lucy left home and moved in to a small community home for people with a learning disability. She now lives in a four-bedroomed house run by her local authority with three other people who also have a learning disability. She attends a local resource centre run by the local authority from Monday to Friday. She attends college once a week to update her catering course; she hopes this will enable her to leave the resource centre as she hopes to find a full time job in a hotel. In addition, she now has a full social life and a boyfriend, and visits her family about once a month at her old home.

Activity 22.1

Consider Case example 22.1 and then attempt to answer the following questions from your existing knowledge base concerning learning disability.

- Do you think Lucy has a learning disability.
- Regardless of your decision as to whether or not Lucy has a learning disability, identify those factors that led you to arrive at this conclusion.

For example, what criteria should be used in deciding whether someone has a learning disability? Surely it is the case that such a decision cannot be arbitrary, with wide variation in decisions. Clearly, in order to be able to say whether or not someone has a learning disability suggests a need for some form of reliable criteria, against which individuals can be measured. The most common criteria for identifying learning disability are social competence and intellectual ability.

SOCIAL COMPETENCE

Mittler (1979) has suggested that most countries have used criteria based on social competence that include the ability of an individual to adapt to changing demands made by society. This, of course, sounds relatively straightforward: one simply identifies people who are socially incompetent and who do not respond well to changing societal demands. On the basis of an individual performing significantly below what might be considered as 'normal', one may presumably say that they might have a learning disability. However, there are a number of problematic issues to consider in relation to the criterion of social competence.

First, social incompetence is to be found in a wide cross-section of people, and not just those with a learning disability. Consider, for example, people with chronic mental health problems.

Second, there is an issue here of expectation and the notion of a self-fulfilling prophecy. Assume, momentarily, that an individual is identified as having a learning disability, on the basis of measured social incompetence. Is it the case that this individual genuinely has a learning disability, or is the social incompetence an artefact of the hospital setting in which this individual has spent his formative years? Such a finding is not beyond the realms of credibility. It is only relatively recently that the large learning disability hospitals have been closing. Thousands of people with a learning disability were segregated from society and led very devalued lives. Opportunities for the development of social competence were few and far between, and even when opportunities arose, they were often perverted attempts to create some kind of social reality in an institutional setting. In short, the expectations of people in these environments were low, and therefore it is not unreasonable to assume that their development of social competence in such environments was reduced.

A further problem in using the criterion of social competence is being able to separate out causes of poor social competence other than learning disability. For example, there may be problems of communication, hearing and vision not necessarily involving a learning disability. Despite the criticisms made in this section, social competence remains a globally used criterion for the identification of a learning disability.

INTELLECTUAL ABILITY

Some would argue that intelligence is an obvious criterion upon which to judge whether or not someone has a learning disability. An immediate problem with this is being able to decide just what intelligence is. This chapter does not have sufficient space to explore this issue, so it is assumed that intelligence is something to do with the ability to solve problems, and that this ability, or absence of it, can be measured.

One way of measuring intelligence is by using intelligence tests. These test have been used since the turn of the century. They serve the purpose of enabling one to compare the ability of one individual to complete a range of standardised tests, against a large representative sample of the general population. The sample with which an individual is compared will be of a similar chronological age. The score that an individual attains can be converted into a percentile, in order that one may understand how this individual compares with others in the general population. Normally, this figure is converted to an intelligence quotient (IQ) that has been, and still is, used as means for identifying learning disability. The intelligence test seeks to compare the mental age of an individual against their chronological age, which is achieved by using the following formula:

$$\frac{\text{Mental age}}{\text{Chronological age}} \times 100 = \text{IQ}$$

In the above formula, chronological age refers to the actual age of an individual and mental age refers to the developmental stage that an individual has reached, in comparison to others of a similar age. If the sum of the number reached by dividing mental age by chronological age is multiplied by one hundred, one arrives at the IQ. Clearly, given the nature of this formula, the IQ would progressively diminish if one were to continue using it throughout an individual's life; therefore the formula is only of use until the chronological age of around 18. For the student who wishes to study both the concept and history of IQ, Gross (1991) is recommended. Given that intelligence is present in the population and is evenly distributed, it is possible to measure how far an individual moves away from what constitutes 'normal'. This so-called normal distribution of intelligence in shown in Figure 22.1.

The use of intelligence tests has appeared to be a favourite pastime of psychologists, especially in the 1950s, 60s and 70s. It has to be said that there are many limitations in the use of such tests, including cultural bias, poor predictive ability and an uncomprehensive relevance for the identification of learning disability. Once again, despite the range of criticisms one may construct concerning the use of intelligence tests, they do, if used appropriately and by properly trained technicians, provide a relatively objective measure of the intellectual ability of an individual. Such a measure, if used in conjunction with other criteria such as social competence, may enable the identification of a learning disability.

TERMINOLOGY

'Learning disability' is a term with contemporary usage in the UK to describe a group of people with significant developmental delay that results in arrested or incomplete achievement of the 'normal' milestones of human development. These milestones relate to intellectual, emotional, spiritual and social aspects of development. Significant delays in one or more of these areas may lead to a person being described, defined or categorised as having a learning disability. The causes of learning disability are multifactorial, and some causes will be outlined below. It should be remembered that the term 'learning disability' is not one that is used internationally, nor is it a term that has been used for very long in the UK. Until recently, the term mental handicap was much more frequently used, but was replaced because it was felt that it portrayed a negative image of people with disability. A relatively recent study by Nursey et al (1990) demonstrated that parents and doctors had preferences in the words that they chose to use when referring to people with learning disability. The study was conducted using a questionnaire, and established that both parents and doctors preferred the term 'mental handicap' or 'learning difficulties.' However, it is interesting that doctors were more inclined to accept the descriptions 'dull', 'backward' and 'developmentally delayed.' Some other terms are given in Activity 22.2.

In the USA, the term 'mental retardation' is widely used for the classification of learning disability. This system is based upon the Classification of Mental and Behavioural Disorders (World Health Organization 1993), in which 'mental retardation' refers to:

Activity 22.2

The following terms are also used to describe people with a learning disability:

- Learning difficulty
- Mentally subnormal
- Mentally retarded
- Mentally impaired
- Spastic
- Idiot
- Imbecile
- Moron
- Cretin
- Benny

- Are you aware of other terms that have general usage?
- Which of these terms do you think is the most acceptable to people in general?
- Do you think that any of the terms used are capable of creating a negative image of this group of people?

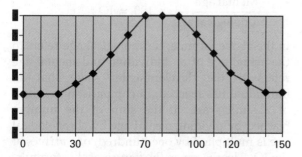

Figure 22.1 The normal distribution of intelligence (IQ).

a condition of arrested or incomplete development of the mind, which is especially characterised by impairment skills manifested during the developmental period which contribute to the overall level of intelligence, i.e. cognitive, language, motor and social abilities.

The World Health Organization organises the degree of disability (retardation) according to how far an individual moves away from the normal distribution of IQ for the general population, as discussed above. In learning disability, one of the problems in deciding which term to use is the possibility that the term may become used as a label that conjures up a negative image. The use of labels for people with a learning disability has in the past served as a way of segregating this group from society at large. For further information concerning the history of labelling in learning disability, the reader should refer to Williams (1978) Ryan & Thomas (1987) and Hastings & Remington (1993). Clearly the sustained use of a label, coupled with any subsequent negative imagery, has the ability to create a group of people who become perceived as deviant and therefore become devalued citizens. Wolfensberger (1972) has demonstrated the very real and negative effects that occur to people when they become marginalised as deviants; he has described eight social role perceptions of people with a learning disability, outlined below.

1. Subhuman

Throughout history and different cultures, it has often been the case that people with a learning disability have been viewed as subhuman. One does not have to search very far back in literature for evidence of this belief. For example, in relation to absolute, complete or profound idiocy, Tredgold and Soddy (1956) said:

In this condition we seen humanity reduced to its lowest possible expression. Although these unfortunate creatures are, indeed, the veritable offspring of *Homo sapiens*, the depth of their degeneration is such that existence – for it can hardly be called life – is on a lower plane than that of even the beasts of the field, and in most respects may be described as vegetative.

Bannerman & Lindsay (1994) provided discussion on the eugenics movement of the latter half of the 19th and the beginning of the 20th centuries, in which segregation and the search to prevent deterioration of the human race were seen as very important. As Mittler (1979) stated:

The late Victorians were so haunted by the spectre of a declining national intelligence that they pursued a ruthless segregationist policy which led to many thousands of people being identified as mentally handicapped and incarcerated in asylums and colonies. The fact that their names were later changed to hospitals does not alter the fact that they were sited and designed to meet the needs of the time to segregate the handicapped from the rest of society and to do everything possible to prevent them from multiplying.

Further evidence of this perception of people with a learning disability can be found in this century that included the attempts to rid Nazi Germany of people with a learning disability (Independent Television Corporation 1993):

Defective people must be prevented from propagating equally defective offspring ... For, if necessary, the incurably sick will be pitilessly segregated – a barbaric measure for the unfortunate who is struck by it, but a blessing for his fellow men and posterity.

This perception was even reinforced in material for schoolchildren. Consider the following mental arithmetic problem that was set for German children in 1936 (Independent Television Corporation 1993):

A mentally defective person costs the republic 4 Reichmarks per day, a cripple 5.50 Reichmarks ... 300,000 persons are being cared for in public mental institutions. How many marriage loans at 1000 Reichmarks per couple could be annually financed from the funds allocated to these institutions?

2. Sick

With the development of the NHS in the latter half of the 20th century came the inevitable medicalisation of learning disability. This resulted in hospital provision being seen as the most appropriate way of caring for people with a learning disability. A natural consequence was the development of a whole 'adult' nursing-oriented approach to caring for people, based upon the medical model of care.

3. A holy innocent

Once again throughout history, a consistent perception of people with a learning disability is that they are innocent from original sin and somehow enjoy some form of special relationship with the deity, perhaps as recompense for their disability.

4. An eternal child

This is probably the most commonly encountered perception of people with a learning disability. In a sense, such a perception has the ability to prevent people with a learning disability from being allowed to 'grow up'. This often manifests itself by carers not allowing adults with a learning disability to take risks or make their own choices, or even by their being given childlike clothes or toys that are inappropriate to their age.

5. An object of pity and burden of charity

Because the person with a learning disability is perceived as not enjoying the 'normalcy' of being human, it is common to find people who feel pity for them. This pity is experienced with such intensity that they are ascribed the need for charity – to be looked after. In some countries, there is an historical involvement of the Church in the care of people with a learning disability, which is evidenced by charitable homes caring for them.

6. An object of ridicule

There is some historical evidence that people with a learning disability were used as 'fools' and jesters in court entertainment during the mediaeval period (Williams 1985). Such a perception of people who are in some way stupid, 'thick' or incompetent is still prevalent in our own society; and it is often thought not inappropriate to ridicule such individuals.

7. A menace

Even today, people with a learning disability are perceived as a menace. It is common to find community initiatives for the relocation of people with a learning disability from hospital to community settings beset with problems of neighbour complaints. These complaints typically concern a drop in the value of their own property or people 'wandering around' who may get into trouble with the police.

8. An object of dread

It is still a fact that, because of the perception of learning disability, a child either born or diagnosed as having a learning disability is regarded as a punishment. Prospective parents view with dread the possibility of having a child with a learning disability. As Bannerman & Lindsay (1994) have said: 'A family's investment in and expectation of their children is often very high and the arrival of a child with a disability may be the end of dearly held dreams about what that child would achieve in life.'

It is perhaps apparent that people with a learning disability are not perceived in the same way as other citizens within society, which may partly be accounted for by the images and attitudes that society holds toward this group of people, which is in part brought about by the effects of labelling and the creation of a deviant group. As human beings, we still have a long way to go before we arrive at the unconditional valuing of all human life, regardless of the level of disability.

HISTORICAL OVERVIEW OF LEARNING DISABILITY

Tracing the origins of learning disability is actually quite difficult, because in centuries past, learning disability has been conflated with problems of mental health. Indeed, prior to the 19th century, people with a learning disability were often cared for in the same institutions as those who were mentally ill. This section concentrates only upon a brief overview of the history of learning disability during the 20th century. In 1904, a Royal Commission was set up to advise on the needs of the 'mentally defective' population. Bannerman & Lindsay (1994) have distilled the four major recommendations from this Commission, that:

- people who were mentally defective needed protection from society and indeed themselves
- all mentally defective people should be identified and brought into contact with caring agencies
- mentally defective people should not be condemned because of their condition
- a central organising body should be established to work with the local caring agencies who would be responsible for the care of individual people.

This commission resulted in the 1913 Mental Deficiency Act. This Act introduced compulsory certification of 'defectives' admitted to institutions, and clearly served to segregate people with a learning disability from society at large. However, it must be acknowledged that at this time there was still a eugenics movement originating from the mid-19th century, which extended well into the 20th century. This desire to segregate people with a learning disability from the rest of society resulted in large numbers of institutions being built. Despite the issue of segregation in the 1913 Act, it is possible to find something positive – the demarcation of learning disability from mental illness. Above it was said that, up until this time, people with mental health problems and learning disabilities were often cared for in the same institutions. It is interesting to note that the Act placed the management and responsibility for the care of people with a learning disability with the local authorities. It is interesting that the asylums that developed during the end of the 19th and beginning of the 20th century, did not become hospitals as we know them today until the emergence of the NHS in 1948. In a sense, the NHS, as a major provider of care for people with a learning disability, occurred almost by chance. This shift in responsibility and the subsequent model of care has led to continuing argument as to the most appropriate agency and model for care provision, namely a social or a health model of care.

The next major piece of mental health legislation to affect people with a learning disability was the 1959 Mental Health Act. This Act replaced previously-used terminology with the terms 'mental subnormality', 'severe mental subnormality' and 'mental or psychopathic disorder'. The Act required local authorities to provide both day and residential care for people with a learning disability, and also made provision for voluntary attendance at a hospital rather than compulsory certification. However this Act, whilst providing new definitions, still perpetuated the apparent need for mental health legislation for people with a learning disability.

During the 1960s, a series of scandals was reported concerning the care of people with a learning disability in the large hospitals. In 1971, the then labour government published an extremely significant document in the history of learning disability, known as 'Better Services for the Mentally Handicapped' (DHSS 1971). This document promoted a model of community care with a significant reduction in the provision of hospital beds and a corresponding increase in local authority provision. This shift in the responsibility for the provision of care resulted in the Griffiths Report (Griffiths 1988), the documents 'Caring for People' (Department of Health 1989a) and 'Working for Patients' (Department of the Health 1989b) and the 1990 National Health Service and Community Care Act. This series of reports, White Papers and subsequent legislation evidences the final move from hospital care to the provision of community care for people with a learning disability. The National Health Service and Community Care Act 1990 also made the local authorities responsible for acting as lead in the provision of care packages for people with a learning disability.

For a comprehensive analysis of current legislation and its impact on the ways in which care is provided, the reader is advised to consult Malin (1994). Those readers with a special interest in the historical study of learning disability might care to read Lazerson (1975) which presents a fascinating historiography of learning disability in the USA. An excellent review of the history of learning disability in the UK can be found in Bannerman & Lindsay (1994).

Having now identified what is meant by the term learning disability and briefly explored its history the next section will explore two different theoretical approaches that have been used to theoretically explain its nature.

TWO THEORETICAL APPROACHES TO UNDERSTANDING LEARNING DISABILITY

Clarke (1986) has said that:

learning disability has been a source of speculation, fear, scientific enquiry for hundreds of years. It has been regarded in turn as an administrative, medical, eugenic, educational and social problem.

The manner in which learning disability has been catered for throughout history has, to some extent, reflected the dominant theoretical perspective used at a particular time in order to understand it. This next section provides a brief overview of two different theoretical perspectives that are commonly associated with learning disability.

A SOCIOLOGICAL PERSPECTIVE

Kurtz (1981) has provided us with a short, but nonetheless powerful, chapter on a sociological approach to understanding learning disability. He suggests that individuals within any society are incumbents of the status that is attached to the role that they occupy in that society. He cites Guskin (1963), who had noted that people with a learning disability play a very generalised role. This role, it is suggested, emphasises the inability of a person with a learning disability to adequately undertake functional activities that are everyday experience for most people, such as going to work, taking care of oneself, behaving in an acceptable way and managing one's own finances. The point here is the suggestion that the person with a learning disability could not adequately perform these activities. Of particular interest to this approach was the question of whether or not one could identify the causation of such inability. Put simply, was the inability caused by the learning disability, or was it a consequence of behaving in the ways that people expected. Guskin (1963) suggested that:

one could hypothesise non achievement orientation, dependency behaviour, and rebelliousness as patterns of behaviour determined by previous and present

interactions with people who have role concepts of the defective emphasising inability, helplessness, and lack of control, respectively.

Kurtz (1981) argued that because of the ways in which learning disability had been perceived, two important images had emerged of such individuals in the USA, those of:

- the person with a learning disability as a sick person
- the person with a learning disability as a developing person.

He suggested that the first of these images was chiefly held by the medical profession, whilst the second was held by educators, psychologists and possibly parents. In conclusion, this sociological approach to learning disability focuses on the role of this group of people within society. It is suggested that, because of the images that society holds toward them, expectations for their role are limited. Dexter (1958) has argued that it is in this sense that learning disability is a creation of society. The student who wishes to pursue this perspective, but wishes for a simpler text than those referred to in this section, should refer to Petrie (1994).

A PSYCHOLOGICAL PERSPECTIVE

Psychology is concerned with the study of human behaviour, and as some human behaviour is deemed abnormal, a branch of study known as abnormal psychology has developed, which is concerned specifically with the study of abnormal behaviour. Paradoxically, like learning disability, abnormal behaviour is difficult to define, so there is a need to identify criteria in order to distinguish abnormal from normal behaviour (Atkinson et al 1990). Generally speaking, abnormal behaviour is identified by:

- deviation from statistical norms
- deviation from social norms
- maladaptive behaviour
- personal distress.

This chapter has already outlined how intelligence tests are used to establish whether people deviate from statistical norms in relation to their measured intelligence. Now consider Case example 22.1

Case example 22.2

Oliver is a little 3½-year-old boy with winning ways. He has an infectious smile and laugh, dark blue eyes and is a little shy. His mother reports a normal and uneventful pregnancy, as well as a normal delivery without any complications. His development up until 6 months of age was within normal parameters. His mother describes him as a 'happy, placid baby with no problems connected with feeding'. At 6 months old, he contracted encephalitis, as a result of which he was hospitalised for approximately 3 weeks.

'It was then that I lost my little boy, you go like – through a bereavement; you feel like you have lost them but we are getting him back now', says his mother.

After leaving hospital, Oliver was left brain damaged, deaf, blind, paralysed down the right side of his body and with severe epilepsy. His mother was subsequently told that there was very little that could be done for him, and that it was likely that he would be profoundly disabled for the rest of his life. At the age of 6½ months Oliver was essentially paralysed, blind, deaf and having repeated seizures. His mother clung to the belief that no matter how profound his disability, he was still capable of learning. She set about providing as much stimulation for

her child as she could, including building a small sensory room under the stairs. This little room has a fan, laser lights, different articles that hang from the ceiling, as well as a small record player so that Oliver could listen to his favourite songs. His development over the last 3 years has been remarkable.

Despite the gains that he has made, Oliver presents significant challenges to both his mother and the statutory caring agencies in the management of his behaviour. He will, on a daily basis, spend prolonged periods of time screaming and engaged in self-harming behaviour, manifested by him picking, scratching and pinching the skin on his arms, legs, hands and back of his neck. This has occurred with such intensity in the past that this little boy already has very deep and permanent scars. His epilepsy has improved but he still has a number of seizures on each day, which sometimes result in double incontinence. This causes problems in the family, as accidents occur on the carpets. Oliver's sleep pattern is very irregular, and he will sometimes go for long periods without sleeping properly. This causes a great strain on his mother, who is very tired but remains defiant, against all odds, to get the best for her son.

(above) and 22.2 and identify whether deviation from statistical norms for social behaviour, maladaptive behaviour and personal distress is present.

In the USA, a category system has been used for the identification of abnormality. This is outlined in the 'Diagnostic and Statistical Manual of Mental Disorders', 3rd edn, and approximates to the international system of the World health Organization, identified earlier in this chapter. The system comprises a number of diagnostic categories, which are themselves composed of subclassifications. Using this system, an individual is evaluated against a number of dimensions, from which developmental disorders, such as learning disability, can be identified.

An alternative way of understanding the term 'learning disability' from these two perspectives is to conceptualise it as a state of health made up of a number of dimensions of being. Figure 22.2 portrays learning disability as a complex state of being, incorporating a number of dimensions. Each of these dimensions has the ability to affect the health of those people with a learning disability. It can be seen that each of these

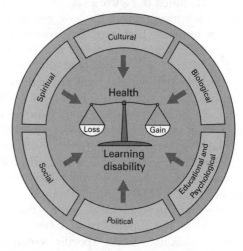

Figure 22.2   Learning disability as a state of health.

dimensions has the potential to affect health, and may result in its loss, gain or maintenance. The two theoretical perspectives outlined above, whilst useful in understanding learning disability at a formal level of theory, do not help people to understand learning disability at a more substantive level. In addition, undimensional perspectives often exclude a wider understanding of the phenomenon of learning disability. It must be reinforced that the term 'health' is used here in its widest sense, and, because of this, it is useful as a means for understanding the nature of learning disability. The next section of this chapter briefly explores the causation of learning disability.

CAUSES OF LEARNING DISABILITY

Learning disability is not an illness and cannot therefore be cured by medical or nursing intervention. However, the condition of learning disability can be greatly ameliorated by appropriate support and care. Learning disability can sometimes be traced to something particular, although it has to be said that this is not always the case. Known or unknown causes of learning disability can occur during the pre-, intra- and post-natal periods of human development, as illustrated in Figure 22.3.

It is not surprising, given the long gestationary period in humans, that a major proportion of learning disability results from the pre-natal period. It should be remembered that, during this period, the embryo and fetus are particularly vulnerable to damage from a variety of factors. Equally, all of the possible complications and trauma that surround birth make the infant particularly vulnerable to peri-natal (up to 28 days after birth) causes of learning disability. Last, the growing child is a vulnerable member of society who, without careful attention to both physical and psychological care, may be susceptible to the possibility of developing a learning disability. Some specific conditions

associated with learning disability are shown in Table 22.1.

A high proportion of learning disability used to be recorded as being idiopathic (of unknown cause), for example, by some unknown effect of birth trauma. Recent advances in the use of non-invasive methods of imaging the brain, whilst still in utero, have helped us to understand how a reduction in bloodflow in the brain can result in learning disability. Some types of learning

Table 22.1 Some examples of the causes of learning disability at different periods in human development

	Possible cause	Possible example
Pre-natal	Chromosome abnormality	Down's syndrome
	Damaged genes	Recessive phenylketonuria
		Dominant tuberose sclerosis
	Illness during pregnancy	Toxaemia
	Environment and nutrition	Substance abuse
	Infections	Rubella, toxoplasmosis
Peri-natal	Developmental abnormality	Prematurity
	Birth injury	Cerebral palsy
Post-natal	Infections	Encephalitis
	Physical	Non-accidental injury
	Toxins	Heavy metals (e.g. lead), drug reactions
	Deprivation	Maternal deprivation
	Trauma	Road accident

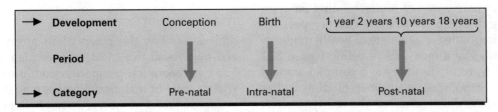

Figure 22.3   Categories of causation of learning disability, with the associated period of development.

disability cases were in the past presumably labelled as learning disability caused by birth trauma, whereas in fact, they may have been the result of pathological disorder prior to birth. Clearly, developments such as these challenge long held beliefs concerning the causation of learning disability (Rutter 1995). In addition, work in the study of genetics is providing new insights into a wide variety of disorders that were previously recorded as idiopathic.

INCIDENCE AND PREVALENCE OF LEARNING DISABILITY

Calculating the incidence of learning disability is extremely difficult, because there is no way of detecting the vast majority of infants who have a learning disability at birth. Only the obvious manifestations of learning disability at birth, for example Down's syndrome, can be detected. In this example, the physical characteristics of Down's syndrome enable an early diagnosis and the ability to calculate the incidence of this disorder. Where there is no obvious physical manifestation, one must wait for delay in a child's development to ascertain whether he has a learning disability.

It is more appropriate, therefore, in learning disability to talk about prevalence. Prevalence is concerned with an estimation of the number of people with a condition, disorder or disease as a proportion of the general population. If one uses the IQ as an indicator of learning disability, one is able to calculate that 2–3% of the population have an IQ below 70, which represents a large segment of society. Given that a large number of people with such an estimated IQ never come into contact with a caring agency, it is more common to refer to the 'administrative prevalence', i.e. the number of people who are provided with some form of service from caring agencies. On this basis, there is a general consensus that the overall prevalence of moderate and severe learning disability is approximately 3–4 per 1000 of the general population (see for example Open University 1987, Department of Health 1992). Such a prevalence would appear to be universally common; for example, Craft (1985) suggests that international studies have identified a prevalence for severe and moderate learning disability of 3.7 per 1000 population. In the UK, it has been further calculated that, of the 3–4 per 1000 population with a learning disability, approximately 30% will present with severe or profound learning disability. Within this group it is not uncommon to find multiple disability, including physical and/or sensory disability as well as behavioral difficulties. It is this group of people who require lifelong support in order for them achieve and maintain a valued lifestyle.

It will be remembered that above it was said that people use different criteria, or benchmarks, as to what constitutes learning disability. This different use of terminology has implications for calculating incidence and prevalence. It should be acknowledged that there is some controversy associated with being able accurately to identify the incidence and prevalence of learning disability. Some would argue that not being able to calculate prevalence accurately is unimportant, as the epidemiological study of learning disability creates labelling, and that this perpetuates inappropriate models of care that are developed outside the ordinary services that are available for ordinary people. One problem – among many others – with this line of argument is that, without careful epidemiological studies in this area, it is inherently difficult to know how best to target resources for those who may need them. It has oft and long been complained that people with a learning disability are not afforded the same rights as other citizens. Careful measurement of prevalence provides one way of ensuring that people with special needs are provided with specialist resources when they are required.

THE ROLE OF THE LEARNING DISABILITY NURSE

In a sense, the role of the learning disability nurse is no different from that of other nurses in other specialties of the family of nursing. A modification of what Henderson (1966) said of the role of the nurse is that:

The function of the nurse for people with a learning disability is to skilfully assist the individual and his/her family, whatever the disability, in the acquisition, development and maintenance of those skills that, given the necessary ability, would be performed unaided; and to do this in such a way as to enable independence to be gained as rapidly and fully as possible, in an environment that maintains a quality of life that would be acceptable to fellow citizens of the same age.

The nurse in learning disability works within a multidisciplinary team in a variety of settings. For example, nurses within this specialty can be found working in learning disability hospitals, community learning disability teams, community homes run by local authorities or NHS Trusts and special schools, as well as the private and voluntary sectors. The nurse in learning disability is becoming increasingly specialised in caring for people with a learning disability who have very special needs. These include:

- people with a profound learning disability and/or multiple physical, sensory, motor disabilities
- people with a learning disability who also have a mental health problem
- people with a learning disability who present their carers with behavioural problems
- people with a learning disability who have offended in law.

There now exists a range of post-registration courses so that nurses in learning disability can specialise in meeting the very specific needs of these people. Regardless of the context or setting in which the learning disability nurse works, or the specific needs of the person or people being cared for, the nurse will need to develop a number of skills. These skills can then be exercised in order to promote an independent and valued lifestyle for people with a learning disability. Specifically the role of the learning disability nurse is to promote:

- the health of the person with a learning disability

- communication and interpersonal skills, including alternative methods of communicating
- independence through teaching life skills
- advocacy and self-advocacy through advocacy programmes
- the philosophy of normalisation
- the rights, risks and responsibilities associated with being a citizen
- dignity and respect
- leisure, recreation and stimulation
- meaningful work opportunities
- lifelong learning
- working in partnerships with families
- harmonious working relationships within the multidisciplinary team for the enhanced care of a person with a learning disability.

If nurses in learning disability are able to fulfil such a role, they are clearly able to make an important contribution to the achievement of optimal health, as discussed above. The last section of this chapter will briefly explore the care-planning process in learning disability, and the contribution that the nurse may make.

Activity 22.3

Spend some time studying Case example 22.2 above. having read the case history, attempt to identify what you think the role of a community learning disability nurse would be for Oliver and his family. If possible, discuss any conclusion reached with a community nurse in learning disability.

CARE-PLANNING IN LEARNING DISABILITY

It is not uncommon in learning disability, because of the range of disciplines and agencies involved in providing care, to find a variety of terms and types of care plans. Each of these different types of care plan share both similarities and differences. Central to all, however, is a desire to articulate in writing a meaningful plan of care that will enhance the quality of life of the person with a learning disability. Different names that may be encountered for care plans include individual programme plans (IPPs), collaborative care plans (CCPs), integrated care plans (ICPs) and nursing care plans (NCPs).

Regardless of the origin or the type of care plan that is being used, it is important that the nurse recognises her role and contribution to the care-planning process and any subsequent documentation. There are numerous ways of looking at how and what the contribution of the nurse should be. Some form of framework should be adopted by nurses in order to provide a meaningful direction for the planning of care, and in nursing, it is common to find a model of nursing directing this activity. Care-planning should be based upon careful assessment of need, construction of a care plan for interventions by the nurse, competent execution of those interventions and finally careful evaluation of their outcomes. It is imperative that the person with a learning disability and/or the carers are actively involved in the care-planning process. Roper et al (1986) provided a useful development model that could be adopted by nurses in the care-planning process, especially in the field of learning disability nursing. The model comprises:

- factors, for example environmental, that influence activities of daily living
- activities of daily living, for example communicating, breathing and expressing sexuality
- the notion of a continuum of dependence to independence for each of the activities of daily living.

These three components of the model are contextualised within the lifespan of an individual, and direct or inform the individualised nursing care that should be offered to an individual. A useful discussion of the care planning process and the contribution of the nurse to this area can be found in Sines (1988). Alternatively, students who wish to explore the use of a nursing model in learning disability in greater breadth should refer to Barber (1987). The National Health Service and Community Care Act (1990) made provision for care managers who would oversee the assessment and coordination of care for individuals with a learning disability living in the community, and a number of learning disability nurses now occupy such roles. Their function is not to provide 'hands-on' care but rather to coordinate it. Although this initiative is a timely development, it is not at all clear whether nurses who occupy such roles are using their specialist knowledge and skills to the fullest extent.

CONCLUSION

This chapter set out to provide an overview of learning disability and the specialty of nursing in this field. The future role of the learning disability nurse will clearly develop in a context very different from the one with which many nurses are familiar. This should not be seen as a threat but rather as a challenge. The environments in which nursing will take place in the future will be different for all specialties of nursing. The learning disability nurse has had to confront the change to a clearly-focused community approach sooner than have many of her colleagues in other nursing specialties. It is also clear that the nurse in learning disability is to become more specialised in caring for people with very special needs, as discussed above. Equally, it is becoming clear that the nurse in the field of learning disability has a duty to develop researched-based practice that is able to demonstrate the benefits of her interventions. There is a need to move from the rhetoric of the past to a demonstrative practice base relevant to today and the future. In other words, learning disability nursing must move to an era when what we say we do for or with people with a learning disability is matched by the highest possible standard of research-based practice, demonstrating that the intervention of the nurse has resulted in health maintenance and/or improvement.

Summary

The prevalence of learning disability, as assessed by the number of people receiving care for this condition, is estimated to be 3–4 per 1000 population. This is probably, however, not completely accurate, not only because some of those affected will not seek help, but also because of the initial difficulty of defining learning disability, as criteria of social competence and intellectual ability may be hard to apply.

The understanding of learning disability may be enhanced by both sociological and psychological approaches, and learning disability is undoubtedly a complex state, incorporating a number of dimensions, all of which may affect the health of the individual. In some cases, physical factors also play a part, some of which may be amenable to treatment.

The role of the learning disability nurse is ultimately, as in other nursing specialties, to enable the individual to develop his skills and increase his independence, thus achieving the best possible lifestyle. The nurse's contribution to planning, executing and evaluating care will be in conjunction with other members of the multidisciplinary team. As a result of this, the person with a learning disability will be better able to reach his full potential.

REFERENCES

Atkinson R L, Atkinson R C, Smith E E, Bem D J, Hilgard E R 1990 Introduction to psychology, 10th edn. Harcourt Brace Jovanovich, London

Bannerman M, Lindsay M 1994 Evolution of services. In: Shanley E, Starrs T (eds) Learning disabilities, a handbook of care. Churchill Livingstone, Edinburgh, pp 19–39

Barber P (ed.) 1987 Mental handicap: facilitating holistic care. Using nursing models series. Hodder and Stoughton, London

Beck C M, Rawlins R D, Williams S R 1988 Mental health psychiatric nursing – a holistic life cycle approach. CV Mosby, London.

Clarke D 1986 Mentally handicapped people, living and learning. Baillière Tindall, London

Craft M 1985 Classification, criteria, epidemiology and causation. In: Craft M, Bicknell J, Hollins S, Mental handicap: a multidisciplinary approach. Baillière Tindall, London, pp 75–88

Department of Health 1989a Caring for people: community care in the next decade and beyond. Cmnd 849. HMSO, London

Department of Health 1989b Working for patients. Cmnd 555. HMSO, London

Department of Health 1992 Social care for adults with learning disabilities. Mental Handicap LAC (92) 15. HMSO, London

Dexter L 1958 A social theory of mental deficiency. American Journal of Mental Deficiency 62: 920–928

DHSS 1971 Better services for the mentally handicapped. HMSO, London

Griffiths R 1988 Community care: agenda for action. HMSO, London

Gostin L 1985 The law relating to mental handicap in England and Wales. In: Craft M, Bicknell J, Hollins S, Mental handicap: a multidisciplinary approach. Baillière Tindall, London, pp 58–72

Gross R D 1991 Psychology: the science of mind and behaviour. Hodder and Stoughton, London

Guskin S 1963 Social psychologies of mental deficiency. In: Ellis N (ed.) Handbook of mental deficiency. McGraw-Hill, New York

Hastings R P, Remington S 1993 Connotations of label for mental handicap and challenging behaviour: a review and research evaluation. Mental Handicap Research 6(3): 237–249

Henderson V 1966 The nature of nursing. Macmillan, London

Independent Television Corporation 1993 Fuhere: seduction of a nation. Independent Television Corporation, London

Kurtz R 1981 The sociological approach to mental retardation. In: Brechin A, Liddiard P, Swain J, Handicap in a social world. Hodder and Stoughton, in association with The Open University Press, Suffolk, pp 14–23

Lazerson M 1975 Educational institutions and mental subnormality: notes on writing a history. In: Begab M, Richardson S A, The mentally retarded and society: a social science perspective. University Park Press, Baltimore

Malin N 1994 Development of community care. In: Malin N (ed.) Implementing community care. Open University Press, Buckingham, pp 3–30

Mittler P 1979 People not patients: problems and policies in mental handicap. Methuen, London

Nursey N, Rhode J, Farmer R 1990 Words used to refer to people with mental handicaps. Mental Handicap 18(1): 30–32

Open University 1987 Mental handicap: patterns for living. Open University Press, Milton Keynes

Petrie G 1994 Social causes. In: Shanley E, Starrs T (eds), Learning Disabilities, a handbook of care. Churchill Livingstone, Edinburgh, pp 83–91

Roper N, Logan W, Tierney A 1986 Nursing models: a process of construction and refinement. In: Kershaw B, Salvage J, Models for nursing. John Wiley & Sons, Chichester

Rutter M 1995 The roots of mental handicap. Medical Research Council News: 20–23

Ryan J, Thomas F 1987 The politics of mental handicap. Free Association Books, London

Sines D, 1988 Towards integration: residential care for people with a mental handicap in the community. Harper & Row, London

Tregold R F, Soddy K 1956 A text book of mental deficiency, 9th edn. Baillière, Tindall and Cox, London

Williams P 1978 Our mutual handicap: attitudes and perceptions of others by mentally handicapped people. Campaign for Mentally Handicapped People, New York

Williams P 1985 The nature and foundations of the concept of normalisation. In: Kracos E (ed.), Current issues in clinical psychology. Clinical psychology 2. Plenum, New York, pp 25–30

Wolfensberger W 1972 The principle of normalisation in human management services. National Institute of Mental Retardation, Toronto

World Health Organization 1993 Describing developmental disability. Guidelines for a multiaxial scheme for mental retardation (learning disability), 10th revision. WHO, Geneva

---

FURTHER READING

Alaszewski A 1986 Institutional care and the mentally handicapped: the mental handicap hospital. Croom Helm, London

Audit Commission for Local Authorities, England and Wales 1986 Making a reality of community care: a report by the Audit Commission. HMSO, London

Ayer A, Alaszewski A 1984 Community care and the mentally handicapped services for mothers and their mentally handicapped children. Croom Helm, London

Beardshaw V 1981 Conscientious objectors at work: mental hospital nurses – a case study. Social Audit, London

Blunden R, Allen D (eds) 1987 Facing the challenge: an ordinary life for people with learning difficulties and challenging behaviour. King's Fund Centre, London

Deacon J J 1974 Tongue tied: fifty years of friendship in a subnormality hospital. MENCAP, London

DHSS 1984a Helping mentally handicapped people with special problems. HMSO, London

DHSS 1984b Mental handicap: progress, problems and priorities. Cmnd 4663. HMSO, London

DHSS 1985 The role of the nurse for people with a mental handicap. Ref. CNO 855. HMSO, London

English National Board for Nursing, Midwifery and Health Visiting 1985 Caring for people with a mental handicap: a learning package for nurses. ENB, London

Wright K, Haycox A, Leedham I 1994 Evaluating community care: services for people with learning difficulty. Open University Press, Buckingham

Malin N (ed.) 1994 Implementing community care. Open University Press, Buckingham

Reid A 1982 The psychiatry of mental handicap. Blackwell Scientific Publications, Oxford

Shanley E, Starrs T 1994 (eds) Learning disabilities, a handbook of care. Churchill Livingstone, Edinburgh

Owens G, Birchenall P 1979 Mental handicap – the social dimensions. Pitman, London

Todd M, Gillbert T 1995 Learning disabilities, practice issues in health settings. Routledge, London

23

Mental health

Robert Newell

The individual with mental health problems is nowadays viewed not so much as a patient suffering from an illness, but as a person with difficulties that need to be tackled in order to achieve as full a life as possible. The aims of the chapter are:

- to consider the historical development of care for individuals with mental distress
- to outline various approaches to the study and classification of mental health and illness
- to review pharmacological, physical and psychological treatments of mental illness
- to discuss the role of the mental health nurse as therapist and educator, and as a member of the multidisciplinary team.

MENTAL HEALTH OR MENTAL ILLNESS?

Psychiatry and mental health care have undergone great changes in the UK during the past century. Today, treatment will involve a range of ideas that emphasise the psycholgocial and social needs of clients, and is most likely to occur in the communities in which clients have to face their difficulties, rather than in a remote institution. Apart from this shift towards social care, the great debate in psychiatry and mental health care has covered the appropriateness and effectiveness of treatment. Treatments have come and gone during the latter part of the 20th century, as some, such as major tranquillisers and behaviour therapy, have demonstrated their effectiveness and resulted in important changes in the well-being of mentally distressed people, whilst others, such as insulin coma, institutionalised care and psychoanalytical treatment have been shown either to be detrimental to clients or to confer little or no benefit. One significant development has been the rise in importance of the mental health nurse, and the enlargement of her role in care and treatment of those experiencing mental distress.

To describe those suffering from psychological distress as being mentally ill has become increasingly unfashionable, except in the medical profession. Nurses, in particular, have preferred to speak of 'people with mental health problems' and to describe themselves as 'mental health nurses'. Certainly, there is little evidence for an organic basis for many so-called mental illnesses, and some critics of psychiatry have preferred to separate these difficulties, which are sometimes referred to simply as 'problems with living', from mental problems that *do* have obvious organic causes, such as dementia and drug-induced and toxic states.

In this chapter, the term 'mental distress' is used to refer to people who are in contact with mental health care services, regardless of whether their difficulties might be expected to have a physical cause. Occasionally, where it is clear from the context that clients have been given a formal diagnosis, the term 'mentally ill' is employed.

Once again, no assumption is made about physical or other origins of their complaints, since, in psychiatry and mental health nursing, the issue of diagnosis has itself been a matter of debate over many years.

HISTORICAL PERSPECTIVE

There are references to both mild and severe mental distress in the Bible, whilst, from Eastern culture, de Silva (1985) has interpreted many Buddhist teachings as being instances of behaviour therapy. Reports of attempts at psychosurgery date to pre-history, although it is clearly impossible to ascertain whether these crude operations would have been carried out for conditions that would today be regarded as mental illness.

In the UK, medical care began to become systematised in the 16th century. However, a wide range of practitioners, with varying levels of training and knowledge, were in practice. Siraisi (1990) gives a comprehensive account of such early medical training and practice. Inevitably, those best able to pay received the attention of the most rigorously trained practitioners. At this time, practitioners made little distinction between disorders of body and mind, and similar treatments were likely to be applied to people suffering from physical illnesses and mental distress. These treatments were often both ineffective and unpleasant, involving blood-letting and purging.

Diagnosis of differing mental illnesses was rudimentary. The major distinction was between mania and melancholia (Foucault 1967), the former being regarded as the more severe of the two complaints, characterised by unpredictable and violent behaviour, whilst the latter was a milder state, usually involving depression, but often accompanied by delusions and hallucinations. It appears that a diagnosis of melancholy may have been simply a general label applied to rule out more severe mental difficulties, much as the term neurosis came to be used during the early and middle part of the 20th century.

Towards the end of the 17th century, incarceration of the mentally ill in public and private 'madhouses' became the dominant mode of care

(Busfield 1986). The standard of care in these institutions was apparently uniformly poor, consisting of inadequate physical surroundings and diet, erosion of liberty and harsh treatments. This state of affairs continued until the end of the 18th century, with proprietors of establishments for those suffering mental distress often having few or no qualifications or experience. More unfortunate still, the prevalent view of madness, which owed much to the work of the 17th century physician Thomas Willis, was that major mental distress resembled an animal state. This view lent a spurious authority to harsh treatments, including flogging, restraint and immersion.

At the end of the 18th century, however, philosophical changes in Europe came to emphasise the importance of the rationality of human beings. This, in turn, had consequences for the treatment of mental illness, as the popularity of analogies between mad people and animals waned. In the UK, William Tuke and his family, wealthy Quakers living and working in York, played a key role in changing the way in which mentally ill people were treated (Tuke 1813). Quakers have a long history of charitable works, based upon their religious belief that God is to be experienced through our experience of others, and that the basis of the divine exists in everyone. This means that they must be treated fairly, with kindness and as rational beings. As a result of dissatisfaction with mental health care, Tuke, in 1795, set up The Retreat in York, an institution founded on 'moral' treatment. Moral treatment is based on the notion that mentally ill people have control over their behaviour and can, with the help and example of others, exercise that control, with a resulting improvement in their mental well-being.

Records of The Retreat show that these tactics worked well. Critics of moral treatment (Foucault 1967) suggest that its proponents merely replaced one form of coercion of the mentally ill with another, and have even asserted that this moral coercion was actually worse than physical restraint, since it was more subtle, and therefore more difficult to resist and more undermining to a sufferer's individuality. The two weaknesses of this critique are that the restraint that moral treatment sought to replace was extraordinarily barbaric and brutalising, and that, in advocating self-restraint, moral therapists expected no more than was expected of other members of the population.

RISE OF MEDICAL TREATMENTS

Many authors have argued that medical interest in mental distress grew in direct relationship to perceptions by doctors that care of mentally ill people would lead to an increase in their power and income. However, the increase of medical interest in mental distress represented, at most, a shift in emphasis, and Roth & Kroll (1986) have argued that critics of medicine and psychiatry have misinterpreted historical accounts of the growth of medical care in line with their political beliefs.

Whatever the merits of medicalisation of mental distress, its power to change people's experience of such disorders was immense. For nurses and attendants dealing with the mentally ill, the application of physical treatments represented a time of unparalleled change. Previously intractable cases apparently underwent cure or dramatic improvement to their condition, whilst disruptive patients become obediently pliable. Nor were those working with mentally ill people the only ones to benefit. The new physical treatments brought hope to patients and their relatives. As a result, many patients benefited indirectly, responding to the air of optimism that became current within the large institutions. Finally, the introduction of physical interventions, even when these were of dubious value, created an atmosphere in which further research began to take place, leading to powerful and effective treatments. However, this progress was often won at the expense of patients who were subjected to ineffective procedures that had little value other than rendering them socially acceptable by reducing their behavioural repertoire to such an extent that they become little more than automata.

Despite these difficulties, the medical treatments were not all ineffective. In particular, two new groups of drugs – anti-depressants and major tranquillisers – changed the face of psychiatry and mental health nursing in the space of a few years. The new drugs often had unpleasant or dangerous side-effects, but they exerted a powerful influence on mood and behaviour. The chief consequences were that patients were less often admitted to hospitals, and, if they were admitted, were discharged back into the community with greater rapidity. It has been argued that drugs have been used as a method of exerting social control over mentally ill people. The powerful counter-argument claims that the use of psychotropic drugs has greatly decreased the stigma attached to mental illness by keeping mentally ill people in touch with the community. Critics, however, have pointed to the long-term effects of the use of psychotropic drugs as being a serious drawback. Whilst this is certainly true, with tardive dyskinesia (uncontrolled muscular movements) being the most frequently cited example, this is simply an argument for greater care in prescribing, rather than a blanket criticism of the use of drug treatments, and the risks must once again be weighed against the undoubted benefits of drug interventions.

Approaches to mental health in the UK today often combine a range of approaches to the client. Medical treatments continue to dominate, particularly in mental distress that is sufficiently severe to warrant referral to a pyschiatrist. However, insights into mental difficulties have made inroads into this so-called 'medical model' of psychological care. Society is more psychologically minded than it was 20 years ago, and public knowledge of mental distress and its treatments is greater. In particular, a series of findings in the 1960s and 1970s (e.g. Brown & Harris 1978) highlighted the role of social circumstances in the genesis and maintenance of mental distress and major mental illness. This had considerable influence on clinical practice, and has informed elements of the general public. The current state of care for major mental illness continues to be dominated by medicine and its traditional treatments, but significant inroads have been made into this domination by those who pursue psychosocial models of care. These attempts at more integrated approaches are often called 'eclectic' models of care and will typically involve a team of professionals, including psychologists, occupational therapists, counsellors and nurses, as well as psychiatrists.

IMAGES OF MENTAL ILLNESS: FEAR AND STIGMA

There can be no doubt that mental distress, particularly when severe, gives rise both to fear and stigma. Mental distress continues to be associated, in the public mind, with unpredictability, violence and bizarre behaviour, whilst, in reality, those experiencing mental distress are much more likely to be quiet, withdrawn and fearful of others. On the rare occasions when disturbed or frightening behaviour does occur, it is taken to be potent evidence both for the dangerous nature of mentally distressed people and for the need to ensure their increased supervision, usually in institutions. Most recently, this has become a political weapon for those who lament the rise of community care, using mentally distressed people as pawns in the debate.

Activity 23.1

Use your local library to gather as many accounts of the 'Hungerford Massacre' (Michael Ryan's apparently unprovoked killings) as possible.

- Is Ryan mentally ill or not?
- How do you know this from the media representations of him?
- What do accounts of this kind imply about mentally ill people?

At the same time, it is often argued that examples of violent behaviour are not, in fact, caused by mental illness, but are simply the actions of bad people. This madness/badness debate seems to surface when the behaviour is of a kind that society would prefer to see punished rather than treated. Peter Sutcliffe, the so-called Yorkshire Ripper, is an obvious example. Regardless of his sanity or otherwise, there was a tremendous desire, supported by the national press, for him to be punished. Unfortunately, the media often reports such issues in contradictory ways, both demanding punishment and offering the behaviour of people like Sutcliffe as examples of the dangerous nature of mental illness. The portrayal of mentally ill people as frightening, dangerous and often homicidal is further reinforced in fiction. Given the power of the media, it is not surprising that members of the public have such confused and inaccurate ideas about mental distress.

APPROACHES TO DEFINITIONS OF MENTAL HEALTH AND ILLNESS

The main approaches to mental health are summarised in Table 23.1.

MEDICAL FORMULATIONS OF MENTAL DISTRESS

The dominant view of mental distress in our society is medical. According to this account of psychological disorder, individuals' emotional difficulties may be regarded as being similar to physical disorders. Although it is unfashionable to admit to this view today, even among doctors, an examination of the way in which mental distress is treated reveals the prevalence of this analogy to physical disorder. The majority of individuals complaining of mental disorder are treated in general practice settings, and many never get beyond treatment from their GP, who will usually prescribe medication. This in itself indicates a belief that the person's distress can be dealt with in much the same way as can a throat infection. For those people who move beyond care from their GP through referral to a psychiatrist, the position is not much better, prescription of medication still being the most common element of treatment. Implicit in this act of prescription is the belief that mental distress is a result of some physical malfunctioning, which medication or other physical treatments seek to remedy. Nevertheless, there remain many complaints in which such physical changes have not been found, or in which, if they are present, it is difficult to distinguish whether they are a cause or an effect. Even in those cases where a chemical *cause* is demonstrable, the effect of purely physical treatments has often been weak.

At its simplest, the medical view of mental distress asserts that difficulties with emotion, thinking or behaviour are symptoms of some physical or (more rarely) psychological *cause*. However, the main problem for this medical account is that there is very often an absence of both signs and causes in the traditional physical sense. There are no physical tests that can reliably tap some physical changes in response to physical causes. In most of the physical ailments from which this cause–symptom view of mental distress is derived, such 'objective' evidence would be required before arriving at a diagnosis. Not so in

Table 23.1   Characteristics of main approaches to mental health

Approach	Characteristics
Medical model	Uses the same general approach as for physical medicine. Stresses the role of physical causes of mental distress. Emphasises drug treatment
Sociological approach	Emphasises the role of society in creating and contributing to mental distress. Stresses the importance of labelling of mentally ill people as deviant
Cognitive–behaviourism	Stresses the role of learning in contributing to both difficulties and their resolution. Does not acknowledge differences in the causation of problematic and non-problematic experiences
Psychoanalysis	Asserts that mental distress is symptomatic of unconscious internal conflicts, usually from childhood
Humanism	Emphasises human needs, particularly for esteem and self-actualisation. Distress is consequent upon thwarting of these needs
Anti-psychiatry	Sees mental distress as a sane response to an insane world. Suggests that mental illness is an experience to be lived rather than a problem to be solved

psychiatry. This difficulty in establishing the presence of causative agents has led to a barrage of criticisms from quite different quarters. On the one hand, behaviourists have argued that, where no physical cause can be found for difficulties in behaviour or mood, it would be best to avoid the use of the illness model, in favour of one that emphasises the way in which people learn through their interactions with others. From the opposite camp, labelling theorists and anti-psychiatrists argue that, in the absence of physical causes, the use of the illness model is a way of exerting social control over individuals who offend society's norms.

THE SOCIOLOGICAL APPROACH

Sociology as a discipline has made major contributions to the well-being of mentally distressed people. In particular, sociologists bring to the study of mental distress the notion of deviance, labelling and institutionalisation. According to deviancy theory, individuals who break rules of behaviour within society are seen as deviant, and stereotypical responses are brought to bear. These usually involve some kinds of sanction, which attempt to bring deviant activities back within the normal limits tolerated by society. Scheff (1967) described how this process applies to mentally distressed people in ways that affect major areas of their lives. Liberty may be curtailed and treatment given under compulsion, whilst at a less severe level, simple tasks, such as driving a car, managing financial affairs or deciding what to eat for dinner, may be taken as being beyond one's capabilities. At the heart of these elements of deviancy theory is the idea of labelling. At the point at which a person is labelled as suffering from a mental illness, others respond not to the person, but only to the label. People with mental distress then become part of a group, to which general rules are applied. It is easy to see other marginalised groups to whom labelling has been applied, for instance people with physical disabilities and learning disabilities, and people from ethnic minorities.

However, the case of mental illness is different, since many critics have argued that the label is *all*

that exists. Mental health professionals are thought to have constructed an elaborate diagnostic structure that is based on the need to exclude from society those who offend its norms (Szasz 1962). Whilst it is tempting to see such an idea as fanciful, given the amount of obvious unhappiness experienced during mental distress and the influence of treatments upon such distress, it is worth remembering that studies have demonstrated the fragility of many ideas about diagnosis. The most famous of these is the work of Rosenhan (1973), who introduced a number of pseudo-patients into American mental health facilities, all of whom were diagnosed as suffering from mental illness. This has been taken as offering evidence that health professionals are incapable of diagnosing with accuracy, although it could equally be argued that they are simply capable of being deceived! Most important, however, for labelling theory, was the finding that behaviour by the pseudo-patients following diagnosis was invariably interpreted as being indicative of mental illness, despite the fact that the pseudo-patients were under instruction to behave normally after their initial interviews. Staff were unable to decide between 'ill' and 'normal' behaviour, even in the absence of deliberate deception, indicating the power of the label to influence perception.

Much less contentious is the finding that institutionalised patients display a variety of behaviours that are the direct consequence of the surroundings in which they live, rather than of the illness from which they are assumed to suffer. In a now-classic work, Goffman (1961) demonstrated the effects of a variety of 'total institutions', including mental hospitals, on the behaviour of their residents. His work has indirectly contributed to the movement away from institutional care and an understanding of what is needed for the rehabilitation of institutionalised people.

COGNITIVE–BEHAVIOURAL FORMULATIONS

Cognitive–behavioural formulations of mental distress have their origins in academic psychology. In particular, they owe a debt to behaviourists, who assert, in their purest form, that internal events, such as thoughts, are incapable of either study or objective verification. Much of the early behavioural work was carried out with animal learning (Walker 1984), and, indeed, many early models of human distress were based upon such work. Behaviourists assert that human distress is caused by inappropriate learning. Humans either learn faulty associations between events (usually through repeated chance pairings of these events) or are inadvertently rewarded by those around them for behaviours that will later cause them distress. These two forms of learning are respectively referred to as classical and operant conditioning, and are believed to govern much of a person's behaviour.

Although strict behaviourists deny the relevance of thoughts to behaviour, one group, associated with the late B F Skinner, makes a much more far-reaching claim. This group, the radical behaviourists, claims that thoughts, whilst existing, are subject to the same rules of association and reinforcement that govern overt behaviour (Jaremko 1986). As a result, it is possible for certain thoughts and patterns of thought to become reinforced and to increase in frequency and intensity. Some such patterns are not useful and cause distress.

Modern behaviourist accounts usually consider thoughts, and are referred to as cognitive–behavioural models. There are two basic approaches. The better known is that of Aaron Beck (1976), who combined psychoanalytical insights with behavioural approaches to treatment to derive a picture of human cognition based on the notion of automatic negative thoughts. These thoughts, according to Beck, contributed to the development and maintenance of psychological distress. Beck argued that it was the repetitive patterns of thought, rather than emotion or behaviour, that were chiefly responsible for human distress, particularly depression.

Until recently, this approach lacked a coherent theory of how certain thoughts came to have the power to affect behaviour and emotion. The second approach in cognitive behaviourism, unlike Beck's account, is derived from careful examination of the thought processes of many people under controlled conditions, using experiments derived from modern information-processing theory. The aim of this approach, which has elements in common with radical behaviourist accounts, is to find basic elements of human cognitive experience and to apply these to mental distress (Brewin 1988).

PSYCHODYNAMIC INTERPRETATIONS

The psychoanalytical tradition has had enormous influence on mental health care in the 20th century. Freud developed, almost single-handed, an account of human experiences based upon his clinical observations and reflections. It is impossible even to attempt to do justice to so vast a canon as Freud's in a brief introduction to the subject. However, the central tenet of psychoanalytical thought is the idea of unconscious conflicts giving rise to behaviours and conscious feelings that attempt to resolve these conflicts. Unconscious feelings, often of a sexual nature, cause anxiety, which the individual seeks to lessen through the use of defence mechanisms. These mechanisms are habits of thinking and behaviour. As well as being attempts to lessen unconscious conflict, the mechanisms also *reveal* the underlying conflicts, at least to the trained eye of the psychoanalyst. Whilst Freud initially worked with hysteria, and did not involve himself in the treatment of people suffering from psychoses, later writers have sought to broaden his ideas to include an examination of these more severe mental problems.

Quite early in the history of psychoanalysis (Jones 1955), a number of Freud's followers argued about the basic elements of his approach, particularly his insistence on the prime importance of sexuality as the governing cause of unconscious conflict. Chief among these early dissidents were Carl Gustav Jung and Alfred Adler, both of whom went on to develop their own schools of psychotherapy. Later followers of Freud have also attempted to revise his ideas and, although reducing the long therapy sessions associated with psychoanalysis, have remained close to its central doctrines.

Whilst it is true that the influence of Freud has been incredibly far-reaching, it is doubtful whether all, or even most of it, has been benign. The two chief criticisms of Freudian accounts of human experience relate to their status as scientific theories (Cioffi 1978) and the effectiveness of their treatments (Eysenck 1952).

HUMANISM

Independently of both psychoanalytical and behavioural accounts of human behaviour, a movement in psychology arose that emphasised that uniqueness of individual human experience, drawing on the work of Abram Maslow. Maslow (1968) postulated the existence of a basic hierarchy of human needs, which individuals attempted to realise in order to reach their full potential. According to Maslow, people work through various levels of the hierarchy, beginning at the level of fulfilment of basic physical needs, and passing through needs for safety, love and belonging, esteem needs, cognitive needs and aesthetic needs, until they reach a stage of becoming self-actualised, through the fulfilment of self-actualisation needs, which relate to the desire to maximise one's human potential. Some descriptions of Maslow's hierarchy omit cognitive and aesthetic needs. Maslow asserts that people do not achieve higher order needs until lower order ones have been satisfied. However, we can easily think of examples that refute this assertion (for example members of a religious order who forgo all but the most basic physical needs in order to attempt to attain spiritual fulfilment). In health care, people who themselves go without food or heat in order to afford to care for beloved pets provide an obvious example of the need for affection and belonging outweighing the desire for physical satisfaction and safety.

The therapeutic work of Carl Rogers (1951), another member of this 'third force' psychology, merits discussion. Rogers' theory is once again a need theory, suggesting that humans have basic needs for 'positive regard' (the need to be seen positively by others and, by extension, by ourselves) and self-actualisation (development and growth as a human being). Difficulties arise when these needs are thwarted, giving rise to conflicts such as those seen in mental distress. The chief difficulties with humanistic theories concern lack of precision in definition of terms and lack of investigation of the various claims made.

ANTI-PSYCHIATRY

Of all the critics of traditional models of mental distress and illness, Laing and the anti-psychiatrists have been the most radical. Laing began his therapeutic life as a psychiatrist and developed the view that the supposedly insane discourse of his schizophrenic patients was, in fact, comprehensible. With his co-workers, Esterson and Cooper, Laing (Laing & Esterson 1964) attempted to demonstrate how his patients were led to express themselves in the way they did, as a response to particular patterns of interaction that put them into an untenable position from which madness was the only rational escape. In later formulations of his ideas, Laing came to regard madness as both a sane response to an insane society and a rite of passage into a world of more authentic experiences than those within the constraints of the insane world.

According to Laing, the traditional role of the psychiatrist is, in many ways, as a gatekeeper of accepted norms of experience. By contrast with this traditional role, Laing (1967) saw psychiatrists as having the potential to adopt a priest-like function, facilitating the passage of the 'mad' person through a personal journey of discovery, from which he would emerge more whole. It is easy, 30 years on, to dismiss the ideas of Laing and his followers as a product of a particular period in history, characterised by a rise in popularity of Eastern and other mystic religions and use of mind-expanding drugs. Unfortunately, this is seriously to underrate the importance of Laing's work. Although many relatives of people with severe mental illness found his ideas unpalatable and offensive, many sufferers were themselves drawn to Laing's ideas, probably because they invested the experiences of mentally ill people with validity and worth. This respect for the internal experiences of others alone was a major departure from much previous thought within mental health care. Added to this, Laing emphasised the importance of caring for damaged individuals with respect, within sympathetic, small care settings, rather than in impersonal institutions. This emphasis, which now seems almost intuitive, again represented a considerable contribution to mental health care.

Activity 23.2

'Despite press accounts to the contrary, most mentally ill people, however disturbed, are safe to be with. By contrast, "well" members of society engage in violent acts. Nations also enact these violences in their foreign economic policies and wars.'

In view of this, examine why we insist that mentally ill people should share our sense of reality, and argue the case that it is not the mentally ill individual but society that is insane.
   You may wish to do this exercise with a colleague, taking opposing views.
(Laing 1967 could provide a source of ideas for this debate.)

CLASSIFICATION OF MENTAL DISTRESS

DIAGNOSTIC VERSUS INDIVIDUALISED APPROACHES TO CARE

In essence, diagnosis in mental distress involves eliciting from clients a series of symptoms and signs that allows the clinician to categorise the client with other individuals who have been demonstrated to show similar symptoms and signs in the past (Table 23.2). It allows the clinician to prescribe a regimen of care based on the successful use of that regimen with previous

sufferers who meet the same criteria. In physical treatment of mental distress, this will involve the use of drug treatments or other physical interventions such as electroconvulsive therapy (ECT). In the case of psychological interventions, most particularly psychoanalysis, symptoms are seen as being caused by underlying psychological, rather than physical, causes which groups of clients share. Psychological interventions are aimed at resolving these unconscious conflicts. Not surprisingly, many critics (Eysenck 1985) have noted that the use of notions of symptom, cause and diagnosis are little more than metaphors when they rely on a body of knowledge that, unlike the physical, has not been adequately demonstrated through structured observation and experiment.

By contrast with diagnosis, which, in the main, seeks to group people together through the features that they share in common, functional analysis chiefly aims to help us to understand what makes one individual with a particular set of difficulties different from another whose problems are superficially similar (Table 23.2). Functional analysis is associated with behaviour therapy and its variants, and stems from the belief that the causes of an individual's difficulties are most likely to be found in that person's external and internal environment – in other words, in what he does, thinks and feels. Most crucially, proponents of functional analysis assert that the person's particular interactions with the world around him maintain his healthy or unhealthy behaviours. The task of functional analysis is to discover which events give rise to and maintain mental distress. Thus, the treatment of one person with 'agoraphobia' would be quite different in its details from that of another, whilst in a more medically oriented approach,

Table 23.2	Diagnosis and functional analysis
Diagnosis	**Functional analysis**
Focuses on similarities within groups	Focuses on differences between individuals
Is chiefly associated with the medical model	Is chiefly associated with the cognitive–behavioural model
Is mainly associated with physical/drug treatment	Is mainly associated with psychological treatment
Is good at guiding organisation of care	Is good at guiding individual care
Ensures comparability between research projects	Does not allow for easy comparison between projects

only a choice of a very few drug treatments would be available. The chief criticism of functional analysis has been that it has little to say about underlying causes of distress. However, supporters of functional analysis feel that this criticism is based once again on inappropriate metaphors with physical disease. Appeals to underlying pathology, whether physical or psychodynamic, are not seen as necessary in explaining and addressing people's difficulties.

It may be thought, from the above, that functional analysis, or some other individualised approach to care, such as a nursing model used in conjunction with the nursing process, has much to offer mental health nursing, whilst diagnosis is a comparatively sterile exercise, chiefly useful only in approaches to mental distress based on physical models. However, there are important reasons for resisting the urge to concentrate on individual approaches alone. First, individualised approaches such as functional analysis are of little use in the administrative organisation of care. Second, in order for the effectiveness of interventions to be established, research must be undertaken. This requires some kind of attempt to establish comparability between studies undertaken using different treatments in different settings. Diagnostic categories provide benchmarks for us to use in undertaking and evaluating research in mental health.

The classification system 'Diagnostic and Statistical Manual 4' (DSM4) and other international systems arose in response to poor comparability between diagnoses in different clinical areas and different countries. This lack of uniformity led to lack of confidence in psychiatric diagnosis (Clare 1976) and even, during the 1970s, to criticism of the validity of psychiatry as a branch of health care. Additionally, it was extremely difficult to compare research studies from different settings. DSM4 and its forerunners attempt to standardise the criteria by which diagnostic labels are applied to clients, essentially through describing various symptoms and in which complaints they are present, and then applying a checklist procedure. If the required symptoms, or a sufficient sub-set of them, can be seen in an individual, that individual may then be validly given a particular diagnosis. Stringent criteria are applied to enable the clinician to decide between similar, competing diagnoses.

NEUROSES AND PSYCHOSES

Within mental health care, perhaps the most enduring classification has been into neuroses and psychoses. Although not always referred to in this way, there has been an abiding sense of a difference between those who do and do not share our sense of what constitutes reality. Clients described as neurotic essentially share our view of life. We have all experienced feelings of anxiety, depression, anger, fear and so on. It is only a slight step to translate these feelings into the more severe manifestations shown by clients suffering from difficulties such as agoraphobia, obsessions and compulsions, and difficulties of anger control. By contrast, those described as psychotic may not share our most basic beliefs about the way the world operates. Thus, people experiencing schizophrenia may believe special messages are being transmitted through the television, that their neighbours are poisoning them by sending special gas through the walls, or that they have a secret message from God or from flying saucers. Likewise, clients suffering from bipolar depression, which is characterised by swings of mood between extreme depression and elation, may, in the manic phase, believe that they have great wealth, and spend vast amounts of money, whilst, in the depressed phase, they may believe their insides are rotting inside them. The defining characteristic of psychotic delusions of this kind is that they are not amenable to change via rational debate. Additionally, so-called psychotic states are typically more severe in their effect on the sufferer.

The main difficulty with this categorical approach is that it is easy to provide examples that do not readily fit into either category. One example is the case of clients with obsessive compulsive disorder. These people carry out ritualised activities in order to ward off fears, often of contamination. Most recognise their fears as irrational, but are unable to resist the urge to ritualise, whilst a small sub-group report strong belief that the contamination they fear will, in fact, occur if they do not ritualise (Salkovskis & Warwick 1985). Since the ritual typically has little to do with the feared event, sufferers cannot fairly be said to share our view of reality. However, they can be persuaded to abandon both their rituals and beliefs. Similarly, Newell & Shrubb (1994) were able to demonstrate that cognitive–behavioural intervention was able to change the beliefs of two individuals with body dysmorphic disorder (the strongly held belief that a bodily feature or function is offensive to others). They could not be dissuaded from their beliefs prior to treatment, a defining characteristic of delusion, and might more properly have been classified as 'psychotic'.

These two examples illustrate a peculiar difficulty with categorical approaches to psychosis and neurosis. If, by the use of psychological manoeuvres such as debate, we succeed in changing the view of people classified as psychotic critics may argue that they could not have been 'truly' psychotic to begin with, since it should have been impossible to change their beliefs. This kind of circular argument has beset psychological treatments of psychoses since the 1960s, when critics made such a claim in regard to the case histories published by Laing & Esterson (1964). It may be that a dimensional, rather than categorical, approach to the distinction between psychosis and neurosis has more to offer both the clinician and the researcher.

THERAPEUTIC APPROACHES

DRUG TREATMENTS

As noted above, the introduction of effective drug treatments to psychiatry transformed the lives those suffering from mental distress. The most significant therapeutic innovation was undoubtedly the use of the major tranquillisers. These drugs, sometimes referred to as neuroleptics, fall into two chief groups: phenothiazines and butyrophenones. They are chiefly used in the psychotic illnesses, particularly schizophrenia, although they can be used to control unwanted

behaviours in almost any situation, even though the ethics of their use simply to control behaviour is dubious. The major tranquillisers are believed to act in treatment of schizophrenia by blocking transmission of dopamine, a neurotransmitter thought to be implicated in the odd beliefs and sensations that characterise the illness. When given by injection as a long-acting preparation, major tranquillisers seem to exert a powerful and lasting force in inhibiting the distressing symptoms of schizophrenia, and help to enable sufferers to live a relatively normal life in the community. Although this represents a huge improvement in the care of schizophrenia, two major difficulties should be noted. First, a number of individuals do not remain stable on these powerful drugs, and, second, the drugs themselves give rise to profound side-effects, for which further medication must be taken. This can often lead to difficulties with clients' adherence to treatment.

Anti-depressants also fall into two main groups – tricyclics and monoamine oxidase inhibitors (MAOIs) – although there are more modern variants. Like the major tranquillisers, these drugs work on chemical messengers in the brain: noradrenaline and serotonin. Although their mode of action is quite different, both tricyclics and MAOIs have the effect of enhancing the transmission of chemical messengers. Whilst there is evidence that these drugs do indeed have considerable effect in lifting mood, both groups are associated with serious side-effects, again lessening the likelihood of client adherence. This is particularly the case with MAOIs, for which a special diet is required. Furthermore, the use of these drugs in isolation leaves issues in the client's life, which may have contributed to the depression, untouched.

Benzodiazepines are the most widely prescribed psychoactive drugs, and have a range of uses, from anxiety reduction to help with sleeping problems. The anxiolytic action is apparently through action on the chemical transmitter gamma aminobutyric acid (GABA). Gray (1982) has produced a powerful animal model of this action. In humans, benzodiazepines certainly produce a short-term reduction in anxiety. However, the chief difficulty is that tolerance to the drug occurs, increasing amounts being required to give relief from anxiety, with a consequent high risk of dependence. Current prescribing policies for benzodiazepines recognise this difficulty, but there are, unfortunately, still many inappropriate prescriptions of the drug and many benzodiazepine-dependent people.

PHYSICAL TREATMENTS

ECT remains a highly controversial treatment. It was once used indiscriminately and at high frequency for a huge variety of complaints. As a result, it came to be seen as little more than a method of social control. Additionally, its reputation as a dangerous, frightening treatment, with impairment of memory as a side-effect, led to fear among patients and the public alike. However, much of the controversy that still surrounds ECT today is based on misunderstanding of how it is currently practised. ECT is now a highly specific treatment for use as a final resort in certain kinds of depression, where its usefulness is well documented (Buchan et al 1992). A brief electric shock is passed through the brain, but no pain is felt by the patient, who is given a general anaesthetic. The risks associated with ECT are similar to those associated with any anaesthetic, and the main side-effect is of short-term memory loss. Although safeguards concerning the use of ECT are important, since it is an invasive procedure whose mode of action is unknown, it should also be regarded as a potential lifesaver in severe depression.

Psychosurgery is little used today. It is highly regrettable that this form of intervention was once widely used in mental health care, to little good effect, particularly in the USA. Its chief use today the UK is in a few intractable cases of obsessive–compulsive disorder. Sufferers from this disorder who are severely affected and do not respond to cognitive–behaviour therapy (the treatment of choice) are so handicapped by their rituals that they are unable even to approximate to a normal life. Psychosurgery often represents their only hope. Even so, protocols regarding its use are now extremely strict, and only a few national centres offer the treatment.

PSYCHOLOGICAL TREATMENTS

Psychological approaches to the treatment of mental distress are generally supposed to have a high profile in mental health care. This is, in fact, only so if one considers those who are referred to some specialist service. The majority of people experiencing mental distress are dealt with in general practice, with care often amounting to little more than prescription of medication or simple advice-giving by the GP. Nevertheless, psychological approaches have had a great deal of impact on mental health work and, within the specialist services, it would be very unusual to find a mental health team that did not possess a heavy commitment to psychological interventions. Very often, a nurse will be closely involved in these interventions, so they are discussed in more detail below, as part of our examination of nursing roles. Table 23.3 summarises the main features of several key psychological approaches to treatment.

NURSING ROLES IN MENTAL HEALTH AND ILLNESS

Mental health nurses (Registered Mental Nurses) often regard the creation of relationships with their clients as the core of their work. Although nurses have, in recent years, undertaken courses in particular forms of therapy, these specific interventions are firmly grounded in the relationships nurses build with their clients. Indeed, some nurses reject the specific role of therapist, fulfilling many roles in their relationships with any given client.

SETTINGS FOR CARE

Although many of these relationships are still built within the context of the hospital, such institutional care is the exception rather than the norm. The most acutely distressed clients are still cared for as inpatients, either because there are severe concerns about their ability to care for themselves, or about their desire to harm themselves or others, or because the nature of their

Table 23.3 Major psychological approaches to mental distress

Approach	Features
Psychodynamic psychotherapy	Derived from psychoanalysis Involves eliciting and examining underlying conflicts Little evidence of effectiveness Little practised by nurses Remains an influential theoretical approach in psychiatry
Humanistic therapies and counselling (client-centred approach)	Based on the work of Carl Rogers Emphasises qualities of the therapist (warmth, empathy, respect) Emphasises human uniqueness and growth Influential and widely practised by nurses Little evidence of effectiveness in serious mental distress
Cognitive–behaviour therapy	Derived from conditioning theory and cognitive psychology Emphasises present problems and learning coping tactics Widely applicable and effective in serious mental distress Not yet widely accepted among nurses
Groupwork	Can be practised for any of the above therapies, sharing their therapeutic approaches and strengths and weaknesses Can involve simple support Very popular in mental health settings Has been practised by nurses (and others) with little training and support
Complementary/alternative therapies	Not specifically psychological Many different approaches, but all emphasise the 'whole' person Little evidence of effectiveness Widely practised but unregulated Rapidly increasing in popularity in nursing

treatment requires close observation. For most, however, a stay in hospital will be very brief. In consequence, much mental health nursing is carried out either in general practice clinics, community mental health centres or clients' own homes. Care in the community is thought to disrupt the individual's life much less than is admission to hospital, and continuing to carry on a normal life also helps in confronting problems *where they occur*. Thus, community mental health nursing is at the core of the role of the mental health nurse. Even for those still working in inpatient settings, preparation for discharge will be a significant part of care-planning.

The development of the role of the community psychiatric nurse (CPN) was almost entirely a consequence of the greater effectiveness of drug treatments for mental illness. The early role of the CPN consisted almost entirely of following-up early discharges, and monitoring and advising about the effects and side-effects of the new medications. Their current therapeutic and pre-ventive roles have developed from these origins (Simmons & Brooker 1986).

NURSING ROLES IN MEDICAL MODELS OF CARE

Despite the rise of other approaches to mental distress, the role of medicine remains dominant. Yet, even within this context, the nurse occupies a number of key roles, both in hospital and the community. Many of these roles were not specifically sought by nurses, but evolved as the mental health nurse role evolved from that of attendant. Mental health nurses perform a clinical administration function, being involved in admission, transfer and discharge of clients, and maintaining adequate records of the client's care. Additionally, in hospital, the nurse will still be primarily responsible for the safety of the client. With the disturbed person, in particular, remnants of the custodial role thus remain. Perhaps most important for the medical aspect of care is that the nurse is expected to monitor the client's behaviour closely, so that effects of the medication on the client's behaviour can be adequately assessed.

In this way, the nurse begins to act as a case manager, although this is typically a role formally reserved for a doctor, particularly where medical approaches to mental distress prevail. Often, however, the case manager role is greatly expanded, most noticeably in the community, where the nurse is often formally acknowledged as being responsible for overall coordination of care. This will involve at least the organisation of services appropriate to the client's needs, and, increasingly, decisions about admission and discharge from the caseload. The nurse is, therefore, responsible for most of the important decisions about management of clients.

THE NURSE AS THERAPIST

Perhaps the oldest and most general nursing role of the nurse as a provider of therapy (rather than custody) involves the use of diversion. This may simply involve helping individuals to keep occupied, whilst the drugs that are expected to alleviate their symptoms have a chance to act. However, it is more likely that diversional work will also include some other aspect of care. For example, the nurse may use a game of cards to assess aspects of the client's behaviour and cognition, by observing interactions with others, the ability to remember which cards have been played, the level of interest in the game and so on. In even more structured settings, diversional activities may form part of therapeutic interventions involving training in social interactions or opportunities to express feelings or recall emotionally charged information.

Mental health nursing always involves the use of interpersonal skills to engage the client, gain information, respond to emotions and help in initiating behaviour change. In counselling, these skills are used in a more structured way, usually in the context of a formal, developing and helping relationship (Egan 1990), in which the nurse helps the client to explore her emotions and behaviours.

Sometimes, the goal of such counselling can be simply support, helping the client overcome some crisis, in much the same way as a good friend might, but with greater detachment from the client's situation than a friend might be able to offer. More often, the nurse is involved in helping the client to move beyond her problems, acting as a 'sounding board' against which the client tests out her feelings about her difficulties and her proposed solutions. The nurse may go so far as to offer the client interpretations of her behaviour, for example, by drawing to her attention times in the past when she has felt or behaved in a similar way. Here, the aim is to give the client greater insight into her behaviours and feelings.

Many organisations offer training in counselling, often based on the work of the humanistic psychologist Carl Rogers (1951). This form of counselling, usually called client-centred therapy, is based on Rogers' beliefs about the need for positive regard and self-actualisation, and involves the therapist in showing the client respect, warmth and empathy, which, in turn, help the client to find her own solutions to her difficulties. Training in this form of counselling aims to equip the nurse to be better able to demonstrate her own personal qualities that show warmth, respect and empathy for the client. Until recently, counselling in the UK was unregulated, so there was little guarantee that any particular training truly equipped people who underwent it to offer treatment. The situation is now slightly improved, with the introduction of a register for therapists and counsellors. Unfortunately, since the effectiveness of these types of counselling is extremely difficult to demonstrate, it is by no means certain that registration offers any protection for the public. Prospective clients will know, through certification, that a counsellor has been trained and receives supervision, but will not know whether the method of counselling that she has been trained to offer in fact leads to any improvement for its clients in general, or for the particular difficulties any given individual brings to the counselling situation.

Whilst client-centred (or Rogerian) approaches to counselling are the most common among nurses and other mental health professionals, there are some who offer a form of therapy based on the works of Freud. Psychodynamic psychotherapy is, in essence, a briefer, less intensive version of traditional psychoanalysis. In this form of intervention, the therapist attempts to uncover and interpret to the client his unconscious internal conflicts that are thought to give rise to current difficulties, by careful examination of the client's behaviour during therapy sessions and his relationship with the therapist. This can take a considerable length of time. Few nurses are trained in this technique, although some have attended courses that typically aim to offer an introductory appreciation of what is involved in psychodynamic psychotherapy.

Cognitive–behaviour therapy is a comparatively new approach, characterised by an emphasis on the client's problems in the present, and concentrating on maintaining factors rather than attempting to find supposed causes in the past. During therapy, clients are taught to recognise unproductive thoughts and behaviours that give rise to difficulty, to challenge them and to practise new and more adaptive behaviours. Two key elements of treatment are the notions of exposure and experiment. Clients are encouraged to expose themselves, in a gradual way, to situations that cause anxiety, taking advantage of the body's natural tendency to cease to respond to frightening situations. Whilst in these situations (for example flying, or speaking in social situations), clients experiment with new ways of thinking and behaving that they have learnt during their therapy sessions.

Cognitive–behaviour therapy represents a major departure for both clients and mental health nurses. For the client, it is the first form of treatment that has made a continuing commitment to evaluation of its effectiveness and which has demonstrated that effectiveness across a wide range of client difficulties. Rachman & Wilson (1980) offer an excellent review of the major outcome studies of cognitive–behaviour therapy, psychodynamic therapy and Rogerian therapy. The consensus today is that cognitive–behaviour therapy has a massive contribution to make to the alleviation of client distress.

For nurses, the chief influence of cognitive–behaviour therapy is that it offered nurses their first opportunity to act as autonomous therapists in mental health. Using the technique, nurses were trained to undertake all stages of therapy, from referral and assessment through to discharge and follow-up. Moreover, trained nurse behaviour therapists, as they came to be called, were shown to be as successful in their treatment of clients as psychiatrists and psychologists using similar techniques (Marks et al 1977).

Counselling, psychodynamic psychotherapy and cognitive–behaviour therapy might all be practised on a group therapy basis, although the aims of each form of group intervention would be different, reflecting the underlying philosophies of the different approaches. Typically, group analytical psychotherapy and some forms of group counselling attempt to use processes observed within the group to help group members come to an understanding of the way in which they interact with others and the relationship of these interaction patterns to more deep-seated personal difficulties. By contrast, cognitive–behavioural group treatments tend to focus on specific problems, and are generally little different from individual treatments, with the obvious savings in time and resources. In such groups, group members will be encouraged to offer their experiences in order to help each other find appropriate coping tactics. This supportive element is common to most groupwork, apart from the strictest forms of group analysis, and some groups may have mutual support as their only aim. In these groups, the chief job of the nurse as therapist is to facilitate this mutual support among group members. Indeed, support groups of this kind are an area in which nurses have been involved for many years. This was often with minimal training, experience or supervision, but, fortunately, it is now recognised that facilitation of supportive group work is a highly skilled nursing role that requires training and support.

Not all therapies offered by nurses are oriented towards counselling and psychotherapy. It is worth noting that, in recent years, nurses have responded to the growth in popularity of alternative and complementary therapies, such as massage, reflexology, acupressure, naturopathy and aromatherapy. For example, training in massage or relaxation techniques may form part of a stress management package, whilst aromatherapy has been offered as an intervention to decrease agitation and anxiety amongst cognitively impaired elderly people. Effectiveness of the complementary therapies remains a matter of considerable debate in health care generally, and the mental health field shares that debate. To date, there is no evidence to support the effectiveness of the complementary approaches as main treatments for mental distress. There is currently no requirement for practitioners of most complementary therapies in the UK either to be registered or to undertake any formal training, so that the complementary therapies are, effectively, unregulated. As a result, considerable care is necessary both for the nurse seeking training in such a therapy and the client seeking treatment.

THE NURSE AS AN EDUCATOR

Nurses have increasingly expanded their remit, so that they are no longer involved only in the treatment of mental distress, but also in the

Activity 23.3

Sharon is 22 years old. Last year, during her final year at university, she developed a virus and was away from the university for several weeks. When she returned to classes, she found she was behind with her work and also that she felt both physically tired and isolated from her fellow students. She came to feel anxious whenever she entered classes. As a result, she started to avoid university. At first, her friends used to call, but Sharon was either too tired to communicate with them or too nervous in their company to tolerate them for long. Now she gets frightened if she goes out at all, and finds even brief walks exhausting. Although there is no physical evidence, she is terrified that she has some dread disease, and repeatedly visits her doctor to seek reassurance.

- How did Sharon come to be affected in this way?
- We all know how it feels to be upset and alone. Using your knowledge of this, say how Sharon feels.
- What can be done?

prevention of such distress, both for individuals and for communities. At the forefront of these educative roles have been community mental health nurses. Their focus on work in the community has led them to work in GP clinics, in schools and in industry. At one level, this has simply been the offer of liaison work or counselling of individuals and groups. However, with increasing frequency, nurses have initiated approaches that, rather than being a response to an expressed need by the community, have anticipated such a need and attempted to respond proactively, before problems develop. Thus, community mental health nurses may be found educating the public on mental health issues by giving talks in schools, advising about stress in general practice 'well person' clinics or initiating and running stress management workshops in industry. Additionally, mental health nurses are valued members of committees and community groups, helping to define the responses of public bodies to mental health issues.

EVALUATING MENTAL HEALTH NURSING

One compelling difficulty for mental health nursing is the lack of studies indicating the effectiveness or otherwise of what mental health nurses do with clients. Although this is a problem common to nursing as a whole, it is particularly acute in mental health nursing, both because of the lack of clear definition of mental health nursing skills and the small number of outcome studies that have been undertaken. Two fields in which much work has been done are behaviour therapy nursing (see above) and community psychiatric nursing. Studies of the effectiveness of the CPN, however, remain mixed. In particular, Gournay & Brooking (1994) found no difference in outcome between clients seen by CPNs and those seen only by their GP.

Part of the problem lies in defining what mental health nurses do, and part in isolating that activity from the interventions of other members of the health care team. However, these are challenges that mental health nursing will have to face if it wishes to demonstrate its effectiveness, particularly in the market climate of health care.

FUTURES IN CARE

COMMUNITY PERSPECTIVE

Closure of mental hospitals has been a continuing trend throughout the latter half of the 20th century. As we have seen throughout much of this chapter, the combination of new, powerful treatments and awareness of the social effects of institutionalisation, coupled with the aspirations of nurses to assume new roles, has led to a gradual move towards emphasis on the community care of people experiencing mental distress. Successive government reports have stressed the need for this community-based approach. Most recently, this has become formalised by the government document 'Caring for People' (DHSS 1989), which sets out the methods by which hospital closure and community provision are to be achieved.

However, support for the initiative has not been universal. As well as unease among communities about having long-stay psychiatric hospital patients relocated into their midst, user and care groups have campaigned vociferously against hospital closures, often claiming that closure will result in increased burden upon families.

The plight of mentally distressed people among the nation's prison population and homeless has also given rise to heated debate, and nurses are currently developing roles to address the needs of homeless people experiencing mental distress. However, there is no clear evidence that these problems, although undoubtedly severe, are related to hospital closure and community care. For example, Pilling (1991) notes that very few individuals were untraceable following discharge into the community.

CHANGES TO THE ROLE OF THE MENTAL HEALTH NURSE

It is uncertain how changes in policy will affect the role of the mental health nurse. Clearly, many more will work in the community, rather than in hospital settings, but the nature of that

Activity 23.4

One element of caring for people with psychological difficulties is the effect it has on carers.

- Imagine you are married to someone with such severe depression that they believe they are responsible for all the world's troubles. What effect will their problems have on *you*?
- Most of us have had to comfort friends or relatives who are upset. Think of the last time this happened to you. How did *you* cope with the effect of your friend's distress on you?

work continues to be defined. In particular, the work of the CPN will undoubtedly come under closer scrutiny, particularly if elements of mental health care become incorporated into the roles of other members of the primary health care team, such as practice nurses. A great deal of CPN time currently involves working with people suffering from minor mental distress, despite a lack of evidence of the usefulness of such intervention (Gournay & Brooking 1994). CPNs have, in recent years, achieved considerable status as autonomous, expert practitioners, yet without effective evaluation of their work. In the future, both the increase of mental health care in the community and in the number of different individuals involved in such care will place pressure upon CPNs to both define and evaluate their continuing role.

Mental health care faces considerable challenges in the future. In particular, examination of the needs of ethnic minorities, women, older people, children and offenders with mental health problems have only begun to be addressed. For nurses, opportunities for continuing education, evaluation of clinical practice and clinical supervision remain rudimentary. The Butterworth Report (Department of Health 1994) focuses on these challenges and highlights the need for a flexible response to future mental health needs and the role of nurses in rising to these opportunities. The report makes some 42 recommendations, of which the most important for future mental health nursing are summarised in Figure 23.1. A key element in NHS reforms has been the recognition that service users and carers have an important role in determining the care

- An improvement in the understanding of racial and cultural needs
- The establishment of research
- Representation and participation of service users
- Links with the criminal justice system
- A focus on work with severe mental illness
- Availability of mental health nursing skills to the primary health care team
- Establishment of clinical supervision
- Development of a framework for good practice

Figure 23.1 Synopsis of the key recommendations of the Butterworth Report.

they receive. As a result, nurses have seen the necessity for helping users to exercise that right to involvement. Of all the challenges likely to be presented to the mental health nurse in the future, this expansion of their relationships with clients and carers is perhaps most crucial, and represents a culmination of the shift in the role of the mental health nurse from custodial attendant to partner in care.

Summary

Until the 19th century, people with mental health problems were subjected to a bizarre range of physical treatments, in the hope of achieving a cure. Philosophical changes then came to emphasise the rational humanity of the individual with mental distress, and management today highlights the psychological and social needs of clients, while also employing pharmacological means of treatment.

The dominant view of mental distress is still medical, but there are several other important approaches to understanding mental health and illness – sociological, cognitive–behavioural, psychodynamic, humanistic and anti-psychiatric – which this chapter outlines. The classification of mental distress is also discussed.

The role of the mental health nurse has, over recent decades, undergone both a development and a broadening. From a primarily custodial role, which differed little from the traditional work of asylum attendants, the role has progressed towards active involvement in care, taking ever greater responsibility for decision-making. At the same time, mental health nurses have moved into different areas of work, whilst maintaining an emphasis on the building of relationships with clients. Mental health nurses now act as case managers and therapists, and increasingly recognise the need for high quality education, research and policy-making. For the future, this focus will need to increase further, emphasising continuing acquisition of skills and evaluation of mental health nursing practice.

REFERENCES

Beck A T 1976 Cognitive therapy and the emotional disorders. International Universities Press, New York

Brewin C 1988 Cognitive foundations of clinical psychology. Lawrence Erlbaum Associates, Hove and London

Brown G W, Harris T 1978 The social origins of depression: A study of psychiatric disorder in women. Tavistock, London

Buchan H, Johnstone E, Mcpherson K, Palmer R L, Crow T J, Brandon S 1992 Who benefits from electroconvulsive therapy? Combined results of the Leicester and Northwick Park trials. British Journal of Psychiatry 160: 355–359

Busfield J 1986 Managing madness. Hutchinson, London

Cioffi F 1978 Freud and the idea of a pseudo-science. In: Borger R, Cioffi F (eds) Explanation in the behavioural sciences. Cambridge University Press, Cambridge, pp 471–499

Clare, A T 1976 Psychiatry in dissent. Tavistock, London

Department of Health 1994 Working in partnership: a collaborative approach to care (Report of the Mental Health Nursing Review Team; the Butterworth Report). HMSO, London

DHSS 1989 Caring for people: community care in the next decade and beyond. HMSO, London

Egan G 1990 The skilled helper: a systematic approach to effective helping. Brooks/Cole, Pacific Grove, California

Eysenck H J 1952 The effects of psychotherapy: an evaluation. Journal of Consulting Psychology 16: 319–324

Eysenck H J 1985 Decline and fall of the Freudian Empire. Penguin, Harmondsworth

Foucault M 1967 Madness and civilisation: a history of insanity in the age of reason. Tavistock, London

Goffman E 1961 Asylums: essays on the social situation of mental patients and other inmates. Anchor, New York

Gournay K, Brooking J 1994 Community psychiatric nurses in primary health care. British Journal of Psychiatry 165: 231–238

Gray J 1982 The neurophysiology of anxiety: an enquiry into the functions of the septo-hippocampal system. Oxford University Press, Oxford

Jaremko M E 1986 Cognitive–behaviour modification: the shaping of rule-governed behaviour. In: Dryden W, Golden W L (eds) Cognitive–behavioural approaches to psychotherapy. Harper & Row, London

Jones E 1955 The life and work of Sigmund Freud, vol. II. Hogarth, London

Laing R D 1967 The politics of experience. Penguin, Harmondsworth

Laing R D, Esterson A 1964 Sanity, madness and the family. Penguin, Harmondsworth

Marks I M, Hallam R S, Connolly J, Phillpott R 1977 Nursing in behavioural psychotherapy. RCN, London

Maslow A H 1968 Towards a psychology of being. Van Nostrand, New Jersey

Newell R, Shrubb S 1994 Attitude change and behaviour therapy in body dysmorphic disorder: two case reports. Behavioural Cognitive Psychotherapy 22: 163–169

Pilling S 1991 Rehabilitation and community care. Routledge, London

Rachman S J, Wilson G T 1980 The effects of psychological therapy, 2nd edn. Pergamon, Oxford

Rogers C R 1951 Client-centred therapy. Houghton-Mifflin, Boston

Rosenhan D L 1973 On being sane in insane places. Science 179: 250–258

Roth M, Kroll J 1986 The reality of mental illness. Cambridge University Press, Cambridge

Salkovskis P M, Warwick H M C 1985 Cognitive therapy of obsessive–compulsive disorder: treating treatment failures. Behavioural Psychotherapy 13: 243–255

Scheff T J (ed.) 1967 Mental illness and social processes. Harper & Row, New York

de Silva P 1985 Early Buddhist and modern behavioural strategies for the control of unwanted intrusive cognitions. Psychological record 35(4): 437–443

Simmons S, Brooker C 1986 Community psychiatric nursing. Heinemann, London

Siraisi N G 1990 Medieval & early renaissance medicine. Chicago University Press, Chicago

Szasz T S 1962 The myth of mental illness. Penguin, Harmondsworth

Tuke S 1813, Reprinted 1964 Description of The Retreat at York. Dawsons, London

Walker S 1984 Learning theory and behaviour modification. Methuen, London

FURTHER READING

Bandura A 1977 Social learning theory. Prentice-Hall, Englewood Cliffs, New Jersey

Brooker C (ed.) 1990 Community psychiatric nursing: a research perspective. Chapman & Hall, London

Brooking J 1986 Psychiatric nursing research. John Wiley & Sons, Chichester

Freud S 1976 Introductory lectures on psychoanalysis. Penguin, Harmondsworth

Hawton K, Salkovskis P M, Kirk J, Clark D M 1989 Cognitive behaviour therapy for psychiatric problems. A practical guide. Oxford University Press, Oxford

Marks I M 1987 Fears, phobias and rituals. Oxford University Press, New York

Masson J 1989 Against therapy. Fontana, London

Silverstone T, Turner P 1974 Drug treatment in psychiatry. Routledge & Kegan Paul, London

Williams J M G, Watts F N, MacLeod C, Mathews A 1988 Cognitive psychology and emotional disorders. John Wiley & Sons, Chichester

Index

D